Trauma Rehabilitation

Trauma Rehabilitation

Lawrence R. Robinson, MD
Professor and Chair
Department of Rehabilitation Medicine
University of Washington School of Medicine
Seattle, Washington

Director
Electrodiagnostic Service
Department of Rehabilitation Medicine
Harborview Medical Center
Seattle, Washington

LIPPINCOTT WILLIAMS & WILKINS
A **Wolters Kluwer** Company
Philadelphia • Baltimore • New York • London
Buenos Aires • Hong Kong • Sydney • Tokyo

Acquisitions Editor: Robert Hurley
Developmental Editor: Scott Scheidt
Project Manager: Nicole Walz
Senior Manufacturing Manager: Ben Rivera
Marketing Director: Sharon Zinner
Design Coordinator: Holly McLaughlin
Production Services: Laserwords Private Limited
Printer: Edwards Brothers

© 2006 by Lippincott Williams & Wilkins
530 Walnut Street
Philadelphia, PA 19106

Library of Congress Cataloging-in-Publication Data

Trauma rehabilitation / [edited by] Lawrence R. Robinson. -- 1st ed.
    p. ; cm.
  Includes bibliographical references and index.
  ISBN 0-7817-6284-7 (alk. paper)
  1. Wounds and injuries--Treatment. 2. Wounds and injuries--Patients
--Rehabilitation.   I. Robinson, Lawrence R. (Lawrence Russell),
1956-   .
  [DNLM: 1. Wounds and Injuries--rehabilitation.   WO 700 T77686
2006]
  RD93.T69615 2006
  617.1'03--dc22
                                            2005017353

Care has been taken to confirm the accuracy of the information presented and to describe generally accepted practices. However, the authors, editors, and publisher are not responsible for errors or omissions or for any consequences from application of the information in this book and make no warranty, expressed or implied, with respect to the currency, completeness, or accuracy of the contents of the publication. Application of this information in a particular situation remains the professional responsibility of the practitioner.

The authors, editors, and publisher have exerted every effort to ensure that drug selection and dosage set forth in this text are in accordance with current recommendations and practice at the time of publication. However, in view of ongoing research, changes in government regulations, and the constant flow of information relating to drug therapy and drug reactions, the reader is urged to check the package insert for each drug for any change in indications and dosage and for added warnings and precautions. This is particularly important when the recommended agent is a new or infrequently employed drug.

Some drugs and medical devices presented in this publication have Food and Drug Administration (FDA) clearance for limited use in restricted research settings. It is the responsibility of health care providers to ascertain the FDA status of each drug or device planned for use in their clinical practice.

The publishers have made every effort to trace copyright holders for borrowed material. If they have inadvertently overlooked any, they will be pleased to make the necessary arrangements at the first opportunity.

To purchase additional copies of this book, call our customer service department at (800) 639-3030 or fax orders to (301) 824-7390. International customers should call (301) 714-2324. Lippincott Williams & Wilkins customer service representatives are available from 8:30 AM to 6:00 PM, EST. Visit Lippincott Williams & Wilkins on the Internet at LWW.com.

10 9 8 7 6 5 4 3 2 1

Dedication

To our patients, who continually teach us; to
our students, who continually challenge us; and
to our families, who continually support us.

CONTRIBUTORS

Barbara Beach, Med, CRC
Director of Rehabilitation Services
Department of Rehabilitation Medicine
University of Washington Medical Center
Seattle, Washington

Kathleen R. Bell, MD
Professor
Department of Rehabilitation Medicine
University of Washington School of Medicine
Seattle, Washington

Medical Director, Brain Injury Rehabilitation
Department of Rehabilitation Medicine
University of Washington Medical Center
Seattle, Washington

Charles H. Bombardier, PhD
Professor
Department of Rehabilitation Medicine
University of Washington School of Medicine
Seattle, Washington

Attending Psychologist
Department of Rehabilitation Medicine
Harborview Medical Center
Seattle, Washington

Diana D. Cardenas, MD, MHA
Professor
Department of Rehabilitation Medicine
University of Washington School of Medicine
Seattle, Washington

Chief of Service
Department of Rehabilitation Medicine
University of Washington Medical Center
Seattle, Washington

Joseph M. Czerniecki, MD
Professor
Department of Rehabilitation Medicine
University of Washington School of Medicine
Seattle, Washington

Interim Director
Department of Rehabilitation Medicine
VA Puget Sound Health Care System
Seattle, Washington

Sureyya Dikmen, PhD
Professor
Department of Rehabilitation Medicine
Adjunct Professor
Departments of Neurological Surgery and Psychiatry
    and Behavioral Sciences
University of Washington School of Medicine
Seattle, Washington

Dawn M. Ehde, PhD
Associate Professor
Department of Rehabilitation Medicine
University of Washington School of Medicine
Seattle, Washington

Clinical Psychologist
Department of Rehabilitation Medicine
Harborview Medical Center
Seattle, Washington

Joyce M. Engel, PhD, OTR/L
Professor
Department of Rehabilitation Medicine
University of Washington School of Medicine
Seattle, Washington

Peter C. Esselman, MD
Associate Professor
Department of Rehabilitation Medicine
University of Washington School of Medicine
Seattle, Washington

Chief
Department of Rehabilitation Medicine
Harborview Medical Center
Seattle, Washington

David C. Grossman, MD, MPH
Professor
Department of Health Services and Pediatrics
University of Washington School of Medicine
Seattle, Washington

Medical Director, Preventive Care
Center for Health Studies
Group Health Cooperative
Seattle, Washington

Joyce S. Hedges, MS, CCC-SLP
Staff Speech Pathologist
Department of Rehabilitation Medicine
Harborview Medical Center
Seattle, Washington

Jeanne M. Hoffman, PhD
Assistant Professor
Department of Rehabilitation Medicine
University of Washington School of Medicine
Seattle, Washington

Attending Psychologist
Department of Rehabilitation Medicine
University of Washington Medical Center
Seattle, Washington

Mark P. Jensen, PhD
Professor
Department of Rehabilitation Medicine
University of Washington School of Medicine
Seattle, Washington

Attending Psychologist
Multidisciplinary Pain Center
University of Washington Medical Center
Seattle, Washington

Gregory J. Jurkovich, MD
Professor
Department of Surgery
University of Washington School of Medicine
Seattle, Washington

Chief of Trauma Services
Department of Surgery
Harborview Medical Center
Seattle, Washington

Lynn K.N. Krog, RN, BSN
Trauma Rehabilitation Coordinator
Department of Rehabilitation Medicine
Harborview Medical Center
Seattle, Washington

Terry Massagli, MD
Associate Professor
Department of Rehabilitation Medicine
University of Washington School of Medicine
Seattle, Washington

Pediatrics Director
Physical Medicine and Rehabilitation Residency
    Training Program
Children's Hospital & Regional Medical Center
Seattle, Washington

Tiffany G. Megargee, MA, OT, CHT
Occupational Therapist
Clinical Specialist
Department of Rehabilitation Medicine
Harborview Medical Center
Seattle, Washington

Paula J. Micklesen, BS
Electroneurodiagnostic Technician
Department of Rehabilitation Medicine
Harborview Medical Center
Seattle, Washington

Charles N. Mock, MD, PhD
Associate Professor
Departments of Surgery and Joint Appointment in
    Epidemiology
University of Washington School of Medicine
Seattle, Washington

Director
Harborview Injury Prevention and Research Center
Harborview Medical Center
Seattle, Washington

Dana Y. Nakamura, OT, CLT
Clinical Specialist, Occupational Therapy/Burns
Department of Rehabilitation Medicine
University of Washington Burn Center
Harborview Medical Center
Seattle, Washington

David R. Patterson, PhD
Professor
Department of Rehabilitation Medicine
University of Washington School of Medicine and
    Harborview Medical Center
Seattle, Washington

Mary Pepping, PhD
Associate Professor
Department of Rehabilitation Medicine
University of Washington School of Medicine
Seattle, Washington

Director
Neuropsychology Testing Services and Outpatient
    Neurorehabilitation Program
Department of Rehabilitation Medicine
University of Washington Medical Center
Seattle, Washington

Melissa Porras-Monroe, BS
Manager, Acute Care
OT/PT/SLP
Harborview Medical Center
Seattle, Washington

Ellen Foisie Robinson, PT, ATC
Clinical Faculty
Department of Rehabilitation Medicine
University of Washington School of Medicine
Seattle, Washington

Clinical Specialist, Physical Therapy
Department of Acute Rehabilitation Therapy
Harborview Medical Center
Seattle, Washington

James P. Robinson, MD, PhD
Clinical Associate Professor
Department of Rehabilitation Medicine
University of Washington School of Medicine
Seattle, Washington

Lawrence R. Robinson, MD
Professor and Chair
Department of Rehabilitation Medicine
University of Washington School of Medicine
Seattle, Washington

Director
Electrodiagnostic Service
Department of Rehabilitation Medicine
Harborview Medical Center
Seattle, Washington

Pamela A. Palmer Smith, PhD, RN
Clinical Assistant Professor
Department of Biobehavioral Nursing and Health Systems
University of Washington School of Nursing
Seattle, Washington

Manager, Trauma Rehabilitation Unit
Department of Rehabilitation Medicine
Harborview Medical Center
Seattle, Washington

Elizabeth L. Spencer Steffa, OTR/L, CHT
Clinical Instructor
Department of Rehabilitation Medicine
University of Washington School of Medicine
Seattle, Washington

Therapist
Highline Hand Therapy
Burien, Washington

Pam L. Stockman, OTR/L
MOT Advisory Board Member
School of Occupational Therapy
University of Washington School of Medicine
Seattle, Washington

Occupational Therapist
Department of Rehabilitation Medicine
University of Washington Medical Center
Seattle, Washington

David B. Weiss, MD
Acting Instructor
Department of Orthopaedics and Sports Medicine
University of Washington School of Medicine
Seattle, Washington

Acting Instructor
Department of Orthopaedic Trauma
Harborview Medical Center
Seattle, Washington

Rhonda M. Williams, PhD
Assistant Professor
Department of Rehabilitation Medicine
University of Washington School of Medicine
Seattle, Washington

Clinical Psychologist
Rehabilitation Care Services
VA Puget Sound Health Care System
Seattle, Washington

PREFACE

Trauma is the most frequent cause of disability in young adults and children. But until now, information on the rehabilitation of trauma patients has been scattered. *Trauma Rehabilitation* provides the first complete text on trauma rehabilitation, with important information on current developments, for anyone interested or involved in the field.

This book will serve as the single most comprehensive source of information relevant to trauma rehabilitation, ranging from acute care to long-term management. The reader will learn about the epidemiology of trauma and how trauma systems are organized. Excellent chapters address the prevention of trauma and early interventions before the patient reaches the trauma rehabilitation facility. Common long-term issues for trauma patients, such as pain, substance abuse, and multiple musculoskeletal trauma, are also well covered.

The authors of this text are expert health care professionals devoted to trauma care at the University of Washington. Many are nationally and internationally known, cutting-edge researchers in their field. The wide-ranging team of trauma professionals contributing to this text includes physiatrists, surgeons, pediatricians, psychologists, nurses, therapists, and other professionals. My sincere gratitude is extended to all of them.

I recommend this text with pride as a must for all those involved in treating individuals affected by trauma. No matter whether you are a physician, psychologist, nurse, therapist, or administrator, I think you will find this book worthwhile.

LRR

CONTENTS

1

Trauma Rehabilitation: An Introduction

Lawrence R. Robinson

This book covers the field of trauma rehabilitation, which is the rehabilitation of injury caused by physical trauma. Trauma is damage to the body caused by an exposure to environmental energy that is beyond the body's resilience. Trauma is the most common cause of death for individuals between the ages of 1 and 44 years in the United States and is the third most common cause of death for individuals of all ages in the United States. Trauma is also a very common cause of significant disability, particularly in younger, productive working-age adults and is of special concern to rehabilitation teams.

Although rehabilitation medicine has its roots in the treatment of the individual disabled by trauma, there is no textbook that specifically deals with the many aspects of treatment of such individuals currently available. This book will fill that gap. It is the goal of this book to cover the rehabilitation of trauma-related disability in a broad sense. Today's rehabilitation professional treating patients disabled by trauma, namely, the *rehabilitation traumatologist,* should be well versed in the entire spectrum of trauma, not simply what happens during a patient's stay in the inpatient rehabilitation unit.

WHAT THE WELL-VERSED REHABILITATION TRAUMATOLOGIST SHOULD KNOW

The knowledge base of the *rehabilitation traumatologist* should include an understanding of epidemiology,

systems of care, acute care treatment, and quality improvement, as well as the core principles of rehabilitation of common traumatic conditions. It is the intention of the authors of this book that the text covers these materials.

Rehabilitation professionals treating traumatically injured individuals should be well versed in the epidemiology of trauma and trauma-related disability, and should be aware of the risk factors for trauma-related disability. Such knowledge arms the members of the rehabilitation team with important data about the population they are serving, as well as with information about risk factors that can be addressed to prevent further injury and/or disability. A select few may also participate in injury prevention programs in their communities.

Rehabilitation traumatologists should know how the acute trauma care system is organized to provide the best possible care and what is required for a level I, II, or III trauma designation. They should be familiar with injury severity scores and how these early measures predict outcome and risk of later disability. Such knowledge enhances the ability of traumatologists to participate more meaningfully in the system of trauma care, including accreditation, development of standards of care, and quality improvement.

It is also important to know how to best participate in the care of patients at the acute stage of their injury while they are in the intensive care unit or on the acute care service before they are admitted to the inpatient rehabilitation unit. There are a number of interventions, if appropriately applied early, that will reduce or prevent later disability, identify rehabilitation needs early on, and allow for optimal functioning of the acutely injured individual. It is vital for rehabilitation traumatologists to educate acute care teams about early rehabilitation interventions that can gradually be incorporated into the standards of care. Screening, tracking, and triaging of traumatically injured patients are also important roles of the rehabilitation team.

Traumatically injured patients that come to the inpatient or outpatient rehabilitation service present many unique features. First, patients with traumatic injuries are generally younger than those with other types of disabilities. Their youth brings into play several concerns not present in an older population of disabled patients, such as return to work, fertility, caring for young children, and a different set of psychological problems.

There are other concerns generally exclusive to disability caused by trauma. For example, in patients with traumatic spinal cord injury (SCI), there will often be additional concerns about spinal stability or other superimposed injuries (for example, traumatic brain injury [TBI], other fractures, or peripheral nerve injuries) that are not necessarily germane to individuals with nontraumatic myelopathy. Similarly, individuals with TBI clearly have different types and sites of pathology compared to individuals with nontraumatic brain lesions, such as stroke or tumor, and thus their needs are quite different. Traumatic amputations present challenges that are different from those of vascular amputations; the former patients will often be more physically active, have more vocational concerns, and will usually have a longer life span after amputation. Patients with traumatic peripheral nerve lesions have very different pathophysiology and require very different treatment compared to those with nontraumatic focal neuropathies. Patients with multiple musculoskeletal injuries have special concerns regarding weight bearing, timing of rehabilitation, and return to work.

Adjustment to disability after trauma is another area the rehabilitation team needs to be well versed in. There is a unique adjustment required to the unexpected losses caused by trauma. Often there is loss of, or injury to, friends and relatives, as well as the injury to the patient himself or herself, to contend with. There are a variety of management approaches to posttraumatic stress disorder, as well as normal and maladaptive responses to trauma.

The management of pain after trauma-related disability can differ from pain management in conditions not caused by trauma. Patients with traumatic neurologic injuries, for example, may have neuropathic pain that is often not amenable to usual methods of pain treatment. Traumatic amputees may have phantom limb or stump pain that limits their functioning. Management of pain after burns can be especially difficult. Pain treatment after trauma also interweaves the psychology of trauma with the psychology of pain control.

Many traumatically disabled patients become further disabled because of problems with substance abuse. It would be naïve to think that the individual with a traumatic brain injury from alcohol abuse who returns to his or her same environment would be cured of substance abuse. Thus, the rehabilitation traumatologist needs to be aware of how to recognize substance abuse and which interventions may be useful in addressing this problem.

The approach to pediatric patients disabled by trauma is also unique. The issues surrounding screening for rehabilitation needs, educational goals, and parental involvement differ from those encountered with either nontraumatically disabled children or traumatically injured adults.

Finally, rehabilitation professionals should be well versed in maintaining a high-quality system of care. They should know how to measure the quality of the rehabilitation program and intervene when measurements call for a change. Rehabilitation traumatologists should know about prevention of trauma and hopefully become personally involved in trauma prevention programs.

DEFINITION OF TRAUMA

The word *trauma* comes from the ancient Greek word τραυμα, which refers to physical injury. Trauma, or injury, can be defined as damage to the body caused by a sudden exposure to environmental energy that is beyond the body's resilience. The energy involved can be in a number of forms. Mechanical energy is the most common form, accounting for the great majority of all injuries (1); examples include motor vehicle crashes, gunshot wounds, and falls. Less commonly, traumatic injury can result from exposure to other forms of energy, including heat (e.g., burns), electricity (electrical injuries), or ionizing radiation. Not all health care providers, however, would typically classify the latter types of injuries as trauma.

HISTORY OF TRAUMA CARE

The recorded history of trauma care dates back to ancient times. There are reports of the surgeons of ancient Egypt dressing wounds, performing amputations, and removing foreign bodies that date back to approximately 3500 BC. In the 5th century BC, in the times of Hippocrates, the Greeks described the treatment of fractures, dislocations, and wounds.

Most modern principles of acute trauma care, however, are a product of advances in the 20th century (2). Many advances in trauma care are a result of lessons learned in warfare. It was during World War I, for example, that intravenous infusion of fluids was introduced; initially seawater was used for this purpose. Later, better substitutes were developed and physicians developed an understanding of the contribution of fluid volume loss to shock after hemorrhages and burns.

During World War II, considerable funding was devoted to medical science in order to treat injured soldiers more effectively. Moreover, developments of new technologies that were originally designed for battle, such as sonar, computers, radar, and nuclear science, later spawned offshoots that aided medical science.

During the Korean War, the helicopter was introduced as a method for rapidly transporting the wounded from the battlefield to Mobile Army Surgical Hospital (MASH) units. At the MASH unit, the patient could be stabilized, transfused if necessary, and prepared for transport to a larger hospital some distance away. Also during the Korean War, the use of antibiotics was expanded and a better understanding of the pathophysiology of hypovolemic shock and renal failure was developed. During the Vietnam War, members of the Walter Reed Army Institute of Research Trauma Study Section, stationed in Vietnam, advanced further understanding of the physiologic changes after combat trauma.

HISTORY OF REHABILITATION OF TRAUMA

The history of rehabilitation medicine has been reviewed elsewhere, and so will be reviewed only briefly here (3). With the advent of World War I, it was recognized that some physical agents could be useful for treating combat casualties. This observation ultimately stimulated the development of the American Congress of Physical Therapy in 1921 by the American Medical Association (AMA) for physicians interested in use of physical agents for diagnostic or therapeutic purposes. Although radiologists were initially part of the group of physicians interested in the use of physical agents, radiology soon become a separate specialty. Physicians interested in the use of physical agents were initially described as physical therapy physicians until Frank Krusen, MD, from the Mayo Clinic coined the term *physiatrist* in 1938; this term was formally adopted by the AMA in 1946.

With the advent of World War II and the occurrence of many combat disabilities, the focus of rehabilitation medicine broadened from physical modalities to functional activities, such as ambulation and activities of daily living. The field also became more comprehensive with attention to the individual's physical, mental, emotional, vocational, and social functioning. It was during and after this time that a shift in the understanding of the influence of activity on injury occurred. For example, Howard A. Rusk, MD, an army physician, designed a controlled experiment in which patients in one barracks were engaged in rehabilitative activities while patients in a second barracks had the usual bed rest. The benefits of early and aggressive rehabilitation were so obviously and vastly superior to passive convalescence that the armed services soon ordered this approach at all of its medical installations (4).

The American Board of Medical Specialties (ABMS) subsequently established the American Board of Physical Medicine in 1947 (which later became the American Board of Physical Medicine and Rehabilitation). Since that time, physiatry has played important roles not only in the rehabilitation of individuals disabled by disease (e.g., poliomyelitis), but also in the lives of veterans returning from the Korean and Vietnam wars with disabilities from trauma and of traumatically injured civilians.

SPECIAL NEEDS OF THE INDIVIDUAL DISABLED BY TRAUMA

The individual with disability from trauma has special needs compared with other disabled individuals requiring rehabilitation. In addition to needs specific to each disability, there are needs generic to many trauma patients. In many cases, the individual has multiple injuries. Some of these may be hidden or as yet undiscovered and the rehabilitation team needs to be on the lookout for fractures or other injuries of this nature. For instance, a patient with thoracic-level paraplegia who would typically have the ability to breathe independently might require ventilatory support due to a superimposed flail chest.

The presence of multiple injuries also increases the need for better coordination of care as more specialists become part of the care team and multiple injuries are treated simultaneously. The rehabilitation professional has a key role in coordinating this care with an eye toward improving functioning as a whole.

The traumatically injured tend to be much younger than the average rehabilitation patient. While the average age of patients in most inpatient rehabilitation units in the United States is mid-60s, the average age in trauma rehabilitation units is mid-40s. Although younger patients may have a better medical prognosis, they also have many issues that require more care than do older or geriatric patients. Return to work is a significant issue for many traumatically injured individuals. Many of them also have psychosocial issues more commonly seen in younger people. They have younger families and responsibilities to spouses and children. Sexuality and fertility are often prominent issues.

IMPORTANT COMPONENTS OF A TRAUMA REHABILITATION TEAM

The trauma rehabilitation team needs to be well coordinated and comprehensive in order to meet the needs of the traumatically injured individual. Strong contributions are required from a wide variety of health professionals including rehabilitation nurses, occupational therapists, physical therapists, psychologists, social workers, speech pathologists, vocational counselors, pharmacists, respiratory therapists, orthotists and prosthetists, therapeutic recreation specialists, and a variety of acute care services. In addition, ongoing plans for program evaluation, quality improvement, and accreditation are required to maintain high standards of care.

WASHINGTON DEPARTMENT OF HEALTH CRITERIA FOR STATE CERTIFICATION OF TRAUMA REHABILITATION SERVICES

In an effort to develop standards for trauma rehabilitation teams, in the early 1990s, the Department of Health in the state of Washington developed criteria for state certification of trauma rehabilitation services. These criteria parallel those for acute care trauma service designations. Certification criteria for trauma rehabilitation services are written into law as part of the Washington Administrative Code (WAC) and attempt to distinguish between three different levels of trauma rehabilitation care: from the most comprehensive (level I) to less comprehensive (level III). Full descriptions are provided in the appendix. Briefly they are as follows.

LEVEL I CRITERIA

Provide comprehensive inpatient and outpatient rehabilitation treatment to trauma patients regardless of the level of severity or complexity of disability. These facilities serve as regional referral centers for patients, physicians, and other health care professionals in the community and outlying areas and have ongoing structured programs for research, education, and outreach. Level I pediatric trauma rehabilitation services provide this same level of care to pediatric trauma patients.

LEVEL II CRITERIA

Provide comprehensive inpatient and outpatient rehabilitation treatment to trauma patients with any disability or level of severity or complexity within the services capabilities and delineated admission criteria.

LEVEL III CRITERIA

Provide a community-based program of coordinated and integrated outpatient treatment to trauma patients with functional limitations who do not need or no longer require comprehensive inpatient rehabilitation.

It is hoped that these criteria, along with the development of more units specializing in trauma rehabilitation, will result in increased expertise in trauma rehabilitation over time. It has been documented that hospitals that care for acutely injured trauma victims more commonly have better outcomes than those facilities that see trauma infrequently (5). Similarly, it is likely that rehabilitation teams that see trauma injuries more commonly will have better outcomes than those who see traumatically injured individuals less commonly.

THE FUTURE NEEDS OF TRAUMA REHABILITATION

The field of trauma rehabilitation is still evolving and improving, and there are many areas for future research and improvement. As with much of rehabilitation, the specific treatments and therapies applied are based upon training and experience, but much of what rehabilitation professionals do has not yet withstood an examination based upon randomized controlled trials. It is not realistic to expect that the complex series of events we call rehabilitation can be fully tested using this approach. Nevertheless, it will be important over time, as scientific evidence is developed, that our treatment approaches be based upon the evidence. We will need to develop clinical guidelines and standards of care that are based upon the latest available research. For critical areas in which it is unknown what the best approach might be, the field will need to develop creative clinical trials to compare alternative treatments. While we are, in some senses, "behind" the acute care world in clinical trials and a molecular understanding of rehabilitative processes, we are "ahead" of many fields in terms of measuring and focusing on functioning.

ABOUT THE EDITORIAL TEAM

The University of Washington faculty and staff chosen to write this book are especially well suited for this task. Harborview Medical Center, one of the two main teaching hospitals of the University of Washington Academic Medical Center (UWAMC), is the only level I trauma center in a four state region, including Washington, Alaska, Montana, and Idaho. It also has a widely recognized regional burn unit. Hence many patients with severe trauma are seen at Harborview. After initial acute care, patients requiring rehabilitation are often cared for in the rehabilitation unit at Harborview or transferred to one of the other hospitals in the UWAMC, such as University of Washington Medical Center, Children's Regional Hospital and Medical Center, or the Veteran's Administration Puget Sound Health Care System.

REFERENCES

1. Baker SP, O'Neil B, Ginsburg JM, et al. *The injury fact book*. New York: Oxford University Press; 1992.
2. Pruitt BA, Pruitt JH, Davis JH. History. In: Moore EE, Feliciano DV, Mattox KL, eds. *Trauma*. 5th ed. New York: McGraw-Hill; 2004:3–19.
3. Fifty years of physiatry; a special issue. *Arch Phys Med Rehabil*. 1988;69:1–68.
4. Kottke F, Knapp M. The development of physiatry before 1950. *Arch Phys Med Rehabil*. 1988;69:4–14.
5. Nathens AB, Jurkovich GJ, Maier RV, et al. Relationship between trauma center volume and outcomes. *JAMA*. 2001;285(9):1164–1171.

APPENDIXES I–IV: TRAUMA REHABILITATION CRITERIA FROM THE STATE OF WASHINGTON

APPENDIX I

WAC 246-976-830 Designation standards for facilities providing level I trauma rehabilitation service.

1. Level I trauma rehabilitation services shall:
   a. Treat trauma inpatients and outpatients, regardless of disability or level of severity or complexity, who are fifteen years old or older. For adolescent trauma patients, the service shall consider whether educational goals, premorbid learning or developmental status, social or family needs and other factors indicate treatment in an adult or pediatric rehabilitation service;
   b. Have and retain accreditation by the commission on accreditation of rehabilitation facilities (CARF) for hospital-based comprehensive inpatient rehabilitation, category one;
      i. Abeyance or deferral status from CARF do not qualify an applicant for designation;
      ii. If the applicant holds one-year accreditation, the application for trauma care service designation shall include a copy of the CARF survey report and recommendations;
   c. House patients on a designated rehabilitation nursing unit;
   d. Provide a peer group for persons with similar disabilities;
   e. Be directed by a physiatrist who is in-house or on-call and responsible for rehabilitation concerns twenty-four hours every day;
   f. Have a diversion or transfer policy with protocols on an individual patient basis, based on the ability to manage that patient at that time;
   g. In addition to the CARF medical consultative service requirements, have the following medical services in-house or on-call twenty-four hours every day:
      i. Anesthesiology, with an anesthesiologist or certified registered nurse anesthetist (CRNA); and
      ii. Radiology;
   h. Provide rehabilitation nursing personnel twenty-four hours every day, with:
      i. Management by a registered nurse;
      ii. At least one certified rehabilitation registered nurse (CRRN) on duty each day and evening shift when a trauma patient is present;
      iii. A minimum of six clinical nursing care hours per patient day for each trauma patient;
      iv. The initial care plan and weekly update reviewed and approved by a CRRN; and
      v. An orientation and training program for all levels of rehabilitation nursing personnel;

i. Provide the following health personnel and services twenty-four hours every day:
  i. Access to pharmaceuticals, with a pharmacist on-call and available for consultation, with capability to have immediate access to patient and pharmacy databases, within five minutes of notification;
  ii. Personnel trained in intermittent urinary catheterization; and
  iii. Respiratory therapy;
j. Provide the following trauma rehabilitation services with staff who are licensed, registered, or certified, and who are in-house or available for treatment every day when indicated in the rehabilitation plan:
  i. Occupational therapy;
  ii. Physical therapy;
  iii. Psychology, including:
    A. Neuropsychological services;
    B. Clinical psychological services, including testing and counseling; and
    C. Substance abuse counseling:
  iv. Social services;
  v. Speech/language pathology;
k. Provide the following services in-house or through affiliation or consultative arrangements with staff who are licensed, registered, certified, or degreed:
  i. Communication augmentation;
  ii. Driver evaluation and training;
  iii. Orthotics;
  iv. Prosthetics;
  v. Rehabilitation engineering for device development and adaptations;
  vi. Therapeutic recreation; and
  vii. Vocational rehabilitation;
l. Provide the following diagnostic services in-house or through affiliation or consultative arrangements with staff who are licensed, registered, certified, or degreed:
  i. Diagnostic imaging, including computerized tomography, magnetic resonance imaging, nuclear medicine, and radiology;
  ii. Electrophysiologic testing, to include:
    A. Electroencephalography;
    B. Electromyography;
    C. Evoked potentials;
  iii. Laboratory services; and
  iv. Urodynamic testing;
m. Serve as a regional referral center for patients in their geographical area needing only level II or III rehabilitation care;

n. Have an outreach program regarding trauma rehabilitation care, consisting of telephone and on-site consultations with physicians and other health care professionals in the community and outlying areas;
o. Have a formal program of continuing trauma rehabilitation care education, both in-house and outreach, provided for nurses and allied health care professionals;
p. Have an ongoing structured program to conduct clinical studies, applied research, or analysis in rehabilitation of trauma patients, and report results within a peer review process.
2. A level I trauma rehabilitation service shall:
a. Have a quality assurance/improvement program in accordance with WAC 246-976-881;
b. Participate in trauma registry activities as required in WAC 246-976-430;
c. Participate in the regional trauma quality assurance program as required in WAC 246-976-910.
[Statutory Authority: Chapter 70.168 RCW. 98-04-038, § 246-976-830, filed 1/29/98, effective 3/1/98; 93-20-063, § 246-976-830, filed 10/1/93, effective 11/1/93.]

APPENDIX II

WAC 246-976-840 Designation standards for facilities providing level II trauma rehabilitation service.

1. Level II trauma rehabilitation services shall:
a. Treat trauma inpatients and outpatients with any disability or level of severity or complexity within the service's capabilities as defined in (c) of this subsection, who are fifteen years old or older;
b. For adolescent trauma patients, the service shall consider whether educational goals, premorbid learning or developmental status, social or family needs, and other factors indicate treatment in an adult or pediatric rehabilitation service;
c. Delineate criteria for admission based on diagnosis and severity of impairment;
d. Have and retain accreditation by the commission on accreditation of rehabilitation facilities (CARF) for comprehensive inpatient rehabilitation, category one or two;
  i. Abeyance or deferral status do not qualify an applicant for designation;

    ii. If the applicant holds one-year accreditation, the application for trauma service designation shall include a copy of the CARF survey report and recommendations;

e. House patients on a designated rehabilitation nursing unit;

f. Provide a peer group for persons with similar disabilities;

g. Be directed by a physiatrist who is responsible for rehabilitation concerns twenty-four hours every day;

h. Have a diversion or transfer policy with protocols on an individual patient basis, based on the ability to manage that patient at that time;

i. In addition to the CARF medical consultative service requirements, provide the following medical services in-house or on-call twenty-four hours every day:

    i. Anesthesiology, with an anesthesiologist or certified registered nurse anesthetist (CRNA); and

    ii. Radiology;

j. Provide rehabilitation nursing personnel twenty-four hours every day, with:

    i. Management by a registered nurse;

    ii. At least one certified rehabilitation registered nurse (CRRN) on duty one shift each day when a trauma patient is present;

    iii. A minimum of six clinical nursing care hours per patient day for each trauma patient;

    iv. The initial care plan and weekly update reviewed and approved by a CRRN; and

    v. An orientation and training program for all levels of rehabilitation nursing personnel;

k. Provide the following health personnel and services twenty-four hours every day:

    i. Access to pharmaceuticals, with a pharmacist on-call and available for consultation, with capability to have immediate access to patient and pharmacy data bases, within five minutes of notification;

    ii. Personnel trained in intermittent urinary catheterization; and

    iii. Respiratory therapy;

l. Provide the following trauma rehabilitation services with staff who are licensed, registered, or certified, and who are in-house or available for treatment every day when indicated in the rehabilitation plan:

    i. Occupational therapy;

    ii. Physical therapy;

    iii. Psychology, including:

        A. Neuropsychological services;

        B. Clinical psychological services, including testing and counseling;

        C. Substance abuse counseling;

    iv. Social services;

    v. Speech/language pathology;

m. Provide the following services in-house or through affiliation or consultative arrangements with staff who are licensed, registered, certified, or degreed:

    i. Communication augmentation;

    ii. Driver evaluation and training;

    iii. Orthotics;

    iv. Prosthetics;

    v. Rehabilitation engineering for device development and adaptations;

    vi. Therapeutic recreation; and

    vii. Vocational rehabilitation;

n. Provide the following diagnostic services in-house or through affiliation or consultative arrangements with staff who are licensed, registered, certified, or degreed:

    i. Diagnostic imaging, including computerized tomography, magnetic resonance imaging, nuclear medicine, and radiology;

    ii. Electrophysiologic testing, to include:

        A. Electroencephalography;

        B. Electromyography; and

        C. Evoked potentials;

    iii. Laboratory services;

    iv. Urodynamic testing;

o. Have an outreach program regarding trauma rehabilitation care, consisting of telephone and on-site consultations with physicians and other health care professionals in the community and outlying areas;

p. Have a formal program of continuing trauma rehabilitation care education, both in-house and outreach, provided for nurses and allied health care professionals.

2. A level II trauma rehabilitation service shall:

a. Have a quality assurance/improvement program in accordance with WAC 246-976-881;

b. Participate in trauma registry activities as required in WAC 246-976-430;

c. Participate in the regional trauma quality assurance program as required in WAC 246-976-910.

[Statutory Authority: Chapter 70.168 RCW. 98-04-038, § 246-976-840, filed 1/29/98, effective 3/1/98; 93-20-063, § 246-976-840, filed 10/1/93, effective 11/1/93.]

APPENDIX III

WAC 246-976-850 Designation standards for level III trauma rehabilitation service.

1. Level III trauma rehabilitation services shall:
   a. Provide a community based program of coordinated and integrated outpatient trauma rehabilitation services, evaluation, and treatment to those persons with trauma-related functional limitations, who do not need or no longer require comprehensive inpatient rehabilitation. Services may be provided in, but not limited to, the following settings:
      i. Freestanding outpatient rehabilitation centers;
      ii. Organized outpatient rehabilitation programs in acute hospital settings;
      iii. Day hospital programs; and
      iv. Other community settings;
   b. Treat patients according to admission criteria based on diagnosis and severity;
   c. Be directed by a physician with training and/or experience necessary to provide rehabilitative physician services, acquired through one of the following:
      i. Formal residency in physical medicine and rehabilitation;
      ii. A fellowship in rehabilitation for a minimum of one year; or
      iii. A minimum of two years' experience in providing rehabilitation services for patients typically seen in CARF-accredited comprehensive inpatient categories one, two, and three;
   d. Provide the following trauma rehabilitation services by staff who are licensed, registered, or certified:
      i. Occupational therapy;
      ii. Physical therapy;
      iii. Social services;
      iv. Speech/language pathology;
   e. Provide or assist the patient to obtain the following as defined in the rehabilitation plan:
      i. Audiology;
      ii. Chaplaincy;
      iii. Dentistry;
      iv. Dietetics;
      v. Driver evaluation and training;
      vi. Education;
      vii. Nursing;
      viii. Orthotics;
      ix. Prosthetics;
      x. Psychology;
      xi. Rehabilitation engineering for device development and adaptations;
      xii. Respiratory therapy;
      xiii. Substance abuse counseling;
      xiv. Therapeutic recreation;
      xv. Vocational rehabilitation.
2. A level III trauma rehabilitation service shall:
   a. Have a quality assurance/improvement program in accordance with WAC 246-976-881;
   b. Participate in trauma registry activities as required in WAC 246-976-430;
   c. Participate in the regional trauma quality assurance program established pursuant to WAC 246-976-910.
   [Statutory Authority: Chapter 70.168 RCW. 98-04-038, § 246-976-850, filed 1/29/98, effective 3/1/98; 93-20-063, § 246-976-850, filed 10/1/93, effective 11/1/93.]

APPENDIX IV

WAC 246-976-860 Designation standards for facilities providing level I pediatric trauma rehabilitation service.

1. Level I pediatric rehabilitation services shall:
   a. Treat inpatients and outpatients, regardless of disability or level of severity or complexity, who are:
      i. Under fifteen years old; or
      ii. For adolescent trauma patients, determine whether educational goals, premorbid learning or developmental status, social or family needs, or other factors indicate treatment in an adult or pediatric setting.
   b. Have and retain accreditation by the commission on accreditation of rehabilitation facilities (CARF) for hospital-based comprehensive inpatient rehabilitation category one, including the additional designated pediatric program standards required to provide pediatric rehabilitative services;
      i. Abeyance or deferral status do not qualify an applicant for designation;
      ii. If the applicant holds one-year accreditation, the application for trauma

care service designation shall include a copy of the CARF survey report and recommendations;

c. House patients in a designated pediatric rehabilitation area, providing a pediatric milieu;

d. Provide a peer group for persons with similar disabilities;

e. Be directed by a physiatrist who is in-house or on-call and responsible for rehabilitation concerns twenty-four hours every day;

f. Have a diversion or transfer policy with protocols on an individual patient basis, based on the ability to manage that patient at that time;

g. In addition to the CARF medical consultative service requirements, have the following medical services in-house or on-call twenty-four hours every day:
  i. Anesthesiology, with an anesthesiologist or certified registered nurse anesthetist (CRNA);
  ii. A pediatrician;
  iii. Radiology;

h. Provide rehabilitation nursing personnel twenty-four hours every day, with:
  i. Management by a registered nurse;
  ii. At least one certified rehabilitation registered nurse (CRRN) on duty each day shift and evening shift when a trauma patient is present;
  iii. A minimum of six clinical nursing care hours per patient day for each trauma patient;
  iv. All nursing personnel trained and/or experienced in pediatric rehabilitation;
  v. The initial care plan and weekly update reviewed and approved by a CRRN; and
  vi. An orientation and training program for all levels of rehabilitation nursing personnel;

i. Provide the following health personnel and services twenty-four hours every day:
  i. Access to pharmaceuticals, with pharmacist in house;
  ii. Personnel trained in intermittent urinary catheterization; and
  iii. Respiratory therapy;

j. Provide the following trauma rehabilitation services with staff who are licensed, registered, or certified, who are trained and/or experienced in pediatric rehabilitation, and who are in-house or available for treatment every day when indicated in the rehabilitation plan:
  i. Occupational therapy,
  ii. Physical therapy;
  iii. Psychology, including:
    A. Neuropsychological services;
    B. Clinical psychological services, including testing and counseling; and
    C. Substance abuse counseling;
  iv. Social services;
  v. Speech/language pathology;

k. Provide the following services in-house or through affiliation or consultative arrangements with staff who are licensed, registered, certified, or degreed:
  i. Communication augmentation;
  ii. Educational component of the program appropriate to the disability and developmental level of the child, to include educational screening, instruction, and discharge planning coordinated with the receiving school district;
  iii. Orthotics;
  iv. Play space, with supervision by a pediatric therapeutic recreation specialist or child life specialist, to provide assessment and play activities;
  v. Prosthetics;
  vi. Rehabilitation engineering for device development and adaptations;
  vii. Therapeutic recreation;

l. Provide the following diagnostic services in-house or through affiliation or consultative arrangements with staff who are licensed, registered, certified, or degreed:
  i. Electrophysiologic testing, to include:
    A. Electroencephalography;
    B. Electromyography;
    C. Evoked potentials;
  ii. Diagnostic imaging, including computerized tomography, magnetic resonance imaging, nuclear medicine, and radiology;
  iii. Laboratory services; and
  iv. Urodynamic testing;

m. Have an outreach program regarding pediatric trauma rehabilitation care, consisting of telephone and on-site consultations with physicians and other health care professionals in the community and outlying areas;

n. Have a formal program of continuing pediatric trauma rehabilitation care education, both in-house and outreach, provided for nurses and allied health care professionals;

o. Have an ongoing structured program to conduct clinical studies, applied research or analysis in rehabilitation of pediatric trauma patients, and report results within a peer-review process.

2. A level I pediatric rehabilitation service shall:

a. Have a quality assurance/improvement program in accordance with WAC 246-976-881;

b. Participate in trauma registry activities as required in WAC 246-976-430;

c. Participate in the regional trauma quality assurance program as required in WAC 246-976-910.

[Statutory Authority: Chapter 70.168 RCW. 98-19-107, § 246-976-860, filed 9/23/98, effective 10/24/98; 98-04-038, § 246-976-860, filed 1/29/98, effective 3/1/98; 93-20-063, § 246-976-860, filed 10/1/93, effective 11/1/93.]

2

Epidemiology of Trauma-related Disability

Lawrence R. Robinson and Paula J. Micklesen

FREQUENCY OF TRAUMA

TRAUMA AS A CAUSE OF DEATH

Trauma is a very common cause of death and disability. Trauma, specifically unintentional injury, is the most common cause of death in those aged 1 to 34 in the United States, and the second most common cause of death in those aged 35 to 44 (Table 2-1) (1). Trauma accounted for more than 148,000 deaths in the year 2001, including 100,000 fatalities from unintentional injuries, 17,000 homicides, and 29,000 suicides. Motor vehicle crashes (MVCs) were the most common cause, accounting for about 31% of all trauma-related deaths. Firearms caused an additional 19% of trauma deaths (2). For the year 2001, trauma deaths represented nearly 3.5 million years of potential life lost before the age of 65 (1).

Death rates are a poor indicator of the magnitude of the problem, however. First, most injured patients survive. For example, in 2001 there were approximately 157,000 trauma-related deaths, but an additional 29 million reported injuries, and of those injured, 1.6 million were either hospitalized or transferred (1). Thus, for each trauma-related death, there were nearly 200 injuries and 10 patients who required hospitalization. Approximately 25% of those who were hospitalized sustained moderate to severe injuries (Abbreviated Injury Scale [AIS] ≥3) (3).

The causes of nonfatal traumatic injuries differ somewhat from the causes of those that result in death (Table 2-2). Firearms are a relatively frequent cause of trauma deaths (19%), but a much less common cause of trauma-related hospitalizations (2.5%), because most shooting victims do not survive to be hospitalized. Conversely, more victims of falls are hospitalized (36% of trauma hospitalizations), with fewer deaths (9% of trauma deaths) (Fig. 2–1, Table 2-3).

Finally, the impact on society is different for fatalities than it is for injuries. Those disabled by trauma will require a higher level of medical resources. Some will recover to the point of independence and return to work. Others will require a high level of care for the remainder of their lives. For 2001, the aggregate lifetime costs for all injured patients were estimated to be $158 billion (1).

FREQUENCY OF TRAUMA-RELATED NONFATAL INJURY

The survival rates after civilian and military trauma have improved significantly over the last 50 years due to a multitude of advances in trauma prevention, the emergency medical trauma system, and acute care hospitalization. As a result, more trauma victims survive and are admitted to the hospital, many of whom will ultimately require rehabilitation care.

Not all survivors of trauma will, however, require inpatient rehabilitation. Those who are too severely injured will die soon after hospital admission, or be so severely injured (e.g., in a persistent vegetative state) as to be unable to participate in the rehabilitation process. Others will be less severely injured and will either receive sufficient rehabilitative services in other settings (on the acute care service or as an outpatient) or not need rehabilitative

Table 2-1 Ten Leading Causes of Death, United States 2001, All Races, Both Sexes

Rank	<1	1–4	5–9	10–14	15–24	25–34	35–44	45–54	55–64	65+	All Ages
1	Congenital Anomalies 5,513	Unintentional Injury 1,714	Unintentional Injury 1,283	Unintentional Injury 1,553	Unintentional Injury 14,411	Unintentional Injury 11,839	Malignant Neoplasms 16,569	Malignant Neoplasms 49,562	Malignant Neoplasms 90,223	Heart Disease 582,730	Heart Disease 700,142
2	Short Gestation 4,410	Congenital Anomalies 557	Malignant Neoplasms 493	Malignant Neoplasms 515	Homicide 5,297	Homicide 5,204	Unintentional Injury 15,945	Heart Disease 36,399	Heart Disease 62,486	Malignant Neoplasms 390,214	Malignant Neoplasms 553,768
3	SIDS 2,234	Malignant Neoplasms 420	Congenital Anomalies 182	Suicide 272	Suicide 3,971	Suicide 5,070	Heart Disease 13,326	Unintentional Injury 13,344	Chronic Low. Respiratory Disease 11,166	Cerebrovascular Disease 144,486	Cerebrovascular Disease 163,538
4	Maternal Pregnancy Complic. 1,499	Homicide 415	Homicide 137	Congenital Anomalies 194	Malignant Neoplasms 1,704	Malignant Neoplasms 3,994	Suicide 6,635	Liver Disease 7,259	Cerebrovascular Disease 9,608	Chronic Low. Respiratory Disease 106,904	Chronic Low. Respiratory Disease 123,013
5	Placenta Cord Membranes 1,018	Heart Disease 225	Heart Disease 98	Homicide 189	Heart Disease 999	Heart Disease 3,160	HIV 5,867	Suicide 5,942	Diabetes Mellitus 9,570	Influenza and Pneumonia 55,518	Unintentional Injury 101,537
6	Respiratory Distress 1,011	Influenza and Pneumonia 112	Benign Neoplasms 52	Heart Disease 174	Congenital Anomalies 505	HIV 2,101	Homicide 4,268	Cerebrovascular Disease 5,910	Unintentional Injury 7,658	Diabetes Mellitus 53,707	Diabetes Mellitus 71,372
7	Unintentional Injury 976	Septicemia 108	Influenza and Pneumonia 46	Chronic Low. Respiratory Disease 62	HIV 225	Cerebrovascular Disease 601	Liver Disease 3,336	Diabetes Mellitus 5,343	Liver Disease 5,750	Alzheimer Disease 53,245	Influenza and Pneumonia 62,034
8	Bacterial Sepsis 696	Perinatal Period 72	Chronic Low. Respiratory Disease 42	Benign Neoplasms 53	Cerebrovascular Disease 196	Diabetes Mellitus 595	Cerebrovascular Disease 2,491	HIV 4,120	Suicide 3,317	Nephritis	Alzheimer Disease 53,852
9	Circulatory System Disease 622	Benign Neoplasms 58	Cerebrovascular Disease 38	Influenza and Pneumonia 46	Influenza and Pneumonia 181	Congenital Anomalies 458	Diabetes Mellitus 1,958	Chronic Low. Respiratory Disease 3,324	Nephritis 3,284	Unintentional Injury 32,694	Nephritis 39,480
10	Intrauterine Hypoxia 534	Cerebrovascular Disease 54	Septicemia 29	Cerebrovascular Disease 42	Chronic Low. Respiratory Disease 171	Liver Disease 387	Influenza and Pneumonia 983	Homicide 2,467	Septicemia 3,111	Septicemia 25,418	Septicemia 32,238

From National Center for Health Statistics (NCHS) Vital Statistics System. Ten Leading Causes of Death, United States 2001, All Races, Both Sexes. Available at: http://webapp.cdc.gov/sasweb/ncipc/leadcaus10.html. Accessed October 27, 2004.

Table 2-2   Ten Leading Causes of Nonfatal Injury, United States 2001, All Races, Both Sexes, Disposition: Transferred/ Hospitalized

Rank	<1	1–4	5–9	10–14	15–24	25–34	35–44	45–54	55–64	64+	All Ages
						Age Groups					
1	Unintentional Fall 3,124	Unintentional Fall 15,623	Unintentional Fall 18,151	Unintentional Fall 14,317	Unintentional MV-Occupant 66,859	Unintentional MV-Occupant 38,045	Unintentional Fall 34,283	Unintentional Fall 41,878	Unintentional Fall 47,028	Unintentional Fall 373,128	Unintentional Fall 590,426
2	Unintentional Foreign Body 863[b]	Unintentional Poisoning 7,456	Unintentional MV-Occupant 6,029	Unintentional MV-Occupant 7,121	Self-harm Poisoning 36,263	Self-harm Poisoning 32,093	Self-harm Poisoning 33,952	Unintentional MV-Occupant 25,583	Unintentional MV-Occupant 15,567	Unintentional MV-Occupant 26,894	Unintentional MV-Occupant 225,099
3	Unintentional MV-Occupant 762[b]	Unintentional Foreign Body 5,007	Unintentional Struck by/against 4,311	Unintentional Struck by/against 5,716	Unintentional Fall 20,005	Unintentional Fall 22,053	Unintentional MV-Occupant 33,102	Unintentional Poisoning 20,179	Unintentional Poisoning 7,039	Unintentional Overexertion 11,991	Self-harm Poisoning 134,774
4	Unintentional Struck by/against 525[b]	Unintentional Fire/Burn 3,893	Unintentional Pedestrian 3,404	Unintentional Pedal Cyclist 5,420	Unintentional Poisoning 14,295	Unintentional Poisoning 15,855	Unintentional Poisoning 31,195	Self-harm Poisoning 18,699	Self-harm Poisoning 5,295	Unintentional Struck by/against 9,782	Unintentional Poisoning 106,041
5	Other Assault[a] Struck by/against 455[b]	Unintentional MV-Occupant 3,823[b]	Unintentional Pedal Cyclist 2,974	Self-harm Poisoning 5,381	Other Assault[a] Struck by/against 11,918	Other Assault[a] Struck by/against 10,154	Unintentional Other Specified 16,208[b]	Unintentional Other Specified 12,351[b]	Unintentional Struck by/against 4,201	Unintentional Unknown/Unspecified 7,937	Unintentional Struck by/against 63,020
6	Unintentional Inhalation/Suffocation 404[b]	Unintentional Struck by/against 3,748	Unintentional Foreign Body 2,199	Unintentional Other Transport 3,377	Unintentional Struck by/against 11,359	Unintentional Struck by/against 8,928	Other Assault[a] Struck by/against 10,487	Unintentional Struck by/against 6,889	Unintentional Overexertion 4,102	Unintentional Poisoning 6,936	Unintentional Other Specified 53,143*
7	Unintentional Fire/Burn 363[b]	Unintentional Pedestrian 1,887[b]	Unintentional Other Transport 2,052	Unintentional Pedestrian 2,433	Self-harm Cut/Pierce 10,148	Unintentional Other Specified 8,435[b]	Unintentional Struck by/against 7,560	Other Assault[a] Struck by/against 5,514	Unintentional Other Specified 3,949[b]	Unintentional Other Transport 6,069	Other Assault[a] Struck by/against 44,207
8	Unintentional Poisoning 325[b]	Unintentional Drowning/Near Drown 1,574[b]	Unintentional Unknown/Unspecified 1,711	Unintentional Unknown/Unspecified 2,382	Other Assault[a] Firearm Gunshot 10,036	Other Assault[a] Cut/Pierce 7,232	Unintentional Motorcyclist 6,205	Unintentional Motorcyclist 5,081[b]	Unintentional Other Transport 3,141	Unintentional Other Specified 4,455	Unintentional Other Transport 39,647
9	Unintentional Unknown/Unspecified 306[b]	Unintentional Other Bite/Sting 1,428[b]	Unintentional Poisoning 1,016[b]	Unintentional Cut/Pierce 2,031	Unintentional Motorcyclist 8,518	Other Assault[a] Firearm Gunshot 6,799	Unintentional Other Transport 5,866	Unintentional Cut/Pierce 4,822	Unintentional Unknown/Unspecified 2,602	Unintentional Pedestrian 4,022	Unintentional Overexertion 32,759
10	Unintentional Drowning/ Near Drown 272[b]	Unintentional Dog Bite 1,410	Unintentional Unknown/Unspecified 983[b]	Other Assault[a] Struck by/against 1,802	Unintentional Other Transport 7,730	Unintentional Motorcyclist 6,209	Unintentional Overexertion 5,675	Unintentional Other Transport 4,744	Other Assault[a] Struck by/against 1,861	Unintentional Foreign Body 3,376	Unintentional Motorcyclist 29,902

[a] The "Other Assault" category includes all assaults that are not classified as sexual assault. It represents the majority of assaults.
[b] Injury estimate is unstable because of small sample size.
From NEISS All Injury Program, operated by the Consumer Product Safety Commission. Ten Leading Causes of Nonfatal Injury, United States, 2001, All Races, Both Sexes, Disposition: Transferred/Hospitalized (CPSC). Available at: http://webappa.cdc.gov/sasweb/ncipc/nfilead2001.html. Accessed October 27, 2004.

Table 2-3	Distribution of Mechanism of Injury/Death in United States 2001 (Percentage)		
Mechanism	Treated and Released (%)	Hospitalized (%)	Deaths (%)
Fall	26	40	10
Transportation	12	19	29
Poison	1	13	14
Struck by/against	21	6	<1
Cut/Pierce	9	3	1
Overexertion	12	2	<1
Firearm	<1	1	18
Drown	<1	<1	2
Burn	2	<1	2
Other	17	16	24

Modified from WISQARS. Centers for Disease Control and Prevention. Web-based Injury Statistics Query and Reporting System (WISQARS) (2003). National Center for Injury Prevention and Control, Centers for Disease Control and Prevention (producer). Available at: www.cdc.gov/ncipc/wisqars. Accessed September 2004.

services at all. Of the 1.5 million trauma patients hospitalized in 2000, 25% had moderate to severe injuries (AIS ≥3). Thus, it is a "middle" group of individuals who will require rehabilitation services. This fact requires that one takes care in examining trauma injuries statistics, and not equate all trauma victims with those receiving inpatient rehabilitation.

The incidence of major disability due to trauma varies according to the type of injury and disability.

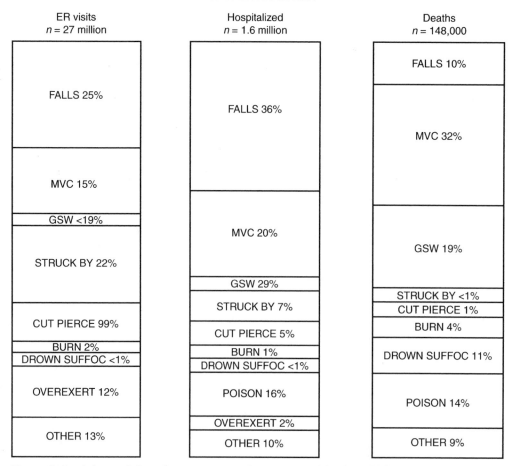

Figure 2–1. Injury etiology for emergency department visits, hospitalizations, and deaths.

Table 2-4	Incidence and Prevalence of Injuries Likely to Cause Major Disability[a]

Injury	Annual Incidence (per million)	Annual Incidence in United States	Prevalence (per million)	Prevalence in United States
Traumatic brain injury	300	90,000 cases	20,000	5,300,000 cases
Spinal cord injury	40	12,000 cases	800	240,000 cases
Traumatic amputation	11	3,300 cases	1,300	390,000 cases
Burns	66	19,800 cases		

[a] Note that the incidence of injury is greater than the incidence of disability. For example, the incidence of TBI is 230,000 cases per year, but only 90,000 are disabled.
From Langlois JA, Rutland-Brown W, Thomas KE. Traumatic brain injury in the United States: Emergency department visits, hospitalizations, and deaths (2001). National Center for Injury Prevention and Control, Centers for Disease Control and Prevention. Available at: http://www.cdc.gov/ncipc/pub-res/TBI_in_US_04/TBI_ED.htm. Accessed September 2004; Facts and figures at a glance—August 2004. National Spinal Cord Injury Statistical Center (NSCISC). Available at: URL: http://www.spinalcord.uab.edu/show.asp?durki=21446. Accessed September 2004; Dillingham TR, Pezzin LE, MacKenzie EJ. Incidence, acute care length of stay, and discharge to rehabilitation of traumatic amputee patients: an epidemiologic study. *APMR.* 1998;79(3):279–287; and Dillingham TR, Pezzin LE, MacKenzie EJ. Limb amputation and limb deficiency: Epidemiology and recent trends in the United States. *South Med J.* 2002;95(8):875–883, with permission.

Musculoskeletal injuries primarily to the upper or lower limbs, including hip fractures in the elderly, constitute 47% of all trauma hospitalizations (approximately 800,000 cases per year), with approximately a third of these in the moderate to severe range (AIS ≥3). Of these, approximately 120,000 go to inpatient rehabilitation, as well as approximately 14,600 with multiple trauma, and an estimated 1,000 cases of traumatic amputation (estimates based on Uniform Data System [UDS] 2003 to 2004 reports, which currently include 70% of inpatient rehab facilities) (4).

Traumatic brain injury (TBI) is the most common neurologic disability, with an incidence of about 300 cases per million (90,000 cases in the United States) and prevalence of 20,000 cases per million in the United States (Table 2-4). Thus there are about 5.3 million individuals in the United States, or roughly 2% of the population, living with disability due to a TBI. Motor vehicle crashes, including those involving bicycles and pedestrians, are the most common cause of hospitalization for head injury, and they account for nearly one-half of all admissions. Falls are the second leading cause of head injury, accounting for another quarter of the total (5). Of the 90,000 estimated to sustain permanent disability from their TBI, approximately 18,000 go to inpatient rehabilitation units (4).

Somewhat less common is disability due to spinal cord injury (SCI) with an incidence of 40 per million. Each year about 12,000 individuals in the United States suffer SCI caused by trauma. Prevalence is about 800 per million with an estimated prevalence of 240,000 in the United States. The most common cause of SCI is motor vehicle crashes, which account for about 40% of all cases. Falls cause another 22%, firearms 25%, and sports- and diving-related incidents are responsible for 12% (6). Approximately 8,700 of individuals with these types of injuries go to inpatient rehabilitation units (4).

Major traumatic amputation is a much less common occurrence in the United States (11 per million) than amputation due to vascular disease or diabetic complications (about 200 per million). However, since individuals with traumatic amputation are generally younger and thus live longer than those with amputation due to other causes, the estimated prevalence of major traumatic amputation is represented to a greater extent at 1,300 per million, while major amputation from other causes is about 2,500 per million; overall about 0.4% of the population has a major amputation.

Major burns requiring hospitalization occur with a frequency of about 66 per million each year. Approximately 1,190 of these cases go to inpatient rehabilitation units each year (4).

Patients with traumatic injuries represent approximately one fourth of the inpatient rehabilitation patient population in the United States. In fiscal year 2003 to 2004, there were approximately 670,000 rehabilitation inpatients in the United States, including many with nontraumatic disorders, particularly stroke. Of the 164,000 injuries with traumatic etiologies, the majority were fractures (73%). TBI accounted for 11%; multitrauma, 9%; SCI, 5%; and burns and traumatic amputations, <1% each (Fig. 2–2) (4).

Patients with hip fractures and other orthopaedic injuries are typically transferred to inpatient rehabilitation fairly soon, and stay only a short time. Many of these patients receive their rehabilitation in community hospitals rather than in level I or II

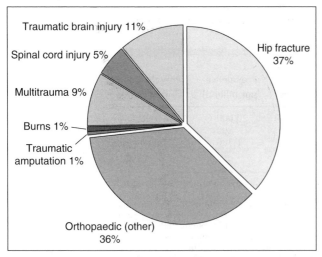

Figure 2–2. Estimated breakdown of patients with traumatic injuries on inpatient rehabilitation units in the United States (based on UDS data).

trauma centers. Patients with burns, multitrauma, and TBI typically arrive at 3 weeks post-injury, and stay for 2.5 weeks. Patients with SCIs typically do not come to rehabilitation until 3.5 weeks post-injury, and have the longest stays, averaging 3 weeks, with even longer inpatient stays for quadriplegia.

INFLUENCE OF AGE AND GENDER

As can be seen from Tables 2-1 and 2-2, the majority of traumatic fatalities are seen in younger individuals, particularly young men, although the majority of nonfatal injuries are in the elderly. Trauma is the most common cause of death for those aged 1 to 34 years. After the age of 35, malignant neoplasms and heart disease increase in frequency and are more common causes of death. However, the risk of traumatic injury does not decline with age, but rather the risk from other causes of death and disability increases more than the risk of injury. The rate of

hospitalization due to trauma increases for 20- to 25-year-olds and then falls slightly, but then increases much more rapidly after the age of 70 (Fig. 2–3). As the population ages, it is expected that the rate of death and disability from trauma amongst the population as a whole will increase.

Throughout most of the adult life span, males are at greater risk of trauma than females (Fig. 2–3). Although this increased risk is most marked in the second and third decades of life, differences remain until age 60. After the age of 70, the risk of trauma to women is greater than for men, particularly as more men die from other causes.

Regarding inpatient rehabilitation patients, those with fractures are mostly female (73%) with an average age of 73 years. Patients with TBI, SCI, and multitrauma are mostly male (65%) with an average age of 50 years (4). As the population ages, there is a greater incidence of trauma due to falls, while the incidence of trauma due to MVC peaks in late adolescence and early adulthood (Figs. 2–4, 2–5).

INJURY BY MECHANISM AND INTENT

The distribution of causes of injury by mechanism and intent are seen in Figure 2–1 and Table 2-3. Intent is generally classified as unintentional (i.e., accidental), intentional (intentionally inflicted either by someone else or by patients themselves), undetermined, or other (e.g., acts of war). Mechanism is classified by what caused the trauma.

The various outcomes seen in Table 2-3 reflect different causes of injury. For those hospitalized (including those most likely to require rehabilitation), the most common causes are falls and transportation. However for trauma fatalities, transportation and firearms are the biggest causes. Although firearms are responsible for 18% of trauma-related deaths, they represent 1% or less of those hospitalized or treated/released, since many die of their wounds. For those

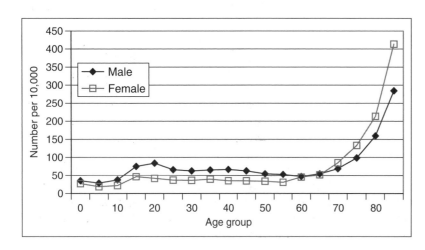

Figure 2–3. Hospitalizations due to injury over the life span.

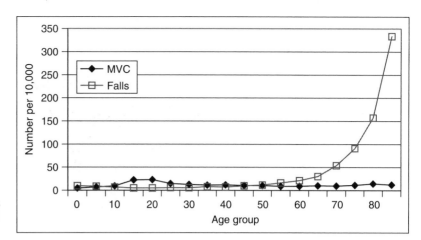

Figure 2–4. Incidence of hospitalizations due to motor vehicle crashes (MVC) and falls over the life span.

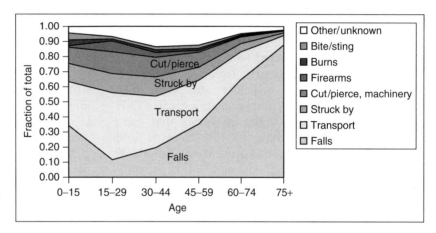

Figure 2–5. Causes of traumatic injury hospitalizations 2001.

interested in trauma prevention, all causes are of interest. However, for those involved in trauma rehabilitation, it is probably the "middle" group that is of most interest; namely, those not fatally injured, but injured severely enough to require hospitalization.

In 2001, 17% of those injured in the United States had injuries caused by either violence or self-harm, most of these from intentional self-poisoning (8%), or from assaults involving blunt trauma, gunshot wounds, or stabbings (6%). The majority (83%) of individuals injured and hospitalized were injured unintentionally (Fig. 2–6).

Falls represent 36% of injury hospitalizations, and nearly 80% of hospitalizations for those over the age of 65. Incidence is highest among elderly women (Figs. 2–3, 2–5, 2–7). Transportation accounts for 20% of injury hospitalizations, with incidence highest among males aged 15 to 30.

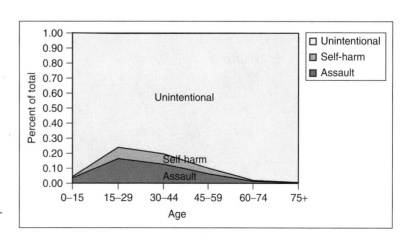

Figure 2–6. Intent of traumatic injury hospitalizations 2001.

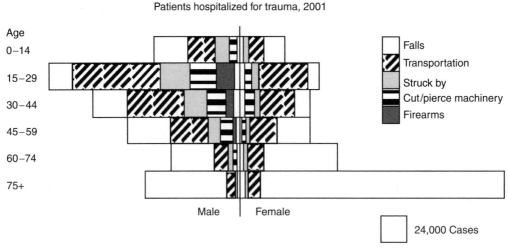

Figure 2–7. Trauma etiologies for patients hospitalized in 2001, with falls in larger numbers of older women, and motor vehicle crashes and firearms in younger men.

Many injuries are related to the workplace. It is estimated that in 2001, there were approximately 4.9 million workplace injuries. Injury rates are highest for mid-sized employers, that is, those with 50 to 249 employees. There were eight industries that each accounted for more than 100,000 injuries and together accounted for 29% of the total (Table 2-5) (7). It is less clear, however, how many of these represent acute injury versus chronic overuse syndromes, or how many represent back and neck strain.

SUMMARY

Trauma is a common cause of death, hospitalization, and disability in the United States. Trauma-related injuries are responsible for a large portion of inpatient admissions to rehabilitation units in the United States, and the number of patients with such injuries is likely to increase as the population ages. It will be important for the specialist in trauma rehabilitation to be familiar with trends in trauma statistics and how these affect the patients treated in the rehabilitation setting.

REFERENCES

1. National Center for Injury Prevention and Control. WISQARS leading causes of nonfatal injury reports. Available at: http://www.cdc.gov/ncipc/wisqars. Accessed 2004.
2. MacKenzie EJ, Fowler CJ. Epidemiology. In: Moore EE, Feliciano DV, Mattox KL, eds. *Trauma*. 5th ed. New York: McGraw-Hill; 2004:21–40.
3. Rice DP, MacKenzie EJ, Jones AS, et al. *Cost of injury in the United States*. San Francisco, CA: Institute for Health and Aging, University of California and the Injury Prevention Center, The Johns Hopkins University Press; 1989.
4. *Annual Inpatient Rehabilitation Facilities Report*. Amherst, NY: Uniform Data System for Medical Rehabilitation; 2003–2004.
5. Sosin DM, Sniezek JE, Thurman DJ. Incidence of mild and moderate brain injury in the United States, 1991. *Brain Injury*. 1996;10:47.
6. National Spinal Cord Injury Statistical Center (NSCISC). Facts and figures at a glance—August 2004. Available at: http://www.spinalcord.uab.edu/show.asp?durki=21446. Accessed September 2004.
7. United States Department of Labor, Bureau of Labor Statistics. *Workplace injuries and illnesses in 2001*. Available at: http://www.bls.gov/iif/oshwc/osh/os/osnr0016.pdf. Accessed 2004.

Table 2-5	Injuries in the Workplace[a]	
Industry	**Cases in 2001**	**Incidence per 100 FTE**
Eating and drinking places	283,700	5.2
Hospitals	285,700	8.2
Nursing and personal care facilities	192,900	13.0
Grocery stores	175,100	7.8
Department stores	145,300	7.7
Trucking and courier services	134,900	8.3
Air transportation, scheduled	116,300	13.6
Motor vehicles and equipment	102,700	10.9

FTE, full time equivalent.
[a] Not all injuries involve acute trauma; many are related to chronic overuse syndromes or back strain.
Adapted from United States Department of Labor, Bureau of Labor Statistics. Workplace Injuries and Illnesses in 2001. Available at: http://www.bls.gov/iif/oshwc/osh/os/osnr0016.pdf. Accessed 2004.

3

Trauma Care Systems in the United States

Gregory J. Jurkovich and Charles N. Mock

TRAUMA AS A HEALTH PROBLEM IN THE UNITED STATES

While injury has been known to be a frequent cause of death in the United States since accurate statistics were first collected more than 150 years ago, its role as leading killer of children and young adults is a phenomenon of the 20th century, and shows little signs of abating. The relative increase in injury as a cause of death is the result of decreases in infectious diseases and the industrialization of society. To be sure, it is also due to an absolute increase in the incidence of trauma, primarily as a result of the introduction of the motor vehicle. Deaths from motor vehicle crashes (MVCs) skyrocketed during the period from 1910 through 1929, rising from an infrequent occurrence to a peak of 30 deaths/100,000 per year during the 1930s and 1940s. During this time, trauma achieved its current status as the leading cause of death in individuals between the ages of 1 and 34 years and the fifth leading cause of death overall. As a result of its effect on these younger age groups, trauma is the leading cause of years of life lost in the American society (1).

There were 157,070 deaths from injury in the United States in 2001 (2). Unintentional injuries accounted for about two thirds of these deaths (101,537 in 2001), with MVC victims, including occupants, pedestrians, and motorcyclists, representing nearly half of those fatalities. Falls, occurring primarily among the elderly, were the second leading cause of death from unintentional injuries. Poison-related deaths were next, followed by burns and

drowning. In 2002, there were 3,482 unintentional drowning and 14,050 burn injuries with 2,670 deaths. Intentional injuries were responsible for slightly more than 50,000 deaths in 2001, of which 60% were from suicide and 40% from homicide. Firearms accounted for 60% of all suicides and 72% of homicides (3).

Although trauma remains the leading killer of young people, the overall trauma mortality rate has gradually decreased in the past two decades. This reduction has been attributed to a decrease in the proportion of workers involved in dangerous occupations, as well as to improvements in the safety of buildings, motor vehicles, and roads, and to improved trauma treatment and injury prevention efforts. Only recently has the prevention of traumatic injury been recognized as a public health issue that requires the involvement of the health care community. Spurred by two sentinel publications by the National Academy of Sciences and the National Research Council (NAS-NRC), awareness of injury as a problem with a greater impact on public health than cancer or cardiovascular diseases has increased. In 1966, the NAS-NRC published a white paper entitled "Accidental Death and Disability: The Neglected Disease of Modern Society" (4). Many have identified this publication as the inaugural event in what has become a sustained effort sponsored by the U.S. government at control of accidental injury. A 20-year follow-up study, entitled "Injury in America: A Continuing Public Health Problem" appeared in 1985, outlining the additional efforts necessary to address the persistent problem of injury (5). Over the past four decades, and especially since the development of the National Center for Injury Prevention and Control (NCIPC) at the Centers for Disease Control and Prevention (CDC), the health care community has assumed a larger role in injury control. Medical and surgical specialists, epidemiologists, statisticians, biomechanical engineers, public health practitioners, and economists have all collaborated to develop a sophisticated interdisciplinary science of injury control (6).

Prevention efforts have been especially effective in improving the safety of motor vehicles. Motor vehicle–related injuries have declined to 20/100,000 per year, their lowest level since the 1920s. Moreover, deaths per mile traveled have declined to the lowest levels ever measured. Improved safety standards for vehicles, better roads, and a moderate decrease in alcohol-related crashes are the dominant contributing factors. Unfortunately, some of the success in combating motor vehicle–related trauma has been offset by increases in death from intentional injury, principally injury related to firearms. Tragically, deaths from firearms now outnumber those from traffic injuries in several of our states.

Hence, despite successes in injury prevention, trauma treatment continues to have an important role in combating the injury epidemic in our country. The most significant advances in the care of injured patients that have occurred in the past 50 years are advances in surgery, anesthesia, imaging technology, and understanding of the basic cellular and genetic response to shock and inflammation. But unique to trauma care is the coordinated societal effort at developing a trauma *system* of care; one that spans the continuum from injury occurrence, notification, transport, emergency and critical care, rehabilitation, and eventual community reincorporation. These advances are highlighted not only in the treatment of individual patients, but also in the establishment of effective systems of prehospital, hospital, and rehabilitative care. This chapter will briefly review these accomplishments and describe the current status of trauma care using the system in one location (Washington state) as an example of trauma care in the country as a whole. We will conclude with an outline of the opportunities for and impediments to further improvements.

HISTORY OF TRAUMA AND EMERGENCY MEDICAL SERVICES

Technological advances in hospital trauma care have been accompanied by a remarkable degree of organization in the delivery of trauma treatment. These improvements in the system of delivering care can be broadly categorized as follows:

1. More rapid prehospital transport;
2. Increased capabilities and training of prehospital care providers;
3. The growth of emergency medicine as a specialty;
4. The development of trauma surgery as a bona fide specialty within general surgery;
5. The creation and promulgation of the advanced trauma life support (ATLS) course;
6. Development of the concept of trauma centers, with a verification system for trauma centers at various levels (I through IV);
7. Regional and state legislative authority for the trauma center franchise.

One of the more significant advances in the organization of trauma treatment is the more efficient transport of injured patients to hospitals afforded by the establishment of emergency medical systems (EMSs) in virtually every community in the nation. A wide appreciation of the importance of the "golden hour" in trauma treatment has led to development of systems of communication and transport that allow rapid conveyance of injured persons to sites of definitive trauma care. More rapid notification and activation of EMS has been achieved by wide adoption of the universal emergency 911 number. While the role of aeromedical helicopters in urban settings remains controversial, there is little argument that their use has been widely adopted and applied to the intermediate transport range (20 to 100 miles) (7,8).

The backbone of this system usually has been community fire departments, with personnel trained at the level of Emergency Medical Technicians (EMTs) and paramedics. Controversies exist as to the efficacy of various prehospital treatments, especially fluid resuscitation for patients in shock. However, there can be little doubt that the increased training for prehospital personnel has improved treatment of problems such as airway obstruction and external bleeding, in addition to providing them with a greater understanding of which patients need to be taken to the hospital most urgently (9).

Physician staffing of the emergency room has also changed. Fifty years ago, for much of the country, emergency care of all types involved a visit to a minimally equipped and staffed emergency room, where a nurse and sometimes an intern would perform an initial evaluation before calling the patient's personal physician. The standard of care has changed in all but the smallest rural hospitals. Recognition of the importance of the early stages of management of many forms of medical emergencies led to the rise of the specialty of emergency medicine. Currently, board certified emergency physicians staff the emergency departments in most community hospitals and many teaching hospitals as well. Trauma training has been a major component of the training of these emergency physicians. Moreover, a greater emphasis on trauma among surgeons has resulted in more senior surgical personnel staffing or being on call for larger urban and teaching hospitals.

Hospitals are no longer considered trauma hospitals unless their capabilities and resources have been verified by an external review and, ideally, designated by a state authority. There now exist approximately 1,200 adult and pediatric trauma centers in the United States, with 190 designated and/or verified as the highest level I trauma centers (10). This represents a doubling of such centers in the last decade of the 20th century (11). Despite this improvement, many states have been slow to develop trauma systems. In 1988, in a review of the status of trauma systems in America, West et al. indicated that only two states had fully organized trauma systems, incorporating the entire state's population. Nineteen had partial coverage by trauma systems and 29 had no formal trauma center designation (12). Since that time, there has been some improvement, but much remains to be done in terms of developing trauma systems to maximally utilize existing facilities and resources.

In this regard it is important to note the contributions of the Committee on Trauma of the American College of Surgeons (ACS-COT). The activities of this committee have contributed to and reflected the growth of trauma as a surgical specialty in the United States. First founded as the Committee on Fractures by Charles Scudder, MD, in 1922, it was the first professional organization emphasizing trauma care as a specialty. It has subsequently grown to be one of the most active components of the American College of Surgeons (ACS). It's activities have included, amongst others, education and verification. In terms of education, it has put forth a series of publications that have been instrumental in advancing trauma care in America. These include *Early Care of the Injured Patient* (13) and *Optimal Resources for Care of the Injured Patient* (14). One of the most outstanding contributions of the COT has been the development of the Advanced Trauma Life Support (ATLS) course (15). ATLS has become the cornerstone of continuing medical education in trauma care for those providing initial care of the injured patient, including surgeons, emergency physicians, and all others who work in emergency rooms. Its international promulgation has been a testimony to its importance.

The *Resources for Optimal Care of the Care of the Injured Patient* outlines the human and material resources needed for each of the levels (I through IV) of trauma centers (14). (See Appendix 1.) It should be understood that this resource is regularly revisited and revised (16). Also, not every state or region uses these exact guidelines for their local definition of the various levels of trauma centers. However, most have adopted these or very similar criteria.

To accompany the guidelines for optimal resources for the care of the injured patient, the ACS-COT has also established a verification process that consists of external site visits for verifying the resources of trauma centers and trauma systems throughout the United States. However, the authority to designate trauma centers rests with the state or regional health care authorities.

Trauma centers are best viewed as part of an overall trauma system that incorporates prehospital care, interhospital transfer, acute hospital care, rehabilitation, and quality assurance. It has been well shown that attention to all of these details can result in improvements in trauma care and outcome (17,18). A consensus conference was held in 1998 to review all available data on the efficacy of trauma systems. This review analyzed three different types of data in support of improved outcomes in trauma centers: preventable death panel studies, studies of effectiveness based on a national trauma registry norm, and large population-based data comparisons. Outcomes for trauma centers are consistently better than those for traditional hospitals, while regions in which a trauma care system has been developed show an even more significant improvement in outcome when compared to areas that lack such systems (19).

The military models of care have also influenced the development of trauma centers and trauma care systems in the United States, as have the physician experience and training accrued during the Korean and Vietnam Wars. The role of the traditional large county teaching hospitals, as well as several important publications that brought to light the large number of preventable deaths following injury, also influenced trauma center development and are well reviewed by Mullins in his introduction to the Skamania Symposium (20). It is important to note that other nations have developed a variety of models for the provision of trauma services involving varying roles for general surgeons, orthopaedists, and emergency physicians (21). The model that has developed in the United States is one that emphasizes the role of the general surgeon/critical care surgeon as the leader of the trauma team, yet incorporates into that team emergency physicians, orthopaedists, neurosurgeons, and anesthesiologists as important colleagues. This model has shown durability for the past 50 years, but is being increasingly challenged by diminishing incidence of penetrating trauma, the pendulum shift to nonoperative management of many blunt internal solid organ injuries, the mandated decreasing work hours of trainees, and the disproportionately poor compensation for trauma care in the United States. Future models will likely take into account these and other factors, and are the active interest of many professional surgical societies at this time.

CURRENT STATUS OF TRAUMA CARE

Arguably, one of the best-developed trauma systems in the United States is to be found in the Seattle area. This system incorporates the spectrum of injury control: prevention, prehospital care, acute hospital care, and rehabilitation. Injury prevention receives considerable attention both from an active Washington Traffic Safety Commission and from the Harborview Injury Prevention and Research Center (HIPRC). HIPRC is a component of the University of Washington and is extremely active in injury-related research and community-based injury prevention programs. One of its best-known activities has been the Seattle helmet promotion campaign, which increased childhood helmet use from near 0% to 60% over a five-year period, with a resultant decrease in the rate of severe head injuries among child bicyclists (22). The organization also has ongoing programs for seat belt promotion, pedestrian safety, burn prevention, decreasing drunk driving, and handgun storage, among others.

In terms of trauma treatment, Seattle has one of the most advanced EMSs in the world. This tiered response to emergencies is run by the Seattle Fire Department, and involves firefighters, police, and EMTs or paramedics (EMT-Ps). Access to the EMS is gained using the enhanced-911 telephone number, meaning that in most areas, the address of the caller is displayed to the central exchange. Trained personnel screen the calls and dispatch appropriate units. First responders consist of EMTs, who are based at 28 fire stations throughout the city. This geographic dispersion allows a 3-minute first response capability. Depending on the nature of the problem, these personnel may treat and transport less seriously ill or injured patients on their own. For more serious problems, they typically call in one of four paramedic units. Oftentimes, both types of units are dispatched simultaneously based on the information provided in the initial 911 call. For example, both units are dispatched for cardiac arrest.

EMTs generally are required to have undergone a 120-hour training course. EMT-Ps in Seattle are required to have undergone a course consisting of 2,000 hours of training and supervised field experience (23). They are trained to perform a variety of prehospital interventions, including intravenous access, endotracheal intubations, cricothyrotomy, and placement of flutter valves for possible pneumothorax. These prehospital interventions are directed by either radio contact with a doctor or standing orders.

This land-based EMS handles almost all trauma in the city of Seattle. Similar units are in place in the suburban towns in the remainder of King County. A single air ambulance service with both helicopter and fixed wing aircraft, Airlift Northwest, is used to transport patients directly from the scene of injuries in remote areas and also to transport patients referred from smaller hospitals throughout the state. This single air-transport service is managed by a consortium of otherwise competing hospitals, an effective self-imposed limitation on resource duplication that is not common in the United States.

There is also a statewide trauma system in place, with hospitals designated as levels I through V based largely on the ACS criteria, but modified specifically by the addition of level V hospitals or clinics in rural or remote regions (14). Figure 3–1 depicts the geographic distribution of the various levels of trauma centers in the state. Harborview Medical Center (HMC) is the only one level I trauma center in the state and receives more than 5,000 trauma admissions per year. While it is unusual in the United States to have only one level I trauma center for an entire state, in Washington this is the only hospital with the resources, education, and research programs that qualifies.

The high volume of admissions to HMC has important implications for patient outcomes. As shown in Figure 3–2, there is growing evidence that the volume of trauma patients cared for is directly related to improved outcome. One important study of outcomes in level I university-affiliated trauma centers of varying volumes of patients demonstrated clear survival advantage for the sickest patients if treated at high-volume trauma centers (Fig. 3–2) (24). The ACS guidelines for trauma centers also suggest that level I trauma centers admit at least 1,200 patients annually, and that 20% of these have an Injury Severity Score (ISS) of 15 or greater, or that each trauma surgeon treats at least 35 patients annually with an ISS of 15 or greater (14). While these recommendations remain controversial (25), the intention is to recognize that higher volumes likely improve experience, preparedness, and outcome, a finding that has been replicated in other technically complex or physiologically challenging patient populations.

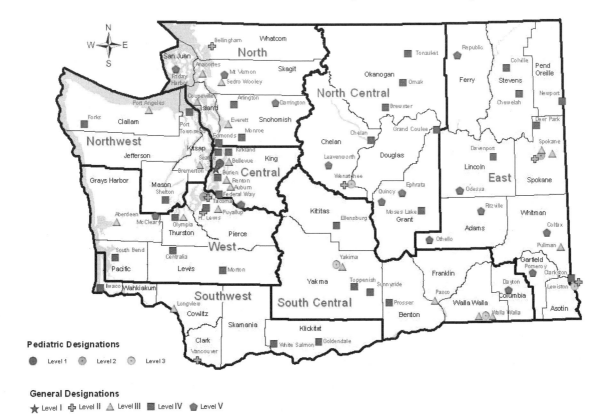

Figure 3–1. Map of the distribution of trauma centers in the State of Washington. From Washington State Department of Health. Office of Emergency Medical Services and Trauma System. Available at: http://www.doh.wa.gov/hswa/emtp/. Accessed 2005.

Funding for trauma system operations in Washington state has been a key to its success. The funding for the trauma center designation process, direct payments to participating hospitals based on the volume they treat, ensuring some payment to physicians for the uninsured trauma victims, and other aspects of the statewide trauma system are essential to keep the system viable. While in most states these funds are typically dependent on yearly allotments from a state legislature, this type of funding source is variable and

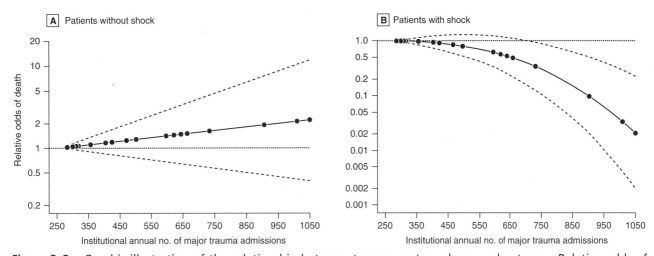

Figure 3–2. Graphic illustration of the relationship between trauma center volume and outcome. Relative odds of death compared with the lowest-volume institution are shown for patients admitted without **(A)** and with **(B)** shock. These estimates are adjusted for New Injury Severity Score, age, and need for massive blood transfusion. The dashed lines are the 95% confidence intervals for the results of the analysis. The solid lines represent the relationship between trauma patient volume (x-axis) and the outcome of interest (y-axis). (From Nathens AB, Jurkovich GJ, Maier RV, et al. Relationship between trauma center volume and outcomes. *JAMA.* 2001; 285[9]:1164–1171, with permission.)

constantly in jeopardy as budget battles invariably arise. Washington state has developed a process of taxation on new motor vehicle licenses to fund a Trauma Care Fund, partially matched by federal dollars, to offset many of these costs (26). This more stable funding source has been essential to the success and viability of the trauma system.

The division of labor among the specialties is as elsewhere in the United States, with the general surgeon as the captain of the trauma team. A member of the general surgery team in the emergency department evaluates all serious trauma. Patients with multisystem injuries are admitted to the general surgery service. Similarly, unstable patients with isolated injuries are usually also admitted to general surgery, resuscitated, and stabilized before eventual transfer to other appropriate services, such as orthopaedics, maxillofacial surgery, or plastics.

There are in-house attending anesthesiologists with a full operating room crew present 24 hours per day. There are in-house chief residents or trauma fellows for general surgery and neurosurgery, capable of initiating operative intervention, with trauma surgeon and critical care attending surgeons on call from home, but within 20-minute response time.

Almost all trauma in the city of Seattle is taken directly to the level I trauma hospital. In the surrounding suburban towns, EMS personnel triage injured persons. Patients with more serious injuries are taken directly to HMC and those with less serious injuries are taken to one of the several suburban level III trauma centers. Triage decisions are based on predetermined plans. In the rural areas of the state, injuries are handled by local EMS departments and by the network of level II, III, and IV trauma centers. Washington state is the only state with level V trauma centers, which primarily are clinics in very remote regions. Depending on the local geography and the level of expertise at each hospital, patients with injuries exceeding local capabilities are transferred to the next highest level of care or directly to HMC. In addition, HMC is the only level I trauma center for a four-state area, including Washington State, Alaska, Idaho, and Montana. HMC receives selected seriously injured patients from these other states as well, primarily for extended intensive care or for subspecialty surgical care.

In addition to the previously noted aspects of acute trauma care, the Washington State trauma system places an emphasis on rehabilitation of the trauma patient. There is a network of rehabilitative services in the Seattle area, including a unit at HMC, a unit at the Children's Hospital and Medical Center in the city, and several units in hospitals in nearby towns. Almost all seriously injured patients receive a rehabilitation consult early on in their hospital course to start planning for necessary rehabilitation services, whether as an outpatient or inpatient on one of the rehabilitation units.

A critical element of the ACS trauma center verification process is the existence and documentation of a quality assurance program. This provision implies that the outcomes of trauma patients are periodically reviewed; that unexpected poor outcomes are discussed by the surgical staff; that corrective action is taken if problems are identified; and that records of this process are kept. The classic weekly surgical morbidity and mortality review forms one of the bases for this quality assurance process. This review is enhanced in trauma centers by a mandatory "trauma council," which consists of a representative for each of the clinical services, plus head nurse of the key trauma-surgical areas (ICU, ER, OR, wards and clinics), and a representative of ancillary services such as respiratory care, blood bank, and trauma registry. These regular meetings with required attendance provide the opportunity to review cross-discipline problems, complications, or concerns, as well as provide a venue for broad dissemination and approval of policy or protocol changes. The meeting is a quality assurance meeting, and its proceedings are held to this legal protection.

All levels of trauma center are required to keep some form of trauma registry. As part of ongoing quality assurance measures, this registry is periodically reviewed for "filters," which are presumed or proven indicators of quality of care or commitment to care. These include items such as response times for the ambulances, times from arrival to the operating room for patients requiring emergency surgery, unplanned repeat operations, and patients with certain diagnoses who do not undergo the usually expected therapies, such as patients with abdominal gunshot wounds who do not receive a laparotomy. The system requires these indicators of quality and safety of care to be reviewed on an annual or on a sentinel basis as needed by the trauma council.

At HMC, all of these elements are in place. Each department carries out its own weekly morbidity and mortality review. In addition, the trauma registry is reviewed regularly for the above-noted audit filters. When problems are discovered by this review, they are discussed at the monthly interdisciplinary trauma council meeting. Moreover, there is a quality assurance process to assess the entire trauma system. This process includes the regional EMS providers and the other trauma center hospitals located in central western Washington state. This Central Region Quality Assurance Committee meets bimonthly to review the function and performance of the trauma system network in the area.

Finally, outcomes assessment involves far more than quality assurance programs and mortality reviews. This field is only now coming into prominence as an important component of medical research (27–29). Until recently, evaluations of patient outcome were limited to mortality, in-hospital complications, and length of stay. Obviously such factors are the *sine qua non* of good medical care. However, they give no indication of patients' long-term functional status. There is a growing body of research on evaluating such functional status, especially from a "patient perceived" vantage point. While still a field largely in its infancy, there is the expectation that trauma centers and trauma systems will be judged on their ability to return injured patients to a functional status, not solely on their overall mortality or survival statistics. The important and critical role of rehabilitation medicine in influencing and affecting these measures of outcome is obvious.

CHALLENGES AND OPPORTUNITIES FACING TRAUMA CARE IN THE UNITED STATES

Despite the advances discussed above in basic science, technology, and trauma system organization, there are serious problems facing trauma care delivery in the United States. A root cause of these problems is the lack of recognition of the importance of trauma on the part of the population as a whole, and the funding priorities of the government. Although more attention has been given to trauma since the National Academy of Sciences labeled injury "the neglected disease" (4), the amount of trauma research funding is far below that of the other major health problems, such as cancer and heart disease, in the United States (1). Following the terrorist attack on the World Trade Center in New York on September 11, 2001, funding for terrorism preparedness has also largely ignored trauma centers and trauma systems, despite the presence of an intact, prepared network of hospitals skilled in providing care for the type of injury most commonly seen in terrorist attacks, namely physical force trauma (30,31).

Even within the existing system, numerous problems arise because of the capitalistic approach of American health care. In many circumstances, this approach results in a mismatch of availability of resources for trauma care. In some areas, too many hospitals want to care for trauma patients. The idea behind the designation of trauma centers is that resources will be concentrated in a few "centers of excellence" that can provide such services as 24-hour-per-day operating rooms and in-house surgical specialties. Too many hospitals competing for relatively too few trauma patients can easily result in wasteful duplication of services and in insufficient volume to maintain clinical expertise at any one of the institutions. Such problems are typical in locations where most patients have health insurance and hospitals vie for their market share.

In locations with large numbers of uninsured trauma patients, particularly in the inner city, the opposite problem exists. There is difficulty in consistently providing the resources to care for such patients. The public institutions that typically provide such care are often in financial difficulty. One of the best examples of this is the near closure of the Los Angeles County Hospital in 1995 (32).

Compounding these institutional difficulties is the lack of willingness on the part of many surgeons to provide trauma care. In a survey of Washington state surgeons, 43% of general and neurosurgeons preferred not to treat trauma patients. Reasons cited for this preference included inadequate reimbursement for primarily nonoperative care of blunt trauma patients, the fact that many trauma patients are uninsured, the after-hours nature of much of trauma care, disruption of elective surgical practice, and perceptions of increased liability risk and increased malpractice premiums (33).

FUTURE DIRECTIONS FOR TRAUMA CARE IN THE UNITED STATES

There are a number of areas that likely will remain focused agenda items for trauma system development and improvement in the United States for the foreseeable future. These include the following (but not complete) listing.

STABILITY IN FUNDING

Perhaps the biggest challenge for trauma care in the United States is to ensure stability in funding (34), both for individual patient care and for trauma system development. As uninsured patients are likely to continue to be a sizable proportion of the trauma patient population, measures to increase and ensure access to medical care for all Americans remain a fundamental component of efforts to improve trauma care in America (35).

STABILITY IN DESIGN

There is currently a mismatch of availability of services and trauma patient needs (36). Moreover, the availability of services frequently changes over time. Thus, greater stability in the design and structure of trauma systems is also needed. Organized trauma systems need to be implemented to cover a wider geographic area and a greater percentage of the population. Obviously this challenge ties in closely with that of funding (12,34).

INFORMATION SYSTEMS

More in-depth information is needed on the extent of the trauma problem in America. Currently, information on trauma deaths occurring in the country is derived from vital statistics registries. Information on motor vehicle–related deaths is available in summary form from the Fatal Accident Reporting System, maintained by the National Highway Traffic and Safety Administration (NHTSA). Information on nonfatal injuries is available from individual hospitals' medical records. There is a need for centralized reporting and linking of these databases, and the development of a National Trauma Data Bank is well underway by the ACS-COT.

FUNCTIONAL OUTCOMES

A greater understanding of the impact of trauma in the lives of survivors is needed. Better recording of functional status at time of discharge, and times to return to work or usual lifestyle, are some examples of what is needed to conduct meaningful outcomes assessment. A greater emphasis on patient perception, safety, and satisfaction with care assessment is also needed.

INJURY PREVENTION

Despite the tremendous successes in lowering the fatality rate from motor vehicle crashes, much remains to be done. Many more lives could be saved each year by increased use of simple, low-cost preventive measures that are already in existence, such as helmets and seat belts. Moreover, a large percentage of motor vehicle–related deaths continues to be caused by alcohol-impaired driving. A greater societal and governmental emphasis on safety and injury prevention is obviously warranted. Moreover, we are still in the very early stages of understanding and developing ways to prevent violence and other intentional injury. The importance of prevention is emphasized by the fact that within a well-functioning trauma system, medically "preventable" deaths in already injured patients constitute only 1% to 5% of all trauma deaths (37). Hence, primary prevention of injuries themselves emerges as the single most important way to lower the overall trauma mortality rate.

PRIORITIES FOR TRAUMA-RELATED RESEARCH

Three recent articles have identified future challenges for trauma treatment research (38–40):

Prehospital interventions. The current controversy of "scoop and run" versus "stay and treat" is overly simplistic. The efficacy of many of the current prehospital interventions remains unknown. Greater research is needed in this sphere, especially in regard to prehospital intravenous fluid resuscitation.

Neurological injury. A major contributor to early trauma mortality is head injury. Many of these deaths occur despite full use of existing therapeutic technologies.

Systemic inflammatory response. Likewise, a major contributor to late trauma mortality is the systemic inflammatory response and associated adult respiratory distress syndrome. This syndrome remains a major source of frustration to trauma surgeons who have undertaken difficult but successful operations, only to have patients eventually succumb to as yet poorly understood complications.

Greater understanding of the scientific basis of neurological injury and the systemic inflammatory response are two of the major challenges facing basic researchers in trauma surgery.

TORT REFORM

Finally, no discussion of the challenges facing any aspect of the American health care system is complete without addressing the need for tort reform. The current system of health care liability hampers the delivery of trauma services and inhibits future development of better trauma systems. Fear of increased liability is one of the frequently cited reasons that many community general surgeons prefer not to care for trauma patients (33). Moreover, the amount of money siphoned off from the medical system by the legal system represents a loss of resources that could be used to improve current trauma systems. Efforts at tort reform have included attempts to impose caps on pain and suffering, increase use of arbitration, limit on lawyers' contingency fees, and restrictions on use of bogus "expert" witnesses. While many members of Congress and the American Trial Lawyers Association (ATLA) continue to vigorously oppose these efforts, malpractice crises in some states have led to the adoption of some or all of these reforms.

REFERENCES

1. Baker S, O'Neill B, Ginsburg M. *The injury fact book.* 2nd ed. New York: Oxford University Press; 1992.
2. National Center for Health Statistics. *Vital statistics: Mortality data.* Atlanta, GA: Centers for Disease Control; 2001. Also available at: http://www.cdc.gov/nchs/.
3. National Center for Injury Prevention and Control. *Injury fact sheets.* Atlanta, GA: Centers for Disease Control; 1999. Also available at: http://www.cdc.gov/ncipc/cmprfact.htm.
4. Committee on Trauma and Shock. *Accidental death and disability: The neglected disease of modern society.* National Academy of Sciences/National Research Council. Washington, DC: National Academy of Sciences; 1966.
5. National Research Council. *Injury in America: A continuing public health problem.* Washington, DC: National Academy Press; 1985.
6. Rivara F, Grossman D, Cummings P. Injury prevention. *N Eng J Med.* 1997;337(8):543–548.
7. Thomas S, Harrison T, Buras W, et al. Helicopter transport and blunt trauma mortality: A multicenter trial. *J Trauma.* 2002;52(1):136–145.
8. Shatney C, Homan S, Sherck J, et al. The utility of helicopter transport of trauma patients from the injury scene in an urban trauma system. *J Trauma.* 2002; 53(8):817–822.
9. Bulger E, Copass M, Maier R, et al. An analysis of advanced prehospital airway management. *J Emerg Med.* 2002;23(2):183–189.
10. MacKenzie E, Hoyt D, Sacra J, et al. National inventory of hospital trauma centers. *JAMA.* 2003;289(12):1520.
11. Bazzoli G, Madura K, Cooper C, et al. Progress in the development of trauma systems in the United States. *JAMA.* 1995;273:395–401.
12. West JG, Williams M, Trunkey DD, et al. Trauma systems: Current status—future challenges. *JAMA.* 1988; 259:3597–3600.
13. Moore E, ed. *Early care of the injured patient.* Philadelphia, PA: B.C. Decker; 1990.
14. American College of Surgeon Committee on Trauma. *Resources for optimal care of the injured patient.* Chicago, IL: American College of Surgeons; 1999.
15. American College of Surgeons Committee on Trauma. *Advanced trauma life support instructor manual.* Chicago, IL: American College of Surgeons; 1997.
16. American College of Surgeons Committee on Trauma. Trauma performance improvement: A how-to handbook. Available at: http://www.facs.org/trauma/handbook.html. Accessed 2005.
17. Mullins RJ, Veum-Stone J, Hedges JR, et al. Influence of a statewide trauma system on location of hospitalization and outcome of injured patients. *J Trauma.* 1996;40(4):536–545; discussion 545–546.
18. Mann NC, Mullins RJ, MacKenzie EJ, et al. Systematic review of published evidence regarding trauma system effectiveness. *J Trauma.* 1999;47(Suppl. 3):S25–S33.
19. Skamania Symposia on Trauma Systems. Evidence, research and action. *J Trauma.* 1998;47(Suppl. 3): S1–S110.
20. Mullins R. A historical perspective of trauma system development in the United States. *J Trauma.* 1999; 47(Suppl. 3):S8–S14.
21. Buckman R, Scalea T, eds. *Trauma quarterly, trauma systems in the world.* Vol. 14 (3). Gaithersburg, MD: Aspen Publications; 1999:191–348.
22. Mock CN, Maier R, Pilcher S, et al. Injury prevention strategies to promote helmet use decrease severe head injury at a level I trauma center. *J Trauma.* 1995;39:29–35.
23. Jetland R. Medic 1—The Seattle system for the management of out-of-hospital medical emergencies. *World Hosp.* 1980;16(1):10–12.
24. Nathens AB, Jurkovich GJ, Maier RV, et al. Relationship between trauma center volume and outcomes. *JAMA.* 2001;285(9):1164–1171.
25. Glance LG, Osler TM, Dick A, et al. The relation between trauma center outcome and volume in the National Trauma Databank. *J Trauma.* 2004;56(3): 682–690.
26. Office of Emergency Medical & Trauma Prevention. *Trauma care fund.* Olympia, WA: Washington State Department of Health; 2003. Also available at: http://www.doh.wa.gov/hsqa/emtp/trfund.htm.
27. MacKenzie EJ, Morris JA Jr, Jurkovich GJ, et al.. Return to work following injury: The role of economic, social, and job-related factors. *Am J Public Health.* 1998;88(11):1630–1637.
28. Mock C, MacKenzie E, Jurkovich G, et al. Determinants of disability after lower extremity fracture. *J Trauma.* 2000;49(6):1002–1011.
29. Jurkovich G, Mock C, MacKenzie E, et al. The sickness impact profile as a tool to evaluate functional outcome in trauma patients. *J Trauma.* 1995;39:625–631.
30. Stein M, Hirshberg A. Medical consequences of terrorism. The conventional weapon threat. *Surg Clin North Am.* 1999;79(6):1537–1552.
31. Centers for Disease Control and Prevention. New classification for deaths and injuries involving terrorism. *JAMA.* 2002;288(13):1584.
32. Cornwell EE, Berne TV, Belzberg H. Health care crisis from a trauma center perspective: The LA story. *JAMA.* 1996;276:940–944.
33. Esposito TJ, Maier R, Rivara FP, et al. Why surgeons prefer not to care for trauma patients. *Arch Surg.* 1991;126:292–297.
34. Trunkey D. Future shock. *Arch Surg.* 1992;127:653–658.
35. Nathens AB, Maier RV, Copass MK, et al. Payer status: The unspoken triage criterion. *J Trauma.* 2001;50(5): 776–783.
36. Nathens AB, Jurkovich GJ, MacKenzie EJ, et al. A resource-based assessment of trauma care in the United States. *J Trauma.* 2004;56(1):173–178; discussion 178.
37. Acosta JA, Yang J, Winchell RJ, et al. Lethal injuries and time to death in a level I trauma center. *J Am Coll Curg.* 1998;186:528–533.
38. Jurkovich GJ, Rivara FP, Johansen JM, et al. CDC injury research agenda: Identification of acute care research topics of interest to the CDC-NCIPC. *J Trauma.* 2004;56:1166–1170.
39. Nathens AB, Rivara FP, Jurkovich GJ, et al. Management of the injured patient: Identification of research topics for systematic review using the delphi technique. *J Trauma.* 2003;54(3):595–601.
40. O'Keefe G, Jurkovich GJ. Measurement of injury severity and co-morbidity. In: Rivara FP, Cummings P, Keopsell TD, et al., eds. *Injury control: A guide to research and program evaluation.* Cambridge, MA: Cambridge University Press; 2001:32–46.

APPENDIX 1 TRAUMA CENTER DISTINCTIONS

The following table is a sample of the differences between the various levels of trauma centers as described by the American College of Surgeons in the 1999 edition of the book, *Resources for Optimal Care of the Injured Patient* (American College of Surgeon Committee on Trauma, 1999 #136). It is not a complete listing. It should be understood that this resource is regularly revisited and revised, and a more current version may be available from the American College of Surgeons Web site, http://www.facs.org/trauma/handbook.html. Also, not every state or region uses these exact guidelines for their local definition of the various levels of trauma centers. However, most have largely adopted these or very similar criteria. Finally, the resources list below represent only a fraction of all the essential (E) or desirable (D) resources for trauma centers.

APPENDIX 2 ISS SCORING

The Injury Severity Score (ISS) is an anatomical scoring system that provides an overall numerical score for patients with multiple injuries, with the intent of quantifying injury severity. Each injury is

Levels	I	II	III	IV
Institutional Organization				
Trauma program	E	E	E	E
Trauma service	E	E	E	—
Trauma program medical director	E	E	E	D
Trauma multidisciplinary committee	E	E	E	D
Trauma coordinator/TPM	E	E	E	E
Hospital Departments/Divisions/Sections				
Surgery	E	E	E	—
Neurological surgery	E	E	—	—
Orthopaedic surgery	E	E	E	—
Emergency medicine	E	E	E	—
Anesthesia	E	E	E	—
Clinical Capabilities (Specialty Immediately Available 24 h/d)				
Published on-call schedule	E	E	E	E
General surgery	E	E	E	D
Published backup schedule	E	E	D	—
Dedicated to single hospital when on call	E	E	D	—
Anesthesia (see Chapter 11)	E	E	E	D
Emergency medicine[a]	E	E	E	—
On-call and Promptly Available 24 h/d				
Cardiac surgery	E	D	—	—
Hand surgery	E	E	D	—
Microvascular/replant surgery	E	D	—	—
Neurologic surgery	E	E	D	—
Obstetrics/gynecologic surgery	E	E	D	—
Ophthalmic surgery	E	E	D	—
Oral/maxillofacial surgery	E	E	D	—
Orthopaedic surgery	E	E	E	D
Plastic surgery	E	E	E	D
Critical care medicine	E	E	D	—
Radiology	E	E	E	D
Thoracic surgery	E	E	D	—
Clinical Qualifications				
General/trauma surgeon (see Chapter 6)				
Current board certification	E	E	E	—
16 h CME/yr	E	E	D	D
ATLS completion	E	E	E	E
Peer review committee attendance >50%	E	E	E	—
Multidisciplinary committee attendance	E	E	E	—
Emergency medicine (see Chapter 7)				
Board certification	E	E	D	—
Trauma education: 16 h CME/yr	E	E	D	—
ATLS completion	E	E	E	E
Peer review committee attendance >50%	E	E	E	—
Multidisciplinary committee attendance	E	E	E	—
Neurosurgery (see Chapter 8)				
Current board certification	E	E	—	—

Levels	I	II	III	IV
16 h CME/yr	E	E	D	D
ATLS completion	D	D	D	D
Peer review committee attendance >50%	E	E	E	—
Multidisciplinary committee attendance	E	E	E	—
Orthopaedic surgery (see Chapter 9)				
Board certification	E	E	D	—
16 h CME/yr in skeletal trauma	E	E	D	D
ATLS completion	D	D	D	D
Peer review committee attendance >50%	E	E	E	D
Multidisciplinary committee attendance	E	E	E	—
Facilities/Resources/Capabilities				
Volume Performance				
Trauma admissions 1,200/yr	E	—	—	—
Patients with ISS >15 (240 total or 35 patients/surgeon)[b]	E	—	—	—
Presence of surgeon at resuscitation	E	E	E	D
Presence of surgeon at operative procedures	E	E	E	E
Operating Room				
Immediately available 24 h/d	E	D[c]	D	D
Personnel				
In-house 24 h/d	E	D[c]	—	—
Available 24 h/d	—	E	E	E
Age-specific equipment				
Cardiopulmonary bypass	E	D	—	—
Operating microscope	E	D	D	—
Thermal control equipment				
For patient	E	E	E	E
For fluids and blood	E	E	E	E
X-ray capability, including c-arm image intensifier	E	E	E	E
Endoscopes, bronchoscope	E	E	E	D
Craniotomy instruments	E	E	D	—
Equipment for long bone and pelvic fixation	E	E	E	D
Rapid infuser system	E	E	E	D
Postanesthetic Recovery Room (SICU is acceptable)				
Registered nurses available 24 h/d	E	E	E	—
Equipment for monitoring and resuscitation	E	E	E	E
Intracranial pressure monitoring equipment	E	E	D	—
Intensive or Critical Care Unit for Injured Patients				
Registered nurses with trauma education	E	E	E	—
Designated surgical director or surgical codirector	E	E	E	D
Surgical ICU service physician in-house 24 h/d	E	D	D	—
Surgically directed and staffed ICU service	E	D	D	—
Equipment for monitoring and resuscitation	E	E	E	—
Intracranial monitoring equipment	E	E	—	—
Pulmonary artery monitoring equipment	E	E	E	—
Respiratory Therapy Services				
Available in-house 24 h/d	E	E	D	D
On call 24 h/d	—	—	E	D
Radiological Services (Available 24 h/d)				
In-house radiology technologist	E	E	D	D
Angiography	E	E	D	—
Sonography	E	E	E	D
Computed tomography	E	E	E	D
In-house CT technician	E	D	—	—
Magnetic resonance imaging	E	D	D	—
Acute hemodialysis				
In-house	E	D	—	—
Transfer agreement	—	E	E	E
Burn Care—Organized				
In-house or transfer agreement with burn center	E	E	E	E
Acute Spinal Cord Management				
In-house or transfer agreement with regional acute spinal cord injury rehabilitation center	E	E	E	E
Rehabilitation Services				
Transfer agreement to an approved rehabilitation facility	E	E	E	E
Physical therapy	E	E	E	D
Occupational therapy	E	E	D	D
Speech therapy	E	E	D	—
Social service	E	E	E	D

Levels	I	II	III	IV
Performance Improvement				
Performance improvement programs	E	E	E	E
Trauma registry				
In-house	E	E	E	D
Participation in state, local, or regional registry	E	E	E	E
Orthopaedic database	D	D	—	—
Audit of all trauma deaths	E	E	E	E
Morbidity and mortality review	E	E	E	E
Trauma conference—multidisciplinary	E	E	E	D
Medical nursing audit	E	E	E	E
Review of prehospital trauma care	E	E	E	D
Review of times and reasons for trauma-related bypass	E	E	D	D
Review of times and reasons for transfer of injured patients	E	E	D	D
Performance improvement of personnel dedicated to care of injured patients	E	E	D	D
Continuing Education/Outreach				
General surgery residency program	E	D	—	—
ATLS provide/participate	E	D	D	D
Programs provided by hospital for				
staff/community physicians (CME)	E	E	E^d	>D
Nurses	E	E	E	D
Allied health personnel	E	E	E	—
Prehospital personnel provision/participation	E	E	E	D
Prevention				
Injury control studies	E	D	—	—
Collaboration with other institutions	E	D	D	D
Monitor progress/effect of prevention programs	E	D	D	D
Designated prevention coordinator-spokesperson for injury control	E	E	D	—
Outreach activities	E	E	D	D
Information resources for public	E	E	D	—
Collaboration with existing national, regional, and state programs	E	E	D	—
Coordination and/or participation in community prevention activities	E	E	E	D
Research				
Trauma registry performance improvement activities	E	E	E	—
Research committee	E	D	—	—
Identifiable IRB process	E	D	—	—
Extramural educational presentations	E^e	D	D	—
Number of scientific publications	E^f	D	—	—

ATLS, advanced trauma life support; CME, continuing medical education; CT, computed tomography; ICU, intensive care unit; IRB, institutional review board; ISS, injury severity score; SICU, surgical intensive care unit; TPM, trauma program manager.

[a]When emergency medicine specialists are not involved with the care of the injured patient, these criteria are not required.

[b]The mechanism to calculate ISS should be through use of AIS 90 and handcoding.

[c]An operating room (OR) must be adequately staffed and immediately available in a level I trauma center. This requirement is met by having a complete operating room team in the hospital at all times, so if an injured patient requires operative care, the patient can receive it in the most expeditious manner. These criteria cannot be met by individuals who are also dedicated to other functions within the institution. Their primary function must be the operating room.

An operating room must be adequately staffed and available when needed in a timely fashion in a level II trauma center. The need to have an in-house OR team will depend on a number of things, including patient population served, ability to share responsibility for OR coverage with other hospital staff, prehospital communication, and the size of the community served by the institution. If an out-of-house OR team is used, then this aspect of care must be monitored by the performance improvement program.

[d]In areas where the level III hospital is the lead institution, these educational activities are an essential criterion. When the level III is in an area that contains other hospital resources, such as a level I or II, then this criterion is no longer essential.

[e]Four educational presentations per year for the program. These presentations must be given outside the academically affiliated institutions of the trauma center.

[f]Publications should appear in peer-reviewed journals. *Index Medicus* listing is preferable. In a three-year cycle, the minimum acceptable number is ten for the entire trauma program. A minimum of one publication (per review cycle) is required from the physicians representing each of the four following specialties: emergency medicine, general surgery, orthopaedic surgery, and neurosurgery.

From Brasel KJ, Akason J, Weigelt JA. The dedicated operating room for trauma: A costly recommendation. *J Trauma.* 1998;14:832–838, with permission.

assigned an Abbreviated Injury Scale (AIS) score ranging from 1 (minor) to 6 (lethal). AIS scores of 3, 4, and 5 are considered serious, severe, and critical, respectively. An AIS score is assigned to each of the injuries in six body regions (head, face, chest, abdomen, extremities (including pelvis), external). However, for ISS calculations, only the highest AIS score in each body region is used. The three most severely injured body regions have their score squared and added together to produce the ISS (Jurkovich, 2001 #170).

An example of the ISS calculation is shown in Table 3-1.

The ISS takes values from 0 to 75. If an injury is assigned an AIS of 6 (nonsurvivable injury), the ISS is automatically assigned to 75. The relationship between ISS and mortality is not linear, but higher scores do generally correlate with increased mortality, morbidity, and hospital stay. Any error in the AIS scoring increases the ISS error, and many different injury patterns can yield the same ISS. Other notable weaknesses of ISS scoring are that injuries to different body regions are equally weighted, and not all injuries are included in the final ISS calculation, as

Table 3-1	Example of the Injury Severity Score (ISS) Calculation		
Region	Injury Description	AIS	Square of Top Three
Head	cerebral contusion	3	9
Face	no injury	0	
Chest	flail chest	4	16
Abdomen	minor contusion of the liver	2	
	complex rupture of the spleen	5	25
Extremities	fractured femur	3	
External	no injury	0	
Injury Severity Score			50

the example above illustrates. Also, since the extent of injuries is usually not appreciated until a full workup has been accomplished, the ISS is not useful as a triage tool.

4

Early Rehabilitation Interventions

Joyce S. Hedges, Lynn K.N. Krog, Tiffany G. Megargee, Melissa Porras-Monroe, and Ellen Foisie Robinson

This chapter will share strategies for the early introduction of rehabilitation interventions. We will demonstrate how these interventions contribute positively to the functional outcomes of trauma patients. The chapter will outline the organizationsof staff and systems, the roles of each member of the team, and treatment guidelines and practices that are critical to early rehabilitation interventions. Rather than provide guidance in an abstract form, we will present the specific organization and practices we have implemented at Harborview Medical Center (HMC) in Seattle, Washington, the only level I trauma center in the four-state area of Washington, Alaska, Montana, and Idaho.

We believe our practices allow for efficient delivery of patient-centered care and that our program is an excellent example of physicians, therapists from all disciplines, and patients and their families working together as a team, toward one common goal—patient success.

PHILOSOPHY OF EARLY INTERVENTION

HMC's primary medical and rehabilitation services have long identified very early rehabilitation intervention as a priority for trauma patients. Involvement of the rehabilitation therapists (occupational therapist [OT], physical therapist [PT], speech-language pathologist [SLP], and therapeutic recreational specialist

[TRS]), trauma rehabilitation coordinator (TRC), and consult physiatry attendings and residents is often initiated as early as the intensive care unit (ICU) setting. All disciplines are active in both the ICU and on the acute care floors. This design allows standards of practices to be consistent regardless of the patient's discharge plan. The benefits of early rehabilitative interventions are multifaceted. Early intervention optimizes functional outcomes, provides thorough patient/family education, and allows opportunity for the ongoing collaboration with bedside nurses to assist in the rehabilitation process. In addition, specific discipline recommendations can be addressed, complications that could hinder a patient from achieving his or her fullest potential are prevented, and early discharge planning and preparation are facilitated.

ACUTE CARE MODEL

SCHEMATIC OF ORGANIZATIONAL CHART

The structure of the rehabilitation department allows for streamlined communication between therapists, trauma rehabilitation nurse coordinator, and physicians within the rehabilitation department and among other medical services. This structure provides the therapists with the support needed to be active on the acute care unit and ICU (Fig. 4–1).

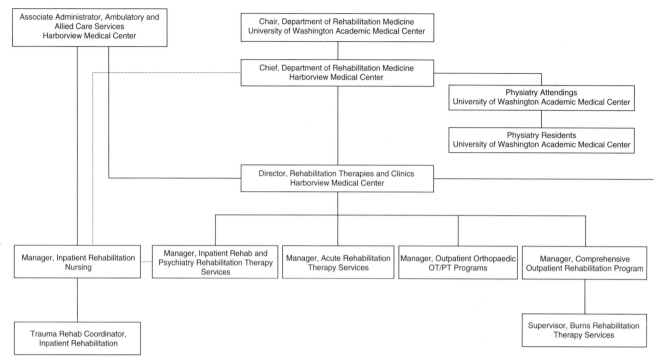

Figure 4–1. Rehabilitation therapies and clinics organizational structure. (Courtesy of the Department of Rehabilitation Medicine at Harborview Medical Center in Seattle, Washington.)

THERAPIES

All the previously mentioned rehabilitation therapists, regardless of which area of the hospital they may work in, are members of the rehabilitation department. Rehabilitation therapies are organized in workgroups rather than along discipline specific lines. A workgroup consists of an OT, a PT, an SLP, and a TRS either within the workgroup or consulting from another workgroup. Each workgroup provides therapy coverage to different medical services of the hospital (Fig. 4–2). Each workgroup has either a manager or supervisor, who may be from any of the disciplines previously mentioned. Each discipline in the workgroup has or can access a clinical specialist or clinical lead who assists the manager/supervisor in providing staff with clinical direction.

On acute care services, the roles of the therapist are defined as follows to allow for optimal patient care. *Occupational therapy* (OT) is responsible for

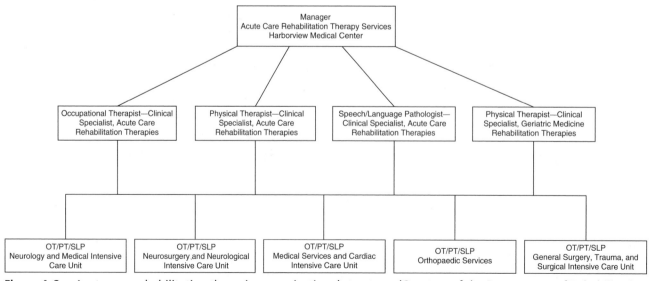

Figure 4–2. Acute care rehabilitation therapies organizational structure. (Courtesy of the Department of Rehabilitation Medicine at Harborview Medical Center in Seattle, Washington.)

Table 4-1	Quick Review of Roles and Responsibilities
Occupational Therapy	• Evaluate functional abilities and provide treatment in the areas of BADL (feeding, grooming/hygiene, bathing, and dressing), IADL (higher level skills such as shopping, cooking, and money management), cognition, functional transfer training, ROM, strength, coordination, and sensorimotor function.
	• Assess the need for and provide interventions in: splinting, positioning, skin protection, edema management, and DME.
Physical Therapy	• Assess musculoskeletal, neurologic, cardiopulmonary, and integument systems.
	• Provide interventions: ROM, strengthening, functional mobility training, patient and family education, assistive devices for ambulation (walkers, crutches, canes, braces), DME recommendations (wheelchairs, scooters, lifts).
Speech-Language Pathology	• Provide assessments of cognitive-communication, language, and swallowing abilities and communication deficits secondary to a central language disturbance, speech intelligibility disturbance, and/or inability to use voice.
	• Interventions include providing guidelines for diet textures, liquid consistencies, and aspiration precautions; maximizing residual speech and language function; providing or suggesting reliable nonvocal/nonverbal communication systems; providing guidelines for communicative interaction and changes to the environment to maximize patient's ability to process information; supply orientation materials that facilitate tracking time, medical care, and goals toward functional communication; educating family/friends/caretakers regarding swallowing, communication, and cognitive-communication issues.

BADL, basic activities of daily living; IADL, instrumental activities of daily living; ROM, range of motion; DME, durable medical equipment

administering assessments and treatment for basic activities of daily living (BADL) and instrumental activities of daily living (IADL), cognition through functional activity, sensorimotor skills, positioning and splinting, patient/family education, and providing assistive devices as indicated. *Physical therapy* (PT) assesses musculoskeletal, neurological, cardiopulmonary, and integumentary systems. Interventions by PT include range of motion (ROM), strengthening, functional mobility training, endurance training, patient/family education, and provision of assistive devices and other durable medical equipment (DME). *Speech-Language Pathology* (SLP) is responsible for assessment of swallowing, communication, and cognitive-communication skills. Interventions for swallowing problems include recommending appropriate food textures, liquid consistencies, and ways to minimize risk of aspiration. Patients are monitored for changes in swallowing function that allow advancement in diet textures and liquid consistencies. A broad spectrum of communication problems can occur with trauma. Communication can be affected by lesions in the speech and language centers of the brain, mechanical problems such as tracheostomy, and ventilators that prevent vocalization and/or cause structural damage to the articulators. Intervention under these conditions involves maximizing residual speech and language function, providing reliable nonvocal/nonverbal communication systems, and educating family/friends/caretakers. Progress is monitored and adjustments are made as the patient improves. Cognitive-communication

deficits are treated with patient/family/caretaker education and provision of guidelines for communicative interaction, and changes to the environment to maximize the patient's ability to process information. When appropriate, patients are supplied with orientation materials that facilitate tracking time, their medical care, and goals toward functional outcomes (Table 4-1).

THE CONSULT TEAM

NURSING UNIT–BASED ORGANIZATION OF ACUTE CARE

Each nursing unit at Harborview Medical Center is a primary unit for a medical service. The acute care rehabilitation therapists are based on each unit. For example, all general surgery patients are cared for on a designated unit, unless a bed is unavailable. OT, PT, and SLP are assigned to a unit, thus to a medical or surgical service. The benefits of this staffing model are enormous. The medical team and discharge planning staff interact with the same therapists, and the same therapists (OT, PT, SLP) work with each other over a period of time, allowing for development of a strong rapport and team behavior. Staff therapists demonstrate a greater investment in developing their skills and contributing to the team with which they work. The use of workgroups throughout the facility has led to the development of consistent standards of practice amongst therapists and paved the way for trusting relationships to develop. Therapists' skills are improved through skill enhancements to various specialty areas, which can be initiated by the therapist or manager. In addition to being assigned to acute care floors, therapists may be assigned to an ICU that is related to the nursing unit on which they work. This practice helps ensure continuity of care for trauma patients, who may have extended ICU stays and multiple system injury.

IDENTIFY THE REHABILITATION CONSULT TEAM

The rehabilitation consult team consists of physicians, nurses, therapists, social workers, psychologists and vocational counselors. Team members make individual contributions to the care of the trauma patient with rehabilitation needs, but the key to a successful plan of care is the coordination of those individual efforts. As with all rehabilitation patients, teamwork is essential. The rehabilitation consult team has the following goals:

- Identify trauma patients with rehabilitation needs within 48 hours of admission
- Identify rehabilitation needs and develop a plan of care to address those needs
- Institute the plan as soon as patient's medical condition allows
- Evaluate the success of the plan and modify the plan as necessary
- Discuss the plan with the patient and family
- Educate others caring for the patient re: rehabilitation team involvement
- Contribute to discharge planning decisions
- Help ensure a timely discharge to most appropriate setting.

Team Members

Physicians

Three physiatry residents, supervised by an attending (faculty) physician, form the core of the physician component of the rehabilitation consult team. These residents are in the second, third or fourth year of the residency program. In addition to consulting on patients throughout the acute care areas of the hospital, these residents also have responsibilities in the outpatient clinic and electromyography (EMG) area. One resident is assigned to take consult calls and triage consults. This resident reviews hospital admissions daily, screening for diagnoses and patterns of injuries likely to benefit from input from the rehabilitation team. Patients for whom the managing team has requested a rehabilitation consult

are usually seen within one day of admission. Patients may also be identified by other members of the team or have referrals initiated by their primary physicians. In our 368-bed medical center, the consult physiatrists generally consult on about 50 patients at any given time, and approximately two thirds of those are trauma patients.

Trauma Rehabilitation Coordinator

The role of the TRC was developed in 1993 in response to Washington state trauma legislation. Recognizing the significant contribution of early rehabilitation interventions to improved functional outcomes for trauma patients, the state of Washington legislated that all level I and II trauma facilities designate a trauma rehabilitation coordinator. The TRC was charged with the task of collaborating with appropriate disciplines and resources to coordinate continuity of trauma patient care from admission through discharge.

In our organization, the TRC is a registered nurse who acts as a sort of "information hub," facilitating effective communication between rehabilitation team members, other professionals involved in the care of the patient, and the patient and family. In addition, the TRC reviews the recommendations of the physiatrists and facilitates implementation of those recommendations, as necessary. The TRC also participates in discharge planning and coordinates transfers to acute care rehabilitation facilities. The TRC's participation includes establishing funding for those admitted to our inpatient rehabilitation facility.

Social Workers

In our organization, social workers are service-based, with those on the neurosurgery, general surgery, orthopaedic, and burn services working most frequently with trauma patients. One social worker is funded by a Spinal Cord Injury Model Systems grant from the National Institute on Disability and Rehabilitation Research (NIDRR). This social worker provides services to all patients with spinal cord injuries (SCIs). Initially the social workers assist patients and their families with social and financial issues that often accompany trauma. Families from out of town may need a place to stay, family conferences might need to be organized to facilitate understanding of the patient's condition, or emergency funds for food might be necessary. Concurrently, the social worker must focus on discharge planning. The patient's source of funding needs to be established, along with an understanding of what the insurance coverage is for various discharge options. Families without commercial insurance typically need help applying for public assistance. Most need direction to identify which facilities are appropriate and are covered by the patient's funding source.

Occupational Therapists

In the acute care setting, occupational therapists evaluate and provide treatment in the areas of BADL (feeding, grooming/hygiene, bathing, and dressing); and IADL (higher-level skills, such as shopping, cooking, and money management). Other areas that OTs assess and provide intervention for include cognition, functional transfer training, sensorimotor functioning, ROM, strengthening, and coordination. The occupational therapist assesses the need for specific interventions such as splinting, positioning, skin protection, edema management, and DME. Such interventions facilitate functional outcomes in patients with traumatic injuries. The occupational therapist also provides family training, and follow-up recommendations as part of the acute care team. The role of OT for patients seen in the emergency department is often to provide splinting, positioning, or ADL assessment in order to initiate treatments for particular traumatic injuries (i.e., severe hand injury), and to facilitate/determine a patient's further treatment needs. OT intervenes early in a patient's ICU stay to prevent further deficits due to joint contracture or skin breakdown, and to initiate functional skill performance when appropriate.

Physical Therapists

Physical therapists are specialists of the musculoskeletal, neurologic, cardiopulmonary, and integumentary systems. They provide examination, evaluation, and diagnosis in these areas. Interventions and education that address patient impairments are then formulated and provided to patients to provide maximal function independence. PTs provide therapy treatments to patients in the intensive care setting, postoperative care hospital wards, and the emergency department. The primary goal of the physical therapist working with a patient in the acute care setting is to initiate rehabilitative techniques that foster early restoration of maximum function mobility and reduce the risk of secondary complications. Roach et al. determined that "the amount of physical therapy that a patient with orthopedic problems receives in an acute care setting is directly related to the degree of improvement in function that occurs during the hospitalization" (1).

Physical therapists also work on the front lines of our hospital in the emergency department. The presence of PTs in the emergency department allows for early intervention. In this setting, therapists evaluate and treat minor trauma such as strains and sprains of the spine and extremities that do not require surgery. They assist with instruction of the care of injuries in the inflammatory response phases. They provide mobility training for patients who do not require hospital admission as well as make recommendations for long-term placements or additional services for patients who may not be able to care for themselves at home. The emergency department PTs triage patients to outpatient therapy follow-up and DME procurement, which may decrease the need for inpatient therapy care and unnecessary admissions to the hospital.

Speech-Language Pathologist

The primary role of the Speech-Language Pathologist (SLP) on the acute care service is to provide diagnostic and rehabilitation services for acquired disorders of swallowing, communication, and cognitive problems as they relate to communication. Patients receiving SLP services are located in various settings throughout the hospital, including the emergency department, observation and short stay departments, intensive care, and acute care floors.

The primary goal of the SLP is to identify problems that affect a patient's ability to communicate effectively with family and caretakers and to take nourishment and fluids safely without secondary complications from aspiration. SLPs provide treatment in the form of

- education and counseling
- therapy for swallowing, communication and cognitive-communication problems
- supplying alternative/augmentative communication for patients without conventional means of communication, such as those who are severely dysarthric, language impaired, nonvocal, ventilator dependent, and/or tracheostomized
- making recommendations for nothing by mouth (NPO) or by mouth (PO) with PO recommendations covering diet textures, liquid consistencies, and aspiration precautions.

The SLP works closely with the medical team and other disciplines to make informed decisions regarding discharge of patients to appropriate settings with adequate therapeutic intervention. Indirect services provided to ensure quality care for the patient include educating staff, keeping current on evaluation and treatment methods for persons with traumatic injury, and participating in quality assurance/management and external and internal review processes.

Therapeutic Recreation Specialists

The primary purpose of therapeutic recreation is to restore, remediate, or rehabilitate areas that will improve patient function and independence as well as reduce or eliminate the effects of illness or disability. In the acute care setting, the therapeutic recreational specialist's role is to assess and provide training for community-integration skills. These skills include pathfinding, problem solving, safety and judgment in high-stimulus areas, transportation training, leisure/community resources, family education, and school re-entry.

REFERRAL PROCESS

Orders

Early intervention begins with initiation of therapy services via the physician orders. For optimal patient outcomes, specific therapy orders must be written as soon as the patient is medically ready. In our hospital setting, nurses are required to complete a patient history/assessment when a patient is admitted. When the organization developed this tool, the rehabilitation therapiists and other providers were asked to provide triggers that would identify therapy needs. Key questions were developed to assist the nurses in determining if a therapy consult/order should be requested from the physician. These questions have been a very successful tool and help provide a consistent approach to ensuring that patients get the ancillary services they require. Nurses and physicians are provided with ongoing education on detecting new disability by both informal and formal mechanisms. At new employee orientation, nurses are provided with education about the role of therapies and how to refer to therapies. Therapists provide nurses with daily reports that contain more detailed explanations about the interventions they provide and the skills that they help patients regain. Medical and surgical acute care residents are given formal education about therapies as part of the team orientation when they rotate onto a new service. During more informal regular rounds, therapists provide education to physicians about therapists' roles, patient progress with therapists, and follow-up therapy needs that patients may have after discharge or transfer.

Once a therapy order is written, therapists have direct interactions with the patient and communicate with both the primary service physicians and, when appropriate, rehabilitation medicine consult physiatrists. In other cases, therapist involvement does not require physiatrist involvement. On acute care units, there are four ways that an order/consult can be written for therapies: (i) the primary medical or surgical service can write orders directly to the therapist without a physiatrist referral; (ii) in the case that the physiatrist is involved prior to therapy involvement, the physiatrist can write orders or consults for therapy involvement; (iii) the physiatrist can contact the primary medical service to request specific therapy orders to be written; or lastly, (iv) when developing clinical pathways, therapies are automatically included, if appropriate. For example, the SCI pathway includes orders that automatically refer to therapies on the appropriate postinjury day, ensuring that the appropriate services are provided in a timely manner. In conclusion, early physician orders for the appropriate therapy services provide the optimal situation for early rehabilitation interventions.

ROUNDS

Primary Team Discharge Planning Rounds

These medical and surgical team rounds may occur at different frequencies depending upon the hospital organization with which one is involved. Ideally, members representing therapies, nursing, discharge planning, utilization review, and physicians should be involved. These rounds provide a forum to discuss upcoming medical plans, pharmacologic issues, functional status, cognitive status, and posthospital discharge settings and follow-up care needs. These rounds can be educational for all involved, as each member of the team serves a specific purpose and all aspects of the patient case can be addressed. This multidisciplinary approach facilitates communication and allows the team to work toward a common goal.

Consult Rounds

Given the number of physiatrists and therapists that provide care in a large medical facility, a central communication system is important to facilitate post-acute care. The rehabilitation team finds that team rounds are useful in the acute care setting. Consult rounds are an interdisciplinary process that includes recommendations from all providers (occupational therapists, physical therapists, speech-language pathologists, rehab psychologists, and social workers) and facilitates transfers from the acute care inpatient units to the inpatient rehabilitation unit. Follow-up patient needs in regard to readiness for inpatient rehabilitation after a subacute care stay, outpatient service requirements, and clinic follow-up can be established at this time.

Relationships with Other Medical and Surgical Services

It is clear that safeguards to ensure that trauma patients who have rehabilitation needs are seen and treated in a timely manner by the rehabilitation consult team are crucial. As noted previously, there are formal processes in place to facilitate referrals and to screen for appropriate patients. However, to make sure that no patient suffers from a delay in the initiation of rehabilitation interventions, informal processes are crucial. All members of the rehabilitation consult team seek to educate our colleagues on other units in the organization concerning our services and how to access them. Much of this education occurs informally in the course of working together on specific patients. It is essential in a teaching hospital setting, where residents turn over frequently, to take advantage of opportunities to formally explain the rehabilitation consult team's makeup and purpose. In pursuit of this goal, we attend monthly resident orientations for all services involved in trauma care. The trauma rehabilitation coordinator is also in a position to identify patients who may have been overlooked. The TRC screens all ICU trauma admissions, attends care rounds, and communicates frequently with caregivers of trauma patients. The TRC alerts the triage physiatry resident to any additional trauma patients who need evaluation and intervention by the rehabilitation consult team.

Rehab Professional Recommendations

As explained previously, our rehabilitation therapists are team and nursing unit based and well known throughout the institution. Their professional expertise is highly respected and their opinions sought. Because of their participation at so many levels of the organization and their high visibility, therapists are in a position to note when patients' conditions improve. Patients who previously could not benefit from rehabilitation intervention, but now can, are quickly identified, and appropriate interventions are instituted. In these cases, therapists can discuss the rehabilitation plan with the primary service, and encourage a consult to the physiatrist or make a referral to the TRC. Therapists may discuss the case with the consult physiatrist directly, especially if there are particular concerns to convey. Therapists may also recommend interventions that the primary physician can order immediately, in order to avoid delays and keep patients progressing in a positive direction.

EVALUATION PROCESS

The therapy disciplines utilize similar general information when evaluating patients (i.e., age, diagnosis), while also addressing specific areas unique to his or her specialty area. All therapists compile a history

and systems review before proceeding to their clinical evaluation and diagnosis. From this information a plan of care and interventions are formulated. Reexaminations are conducted at appropriate intervals, and outcomes are measured. A full reexamination may be completed if there is a change in patient status with new medical problems or new clinical findings or if there is a lack of patient progress. A reexamination may also provide data that identify the need for consultation with another provider (2).

The termination of therapy services is determined by the patient's progress in meeting the therapy goals. Therapy services may be terminated either by discharge or discontinuation of services. Discharge occurs when the patient has achieved the anticipated goals and expected outcomes. Patients may still require periodic follow-up care over their life span to ensure safety and adaptation to disability. For example, patients with SCI may have annual follow-up visits in a seating clinic to review DME needs and make adjustments and changes to wheelchairs based on improvements/decline in physical status. Patients with mild cognitive-communication deficits may require outpatient evaluation and intervention by an SLP who will train them in compensatory strategies and to recommend approaches to return-to-work issues and community re-entry. Discontinuation of services is the process of ending therapy services when the patient declines continued intervention, when the patient is unable to progress toward anticipated goals and expected outcomes because of medical or psychosocial complications, or when financial insurance resources have been depleted. Therapists may also determine that the patient will no longer benefit from treatment and discuss the ending of therapy intervention with the referring physician. If therapy services are terminated, the patient status and rationale for discontinuation are documented in the medical record (2).

OCCUPATIONAL THERAPY EVALUATION

Occupational therapists take a patient history that includes past and present medical conditions, and any precautions that could affect functional outcomes. They also note psychosocial, emotional, vocational, and leisure histories that may affect patients' goals and outcomes. Preexisting problems in any of these areas can overlap with disability from new traumatic injuries and need to be addressed in the evaluation. For example, a patient with underlying diabetes or peripheral vascular disease may have problems tolerating splints or positional devices. A patient with prior pulmonary dysfunction will benefit from instruction in energy conservation techniques during activities of daily living. A patient whose lifework is being a mechanic will be significantly affected by a severe hand injury, both physically and emotionally.

After compiling the available history, OTs review the patient's systems including cardiovascular, pulmonary, skin, musculoskeletal, sensorimotor, lymphatic (edema/fluid control), cognitive, and neurologic. They also incorporate an understanding of patient psychosocial skills, learning needs, and communication abilities.

Occupational therapists use a variety of tests and measures during their clinical evaluations. Joint range of motion, muscle strength, coordination, gross and fine motor control, sensation, circulation, skin integrity, visual perception, and cognitive functioning are a few areas that may be tested.

OTs determine the level of improvement that may be achieved through intervention and the amount of time required to reach that level. These expectations are outlined in short- and long-term goals. The OTs' goals are achieved through their purposeful and skilled interaction with the patient/client, family, and other individuals involved with the care of the person. Therapists incorporate the patient's and family's individual goals into the overall goal setting process and communicate the goals and plan to the patient and family. Therapists strive to take into account all-important elements of a patient's past and present history when formulating goals and setting expectations for outcomes.

For example, an 80-year-old who has a lower extremity fracture, as well as severe upper extremity rheumatoid arthritis, is going to have more difficulty with self-care tasks such as toilet transfers, toilet hygiene, dressing, and bathing. Such a patient would be expected to require more OT treatment over a longer period than a patient with the same fracture but no other underlying medical problem. A patient with an arm injury who works doing heavy construction would likely have different functional goals and desired outcomes than patients who are not required to do heavy lifting in their work. Occupational therapists provide a variety of interventions to assist patients in meeting their goals and improving functional outcomes. These interventions will be described in detail in later sections of this chapter.

PHYSICAL THERAPY EVALUATION

Physical therapists take into account medical history from both the past and the present that may affect functional outcomes. New and baseline disease processes can affect the therapy treatment plans. For example, a newly diagnosed femur fracture or a history of a total knee replacement would affect the evaluation and expectations of the musculoskeletal system. A patient with a history of a stroke (cerebrovascular accident [CVA]) or new traumatic brain injury (TBI) would have different effects on the neurologic system. A degloving injury to an extremity or a history of diabetes would be important information for healing of the integumentary system. Cardiopulmonary injuries such as pulmonary contusion, or chronic medical problems, such as atrial fibrillation, will affect a patient's recovery. How preexisting problems may overlap and affect new trauma injuries needs to be assessed during the evaluation. Information relating to previous level of function, social history, demographics, and health habits is another important part of the evaluation. Smoking history can play a large role in endurance and healing expectations. Activity level prior to admission needs to be assessed to understand how the patient may function given the current injury. If the patient was sedentary before the trauma admission, he or she cannot be expected to walk up and down stairs on crutches with ease after the injury. When taking a patient history, the PT identifies health restoration and prevention needs and coexisting health problems that may have implications for intervention (2).

After organizing the available history, a systems review is performed. Vital signs are taken to assess the cardiovascular and pulmonary systems. Available labs values (e.g., hematocrit, arterial blood gases) provide further information. Skin integrity assessment (e.g., color, scars, edema), gross ROM and strength measurements, and detailed balance and co-ordination testing complete the physical evaluation. A brief work-up of the patient's communication ability, cognition, language and learning style, and level of consciousness needs to be performed, and information from OT and SLP can supplement the physical therapist's basic screening.

Physical therapists use a variety of tests and measures during their clinical evaluations. Joint range of motion, muscle performance, circulation, cranial and peripheral nerve integrity, neuromotor development and motor control, and reflex and sensory integrity are a few areas that may be tested.

On the basis of their evaluation findings, physical therapists will make their diagnosis. A physical therapy diagnosis may differ from the medical diagnosis and is used by the physical therapist to determine the prognosis, plan of care, and appropriate intervention strategies. Therapists make a determination of the level of improvement that may be achieved through intervention and the amount of time required to reach that level. These expectations are outlined in terms of short- and long-term goals. The purposeful and skilled interaction of the PTs with the patient/client, family, and other individuals involved with the care of the person is integral to the achievement of the therapy goals. Therapists strive to take into account all-important elements of a patient's past and present history when formulating goals and setting expectations for outcomes.

For example, an 88-year-old female who suffers a pelvic fracture may be expected to have a worse prognosis for full ambulatory status with a longer recovery period and the need for more therapy intervention than a 21-year-old male who was a college athlete prior to injury. A patient who suffered a stroke in the past with residual weakness, with a new hip fracture and repair, may be unable to ambulate within the limits of weight-bearing restrictions, and may require the use of a wheelchair. The outcomes of physical therapy interventions on the disease or injury are measured in terms of functional limitations or disabilities. PTs provide a variety of interventions to assist patients in meeting their goals and improving functional outcomes. These interventions will be described in detail in later sections of this chapter.

SPEECH-LANGUAGE PATHOLOGY EVALUATION

SLPs review medical records as the initial part of the evaluation. It is of particular interest to SLPs to know the diagnosis, the source of trauma, and whether there was a known brain injury. It is helpful to know if the head injury was open or closed, if the injury to the brain was focal or general, and if there was brainstem involvement or a loss of consciousness, and to know the site or sites of lesions. Other factors that may influence evaluation, treatment, and outcome include secondary complications, time of onset, recovery curve, previous head injuries or illnesses, psychosocial background (family, psychological history, education, and employment), age, previous communication or swallowing problems, prosthetic devices (glasses, dentures, and hearing aids) used prior to the injury, surgical procedures and outcomes, lab values, medications, and medical precautions. Information in the medical chart regarding the patient's complaints, family perceptions and the evaluations, and treatments of other disciplines is also helpful. For the pediatric population, the developmental history, academic performance, and family/living situation are considered.

Areas evaluated by SLPs are primarily focused on swallowing, communication, and cognitive communication, though other areas are often assessed.

Swallowing

Patients appropriate for a swallow evaluation include those with neurological or physical conditions that predispose them to dysphagia, those who are recently extubated and may have laryngeal involvement, those with tracheostomies either with or without ventilatory support, and those with facial fractures. The patient must be arousable and able to sustain wakefulness for an adequate amount of time for reliable testing. The examination includes an evaluation of the structure and function of the oral/facial mechanism, oral phase of swallow, timing of the swallow response, laryngeal excursion during the swallow, and vocal quality before and after taking a test item by mouth. In addition the patient's general behavior, positioning ability, awareness of the environment, and ability to follow commands are assessed. PO trials begin with ice chips and/or water because of their relatively benign nature. The PO trial is completed with a variety of food textures and liquid consistencies. The purpose of the swallow evaluation is to determine aspiration risks and swallowing problems that may impede adequate nutrition, hydration, and ability to take medications; provide guidelines for diet textures and liquid consistencies; and make recommendations for positioning and other aspiration precautions.

The prognosis for swallowing disorders is based on the nature and severity of the problem, underlying etiology of the problem, the age of the patient, the time postonset, associated defects and health history, and the ability to benefit from therapeutic intervention.

Persons with dysphagia are evaluated and recommendations are made for diet texture and liquid consistency. Aspiration precautions are also provided. Radiologic swallowing evaluation is sometimes recommended when the risk of aspiration is unclear from the previously described clinical examination.

Communication/Cognitive-Communication

A communication evaluation includes an assessment of general functional abilities, language, motor speech, reading, writing, and functional use of language. Communication problems arise from a variety of sources ranging from generalized or localized brain damage to structural and/or physiologic changes in the speech mechanism. A patient may present with aphasia or language impairment, a motor speech deficit, or inability to vocalize. Hearing acuity is an important part of auditory processing and may be screened instrumentally or evaluated subjectively. If appropriate, a patient may be referred for an audiological evaluation through the ear, nose, and throat (ENT) clinic. There are a variety of non-standardized and standardized tests used to assess communication. Tests are selected based on the patient's perceived needs including communication needs, positioning, ability to participate, visual acuity and hearing ability, motor function, level of premorbid function, and present level of function. The purpose of the communication evaluation is to establish linguistic competence and a reliable mode of communication. Evaluations generally occur at the bedside. The environment is noisy, and there are multiple distractions. Efforts are made to schedule an evaluation when the patient's condition allows for peak performance, with minimal effects from pain or illness, lack of sleep, or sedating medications.

Communication problems secondary to cognitive impairment fall into the category of cognitive-communication disorders. Cognitive-communication problems may include impaired pragmatics, language disturbances, decreased attention/concentration, reduced memory and new learning, impaired thought processing, reduced mental flexibility and reasoning, disorientation, lack of initiation, impaired planning, and reduced organizing and regulation of behavior. Evaluation of cognitive-communication ability may be similar to a communication evaluation, but the focus will be different. Tests of cognitive communication have to allow a comparison of test performance versus function, have a hierarchy of complexity, present a range of tasks from structured to open-ended and place demands on mental flexibility, sustained attention, and memory, both immediate and delayed.

Based on the medical record review and clinical evaluation, the SLP is able to identify swallowing and/or communication/cognitive-communication problems and their probable causes. This information helps the SLP determine the expected course and rate of recovery and if the patient is amenable to therapeutic intervention.

The plan of care is established based on the needs of the patient, the prognosis for recovery, the environment that is considered most conducive to recovery, the level of intensity of therapy needed, the ability to benefit from therapeutic intervention, and the resources available.

Therapy may be initiated at any point along the continuum of care within the hospital and is determined by the level of need and the potential to benefit from therapy. When the patient is experiencing varying levels of alertness and responsiveness, the intervention that would be most beneficial may be educating the caretaker and providing a plan of care or counseling the patient and family. When the patient is medically stable, intervention may be more direct. Therapeutic interventions provided at this level are basic in that they meet immediate needs such as providing low-tech communication systems for persons without spoken communication or ordering an electrolarynx and providing training for its use. Initiating training of compensatory strategies for communication problems occurs at the acute care level if it is thought to be beneficial and will expedite change.

Evaluations and therapies are directed toward functional outcomes for placement in the least restrictive environment, facilitating the greatest level of independence with as close as possible return to the premorbid level of function.

Termination of service occurs when the patient returns to baseline, reaches the goals of therapy, fails to benefit from therapeutic intervention, or changes in medical status, or if services are refused by the patient or family.

SCREENING TOOLS

Screening tools are essential for early efficient identification of new disability or therapy needs in the acutely injured individual.

Screening Tools Used by Occupational Therapists

Occupational therapists use general ADL evaluations to observe a patient's ability to complete basic or higher-level ADL tasks. Occupational therapists are skilled at assessing specific self-care tasks, and at task analysis and breaking down components of tasks to assess and facilitate completion of tasks. Any number of injuries or diagnoses may affect a patient's independence with daily living skills. Decreased ROM, strength, coordination, cognitive skills, and visual impairment all affect one's ability to complete ADL. The OT will note ROM within functional terms, as many activities of daily living do not require full ROM. The concern for ROM treatment then would be to try and increase ROM that is limiting self-care performance. For example, a significant limit in elbow flexion would affect ability to self-feed and perform oral hygiene (3).

The OT also uses a variety of upper extremity assessment tools. Grip and pinch testing, muscle testing, sensation testing with Semmes-Winstein Monofilaments, two-point discrimination, circumferential or volumetric measurements for edema, nine-hole peg coordination testing, and dexterity testing can all give useful information (4). Research has shown that a grip strength of 20 pounds allows patients to perform most ADL, and a pinch strength of 5 to 7 pounds is useful in accomplishing most daily tasks (5).

Occupational therapists use observational and standardized assessment to screen for visual and perceptual deficits. A patient with traumatic injuries may exhibit any number of visual/perceptual problems such as: visual field cut, diplopia, or figure-ground deficit. The Motor-Free Visual Perception Test-Revised (MVPT-R) (6) is one standardized tool used to screen for these deficits. The test avoids any motor involvement that would influence the assessment of visual perception. It screens five skills: spatial relationships, visual discrimination, figure-ground, visual closure, and visual memory and has been shown to be valid for a variety of populations including adults with brain injury.

Occupational therapists frequently perform a Kitchen Screening to determine a patient's safety, awareness, judgment, visual perception, and physical ability when performing an IADL task. In our setting, a patient must prepare an egg and make a cup of coffee or tea with minimal instruction or cueing from the therapist. We have found this simple screening tool effective for a variety of acute care patients with traumatic injury such as multiple trauma, TBI, or orthopaedic injuries. See Appendix 1 for a sample Kitchen Screen form.

An occupational therapist may use the Hazard Safety Screening instead of or in addition to the Kitchen Screening. The Hazard Safety Screening involves a bathroom and kitchen setup with notable dangers present that the patient needs to identify. This screening was designed to provide information on functional skills and safety awareness in patients who may not be appropriate for a Kitchen Screening. For example, a teenager who does not work in the kitchen at baseline or a person who has not cooked for some time and/or does not have facilities to cook at home may not require a Kitchen Screening, but may benefit from the Hazard Safety Screening.

Another screening tool for occupational therapists that can be useful in the acute care setting is the Kohlman Evaluation of Living Skills (KELS) (7). The KELS is a pen and paper task tool that identifies potential deficits in areas of reading, writing, self-care, safety and health, money management, transportation and telephone, and work and leisure. The KELS can be a helpful tool with various populations, including those from inpatient and acute care units, and for people with brain injury.

Screening Tools Used by Physical Therapists

Balance Screening

Patients who suffer traumatic injuries may have impairments in balance that could endanger them for further injury upon discharge from the hospital. There may be a number of causes of these impairments: vestibular injury, TBI, visual impairments, muscle weakness, or a generalized balance disorder subsequent to prolonged bed rest. Physical therapists provide functional balance testing to help determine the safety of ambulation on level surfaces and outdoor uneven surfaces (stairs, curbs, ramps, and terrain). Balance should also be assessed in settings with various levels of stimulation. Patients should be challenged in noisy or busy environments, as these are the situations they will encounter when they are discharged from the hospital. There are standardized tests to assess risks of falls that therapists can administer in the acute care setting. The Berg Balance Scale (8), the "Get-up and Go" test (9), the physical performance test (10), and the Tinetti test (11) are a few of the most common assessment tools. While the majority of these balance assessments were designed to assess fall risk in elderly patients, components of the examinations can be used to give therapists objective data when measuring balance. Physical therapists can use the results from balance testing to make recommendations for assistive devices and/or safety techniques for home settings.

Pathfinding

Physical therapists may also assist with assessment of safety in the community or home with a pathfinding test. Patients may be able to ambulate safely, but may not be able to locate signs, follow directions, or navigate independently. Difficulties in pathfinding may provide insight into potential difficulties patients could encounter upon discharge from the hospital setting. This information, in conjunction with other therapy screening tests, may provide an indication that a patient requires increased supervision upon discharge to ensure their safety. It may provide information that supervision at home or a supervised medical setting is required. See Appendix 2 for an example of a pathfinding test.

Screening Tools Used by Speech-Language Pathology

SLPs have developed and implemented protocols to provide consistency and to meet the highest standard of care that can be provided with available resources. Ideally, diagnostic tools for evaluation of communication and cognitive-communication function used by the SLP on the acute care service provide a means of acquiring the greatest amount of information in the shortest amount of time. The materials have to be portable and require minimal setup and space. The normative data needs to be based on groups with a wide range of ages and socio-economic–educational background. The tests should be sensitive to mild impairment. Realistically, there are few tests available on the market that meet these criteria, so the SLPs at HMC have put together a portfolio of subtests from a variety of published tests that are found to be adequately reliable and sensitive and are based on reasonable normative data. These test batteries have been reviewed by the entire speech pathology group and discussed in staff meetings before being added to the repertoire of tests. Attempts are made to minimize test redundancy across disciplines. Materials used for formal testing include the following:

- Revised Token Test (12)
- Controlled Oral Word Association Test (COWA) (13)
- Subtests from the scales of Cognitive Abilities for Traumatic Brain Injury (SCATBI) (14)
- Boston Diagnostic Aphasia Examination (BDAE) (15)
- Minnesota Test for Differential Diagnosis of Aphasia (MTDDA) (16)
- Arizona Battery for Communication Disorders (ABCD) (17)

The most frequently used evaluation method for swallowing problems is the standard bedside evaluation. Use of instrumentation has not been necessary because of readily available services of otolaryngology and respiratory care therapists. The need for a Videofluoroscopic Swallow Study has been relatively low due to the nature and short duration of the majority of the swallowing problems seen at HMC on the acute care service.

Screening Tools Used by the Trauma Rehabilitation Coordinator

The trauma rehabilitation coordinator (TRC) sees all trauma patients who are being followed by the consult physiatrists. The TRC reviews the physiatrist's notes for any specific recommendations. The TRC then reviews the patient's orders and care plan from the primary medical or surgical team to see if those recommendations are included. If they are not, the TRC works with the caregivers for that patient to determine the barriers preventing implementation of the recommendations. Sometimes there are medical contraindications, such as a high intracranial pressure (ICP), which would appropriately delay the initiation of physical therapy, for example. If no contraindications are noted, then the TRC works with the primary team to ensure orders

are written and recommendations carried out. The TRC might also communicate directly with therapy or nursing staff to speed up the process. The TRC uses a screening tool to document the patient's injuries, treatment, social history, and family support. See Appendix 3 for a sample form. This informal tool is used to track the patient's progress towards discharge. Whenever possible, the TRC meets the patient and family and explains who the rehabilitation team members are and what their roles are in assisting in the patient's recovery. The TRC assesses the patient and family's understanding of the impact the patient's injuries are likely to have on functional status and provides access to information, as appropriate.

Screening Tools Used by Physicians

The consult physiatrists use a chart admissible screening tool that assists them in documenting the patient's medical history, physical examination, pertinent imaging and lab results, and social history. See Appendix 4 for a sample form. The physiatrist's assessment differs from that of other physicians involved in the patient's care. It is comprehensive in nature and focuses on how the patient's impairments correspond to disability (activity restrictions and limitations) or affect social roles and societal participation. The physiatrist's evaluation is geared toward developing recommendations aimed at ultimately reducing disability, maximizing independence, and enhancing social functioning. See Table 4-2 for a quick reference to screening tools.

Table 4-2	Quick Reference for Screening Tools
Occupational therapy	ADL evaluation, UE tests, MVPT-R, Kitchen Screening, Hazard Safety Screening, KELS
Physical therapy	Balance screening, pathfinding tasks
Speech-language pathology	Interview process, Revised Token Test, COWAT, subtests from the SCATBI, BDAE, MTDDA, ABCD, informal tests
Trauma rehabilitation coordinator	Medical screening, family screening
Physician	Physical examination, lab results, social history

ADL, activities of daily living; MVPT-R, Motor-Free Visual Perception Test-Revised; KELS, Kohlman Evaluation of Living Skills; COWAT, Controlled Oral Word Association Test; SCATBI, Scales of Cognitive Abilities for Traumatic Brain Injury; BDAE, Boston Diagnostic Aphasia Examination; MTDDA, Minnesota Test for Differential Diagnosis of Aphasia; ABCD, Arizona Battery for Communication Disorders.

EARLY THERAPY INTERVENTION

PREPARING THE PATIENT/FAMILY FOR PARTICIPATION IN FUNCTIONAL SKILLS

Trauma patients may spend extended periods in an ICU setting, unable to actively participate in their care. Interventions at this stage can help ensure that patients are prepared for a higher level of activity when they are medically stabilized. Prevention of complications that would inhibit patients from reaching their full potential is the goal of early therapy interventions at this stage of the patient's care.

Positioning/Splinting

Trauma patients may require prolonged periods in bed on bed rest because of medical, surgical, or orthopaedic injuries/issues. Prevention of joint contracture and skin breakdown is key to maximizing long-term functional outcomes and this can be achieved through positioning and splinting interventions.

Bed Positioning

Proper positioning in bed plays a large role in prevention of these complications. Trauma patients are at risk for skin breakdown for many reasons. Patients who are unconscious from a traumatic brain injury or insensate from a spinal cord or nerve injury are unable to protect their skin. Trauma victims are often immobilized on hard backboards for lengthy periods of time while transported from outlying areas to a trauma center. Oxygenation of peripheral tissues may be compromised due to the effects of shock in a hypotensive trauma patient.

Patients should be repositioned frequently with turning and out-of-bed positions to allow for circulation to pressure-bearing areas and improved vascular flow to the skin. Bony prominences are at highest risk for skin breakdown, and close inspection of the head, elbows, ischial and sacral area, and heels should be performed daily. Positioning of the limbs in a neutral position and avoiding severe external rotation of the lower limbs and excessive internal rotation of the upper limbs are crucial to maintaining joint integrity. Avoiding pressure over peripheral nerves that lie near bony prominences, the peroneal and ulnar nerves, for example, will decrease the risk of damage to those structures. Elevation of injured limbs to prevent chronic edema is another important aspect of positioning.

Eachempati et al. (18) found that "most ulcers developed in patients with an ICU stay >7 days" and that "increased age, non ambulatory status, prolonged time without any nutrition and an emergent ICU admission" were the greatest risk factors in development of decubits ulcers. A 1998 study at Inova Fairfax Hospital in Falls Church, Virginia, revealed that 20% of trauma patients hospitalized for more than 2 days developed at least one area of skin breakdown. The most common cause of breakdown was positional pressure (47%), followed by cervical collars (24%) (19). Hospitals have nursing policies and protocols related to turning and positioning patients and the use of cervical collars and other braces, which are designed to prevent skin breakdown. Many also use the Braden Pressure Ulcer Risk Assessment tool to help predict a patient's susceptibility to skin breakdown (20). See Appendix 5 for sample Braden Scale.

A variety of specialty beds are on the market, and can be used to help prevent breakdown on high-risk areas of the body. Members of the rehabilitation consult team can augment the efforts of the nursing staff and play an important role in helping to prevent skin breakdown. Nursing specialists and therapists can act as a team, to consult on patients with skin issues, and can assist in decision-making about appropriate beds or specialized treatments for skin impairments. Rotating beds are used in trauma care to manage patients with spine injuries, who need turning prior to their fixation or bracing, and in patients with acute respiratory distress syndrome (ARDS), who may require rotation to assist with improving their pulmonary function. These beds relieve pressure by providing constant turns, but given the nature of their firm surfaces, require frequent monitoring of the skin, similar to that required with other beds.

It is essential to prevent skin breakdown whenever possible or to at least identify and treat breakdown early and appropriately. A patient's ability to progress with a rehabilitation program can be significantly delayed because of skin breakdown problems. For example, a patient with a spinal cord injury who cannot sit up because of a decubitus ulcer would need to remain on bed rest until the ulcer healed.

Adaptive Positioning

Adaptive positioning devices can also be used to prevent skin breakdown and prevent joint contracture. Several positioning devices have been used with success at our facility. For prevention of breakdown at the occiput or posterior head, egg crate

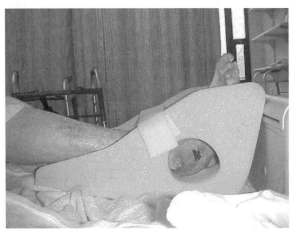

Figure 4–3. Cradle boot, a lower extremity positioning and skin protection device.

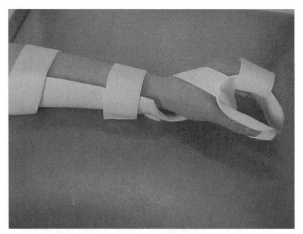

Figure 4–4. Resting hand splint.

foam or Custom foam head positioners with a cutout for the affected area provide options other than the standard pillow. For prevention of breakdown at the heels, a "cradle boot" positioner is used that has cutouts for all bony prominences of the foot and ankle and suspends the distal extremity from the bed, thereby relieving pressure (Fig. 4–3). These devices are ready-made but often need to be customized by trimming or cutting areas based on the patient's size and shape to provide an appropriate fit and the desired relief area. For prevention of breakdown at the elbows, elbow pads are used that come in a variety of sizes and pad the area near the olecranon process and epicondyles, providing pressure relief. Occupational therapists can assess for, provide, or adapt other positioning devices for patients as needed.

Splinting

Splinting becomes important during the acute phase of a patient's treatment to prevent joint contracture, prevent injury, and promote healing. Occupational

therapists are trained in the fabrication of custom splinting devices. A resting hand splint may be fabricated in order to prevent deformity in a patient with mild to moderate hypertonicity post-TBI (Fig. 4–4). Glasgow et al. reported significant positive findings in patients who wore upper extremity splints for 6 to 12 hours per day as compared to those who wore their splints less than 6 hours per day (21). A variety of hand splints or a wrist cock-up splint may be fitted in order to prevent shortening or elongation of tendons due to imbalance post–nerve injury (Fig. 4–5). An elbow extension splint may be required for a patient at risk for an elbow flexion contracture, such as a patient with muscle imbalance after C5 or C6 SCI (Figs. 4–6, 4–7). There are a variety of specific hand injuries that require immediate postoperative splinting as part of an early treatment protocol. For example, a flexor tendon injury that has been repaired may require specialized splinting to enable specific frequent protective exercises to promote appropriate healing. A patient post-TBI may be at risk for ankle joint contracture caused by either high or low muscle tone. Patients' postorthopaedic

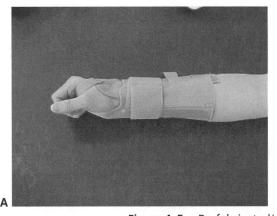

A

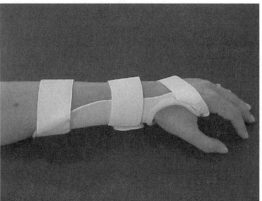

B

Figure 4–5. Prefabricated/custom wrist cock-up splint.

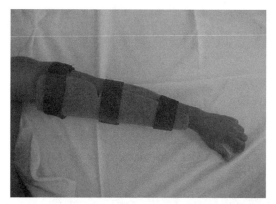

Figure 4–6. Prefabricated elbow extension splint.

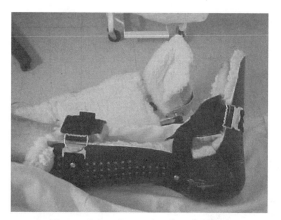

Figure 4–8. Posterior foot splint.

injury may also be at risk if they tend to rest in a plantar-flexed position or if they lack active dorsi-flexion of the ankle. A posterior foot splint should be provided in order to prevent ankle joint contractures in patients with these types of injuries (Fig. 4–8). It has been our experience that splinting as early as possible in the acute stage of a patient's care helps prevent future functional deficits.

Casting

Serial casting is also used as a modality for increasing ROM or preventing contracture, most commonly in the ankles and the elbows, and less commonly in the knees and hands of patients with spasticity. Patients with traumatic brain injury often demonstrate patterns of hypertonicity in their extremities. Most commonly, the lower extremity rests in an extended position with plantar flexion and inversion at the ankle joint, and the upper extremity in a flexed position with a fisted hand (Fig. 4–9). The rationale for serial casting is to improve joint ROM and muscle length in a hypertonic extremity to allow for improved function in

the limb as motor control returns or normalizes. The decision to serial cast should be determined after consultation between the physiatrist, the managing surgical or medical team, and the therapists.

Clinical judgments weighing the pros and cons of casting need to be investigated to ensure an appropriate outcome for the patient. A meta-analysis by Mortenson and Eng found "sufficient evidence (of improved PROM [passive range of motion]) to support use of casts in clinical practice" (22). In support of the safety of PROM on patients with traumatic brain injury, Brimiou et al. found the "PROM did not increase ICP and even tended to decrease ICP in patients with intracranial hypertension" (23). Indications for serial casting are an equinovarus deformity in one or both ankles that cannot achieve a neutral plantargrade position when the knee is extended (24) (Fig. 4–10). Singer et al. reported "support for the short-term efficacy of this intervention (serial casting) in patients with acquired brain injury. Significant gains in ankle motion were demonstrated after casting" (24). Moseley determined that "this study demonstrated that plantar flexion contracture can be reduced with casting

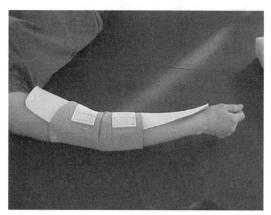

Figure 4–7. Custom elbow extension splint.

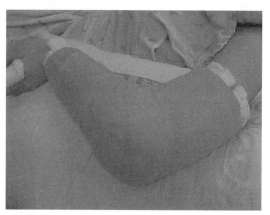

Figure 4–9. Upper extremity bivalved serial cast.

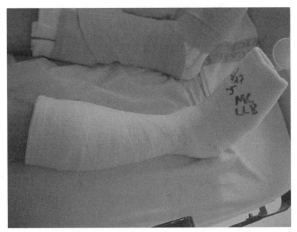

Figure 4–10. Lower extremity serial cast.

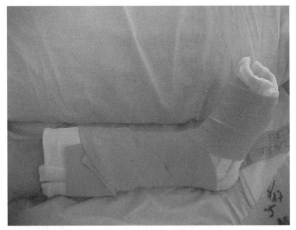

Figure 4–12. Lower extremity bivalved serial cast (on patient).

combined with stretching in individuals with traumatic brain injury, resulting in greater range of dorsiflexion motion" (25). Serial casts can also be bivalved, which renders them removable to allow for close monitoring of the skin or to allow for weight bearing through the extremity to facilitate functional use of the extremity (Figs. 4–11, 4–12). Bivalved serial casts are usually worn for periods on and off with scheduled time allotments determined depending on the patient's level of hypertonicity and response to casting. Serial casting is most successful when all team members are involved in decision-making and are in agreement that the improved joint ROM is a priority in the present rehabilitation goals.

Range of Motion

Range-of-motion exercises should be performed on all joints of patients within the limitations of their

musculoskeletal injuries. Patients with generalized edema after resuscitation will benefit from passive range of motion to avoid joint contracture. Patients with acute fractures that have been stabilized will benefit from ROM activities within prescribed precautions to avoid joint contracture. For example, a patient with a femur fracture who has been stabilized with an intermedullary nail will need to obtain 90 degrees of knee flexion to allow for a functional sitting position in the future. Patients who suffer a wrist fracture and have an open reduction and internal fixation, or patients who may have edema and impaired active movement after systemic trauma, need to receive digit ROM to ensure that future hand function abilities are preserved.

Key joint contractures that affect function in the lower extremity are in the ankles and knees (Fig. 4–13). A lack of dorsiflexion prevents anterior movement of the tibia over the talus, which will make standing impossible. A lack of flexion at the

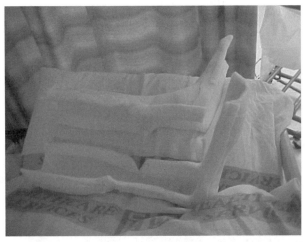

Figure 4–11. Lower extremity bivalved serial cast (off patient).

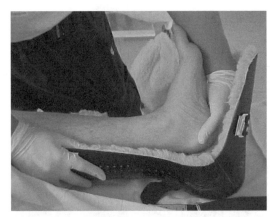

Figure 4–13. Ankle range of motion, posterior foot splint.

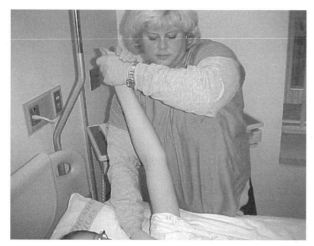

Figure 4–14. Upper extremity range of motion.

knee will make sit-to-stand transfers difficult, and a lack of knee extension prevents normal heel strike and affects the stance phase of gait. In the upper limb, contractures in the shoulders or elbows would prevent patients from completing ADL, dressing, washing, or grooming, and limitations in the hands can decrease efficiency with fine motor tasks, or prevent the ability to perform these skills in any form (Fig. 4–14). If joints become stiff in the early phases of the hospitalization, muscle strengthening later becomes more difficult, as the joints will need to regain ROM before effective strengthening can take place. Occupational therapists and physical therapists work together closely during these interventions. Both disciplines are skilled at joint assessment and the patient treatment plan may be similar for the two disciplines at this phase of patient care.

Continuous Passive Motion

Continuous passive motion (CPM) machines are indicated to prevent stiffness and maintain joint motion after surgical fixation or surgical manipulation or injury of the joint. CPM provides gentle passive ROM of the limb through a specific and controlled amount of joint range. Patients can use the machines for 8 to 10 hours per day. CPM is used for intra-articular fractures of the hip, knee, shoulder, or elbow. CPM applied during the early stages of healing acts to pump blood and edema away from the joint and periarticular tissues (26). The more quickly a joint can gain normal range of motion, the more quickly a patient can regain normal function.

Communication

The SLP provides a communication care plan based on the outcome of the early evaluation results. A written care plan is listed in the evaluation report, and we have found it very effective to also post it over the head of the bed, so all team members are aware of the plan. The care plan provides guidelines for maximizing communication between patient and family and/or caretakers and gives suggestions regarding environments that promote the highest level of cognitive-communication function at which the patient is capable of performing. It states information identifying a patient's most reliable mode of communication and methods for facilitating understanding and expression so that basic needs can be met.

The occupational therapist may also be involved in assessing and implementing treatment for a patient's communication needs in order to facilitate increased independence for the patient. An OT can assess a patient's motor function and cognition to help select a communication device such as a soft touch pad or a sip-and-puff call light system. These systems increase patients' ability to communicate and interact with their environment in the acute stages of their recovery.

Pulmonary Intervention

Trauma patients may have pulmonary compromise for a variety of reasons. Direct lung injury, aspiration, chest wall trauma, neurologic injury that affects the diaphragm and respiratory muscles in the case of spinal cord injury, or central control dysfunction in the case of traumatic brain injury all have implications on the pulmonary function of a patient. Treatment of a patient's pulmonary problems must be approached as a team effort.

Physical therapy is directed toward interventions that maximize gas exchange by improving ventilation, increase chest wall mobility, and increase effectiveness of airway clearance abilities. A bronchopulmonary treatment plan may include forced expiratory technique or active cycle of breathing, incentive spirometry, and assisted coughing. Other exercises include diaphragmatic breathing and lateral costal and segmental costal expansion exercises. Mobilization within patients' activity tolerance while monitoring oxygen saturation via pulse oximetry is another component. Upright positioning of patients is encouraged to improve lung volumes, coughing, and lung compliance (27). Within the physician's medical parameters, PTs can determine supplemental oxygen needs for patients during activity with physician's assistance by assessing oxygen requirements via perceived exertion ratings and vital sign monitoring. Improved pulmonary function may assist patients with quicker progression through their acute care hospitalization. Patient education about breathing strategies, cough techniques, and energy conservation is an important component of pulmonary training as well.

In the ICU setting, the occupational therapist's involvement in providing proper positioning and encouraging upright mobilization/activity can positively affect a patient's pulmonary status. The occupational therapist incorporates endurance training to improve pulmonary function as part of the ADL assessment and treatment interventions. The OT must be aware of a patient's activity tolerance and oxygen needs while working on functional ADL and other activities. The OT can also provide helpful information for the patient and family in teaching energy conservation techniques during functional tasks.

Pulmonary complications are the leading cause of death in patients with cervical spine injuries (28). In addition to being a cause for mortality, these complications can significantly increase a patient's length of stay on acute care. A 3-year retrospective analysis of patients with cervical SCI at our institution showed that the acute care length of stay for patients with pulmonary complications was 21.4 days versus 7.2 for those without complications.

The TRC, in concert with the neuroscience clinical nurse specialist and respiratory clinical specialist, monitors the pulmonary status of acute care patients with cervical spine injuries and recommends interventions to minimize or prevent complications. For intubated patients, their efforts focus on identifying which patients will likely require a longer weaning period and recommending an early tracheostomy. This practice prevents the physical and emotional trauma of repeated failed extubations and allows for a quick transition to an inpatient rehabilitation program where the patient can slowly wean from the ventilator while participating in therapy. For patients who appear to have the ability to wean, a protocol developed in conjunction with the pulmonary medicine department is recommended (Fig. 4–15). These guidelines should include high tidal volumes (up to 15 mL per kg of ideal body weight), because these volumes have been demonstrated to decrease the incidence of atelectasis in patients with SCI (28). Daily weaning parameters and adjusted rates to prevent hypercarbia should also be included. Patients with cervical spinal cord injury who do not require a ventilator must also be closely monitored for pulmonary complications. Respiratory therapists institute a bronchial hygiene protocol aimed at decreasing the possibility that the patient's respiratory status will deteriorate. The protocol may include incentive spirometry, assisted cough, hyperinflation therapies including intermittent positive pressure breathing (IPPB), chest physiotherapy for lobar atelectasis, mechanical insufflation-exsufflation, nasotracheal suctioning, and positive expiratory pressure (PEP) therapy.

Swallow

The swallowing mechanism and function are explained to the patient and/or family/caretakers, and the results of testing are discussed. The patients are informed of the different textures of solids and the consistencies of liquids best suited to meet their swallowing abilities. They are also provided with guidelines for maximizing safety (e.g., chin tuck) while taking food by mouth. The diet recommendations and aspiration precautions are written in the report summary and also posted over the head of the bed.

Patient and Family Education

Trauma is a sudden and unexpected event. For most patients and their families it represents a first-time experience with a significant and potentially life-threatening injury. Family members and friends are often in a state of shock as they struggle to come to grips with the reality of their loved one's condition. As they hover together in the patient's room or in the waiting area, a stream of professionals approach them to share test results or obtain permission for operative interventions. Bedside nurses and social workers assist them as they try to make sense of the rapidly changing pieces of information concerning the status of their loved one's condition. As hours and days pass and it becomes clear that the patient will survive his or her injuries, family members are frequently confronted with new questions. What will be the outcome of their loved one's trauma? Will the person ever be the same again? How long will the patient be in the hospital and where will he or she go next? Though relieved that their loved one's condition has stabilized, family members are often newly overwhelmed by this sense of the unknown. Members of the rehabilitation consult team play a very important role in assisting patients and their families as they navigate this new phase. The patient's primary physician and nurses working with the patient are understandably concerned with the patient's *medical* status. When physiatrists and therapists examine and work with patients they are in a unique position to help patients and their families understand current and potential *functional* status.

Patients and family are provided with both verbal and written information when appropriate. The information may be written by the clinician or may be published literature on the subject that requires explanation.

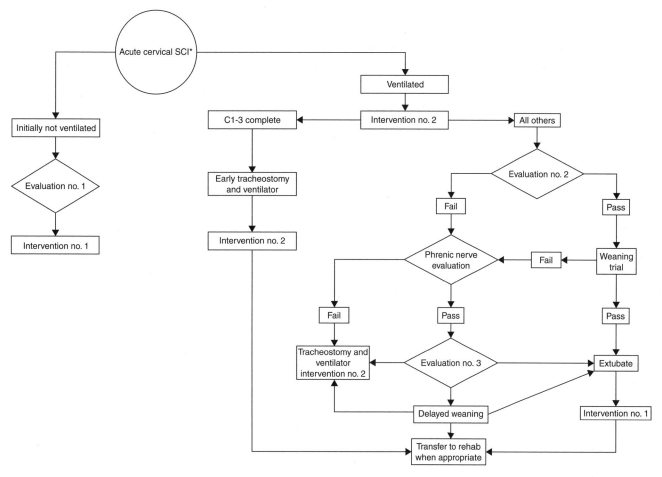

Figure 4–15. Pulmonary protocol.

Evaluation no. 1 (ER assessment)
Chest exam, breath sounds
Spontaneous respiratory pattern
Respiratory rate
Vital capacity
Chest radiograph

Intervention no. 1 (Patients with unassisted breathing)
Bronchial hygiene protocol
DVT/PE prophylaxis
Pneumonia prophylaxis

Intervention no. 2 (Patients with assisted ventilation)*
Evaluate CXR
Recommend ventilator settings
    Mode: A/C assist-control (A/C, AMV)
    Tidal volume: (1) Initially 15 mL/kg IBW
                  (2) If plateau pressure $\geq$ 35 cm H_2O,
                     reduce Vt by 1 mL/kg increments until
                     Pplat <35
                (3) Monitor minute ventilation: RR may
                     need to increase as Vt decreases
                     to prevent hypercarbla
    Respiratory rate: (1) Adjust initial rate to obtain a minute
                     ventilation of 8 and check an ABG
                (2) Titrate A/C rate to maintain PCO
                     36–44 mm Hg
    PEEP: (1) 0–5 cm HO
    FiO: (1) Initial FiO = 1.0
                (2) Wean FiO to keep SpO $\geq$ 92%
                    or PaO $\geq$ 65[†]

Evaluation no. 2
Daily weaning parameters
At $\geq$ 24 hours post surgical stabilization, to "pass" weaning
parameters means to have all of the following:
        NIF < $-$20
        RR $\leq$ 30
        Vt $\geq$ 5 mL/kg
        VC $\geq$ 10 mL/kg
        RSBI <105
        Spontaneous VE $\geq$ 2/3 assisted VE
If weaning parameters are "failed," reassess daily until "pass" or until
phrenic nerve assessment completed

Evaluation no. 3
Daily weaning parameters
Consider additional diagnostic studies, such as: repeat C-spine
MRI, fluoroscopic sniff test, metabolic cart study
Evaluate for other confounders, such as:
    upper airway obstruction, acute or chronic airflow limitation
    (asthma, COPD), poor nutrition, psychological factors, and
    other chronic diseases
Consider a Team Meeting or Patient Care Conference
Consider transfer to MICU service and/or to a RICU bed

*If the patient has ALI/ARDS, management strategy and goals need
to be reevaluated. This strategy could worsen lung injury if applied
to ALI/ARDS.
[†]If there is coexistent brain or myocardial injury, it may be prudent to
keep the SpO $\geq$ 94% or PaO $\geq$ 75.
NIF, Negative Inspiratory Force (may also be called Maximal Inspiratory Pressure); Vt, Tidal Volume; RSBI, Rapid Shallow Breathing Index.

Family members of patients who suffer severe trauma are often interested in contributing to the care of the patient. Instruction in gentle ROM of uninvolved extremities may provide opportunity for family members to touch the patient and assist in their care while maintaining precautions that relate to surgical repair, IVs, tubing, and other lines patients may have during the early phases of their medical care. Instruction in edema control techniques also provides a beneficial opportunity for touching their loved one. Instructing the family members in the appropriate purpose, fit, and wearing schedules for the patient's splints or positioning devices can assist in consistency of care for the patient, as well as giving the family understanding and ownership over these medical interventions. The speech pathologist provides information on a variety of topics related to communication, cognitive-communication, and swallowing. Allowing family members to be involved with patient care early on prepares them for future opportunities when they may assist patients upon discharge from the hospital.

The trauma rehabilitation coordinator checks in with patients and their families to assess how well they understand their condition and the next steps in care. The TRC provides printed information, as necessary, and directs them to the hospital's Patient and Family Resource Center, where they can access the Internet with guidance, if they wish more detailed information. The TRC assesses the possible need for the intervention of other professionals, such as social workers or rehabilitation psychologists.

A specialized resource, which the TRC coordinates, is the Brain Injury Information and Support Group. This group meets once a week and is facilitated by nurses specializing in neuro-trauma, rehabilitation therapists (PT, OT, and speech) and family members of past patients. The group provides a forum for friends and family members of patients who have suffered traumatic brain injury to gain a more extensive understanding of TBI and to share with and learn from others who are going through a similar experience. In existence for more than 15 years, this group has not only helped countless families, it has also provided an opportunity for the facilitators to better understand the perspective of families affected by traumatic brain injury.

PATIENT PARTICIPATION IN FUNCTIONAL SKILLS

Mobilization

Mobility improves pulmonary function, decreases risk of decubitus ulcers, assists with strengthening and decreases risk of muscle atrophy, and improves circulation and cardiac function. Physical therapists assess the safest mobility technique for patients and provide this information to the team so it can be incorporated into the patient plan of care, which allows nursing staff to follow through on the mobility plan safely. Patients with serious disability, such as SCI or TBI will benefit from the expertise of physical therapists with mobility planning. Wang et al. reported that "unnecessary delay in mobilization results mainly from the development of severe respiratory complications and avoidable complications such as pressure sores" when SCI patients were in "nonspecialized units" (29). They emphasized that a "long stay in bed was associated with complications, especially pressure sores" and only if "early operation (for spine surgery) was supplemented by good general medical and nursing expertise to prevent complications, could early mobilization be achieved" (29).

Physical therapists play a large role in mobilization of trauma patients, who may have more complex mobility needs than the average hospitalized patient. After trauma and prolonged intensive care unit stays, patients' impairments in strength and endurance or cardiovascular deconditioning may be too great to allow for aggressive mobility progression. An option for these types of patients is the use of a tilt table. This device provides a supportive surface for a patient to move from the supine position to an upright position. The tilt table allows a partial standing position to encourage weight bearing through the lower extremities in patients who would otherwise be unable to stand (Fig. 4–16). Bohannon and Larkin also showed "increased passive ankle

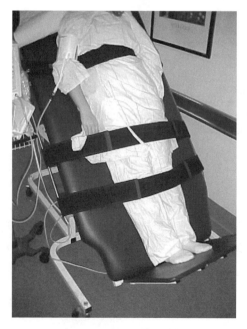

Figure 4–16. Tilt table.

dorsiflexion" in 20 patients treated consecutively to determine the effectiveness of the treatment (30). The tilt table may be used in patients with neurological impairments, as in TBI or SCI, or with patients who have suffered generalized myopathy after trauma, as in patients with critical illness.

Patients who have suffered multiple trauma may also be nonambulatory for a prolonged period of time as they recover. Physical therapy evaluation may be required to provide specialized seating systems and wheelchair assessment. Appropriate size wheelchairs with appropriate support to the injured extremities, trunk, and/or head will allow patients to begin to mobilize out of bed and eventually out of their room. Custom cushion systems and postural supports provide optimal seating positions that decrease the risk of sheering and pressure over bony prominences.

Pressure relief while patients are using wheelchairs is as important as pressure relief strategies for bed positioning. Commonly used pressure relief techniques include the tilt back and the forward lean. Henderson et al. found that "the forward leaning (position) consistently reduced pressures over the ischial tuberosity" (31). Unfortunately, many acutely injured patients cannot achieve this position due to braces and external supports. This study showed that "the sixty-five degree backward tip position reduced pressure, but not to levels considered threshold for pressure ulcer generation" and the 35-degree backward tilt "is of little value in pressure reduction over the ischial tuberosity" (31). Appropriate wheelchairs that allow for a 65-degree or greater backward tilt are important in prevention of pressure ulcers in patients who are in a prolonged seated position. Physical therapists are skilled in the assessment of wheelchairs and can make recommendations that will allow patients' independence as they begin their recovery.

Trauma patients may suffer lower extremity injury that requires an assistive device for ambulation. Physical therapists assess patients' strength, balance, and endurance when selecting the appropriate device. Physical therapists may employ the use of walkers, axillary crutches, forearm crutches, or canes to assist patients with walking activities. An upper extremity injury may require a platform attachment to the device, to allow the patient to use the device without weight bearing on their hand or wrist. The ability to walk is an integral part of a patient's being able to regain independence and a commonly stated goal that many patients have after trauma.

Occupational therapists work to reinforce the mobilization plan for the patient and to assess and train the patient in functional mobilization during ADL. The OT may recommend appropriate adaptive equipment to facilitate independence and safety in toilet/commode transfers, and reinforces appropriate

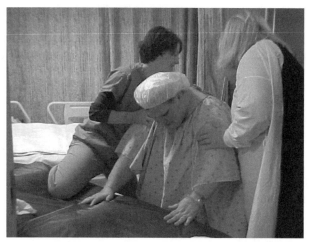

Figure 4–17. PT/OT cotreatment, standing.

use of the assistive device prescribed by the PT, as the patient practices use during functional tasks (Figs. 4–17, 4–18).

Basic Activities of Daily Living

The OT works with patients on the acute care units to assess and instruct in BADL skills. The goal of this treatment is to facilitate functional independence. Depending on the injury the focus may be on increasing the ROM or strength required for ADL, on instructing the patient in appropriate adaptive equipment to facilitate safe and independent self-care, or on compensatory or reeducation methods to facilitate independence in the cognitive skills required for ADL performance. ADL can be a motivating modality to achieve increased functional endurance and independence. For example, a patient will sometimes be more motivated to complete his or her hygiene independently than to perform repetitions of ROM exercises.

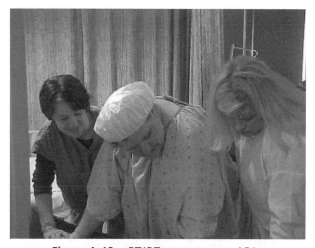

Figure 4–18. PT/OT cotreatment, ADL.

Communication

Communication problems can arise from a variety of sources in the trauma patient. A patient may not be able to communicate due to a brain injury affecting the dominant language and/or speech centers of the brain. Nondominant hemisphere lesions and generalized brain damage may affect a patient's ability to comprehend abstract information, to reason, or to recall important information. Injury to the midbrain may result in an inability to speak or write. The patient may have respiratory problems, resulting in the need for ventilatory support or tracheostomy, making vocalized speech difficult or impossible.

The SLP's goal is to identify the areas of strength in the patient's communication process and to use these strengths to offset the areas of deficit. A patient with quadriplegia who is on ventilatory support or a person with locked-in syndrome may be limited to eye blinking responses. The most basic level of communication of differential blinking for yes/no questions may be used. If their vision, language systems, and memory are intact and they have the endurance, patients may be trained to use an alphabet, word, picture, and/or topic board. Patients with a laryngectomy may be trained to use an electrolarynx. Patients with severe dysarthria may be supplied with a dry erase board if they have the ability to write.

Occupational therapists may also be involved in assessing and implementing treatment for a patient's communication needs. The purpose of their early involvement is to help facilitate increased independence for the patient. An OT can assess a patient's motor function and cognition to help choose a communication device such as a soft touch pad or a sip-and-puff call light system. These systems enable increased ability for patients to communicate and interact with their environment in the early stage of their recovery.

Swallow

When the swallowing mechanism is impaired, choices the patient can make regarding food and beverages are limited. The texture of the food and the consistency of the beverages are dictated by the type and severity of impairment of the swallow. The SLP works closely with the clinical nutritionist to provide modified diets that meet taste preferences while fulfilling the nutrition and hydration needs of the patient. Whether a patient is a self-feeder or needs to be fed is determined during the evaluation process. If the patient is thought to be incapable of following the guidelines, or if the intake would be insufficient for adequate nutrition and hydration, the patient will be offered one-to-one feeding, supervision, or assistance by the nursing staff and aides.

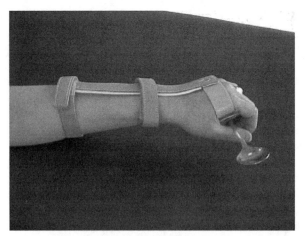

Figure 4–19. Self-feeding, adaptive spoon.

If the patient appears capable of self-feeding he or she will be instructed regarding appropriate food textures, liquid consistencies, and the aspiration precautions to follow. If the SLP finds that the patient is unable to self-feed an OT is consulted to complete a self-feeding assessment and provide training in the use of adaptive equipment, strengthening, or other compensatory techniques to increase independence with self-feeding (Fig. 4–19).

Cognition

Patients with cognitive-communication deficits may have limited awareness and responsiveness to the environment, impaired memory, and/or disorientation. Attention to task and ability to concentrate to perform tasks may be extremely impaired. Some patients have adequate communication skills but very poor verbal memory or recall. Patients who are disoriented may be provided with a sign with the name of the hospital and city on it and a calendar. They are then trained to refer to these sources when answering orientation questions. A patient with advanced communication skills may be given a pad of paper and a pen and asked to journal daily events, important questions to ask other medical team members, and planned activities. Family members are trained to assist with daily orientation and journaling.

The occupational therapist works in assessing and treating cognitive deficits. By observation of functional self-care the skilled therapist can gather information regarding a patient's initiation, thoroughness, follow-through, attention span, concentration, perception, memory, safety judgment, and awareness. The therapist can then provide the appropriate environment, patient, and family training to help facilitate improvement in these skills. As mentioned earlier, the therapist can use kitchen or safety hazard screening tools to help determine a patient's skill and the potential for unsafe behavior. In the acute care setting these assessments are used to help determine discharge and ongoing therapy needs (7,8).

Bowel and Bladder

All patients with spinal cord injuries are seen and evaluated by a consult physiatrist within 24 hours of admission. These patients are subsequently followed closely for the duration of their acute care stay. The physiatrist offers recommendations to the primary service physicians on many areas of management of these complex patients.

Most patients with spinal cord injuries will suffer from some degree of neurogenic bowel or bladder dysfunction. These conditions can lead to significant problems for patients, both early on and long term. In our organization, primary service physicians are often inexperienced in diagnosing these problems and applying appropriate approaches to prevent complications.

Our interventions focus on diagnosing the degree of the bowel dysfunction and recommending appropriate medications and techniques for promoting regular bowel movements.

See Appendix 6 for sample bowel program orders. Patients with neurogenic bowel dysfunction are admitted to an inpatient rehabilitation program for further bowel training.

If the physiatrist anticipates that the patient with SCI will be moving directly from acute care to an inpatient rehabilitation unit, he or she will usually recommend that a Foley catheter be left in place until transfer. A comprehensive assessment of bladder function and a coordinated approach to care will then be initiated on the rehabilitation unit. If a patient has a relatively mild SCI and may not require an inpatient rehabilitation stay, the physiatrist will typically advise the primary service to remove the catheter, observe for ability to urinate within a specified period, and check the patient's postvoid residual, either through catheterization or by means of a bladder ultrasound. If a significant problem with voiding is identified, the patient is often admitted for an inpatient rehabilitation stay to specifically address the neurogenic bladder issues.

The team approach is important in planning and providing for a patient's bowel and bladder needs. As a part of bladder and bowel management, occupational therapists assess a patient's function in mobilizing to the toilet or commode and in motor control for performing toilet hygiene. The OT can help facilitate early mobilization to the appropriate commode or toilet with adaptive equipment, and help coordinate this mobilization to occur at the appropriately scheduled time (bowel program) in coordination with the patient's nurse. The OT can also problem solve and train a patient in the use of adaptive equipment to facilitate increased independence in mobility or toilet hygiene.

Instrumental Activities of Daily Living

There are some patients within the acute care setting who may progress enough prior to discharge to participate in higher-level ADL assessment or treatment. As mentioned in the section on screening tools, the occupational therapist uses functional activity such as cooking to determine a patient's status and abilities and to help determine readiness and appropriateness for discharge.

Patient/Family Education

Instruction of family members in the latter phase of the acute care stay is crucial to assisting with good outcomes. As the patient's condition stabilizes and the hospital stay nears an end, patient and family education begins to focus on understanding the transition to the next level of care. The physiatrist, relying on input from other rehabilitation team members, recommends whether the next level of care will be an acute inpatient rehabilitation unit, a skilled nursing facility, or home with some level of assistance or outpatient therapy. Families and patients are often confused by the factors that affect this recommendation and need help from the team to understand them. This understanding is necessary in order for the family to participate in choosing an appropriate facility or to prepare for the level of participation necessary to transition to home.

Social workers help the family to understand their options. These options are often influenced by the type of insurance coverage patients have, or by the fact that they have none. Therapists explain to the patient and family what their therapy needs will be, how they can anticipate participating in that therapy, and where it can be obtained, if they are going home.

Physical therapists can educate family members to assist with follow-through on active or passive exercise programs, to increase frequency during the day, and assist patients with understanding their precautions to prevent possible injury. Many trauma patients do not recall their ICU stays, and are not familiar with their anatomic injuries. Patients' family members may be overwhelmed and stressed during the ICU phase, and also may not have a full understanding of the injuries. Use of pictures, skeletal models, and written information can help explain precautions and pain issues. Education about their injuries and future outcomes can make the rehabilitation process go smoothly and expedite the transition from hospital-based care to the home setting.

Occupational therapy uses family training toward the end of an acute care stage to ensure that patients continue to improve their functional skills within a safe setting. Families may need to learn how to assist patients with self-care tasks, how to use or encourage patients to use adaptive equipment, how to supervise them to maintain safety, or how to continue therapeutic positioning, splinting, or exercise programs.

The SLP provides patients and family members with information regarding communication, cognitive-communication, and/or swallowing in general. Families are counseled on specific behaviors they may encounter with their family member and given guidelines on how to manage these behaviors and when to contact a health care professional. They are encouraged to work with the rehab team to increase the awareness of deficit experienced by their family member and to encourage and in some cases assist with follow-through with techniques provided to facilitate maximum function.

EARLY PHYSICIAN-RELATED INTERVENTIONS

Physiatrists have expertise in areas that are often outside the scope of everyday practice for other physicians involved in trauma care. Their perspective is long range and they are alert to issues that might appear minor but, if not addressed, could significantly delay transition to the next level of care or even have an effect on the patient's ultimate functional ability.

CHALLENGES AND POTENTIAL BARRIERS TO INTERVENTION

MEDICAL ISSUES/PRECAUTIONS

There are a variety of medical issues or precautions that pose a barrier to early rehabilitation interventions. Some physical barriers are based on the patient's diagnosis. For example, orthopaedic injuries most often require weight-bearing precautions and often limit movement or ROM. Many patients suffer multiple trauma or multiple fractures that limit their active participation in therapy. If patients are not-allowed to bear weight on three or four extremities for the first 6 weeks of their recovery, their active participation in rehabilitation will be limited. Orthopaedic injuries often necessitate structural barriers as well, such as spinal

orthoses, HALO braces, or external fixation. Other spine orthoses include soft cervical collars, Miami J or Aspen collars, TLSO, Minerva, or Jewett braces, which allow a patient's mobilization but may limit their ability to gain full independence.

There are medical complications or issues that potentially create other barriers to early rehabilitation interventions. Patients with multitrauma, who have had periods of time on bed rest, are at high risk for deep vein thrombosis (DVT). If a patient has a known or suspected DVT, they may be placed on bed rest and/or have restricted ROM orders to the involved extremity. Medical barriers also take the form of lines that may be required for patient medical management. Patients with newly placed ventriculoperitoneal (VP) shunts must lie flat postoperatively and are progressed to an upright and out of bed positioning over a 48- to 72-hour period, at the discretion of the surgeon, to allow pressure in the brain to gradually equilibrate. Patients with lumbar drains are also on bed rest and must lie flat at all times. During these periods, therapy interventions are limited to those that can be provided to the patient in bed prior to mobilization.

Patients may have nasogastric tubes for tube feedings or drainage of stomach contents. Precautions must be followed for these patients. To avoid reflux or aspiration, patients must be in reverse Trendellenburg position or have the head of the bed elevated at least 30 degrees while the tube feeding is running. The tube feeding must be turned off before laying a patient flat. Prone positioning must be approached with caution in patients with feeding tubes in the abdomen, to avoid inadvertent removal. Intravenous lines should not be a barrier to providing therapy services, as they can usually be temporarily disconnected for therapy sessions. This is true unless the patient has vasospasms, has just come out of surgery, or is on anticoagulant therapy for a DVT. There are also specific monitoring lines that require specific precautions.

Arterial lines are used with many patients in the ICU to monitor blood pressure continuously and to allow access for arterial blood gas measurements. These lines are placed directly into an artery and require caution when moving extremities. Typically, the joint near the arterial line will be immobilized. For example, a patient with a radial arterial line will have an arm board over the wrist to protect the line and to prevent wrist flexion. ROM to joints with arterial lines should be avoided. Patients may have larger lines into their femoral arteries, usually for dialysis access or monitoring. Hip flexion should be below a 60-degree angle to avoid kinking. Patients may have central lines in place that lead from their arm, neck, or chest into the central vessels near their heart. These lines are sutured in place, but should be noted and watched during ROM activities. All patients in the ICU will be hooked up to monitors that have the capacity to measure the patients' heart rate, respiratory rate, oxygenation, blood pressure, and pulmonary pressure. Such devices allow the therapist to monitor the patient's vital signs and response to treatment. These lines should not be disconnected during treatment in the ICU.

Patients with injuries to the brain may have an intracranial pressure monitor (ICPM), also called a Camino or a Bolt. This device is used to measure pressure inside the head for patients who have incurred a traumatic head injury or have undergone a neurosurgical procedure. Normal ICP is approximately 5 to 10 mm Hg. To avoid impairing cerebral perfusion pressure, therapy interventions may be held on patients with intracranial pressure greater than 20 (to avoid cerebral perfusion pressure [CPP] <70). The therapist should seek advice from nursing and the physician about whether it is appropriate to attempt therapy when ICP levels are high. A ventriculostomy is a tube that is placed in the patient's ventricle to assist with drainage of excessive cerebral spinal fluid (CSF) or blood, and provide decompression to the brain. Both of these medical lines are calibrated by the patient's head position. Changing the position of the head of the bed may have a serious effect on the monitor, and a life-threatening effect on a patient with a ventriculostomy. Most patients with these lines will be confined to bed, and therapy interventions may be limited to those that can be provided to the patient in that position.

Another barrier that presents in the traumatic brain injury population is a surgical craniectomy, used to allow access to the brain for evacuation of blood and decompression of these fragile tissues. Patients with brain injuries that require a craniectomy must wear a helmet at all times when out of bed to protect their brain. Patients who have had a craniotomy have the skull intact, and therefore no helmet is required. OT fits a patient who has had a craniectomy with a helmet as soon as the ICPM and/or ventriculostomy is removed. Patients with craniectomies cannot be mobilized without a helmet. For patient safety, all staff must be aware that the patient cannot be moved out of bed without the helmet on.

Many ICU patients are intubated and on a ventilator. Some will be intubated through an endotracheal or nasotracheal tube, while others may have a tracheostomy. Most therapy treatments can be done around ventilator tubing; however, care needs to be taken. Mobilization and out-of-bed activities can be performed on patients who are ventilated, if their level of alertness, strength, and pulmonary function will allow. Communication with the nurse or respiratory therapist is an integral part of therapy with these patients to determine the best treatment times and options.

Chest tubes are used on patients who have had either partial or complete collapse of the lung, secondary to a pneumothorax or hemothorax. The chest tube is placed between the lung and the chest wall to drain excess fluid from the intrapleural space while providing suction to reinflate the collapsed lung. If a patient's chest tube is connected to "wall suction," all therapy activities must be completed in the room, as that suction cannot be unhooked. Once a patient's chest tube is placed on a portable "water seal," the patient may be mobilized as tolerated. During a therapy session care must be taken to never raise the chest tube drainage collector higher than the patient's chest tube site, as this could cause fluid to drain back into the intrapleural space and cause further lung collapse. Activities that cause this position should be avoided, while techniques to improve pulmonary function can complement the care of patients with chest tubes.

Patients may also require procedures that are barriers to therapy treatment. For example, after receiving a lumbar puncture, a patient generally remains on bed rest for at least six hours. This precaution allows the body time to equilibrate for the loss of CSF pressure. Patients who have an angiogram procedure must be on bed rest and avoid hip flexion for 6 hours after the procedure. Because the procedure is done through the femoral artery, activity or motion too soon after the procedure could cause a rupture or hematoma of the vessel.

If a patient has severe cerebral vasospasm, a physician may put him or her on bed rest. If a patient has been cleared to be out of bed but still has mild vasospasms, specific mobility progression guidelines should be requested from the physician. Patients with vasospasms should not be allowed to go outside to smoke, as smoking increases the vasospasms.

Patients who have undergone a skin graft may have a change in activity or ROM orders, and therapists should communicate with the physicians to ensure that graft sites are not disturbed by therapy intervention.

In the acute care setting, barriers to early rehabilitation intervention take on many forms. Whether the limitations are physical, medical, or procedural, they can affect how interventions are provided. Knowledgeable therapists and team communication ensure that patients can maximize their participation while maintaining patient safety.

PAIN CONTROL

In the acute care setting, patients suffer pain from a variety of causes. Effective control of this pain is key to providing care to these patients. If patients' pain is not controlled, they cannot be expected to perform therapy interventions in a progressive manner. Co-ordination of care for pain control is key for therapists. Communication between physicians, nursing, and pharmacy can help determine the optimal pain control strategy for patients. Scheduling around medication may need to occur. Therapists need to be aware of patients' pain medication schedule and the duration of the medications being used. The use of splints or other forms of bracing to support a painful area, the use of bed features to provide assistance with early mobility, and breathing strategies to decrease pain may also be used to make therapy interventions successful and allow patients to progress through the stages of rehabilitation (32).

LANGUAGE

Treating patients for whom English is a second language is a frequent occurrence in the acute care setting. Some patients do not speak English. Language differences can be a major obstacle to rehabilitation interventions. To gain from the experience of therapy, a patient and family must be able to benefit from education regarding the illness or injury and the impact on daily living. They need to understand the reason for facilitating and/or compensatory strategies. It is necessary for the patient and family to follow through on recommendations to home therapy, outpatient clinic visits, SNF placements, or rehab settings. Without a common language between the patient and clinician the information must be passed through interpreters. The benefit of interpreters is that they provide a means of communication. The drawback is that the interpreter may lack knowledge of the medical system and disorders as well as an understanding of therapeutic intervention. It is essential to have well-trained interpreters with experience in the medical setting and in particular with the needs of patients and therapists.

CULTURAL DIFFERENCES

Cultural differences can make administration of therapeutic evaluation and treatment difficult. Language differences affect communication directly as discussed earlier. Other communication problems may occur with body language and gestures. Some hand gestures widely accepted in the United States may be offensive and have different meanings in other countries. There may be culturally based perceptions of gender that affect a therapist's ability to engage a patient and/or family members in therapeutic activities. Cultures where males are in an authoritative position may have difficulty taking directions from a female therapist. Cultures that have sensitivity in areas of physical exposure may have difficulty receiving training in areas of personal hygiene from a male occupational therapist. Some cultures believe strongly in the responsibility of the family to support the patient whether or not they have adequate resources or understanding of the needs of the patient. Rehabilitative services may be a concept that is unfamiliar within the culture of certain countries, because the financial resources to support such an endeavor may not be available there. It is essential that therapists have some basic understanding and respect for cultural differences and that an effort be made to integrate this understanding and respect into the management of the patient's needs.

SUBSTANCE USE DISORDERS

Nearly half of injured trauma survivors suffer from substance use disorders, particularly abuse of alcohol and stimulants (33). Patients who suffer from these disorders present challenges to all of their caregivers, including members of the rehabilitation consult team. Many of these patients exhibit the effects of withdrawal during their initial days in the hospital. Symptoms of withdrawal, as well as the effects of medical interventions designed to minimize these symptoms, interfere with the ability of physiatrists and therapists to perform a thorough neurologic evaluation. Evaluation and intervention are frequently delayed until the patient's condition stabilizes. A patient's behavior may also pose barriers to therapy treatment. Our facility uses a screening scale to determine a patient's level of impairment when going through alcohol withdrawal. The Clinical Indicators of Withdrawal from Alcohol (CIWA) assessment is completed by nursing staff (34). See Appendix 7 for the CIWA form. The therapy department has determined that it is not appropriate to initiate treatment with these patients until their score on this screening is under 10, as the symptoms they are experiencing at that level are most likely caused by the alcohol withdrawal. A score under 10 allows a truer assessment of mobility and cognitive status without the effects of tremors, instability, or hallucinations caused by the withdrawal.

Patients with substance use disorders may show signs of anxiety or depression. These feelings can interfere with a patient's ability or motivation to participate in therapy.

Patients with substance use disorders often have weaker social support systems than other patients. Or their support systems might be counterproductive, encouraging inappropriate behaviors rather than behaviors that contribute to recovery from their injuries.

Naturally, since substance use is such a common contributor to trauma, members of the rehabilitation consult team in our organization have become skilled at working with patients with substance use issues. Approaching patients nonjudgmentally is helpful. The rehabilitation psychologist or psychiatric clinical nurse specialist is often consulted to offer suggestions to the team and to work directly with the patient, teaching relaxation techniques and other coping mechanisms. The physiatrist reviews the patient's medications, which often include drugs to combat anxiety or agitation. Suggestions are made if other, less sedating drugs might be equally effective. The goal of the team is to work effectively with patients with substance use issues so that they can transition to an intensive rehabilitation setting, where an interdisciplinary approach to treating their substance use can be integrated into their overall rehabilitation program.

PSYCHOLOGICAL ISSUES

Patients recovering from trauma may suffer from any of a number of psychological problems that can affect their ability to fully and actively participate in a rehabilitation program. Most trauma patients are confronted with the need to cope with some degree of loss or change in body image. Some losses, such as paralysis, are obvious and can be anticipated by team members, but many times the losses are subtle. Patients' reactions and ability to cope are not necessarily directly correlated to the degree of loss perceived by others.

Participation in therapy can be helpful for some. Physical exertion and focusing on a task can help relieve anxiety. Providing information about current functional disabilities and assisting the patient in beginning to overcome those disabilities empower and help patients to anticipate a potential positive outcome (35). Some patients are overwhelmed and require interventions such as medications or counseling in order to focus on their recovery. Rehabilitation professionals are in a position to recognize when patients are experiencing more than ordinary levels of stress while adjusting, and to facilitate initiation of these interventions.

It is not unusual for trauma patients to have underlying psychiatric illnesses that may have contributed to their injuries and can significantly affect their recovery. When a patient's injuries are life-threatening, it often takes a while to sort out medications that the patient was taking previously. A delay in reinitiating psychiatric medications might destabilize a patient's mood. Such patients will need special attention from the psychiatry service, as well as rehabilitation psychologists, until medications again take effect. Some patients are injured as a result of a suicide attempt. These patients may need to be restrained to prevent them from further harming themselves, until they no longer experience suicidal urges.

All of these conditions present challenges to rehabilitation professionals. Awareness and sensitivity to the varying degrees of the psychological impact of trauma is the first step in working effectively with recovering trauma patients. Understanding how underlying conditions might affect a patient is another. Rehabilitation professionals are uniquely positioned both to evaluate how trauma patients' coping abilities affect their recovery and to help patients cope more effectively.

DISCHARGE FROM ACUTE CARE

CRITERIA FOR REHAB

When a trauma patient is ready for discharge from acute care, the rehabilitation consult team is also ready with a recommendation for the most appropriate discharge setting. This recommendation is based on how the patient has performed during therapy evaluations. The most common discharge locations are intensive inpatient rehabilitation, low intensity rehabilitation, skilled nursing facility, and home. Several factors influence which setting the team recommends.

The criteria for admission to an acute inpatient rehabilitation unit vary somewhat by region of the country but must conform to Medicare and other federal and state regulations as well as those of appropriate certifying bodies such as the Joint Commission on Accreditation of Healthcare Organizations (JCAHO) and the Commission on Accreditation of Rehabilitation Facilities (CARF). These are the criteria we have developed for patients admitted to our acute inpatient rehabilitation unit. The basic criteria for our unit include the following:

- The patient must be willing and able to actively participate in the rehabilitation program;
- The patient must have goals in at least two of the three major therapy areas (PT, OT, and speech);
- The patient must have the endurance to tolerate at least 3 hours of therapy over the course of a day;

- The patient must demonstrate the ability to carry over new information;
- The patient must be medically stable.

It is essential that patients be medically stable when they begin their acute inpatient rehabilitation program. While our usual goal is to advance patients to the rehabilitation portion of their recovery as quickly as possible, this objective must be balanced against their readiness from a medical standpoint. Medical stability is important for several reasons. Patients who are not feeling well as a result of pain or a fever do not have the energy for active participation. Patients who require numerous interventions from physicians or nurses during the day do not have sufficient time available to fully participate. Patients who are undergoing diagnostic procedures are absent from the unit for extended periods and miss out on therapy sessions. While it is impossible to always rule out ongoing medical issues or to predict which patients might suffer a setback, we make every effort to avoid bringing patients to our rehabilitation unit before they are medically stable. These are the criteria that we have developed that help ensure that patients are medically stable on admission:

- Patients must be afebrile for 48 hours; may have low-grade temperature if a source has been identified and a treatment plan is in place;
- Patients who are ventilator-dependent (e.g., those with high quadriplegia) must be stable on a portable ventilator for at least 48 hours;
- Patients must not require suctioning more frequently than every four hours;
- Patients need to have a stable cardiac rhythm;
- Patients who require oxygen must have adequate blood oxygen saturation on portable oxygen;
- Patients must be off continuous positive airway pressure (CPAP), except for treatment of sleep apnea;
- If a patient has a chest tube, it must be stable to gravity only for at least 48 hours;
- The patient's medical work-up must be complete.
- If a patient has nutritional, pain, or wound issues, they must be manageable and not interfere with therapies.

The consult physiatrists follow patients closely and monitor their medical readiness for participation in rehabilitation. The physiatrist is responsible for checking on the patient on the day of admission to ensure that no events have occurred overnight that could interfere with therapy.

OTHER DISCHARGE SETTINGS

Home

After trauma, returning to the home setting may or may not be possible and is influenced by many factors. The environmental setting can be problematic if the patient has multiple stairs or narrow doorways, or lives in a rural setting where follow-up care may not be available. The patient may require assistance with mobility, shopping, food preparation, and ADL care. If the patient's family or support system is not available to provide this assistance, then discharge to the home setting may not be possible. If a patient is having cognitive problems and needs supervision for safety, this level of support must be available in order for a home discharge to be recommended. If a patient and family can provide appropriate support and have a home that is accessible for the patient, home therapy services can be provided in most cases. These therapy sessions will only be viable if the patient is homebound and does not require daily therapy, as daily home therapy cannot usually be provided.

Outpatient Therapies

If a patient is mobilizing safely and is not considered homebound, therapy services can be provided on an outpatient basis. If a patient requires service from multiple therapy disciplines, a comprehensive outpatient rehabilitation program may be the most ideal therapy setting when it is available. If a patient lives in a rural area and cannot get to therapy conveniently or the recommended therapies are not available, other discharge settings may be more appropriate.

Skilled Nursing Facility/Subacute Rehabilitation

There are times when patients may not be able to transfer to an intensive rehabilitation setting due to orthopaedic precautions, medical issues, low endurance, or decreased level of cognition that may affect their ability to participate defined by the criteria outlined above. In some cases, patients do not have the appropriate home situation or family support to allow them to return to that setting. Skilled nursing facility or subacute rehabilitation settings may be able to provide a level of therapy and nursing care that such patients will benefit from.

There are little differences between these two types of facilities. Some subacute rehabilitation facilities may provide more hours of therapy than a skilled nursing facility. Sometimes both programs are offered in the same facility. Patients and families should tour these facilities to find the one they feel comfortable with. Some facilities may cater to younger adults or children, some may manage patients with mechanical ventilation needs, and some may have better ability to manage patients with complex wound care needs.

Patients who have suffered traumatic brain injuries may not always be alert enough to participate in an acute rehabilitation program when they have completed their acute care hospitalization, and may require placement in a subacute facility until their level of alertness improves. In many instances patients who have multiple injuries might have weight-bearing restrictions that preclude full participation in rehabilitation. For example, a patient with a spinal cord injury may also have an upper extremity fracture. Such a patient would usually require a stay in a less rehabilitation-intensive setting until the upper extremity fracture has healed and the patient is able to use it. Likewise, for a patient with bilateral lower extremity fractures, it makes more sense to invest time and money intensively training the patient in gait skills once they are permitted to bear weight, because they will be using a wheelchair only until their fractures heal.

Transition Back to Inpatient Rehabilitation

Some patients discharged to a skilled nursing or subacute facility will eventually transition directly to home. Others might never improve significantly and will continue to require nursing care. For some patients, however, it is very important that they eventually are admitted to an acute rehabilitation program to ensure the best possible functional outcome.

Temporary placement at skilled nursing facilities often occurs in our setting for patients with traumatic brain injuries, with the anticipation of improvement, and for patients with multiple traumatic injuries whose fractures and medical precautions interfere with rehabilitation. Before discharge to the skilled nursing facility, we explain to patients and their families what the criteria for admission to acute rehabilitation are and why the patient does not currently meet those criteria. We explain why we believe that returning for the acute rehabilitation program is important and we provide information about how to initiate that readmission.

In addition, we keep track of where the patients are discharged to, and call periodically or review notes from return clinic appointments to help pinpoint when the patient might be ready for acute rehabilitation.

We have also forged relationships with many of the skilled nursing facilities in our area. Social workers at those facilities are aware of our admission criteria and refer patients appropriately. Nurse practitioners and physicians from our organization provide medical coverage for many facilities and are in a position to recognize when a patient is ready to benefit from acute rehabilitation.

CHALLENGES TO DISCHARGE

Finances

Patients' potential discharge alternatives are frequently influenced by financial considerations. Social workers and the trauma rehabilitation coordinator assist the team in understanding how a patient's financial situation affects discharge options.

Commercial insurance policies often have specific dollar or day limitations on acute rehabilitation or nursing home benefits. The policy may even exclude rehabilitation completely. Insurance companies frequently only contract with certain facilities, thereby limiting the patient's range of choices. Many commercial insurance companies assign case managers to oversee the care of patients with complex injuries. These case managers must preauthorize transfers to rehabilitation or skilled nursing facilities. Many skilled nursing facilities will accept only a fixed number of patients who are covered by Medicare or Medicaid. If these facilities are full and the patient's resources are limited, it may be difficult to locate a bed in a facility acceptable to the patient and family in a timely fashion.

Obviously, it is important to obtain accurate information about a patient's financial coverage for health care, specifically information that will affect a patient's eligibility for discharge options. Nearly all trauma patients followed by the rehabilitation consult team will need some form of ongoing care after discharge.

In our organization, patients are screened by a financial counselor as soon as possible after admission to determine if they have coverage for health care. If the patient does not have coverage (e.g., commercial insurance, Medicare, Medicaid, or workmen's compensation), they are referred to the health coverage services department. Employees in this department determine if a patient is eligible for public assistance and help the patient or their next-of-kin to apply for assistance.

When a patient is identified as having rehabilitation needs, the patient's social worker and the TRC analyze the patient's health care coverage to determine if it is adequate for the care recommended by the team. They help the patient and family to understand their coverage and what their degree of financial responsibility is likely to be. Obviously, each case is individual, and many are quite complex. It can be challenging but ultimately satisfying to work to ensure that patients receive the care necessary to fully recover from their injurie. Conversely, it can be frustrating when a patient's access to care is denied for financial reasons. Fortunately, solutions can be found for most patients.

SUMMARY

In conclusion, early rehabilitation interventions are crucial to patient care success. Length of hospital stay, patient outcomes, and patient and family satisfaction can all be improved when the appropriate "team" therapy interventions are provided early in the care of traumatic injuries.

Length of stay may be decreased when discharge needs are identified early. Therapists help to determine an adequate source of nutrition for patients and thereby improve their medical condition and energy level. Therapists are often able to identify the mode of communication for patients that will best allow active intervention and interaction to occur. Early mobilization with therapists will prevent a multitude of medical complications that are associated with bed rest, for example, DVT, atelectasis, and muscle atrophy. Family training allows families and patients to be prepared to assist with discharges even if patients require physical assistance or supervision. Therapists may suggest options for patient safety that do not require restraints. When the use of restraints is decreased, patients may be able to discharge to nonhospital settings sooner. By documenting the patient's need for home equipment, therapists can help secure the appropriate financing.

Rehabilitation interventions can improve patient outcomes in many ways. Maximizing patient independence is the focus of therapy intervention. Increasing a patient's physical, mental, and emotional independence can lead to better outcomes. Instructing patients who have long-term disability as a result of their trauma about the power of self-advocacy can prepare them to face the barriers they may encounter in the future. By identifying the patient's follow-up needs early on, the rehabilitation team can assist with setting up therapy services near the patient's home and in securing appropriate coverage for those services. Early and continuous patient and family education throughout the hospital stay leads to improved outcomes, by preventing the saturation of information during the final hour of the patient discharge. Patients learn more effectively by receiving small amounts of education over the course of their recovery and having time to process this information as their hospital stay proceeds.

Therapists assist with improved patient and family satisfaction. Patients appreciate holistic care. Adding skilled therapists as members of the medical team and allowing them to educate and train families in their specialty areas ensure that patients are getting the most thorough and efficient methods of care and training. Early rehabilitation interventions provide patient centered care and contribute to everyone's common goal — *patient success.*

REFERENCES

1. Roach KE, Ally D, Finnerty B, et al. The relationship between duration of physical therapy services in the acute care setting and change in functional status in patients with lower extremity orthopaedic problems. *Phys Ther.* 1998;78(1):19–24.
2. Rothstein JM, ed. Guide to physical therapist practice. 2nd ed. *Phys Ther.* 2001;81(1):9–744.
3. Pedretti LW. *Occupational therapy practice skills for physical dysfunction.* St. Louis, MO: C.V. Mosby Co; 1985.
4. Trumble T. *Principles of hand surgery and therapy.* Philadelphia, PA: WB Saunders; 2000.
5. Falkenstein N, Weiss-Lessard S. *Hand rehabilitation: A quick reference guide and review.* St. Louis, MO: Mosby; 1999.
6. Colarusso RP, Hammill D. *Motor-free visual perceptual test-revised.* Novato, CA: Academic Therapy Publications; 1996.
7. Kohlman Thomson L. *The Kohlman evaluation of living skills.* 3rd ed. Rockville, MD: AOTA, Inc; 1992.
8. Berg K, Wood-Dauphinee S, Williams JI, et al. Measuring balance in the elderly: Preliminary development of an instrument. *Physiother Can.* 1989;41(6):304–311.
9. Mathias S, Nayak USL, Isaacs B. Balance in elderly patients: The "Get-up and Go" test. *Arch Phys Med Rehabil.* 1986;67:387–389.
10. Winograd CH, Lemsky CM, Nevitt MC, et al. The development of a physical performance and mobility examination. *JAGS.* 1994;42:743–749.
11. Tinnetti ME. Performance-oriented assessment of mobility problems in elderly patients. *JAGS.* 1986;34:119–126.
12. McNeil MR, Prescott TE. *Revised token test.* Baltimore, MD: University Park Press; 1978.
13. Benton AL, Hamsher K De S. *Multilingual aphasia examination.* Iowa City, IA: AJA Associates; 1989.
14. Adamovich BB, Henderson JA. *Scales of Cognitive Ability for Traumatic Brain Injury (SCATBI).* Austin, TX: Pro-Ed; 1992.
15. Goodglass H, Kaplan E. *Boston Diagnostic Aphasia Examination (BDAE).* Philadelphia, PA: Lea & Febiger; 1983.
16. Schuell H. *The Minnesota test for differential diagnosis of aphasia.* Minneapolis, MN: University of Minnesota Press; 1973.
17. Bayles KA, Tomoeda CK. *Arizona battery for communication disorders of dementia.* Tucson, AZ: Canyonlands Publishing; 1993.

18. Eachempati SR, Hydo LJ, Barie PS. Factors influencing the development of decubitus ulcers in critically ill surgical patients. *Crit Care Med.* 2001;29(9): 1678–1682.
19. Watts D, Abrahams E, MacMillan C, et al. Insult after injury: Pressure ulcers in trauma patients. *Orthop Nurs.* 1998;17(4):84–91.
20. Bergstom B, Braden BJ, Laguzza A et al. The Braden Scale for predicting pressure sore risk. *Nurse Res.* 1987;36:205–210.
21. Glasgow C, Wilton J, Tooth L. Optimal daily total end range time for contracture resolution in hand splinting. *J Hand Ther.* 2003;16(3):207–218.
22. Mortenson PA, Eng JJ. The use of casts in the management of mobility and hypertonia following briar adults: A systematic review. *Phys Ther.* 2003;83(7): 648–658.
23. Brimioulle S, Moraine JJ, Norrenberg D, et al. Effects of positioning and exercise on intracranial pressure in a neurosurgical intensive care unit. *Phys Ther.* 1997;77(12):1682–1689.
24. Singer BJ, Jegasothy GM, Singer KP, et al. Evaluation of serial casting to correct equinovarus deformity of the ankle after acquired brain injury in adults. *Arch Phys Med Rehabil.* 2003;84(4):483–491.
25. Moseley AM. The effect of casting combined with stretching on passive ankle dorsiflexion in adults with traumatic head injuries. *Phys Ther.* 1997;77(3): 240–247.
26. Namba RS, Kabo JM, Dorey FJ, et al. Continuous passive motion versus immobilization. The effect on posttraumatic joint stiffness. *Clin Orthop.* 1991;267: 218–223.
27. Ciesla ND. Chest physical therapy for patients in the intensive care unit. *Phys Ther.* 1996;76(6):609–625.
28. Mansel J, Norman JR. Respiratory complications and management of spinal cord injuries. *Chest.* 1990; 1446–1452.
29. Wang D, Teddy PJ, Hnderson NJ, et al. Mobilization of patients after spinal surgery for acute spinal cord injury. *Spine.* 2001;26(20):2278–2282.
30. Bohannon RW. Passive ankle dorsiflexion increases in patients after a regimen of tilt table-wedge board standing. A clinical report. *Phys Ther.* 1985;65(11): 1676–1678.
31. Henderson JL, Price SH, Brandstater ME, et al. Efficacy of three measures to relieve pressure in seated persons with spinal cord injury. *Arch Phys Med Rehabil.* 1994;75(5):535–539.
32. Paz JC, Panik M. *Acute care handbook for physical therapists.* Boston, MA: Butterworth-Heineman; 1997.
33. Dunn C. Brief motivational interviewing interventions targeting substance abuse in the acute medical setting. *Semin Clin Neuropsychiatry.* 2003;8(3):188–196.
34. Sullivan JT, Sykora K, Schneiderman J, et al. Assessment of alcohol withdrawal: The revised Clinical Institute Withdrawal Assessment for Alcohol scale (CIWA-Ar). *Br J Addict.* 1989;84:1353–1357.
35. Dewar AL. Challenges to communication: Supporting the patients with SCI with their diagnosis and prognosis. *SCI Nurs.* 2001;18(4):187–190.

APPENDIXES

Appendix 1—Sample Kitchen Screening Form. (From the Department of Rehabilitation Medicine at Harborview Medical Center in Seattle, Washington, with permission.)

Appendix 2—Sample Pathfinding Test. (From the Department of Rehabilitation Medicine at Harborview Medical Center in Seattle, Washington, with permission.)

Appendix 3—Sample Trauma Rehab Coordinator Screening Tool. (From the Department of Rehabilitation Medicine at Harborview Medical Center in Seattle, Washington, with permission.)

Appendix 4—Sample Physiarist Screening Tool. (From the Department of Rehabilitation Medicine at Harborview Medical Center in Seattle, Washington, with permission.)

Appendix 5—Sample Braden Scale. (From Bergstrom N, Braden BJ, Laguzza A, et al. The Braden Scale for predicting pressure sore risk. *Nurse Res.* 1987; 36:205–210, with permission.)

Appendix 6—Sample Bowel Program Orders.

Appendix 7—Clinical Institute Withdrawal from Alcohol (CIWA) Form.

APPENDIX – 1

OCCUPATIONAL THERAPY KITCHEN SCREEN

Length of Activity: Start _____ Stop _____   **Items Prepared:** Fried egg ___ Scrambled egg ___ Coffee ___ Tea ___
Preparation Method: Microwave _____ Electric range _____

Purpose: This screening tool is designed to determine a patient's safety, judgment, and mobility within the kitchen environment. The results of this test are used to assist with general discharge planning.

Procedure: The patient is asked to cook an egg and/or make a cup of coffee or tea. The patient is allowed to either fry or scramble the egg. The patient may either use the electric range or the microwave to prepare the drink.

Patient Performance Areas: *Circle components evaluated

Sensorimotor	*Level of verbal cues:*	*Level of assistance:*
Coorrdination Bilateral Integration Crossing Midline Postural Control ROM Strength Endurance Tactile Auditory		

Cognitive	*Level of verbal cues:*	*Level of assistance:*
Attention Span Initiation Termination Memory Recognition Generalization Following Directions Sequencing Problem solving		

(continued)

APPENDIX – 1 (*Continued*)

Visual/perceptual	*Level of verbal cues:*	*Level of assistance:*
Depth Perception Spatial Relations Figure Ground R-L Discrimination Visual Topographical Orientation (optional)		

Therapeutic adaptations	*Level of verbal cues:*	*Level of assistance:*
Items Used Issued Needed		

Assessment:

Recommendations:

_____ Recommend patient receives 24-hour supervision.

_____ Patient would benefit from outpatient/home O.T. follow-up addressing the following areas:

KEY: *Use terminology to document level of verbal cueing and physical assistance provided

Verbal Cues:	**FIM LEVELS:**

<u>Complete cue:</u> (complete statement or redirection during tasks)
Ex. "Turn off the left burner."
 	
<u>Specific cue:</u> (providing one part of process to complete tasks)
Ex. "What should you do with the egg now?"
 	
<u>Non-specific cue:</u> (feedback that error was made during tasks)
Ex. "Have you forgotten anything?"
 	
* List number and level of cue given to successfully complete.
	No Helper
	IND - Complete Independence (Timely, Safely)
	MI - Modified independence (Independent with Device)
	Helper - Modified Dependence
	SUP - Supervision (Subject = 100% with SUP for safety)
	MIN - Minimal Assistance (Subject = 75% or more; require therapists hands-on)
	    ♦ Stand-by Assist
	    ♦ Contact Guard Assist
	MOD - Moderate Assistance (Subject = 50% or more)
	Helper - Complete Dependence
	MAX - Maximal Assistance (Subject = 25% or more)
	DEP - Total Assistance or Not Testable (Subject less than 25%)

SCORESHEET FOR PATHFINDING 3WH

NAME _____ DATE _____

TIME STARTED _____ TIME COMPLETED _____

2 points = **independent**
1 point = **needs assistance**
0 points = **unable to perform**

I.   Compass Directions

    A. ☐ _____

    B. ☐ _____

II.   Right/Left Discrimination

    A. ☐ _____

    B. ☐ _____

    C. ☐ _____

    D. ☐ _____

III. Reading Room Numbers/Scanning

    A. ☐ _____

    B. ☐ _____

    C. ☐ _____

IV.   1 Step Written Instructions

    A. ☐ _____

    B. ☐ _____

V.   2 Step Verbal Instructions

    A. ☐ _____

    B. ☐ _____

VI.   2 Step Written Instructions

    A. ☐ _____

VII. 3 Step Verbal Instructions

    A. ☐ _____

VIII. 4 Step Written Instructions

    A. ☐ _____

IX.   5 Step Written Instructions

    A. ☐ _____

X.   Map Reading

    A. ☐ _____

TOTAL SCORE = _____ /34

(*continued*)

APPENDIX – 2 (*Continued*)

1. COMPASS DIRECTIONS
   Location: Inside the patient's room
   Procedure: The therapist points North in the compass and says:
   a. "This way is North, please point South."
   b. "This way is North, please point East."

2. RIGHT/LEFT DISCRIMINATION
   Location: Inside the patient's room
   Procedure: Give instructions verbally:
   a. "Point to my right hand."
   b. "Point to my left leg."
   c. "Point to the wall on your left."
   d. "Turn 1/4 turn to your right."

3. READING ROOM NUMBERS AND SCANNING
   Location: Outside patient room 381 on 3 W and facing North up the hallway
   Procedure: Give instructions verbally, one at a time:
   a. "Walk to the second door on your right."
   b. "Find patient room 375."
   c. "Find room 381."

4. ONE STEP WRITTEN INSTRUCTIONS
   Location: Outside room 381
   Procedure: Give patient written instructions:
   a. "Find the shower."

5. TWO STEP VERBAL INSTRUCTIONS
   Location: Outside the double door crossroads
   Procedure: Give patient verbal instructions (simple):
   a. "Walk past the pictures on your left and turn left in the patient lounge."
   Location: Inside the patient lounge
   Procedure: Give patient verbal instructions (simple):
   b. "Before you go back to room 381, point out the office on your right."

6. TWO STEP WRITTEN INSTRUCTIONS
   Location: Outside room 381
   Procedure: Give written instructions:
   a. "Walk past the nursing station."
   b. "Find the fire extinguisher in front of you."

7. THREE STEP VERBAL INSTRUCTIONS
   Location: Outside room 381
   Procedure: Outside room 369, give verbal instructions:
   a. "Go to the end of the hall."
   b. "Follow the hall around to the left."
   c. "Have a seat on the chairs."

8. FOUR STEP WRITTEN INSTRUCTIONS
   Location: Outside room 350 facing the double-door crossroad
   Procedure: Give written instructions:
   a. "Go down the hall."
   b. "Take the first right turn."
   c. "Go down the carpeted hallway."
   d. "Stop at the second public restroom."

9. FIVE STEP WRITTEN INSTRUCTIONS
   Location: Outside the public restrooms
   Procedure: Give written instructions:
   a. "Walk back down the hall."
   b. "Turn left to the elevators."
   c. "Take the elevator to the ground floor."
   d. "Go down the carpeted hallway."
   e. "Go to the hospital main entrance."

10. MAP READING
    Location: Outside room 381
    Procedure: Give patient a map that leads them to the fire extinguisher, and give the verbal instructions:
    a. "Follow the arrows on the map."

APPENDIX – 3

TRAUMA REHAB DATA SHEET

PT NAME: _____ AKA: _____ DOB/AGE: _____

HOSPITAL NUMBER:_____ DATE OF INJ: _____ DATA OF ADM: _____

RACE:_____ PRIMARY LANGAUGE:_____ ADM SERVICE: _____

DX: _____ CONSULT SERVICES: _____

_____   _____

_____   _____

_____   _____

_____   _____

_____   _____

_____   _____

Initial Neuro Exam:

Pupils: Reactivity _____ Equality _____

GCS: at scene: E ___ M ___ V ___   Hypotensive? _____

       in ER   E ___ M ___ V ___   Hypoxic? _____

       p OR   E ___ M ___ V ___

LOCATION: DATE   UNIT   PRIMARY NURSE

               _____   _____   _____

               _____   _____   _____

               _____   _____   _____

               _____   _____   _____

PROCEDURES/STUDIES/COMPLICATIONS:

    DATE   EXPLANATION

    _____   _____

    _____   _____

    _____   _____

    _____   _____

    _____   _____

    _____   _____

    _____   _____

    _____   _____

    _____   _____

    _____   _____

    _____   _____

    _____   _____

ASSESSMENTS:

DATE:						
PULM:						
NEURO:						
SKIN:						
GI/GU:						
CV:						
OTHER:						

(continued)

APPENDIX – 3 (*Continued*)

NAME OF REHAB RESIDENT: _____

SEEN BY:	**DATE:**	**ISSUES/CONCERNS: (UPDATE FOR CHANGES ONLY)**

REHAB MED

P.T.

O.T.

NUTRITION

SOCIAL WORK

SPEECH

REHAB PSYCH

RECH TX

VOC TX

(*continued*)

APPENDIX – 3 (*Continued*)

PATIENT HISTORY (SOURCE: _____)

PMH: _____

_____

_____

_____

SIGNIFICANT OTHERS:

NAME	RELATIONSHIP	PHONE NUMBER	SEEN/GIVEN INFO?

PRE-INJURY LIFESTYLE:

LIVING SITUATION: _____

_____

_____

EDUCATIONAL LEVEL: _____

OCCUPATION: _____

SUPPORT SYSTEM: _____

_____

_____

COPING STYLE/BELIEFS: _____

_____

ALCOHOL/DRUGS/CIGS: _____

OTHER: _____

_____

_____

_____

_____

(*continued*)

APPENDIX – 3 (*Continued*)

REHAB READINESS

TRANSFER READINESS:

IDENTIFIED GOALS	
DISCHARGE PLAN	
MEDICAL STABILITY	
ACTIVITY TOLERANCE	
PARTICIPATION IN LEARNING	
FUNDING	

CONDITION ON TRANSFER:

MEDICAL CONCERNS (e.g., suction, O_2):	ADLs:
MOBILITY/LOCOMOTION:	COGNITION/COMMUNICATION:
STRENGTH/ACTIVITY TOLERANCE:	BLADDER/BOWEL:
PT/FAMILY EXPECTATIONS OF REHAB:	COMPLICATIONS (e.g., skin condition, pain control, behavioral issues, language/cultural barriers, addictions)

REHAB NURSING CARE STATUS:

MAXIMUM _____   MODERATE _____   MINIMUM _____

FINAL DISPOSITION:

DISCHARGED TO: _____

RECEIVING PHYSICIAN: _____

IF TO HOME, HAS RECEIVED: OUTPATIENT APPTS: _____

DISCHARGE INSTRUCTIONS: _____

APPROPRIATE REFERRALS: _____

FOLLOW UP PHONE CALL: _____

APPENDIX – 4

REHABILITATION MEDICINE RESIDENT CONSULT NOTE	PAGE 1 OF 2

DATE:	SERVICE REQUESTING CONSULT:

	PAST MEDICAL HISTORY
CC: **HISTORY OF PRESENT ILLNESS:**	DRINKS/DAY ETOH PPD TOBACCO SUBSTANCE USE **MEDICATIONS** **ALLERGIES** (MEDS AND OTHERS; e.g. LATEX)

PERTINENT IMAGING   **PERTINENT LABS**

REVIEW OF SYSTEMS (CIRCLE +)

CONST: WT LOSS, FEVER, APPETITE, SLEEP

EYES: GLASSES, BLURRED, DIPLOPIA

ENT: HEARING, DENTITION, VERTIGO

CV: CP, DOE, HIN, SYNCOPE

RESP: SOB, PNEUMONIA, ASTHMA

GI: N, V, D, C PAIN, BOWEL PROG

GU: RETENTION, INCONT, UTI, SEXUAL DYSFCN, ICP, FOLEY

MSK: FRACTURES, PAIN, SWELLING, TRAUMA

SKIN: RASH, ULCERS

PRIOR FUNCTION	**CURRENT FUNCTION**
Mobility	Mobility
ADLs	ADLs
Cog/Comm	Cog/Comm

NEURO: WEAK, NUMB, ATAXIA, TREMOR, HA

SOCIAL HISTORY

HOME ARCHITECTURE:

___STEP ENTRY, ___ LEVEL HOUSE
STAIRS, RAILING
LAYOUT

SOCIAL SUPPORT:
EDUCATION:
VOCATION:
AVOCATION:

FAMILY HISTORY

PSYCH: DEPRESSION, ANXIETY, LABILITY, PSYCHOSIS

ENDO: THYROID, DM, HRT

HEME/LYMPH: ANEMIA, BRUISING, LYMPH GLANDS

ALL/IMMUN: ITCHING, HIVES, AUTOIMMUNE D/O

PT.NO.

NAME

D.O.B

UW Medicine
Harborview Medical Center – UW Medical Center
University of Washington Physicians
Seattle, Washington
REHABILITATION MEDICINE

Inpatient Resident Consult Note

(continued)

APPENDIX – 4 (*Continued*)

REHABILITATION MEDICINE RESIDENT CONSULT NOTE   PAGE 2 OF 2

PHYSICAL EXAM

VITALS	ABD	**MENTAL STATUS EXAM**
GEN	RECTAL	ORIENTATION ___/10
HEAD	GU	SERIAL 7/3 ___/5
EYES	SKIN	REGISTRATION ___/3
ENT	PASSIVE ROM	RECALL ___/3
NECK	SPINE/JOINTS	NAMING ___/2
CHEST/RESP		REPETITION ___/1
HEART/CV		3 STEP COMMAND ___/3

NEURO EXAM   **REFLEXES**

READING ___/1

CN

TONE   WRITING ___/1

MOTOR   COPY ___/1
   S Ab / EF / WE / EE / FDP / APB / HF / KE / DF / EHL / PF / KF / HF /H Ab

R   TOTAL ___/(30)

L

SENSORY (pin, proprio)   OTHER:

COORDINATION   CLONUS

BALANCE/TRANSFERS/GAIT   HOFFMANS

ASSESSMENT AND RECOMMENDATIONS

RESIDENT PHYSICIAN NAME AND SIGNATURE	PAGER	DATE

PT.NO.

NAME

D.O.B

UW Medicine
Harborview Medical Center – UW Medical Center
University of Washington Physicians
Seattle, Washington
REHABILITATION MEDICINE
Inpatient Resident Consult Note

APPENDIX – 5

BRADEN SCALE FOR PREDICTING PRESSURE SORE RISK

Patient's Name _____   Evaluator's Name _____   Date of Assessment

SENSORY PERCEPTION ability to respond meaningfully to pressure-related discomfort	**1. Completely Limited** Unresponsive (does not moan, flinch, or grasp) to painful stimuli, due to diminished level of consciousness or sedation. OR limited ability to feel pain over most of body.	**2. Very Limited** Responds only to painful stimuli. Cannot communicate discomfort except by moaning or restlessness OR has a sensory impairment which limits the ability to feel pain or discomfort over ½ of body.	**3. Slightly Limited** Responds to verbal commands, but cannot always communicate discomfort or the need to be turned. OR has some sensory impairment which limits ability to feel pain or discomfort in 1 or 2 extremities.	**4. No Impairment** Responds to verbal commands. Has no sensory deficit which would limit ability to feel or voice pain or discomfort.
MOISTURE degree to which skin is exposed to moisture	**1. Constantly Moist** Skin is kept moist almost constantly by perspiration, urine, etc. Dampness is detected every time patient is moved or turned.	**2. Very Moist** Skin is often, but not always moist. Linen must be changed at least once a shift.	**3. Occasionally Moist:** Skin is occasionally moist, requiring an extra linen change approximately once a day.	**4. Rarely Moist** Skin is usually dry, linen only requires changing at routine intervals.
ACTIVITY degree of physical activity	**1. Bedfast** Confined to bed.	**2. Chairfast** Ability to walk severely limited or non-existent. Cannot bear own weight and/or must be assisted into chair or wheelchair.	**3. Walks Occasionally** Walks occasionally during day, but for very short distances, with or without assistance. Spends majority of each shift in bed or chair.	**4. Walks Frequently** Walks outside room at least twice a day and inside room at least once every two hours during waking hours.
MOBILITY ability to change and control body position	**1. Completely Immobile** Does not make even slight changes in body or extremity position without assistance.	**2. Very Limited** Makes occasional slight changes in body or extremity position but unable to make frequent or significant changes independently.	**3. Slightly Limited** Makes frequent though slight changes in body or extremity position independently.	**4. No Limitation** Makes major and frequent changes in position without assistance.
NUTRITION usual food intake pattern	**1. Very Poor** Never eats a complete meal. Rarely eats more than ⅓ of any food offered. Eats 2 servings or less of protein (meat or dairy products) per day. Takes fluids poorly. Does not take a liquid dietary supplement OR is NPO and/or maintained on clear liquids or IV's for more than 5 days.	**2. Probably Inadequate** Rarely eats a complete meal and generally eats only about ½ of any food offered. Protein intake includes only 3 servings of meat or dairy products per day. Occasionally will take a dietary supplement. OR receives less than optimum amount of liquid diet or tube feeding.	**3. Adequate** Eats over half of most meals. Eats a total of 4 servings of protein (meat, dairy products) per day. Occasionally will refuse a meal, but will usually take a supplement when offered OR is on a tube feeding or TPN regimen which probably meets most of nutritional needs.	**4. Excellent** Eats most of every meal. Never refuses a meal. Usually eats a total of 4 or more servings of meat and dairy products. Occasionally eats between meals. Does not require supplementation.
FRICTION & SHEAR	**1. Problem** Requires moderate to maximum assistance in moving. Complete lifting without sliding against sheets is impossible. Frequently slides down in bed or chair, requiring frequent repositioning with maximum assistance. Spasticity, contractures or agitation leads to almost constant friction.	**2. Potential Problem** Moves feebly or requires minimum assistance. During a move skin probably slides to some extent against sheets, chair, restraints or other devices. Maintains relatively good position in chair or bed most of the time but occasionally slides down.	**3. No Apparent Problem** Moves in bed and in chair independently and has sufficient muscle strength to lift up completely during move. Maintains good position in bed or chair.	

Total Score

From Bergstrom N, Braden BJ, Laguzza A, et al. The Barden Scale for predicting pressure sore risk. *Nurse Res.* 1987;36:205–210, with permission.

APPENDIX – 6

1. ☐ COLACE 250 mg PO BID or

   ☐ 100 mg PO BID

2. ☐ METAMUCIL 1 pkg PO BID or

   ☐ PRN

3. ☐ MILK OF MAGNESIA 30 – 60 cc PO BID PRN

   ☐ MILK OF MAGNESIA 30 – 60 cc PO HS PRN

4. ☐ DULCOLAX suppository 1 PR q day PRN constipation

   * For spinal cord injury patients:

   ☐ DULCOLAX suppository 1 PR q A.M. with digital stimulation q 15 minutes after insertion X 3 – 4 times

5. ☐ FLEETS ENEMA 1 PR q day PRN; may repeat X 1 if no results or

   ☐ other enema choice (specify): _____

   * For spinal cord injury patients: Enemas are avoided due to potential autonomic dysreflexia.

6. ☐ HIGH FIBER DIET

PHYSICIAN SIGNATURE	TIME	DATE

PT.NO.

NAME

D.O.B.

UNIVERSITY OF WASHINGTON MEDICAL CENTERS
HARBORVIEW MEDICAL CENTER – UW MEDICAL CENTER
SEATTLE, WASHINGTON
ADULT BOWEL PROGRAM
STANDING PHYSICIAN ORDERS

APPENDIX – 7

Physician Orders for Alcohol Withdrawal
MD: Check boxes, fill in where applicable or delete orders which are N/A

Assessment:

☑ Ask patient and document about previous ETOH withdrawal, seizures, severity/duration of withdrawal, history of known DT's, and date/time of last drink.

☑ Using CIWA tool, assess severity of alcohol withdrawal on admission.

☑ Perform CIWA score: q 30 minutes until CIWA is <20; q 2 hours if CIWA is 10–20, and q 4 hours if score is <10 and patient is awake. Also perform CIWA 30 minutes after each dose of medication.

☑ Discontinue assessments if CIWA scores are: <10 without medication x 24 hours. Restart scoring and protocol if any symptoms reappear.

☑ Notify HO if CIWA score continues to increase, does not decrease or is >20. Also notify HO if patient becomes oversedated.

Medications:

Administer medication according to the following table. Hold medication if patient is excessively sedated. (MD: check desired medication.)

	☐ **Lorazepam*** (Ativan)	☐ **Diazepam**** (Valium)
If score is >20	Call HO	Call HO
If score is 16–20	Lorazepam 2 mg IV q 4 hours	Diazepam 10 mg IV q 4 hours
If score is 10–15	Lorazepam 1 mg IV/PO q 4 hours	Diazepam 5 mg IV/PO q 4 hours
If score is <10	Lorazepam 1 mg PO q 4 hours PRN	Diazepam 5 mg PO q 4 hours PRN
PRN If breakthrough symptoms occur between scheduled doses give:	Lorazepam 1–2 mg IV/PO PRN q 1 hour *Prior to IV administration, dilute with equal volume diluent, do not exceed rate of 2mg/min.	Diazepam 5–10mg IV/PO PRN q 1 hour **Administer IV into large vein, do not exceed 5mg (1ml)/min.

Patients with known seizures due to alcohol withdrawal should be placed on a fixed schedule X 3 days:

☐ Chlordiazepoxide (Librium) 50 mg PO q 6 hours x 24 hours, then Librium 25 mg PO q 6 hours x 48 hours

☐ Other fixed schedule: _____.

☑ Thiamine 100mg IV/PO daily x 3 days

☑ Multivitamin with Folate 1mg PO/IV daily

☑ Administer Pneumococcal Vaccine 0.5cc IM prior to discharge, if documentation (review Mindscape immunization tab) of prior immunization within 5 years is unavailable. (Best given when afebrile, if possible.)

Labs/IV fluids:

☑ Minipanel, magnesium, and phosphate levels daily x 3

Other:_____.

IV Fluids:_____, add _____ grams MgSO4 per liter x 1 liter

Nursing Care:
(8mEq = 1 gram MgSO4)

☑ Provide calm, quiet, supportive environment. If patient is hallucinating, keep room softly, but well lit.

☑ Refer to social worker if patient expresses interest in alcohol dependency treatment.

MD Signature	Date/Time	RN Signature	Date Time

PT.NO. NAME D.O.B.	**UNIVERSITY OF WASHINGTON MEDICAL CENTERS** HARBORVIEW MEDICAL CENTER - UW MEDICAL CENTER SEATTLE, WASHINGTON **PHYSICIAN ORDERS** **ALCOHOL WITHDRAWAL ORDERS**

(continued)

APPENDIX – 7 (*Continued*)
CIWA: Clinical Indicators and Withdrawal Assessment

Nausea/Vomiting: *Ask about nausea/vomiting*

0   no nausea/vomiting
1   mild nausea with no vomiting
2
3   nausea and vomiting – occasional
4   intermittent nausea with dry heaves
5
6   constant extreme nausea, frequent vomiting/dry heaves

Tremor: *To assess, touch your fingertips to patient's fingertips*

Also assess with arms extended and fingers spread apart.

0   no tremor
1   non *visible*—can be *felt* fingertip to fingertip
2
3   mild visible tremor
4   moderate, with patient's arms extended
5
6   severe tremor when extended
7   severe, even with arms not extended

Paroxysmal sweats: *Observation*

0   no sweat visible
1   barely perceptible sweating, palms moist
2   forehead damp
3
4   beads of sweat obvious on forehead
5
6
7   drenching sweats

Anxiety: *Ask: "Do you feel nervous or edgy?"* *Observation*

0   no anxiety, at ease
1
2   mildly anxious
3
4   moderately anxious or guarded
5
6
7   extremely anxious—equivalent to acute pain state

Agitation: *Agitation persists although reassurance/support offered. Observation*

1   normal activity
2   somewhat more than normal activity
3
4   moderately fidgety or restless
5   agitated
6   very agitated
7   pacing back and forth most of the time, or constantly thrashing about

*Use this tool with the "Physician Orders for Alcohol Withdrawal." Assess as directed per the order sheet.

CIWA scale is located on CIS, and score will be calculated.

Tactile Disturbances: *Ask: "Have you any unusual sensation (i.e. itching, pins/needles, burning, numbness)? Do you feel bugs crawling on or under your skin?"*

0   none
1   very mild itching, pins/needles, burning
2
3   moderate itching, pins/needles, burning, numbness
4   tactile hallucinations or may misinterpret sensations
5   severe hallucinations
6
7   continuous tactile hallucinations

Auditory Disturbances: *Ask: "Are you more aware of sounds? Do they startle you or sound harsh? Are you hearing anything that disturbs or frightens you? Are you hearing things you know are not there?" Observation*

0   not present
1   very mild harshness or ability to frighten
2   mild sensitivity
3   moderate harshness or ability to frighten
4   moderately severe
5   severe hallucinations
6   extremely severe hallucinations
7   continuous auditory hallucinations

Visual Disturbances: *Ask: "Does the light seem too bright or hurt your eyes? Is the color different? Are you seeing anything that you know is not there?" Observation*

0   not present
1   very mild sensitivity
2   mild sensitivity
3   moderate sensitivity
4   moderately severe hallucinations or misinterprets visual images
5   severe hallucinations (sees something that is not there)
6   extremely severe hallucinations
7   continuous hallucinations

Headache, Fullness in the Head: *Ask: "Does your head feel different? Does it feel like there is a band around your head or other unusual sensation?"* (Do not rate dizziness.)

0   not present
1   very mild
2   mild
3   moderate
4   moderately severe
5   severe
6   very severe
7   extremely severe

Orientation/Clouding of Sensorium: *Ask: "What day is this? Where are you? Who am I?"*

0   orientated and can do serial additions
1   cannot do serial additions or is unsure of the date
2   disoriented to date, by not more than 2 calendar days
3   disoriented to date by more than 2 calendar days
4   disoriented to place and/or person

Autonomic hyperdynamic state: Assess also for indication of ↑ temperature, ↑ pulse, ↑ BP, ↑ respiratory rate

5

Multiple Musculoskeletal Trauma

David B. Weiss

With the increase in high-velocity "extreme" sports and activities, as well as the overall increase in the number of automobiles on the road and higher average speeds, the incidence of accidents causing musculoskeletal injuries is on the rise. It is estimated that trauma is the leading cause of death and disability in the United States in individuals from ages 0 to 44 years and overall accounts for $260 billion in direct costs of mortality and morbidity and lost work time (1). Musculoskeletal injuries represent more than 45% of inpatient rehabilitation admissions in the United States (see Chapter 2). Most high-velocity injuries (so-called blunt trauma) result from motor vehicle or motorcycle accidents (MVAs), pedestrians struck by automobiles, or falls from a height. Other causes include industrial accidents, which can involve crushing type injuries (i.e., those in which individuals are caught between a vehicle and a solid object or under falling items or in heavy mechanical equipment) or, less frequently (at least in the civilian population), injuries from blasts. Gunshot wounds or other penetrating-type trauma may cause massive injury (depending on range and type of projectile); however, such injuries frequently are limited to a localized area and less likely to involve multiple extremities.

Musculoskeletal injuries can be divided into two phases: acute and chronic. The acute phase involves the medical evaluation and resuscitation of the patient. Frequently surgery is required to repair injured areas and to stabilize the patient and observe for further problems, often with a short stay in the intensive care unit (ICU). During the acute phase, opportunities for rehabilitation may be limited due to the patient's unstable medical condition but can still play an important role in speeding the recovery and preventing complications as a result of immobility. The chronic phase involves the period after the patient is medically stable but requires significant rehabilitation and therapy services to regain functional capacity and, hopefully, to return to being a productive member of society.

ORTHOPAEDIC INJURIES

Any discussion of injury should be preceded by a brief review of anatomy to ensure that we are all speaking the same language. The bony skeleton serves to provide a structural framework and insertion points for tendons and ligaments. In general, there are two types of bones: cortical and cancellous. Cortical bone is dense and highly mineralized and makes up the shaft section of long bones. It is present in a thinner layer at the ends of long bones and around certain specialized bones such as the calcaneus (cortical shell) and forms the outer and inner wall of the pelvis. Cancellous bone is softer and less structurally solid and contains better blood supply and higher numbers of bony cells. It is present around the joint area (periarticular) at the ends of long bones and in between the walls of the pelvis. Inside the joints there is a smooth, articular cartilage lining the ends of the long bones, allowing almost friction-free interaction at the joint.

Cortical bone can withstand higher compressive and bending forces than cancellous bone. When it breaks, cortical bone frequently has relatively clean fracture lines (although in very high-energy injuries it can splinter and become comminuted). Cancellous bone is more likely to suffer crush or impaction type injuries, and this type of injury can affect future joint function if the cartilaginous surface of the joint is not restored to near normal alignment (2).

The relative availability of blood supply to bones becomes important when determining options for fixation and trying to predict the likelihood that certain fractures will heal. Cortical bone receives primarily an endosteal blood supply (from within the medullary canal); however, when this type of bone is fractured, the overlying periosteal blood supply significantly increases to provide healing factors to the zone of injury. If the periosteum has been injured during the traumatic event (or from the subsequent surgery) the healing will be slower and may not take place, leading to delayed union or nonunion. This situation can significantly delay the functional recovery and will often lead to more surgery to attempt to stimulate healing. Cancellous bone, on the other hand, has a richer blood supply from the medullary artery and is less dependent on the periosteal supply after an injury.

Bone healing can proceed by one of two methods. Primary bone healing occurs when there is direct contact between the two injured bone segments and there is rigid immobilization. Osteons (microscopic units of bone formation with haversian canals and surrounding lamellae) cross between the two segments and re-establish the normal bony architecture. This healing method typically occurs with plate and screw fixation (in simple fracture patterns). Secondary healing occurs when there is micromotion between the fracture fragments and a callus forms around the bone ends to help stabilize them and provide a source of healing factors. This method occurs with casting, bracing, and intramedullary devices (3).

Muscles are attached to bones by tendons. This musculotendinous junction is the weakest part of the construct and hence is the area most likely to be injured in a "muscle strain." Ligaments attach bones to bones—often around joints. Ligaments are susceptible to being stretched (grade 1 sprain), torn mid-substance (grade 2 sprain) or avulsed from their bony attachment—often with a small fragment of bone (grade 3 sprain).

Depending on the location of the injury and the mechanism involved, bones, muscles, tendons, ligaments, or any combination may be injured. The involvement of these various structures has implications for rehabilitation and therapy, as weight bearing, range of motion (ROM), or both may be restricted during the early healing phases. Prolonged immobility can produce fibrosis and contracture, so these competing forces must be appropriately balanced.

METHODS OF FIXATION

The modern orthopaedic surgeon has a wide armamentarium of tools and techniques for treating fractures, each with its benefits and downsides. There is rarely a single accepted technique for a given injury and many factors must be accounted for, including age and activity level of the patient, medical comorbidities, social issues, quality of bone, and presence of tumor or infection. The overall goals, regardless of which technique is chosen, are to stabilize the fracture, repair or stabilize other structures as necessary, provide pain relief, prevent future functional problems, and allow for early mobilization of the patient to prevent further complications.

CASTING

Ancient Egyptian remains have shown evidence of wooden splints applied to heal fractures with successful results. Egyptian texts from the 9th and 10th centuries discuss plaster cast application, and this technique has stood the test of time (4). Modern casting techniques use strong, lighter-weight fiberglass casting tape. This type of cast is often the treatment of choice for fractures in children, because they have excellent healing and remodeling potential. While it is acceptable to treat a number of stable adult fractures in casts, this method has several downsides. Casts provide only relative stability and are not a good choice for unstable fracture patterns. They do not allow for early mobilization, and in a patient with multiple fractures, this immobility can significantly delay any chance at functional rehabilitation. They block the skin and soft tissues, are relatively heavy, and are often not well tolerated. Currently, in multiply injured patients, casts are primarily used to provide temporary immobilization until more definitive fixation can be done, and to provide temporary protection of a surgically repaired area that needs time to consolidate and become strong enough to withstand exercise and/or weight bearing. Typically, patients treated in casts are allowed limited or no weight bearing on that extremity for at least 4 weeks and often longer.

FUNCTIONAL BRACING

Functional bracing is a good alternative to casting because it provides some stability to the injured

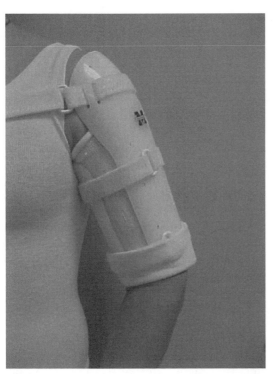

Figure 5–1. Humeral Sarmiento fracture brace.

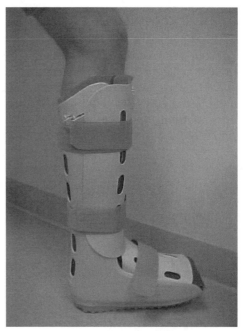

Figure 5–3. Cast boot.

area but frequently allows motion at the adjacent joints. The braces can be removed for hygiene or to evaluate the skin and soft tissues and are lighter and better tolerated than casts. They are most useful in isolated extremity injuries where surgery is not warranted, or in the subacute phase after surgical repair to provide some additional protection to the area while still allowing functional rehabilitation to begin. Examples of functional braces include Sarmiento braces for humerus (Fig. 5–1) or tibia fractures (Fig. 5–2), cast boots for ankle and foot injuries (Fig. 5–3) and Range of Motion knee braces (Fig. 5–4) for distal femur/knee and proximal tibia injuries (5,6). Weight bearing may be allowed with functional braces and range of motion is typically encouraged, although there may be limits set. Custom functional braces are also used for specific regions and injuries; however, discussion of these would necessitate a chapter unto itself.

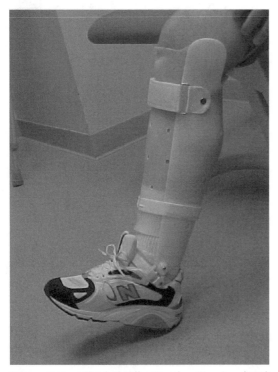

Figure 5–2. Tibial Patellar Tendon Bearing (PTB) Sarmiento fracture brace.

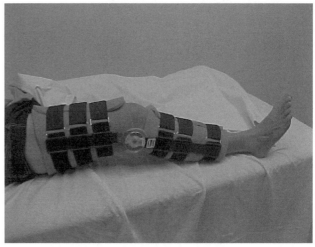

Figure 5–4. Range of Motion knee brace.

EXTERNAL FIXATION

External fixation consists of a series of pins or wires inserted through the skin and into bones and attached to bars or rings. There are two primary uses: temporary and definitive treatment. Temporary external fixation is typically applied when the injury pattern and/or the patient's medical condition does not allow for a more definitive fixation to occur within a few days from injury (Fig. 5–5). Factors that may warrant this type of fixation include soft tissue swelling, damage to the skin or underlying muscle, and the location of the injury (distal tibia fractures almost always get temporary external fixation to avoid soft

tissue complications in the first 1 to 3 weeks after injury) (7). Treatment external fixation may be indicated when the injury pattern or the patient's overall condition does not allow a more involved surgery to place internal fixation, or when it is the surgeon's preference for certain types of fractures (8). There are also external fixators used for lengthening of short bones and correction of deformity using a technique known as the Ilizarov method (also known as distraction osteogenesis).

Regardless of whether the fixator is on for the short or long term, it is always important to evaluate the sites where the pins enter the skin, because the most frequent complication of external fixators is infection. These infections are typically local and may be treated with oral antibiotics; however, they can progress to become deeper abscesses or osteomyelitis and may compromise additional procedures in that region. For this reason, temporary external fixation often spans the area of injury, frequently immobilizing at least one adjacent joint, to avoid putting pins into a region where internal hardware will go later. Treatment external fixation places pins or wires near the fracture site for additional stability, and the goal is to avoid immobilizing any adjacent

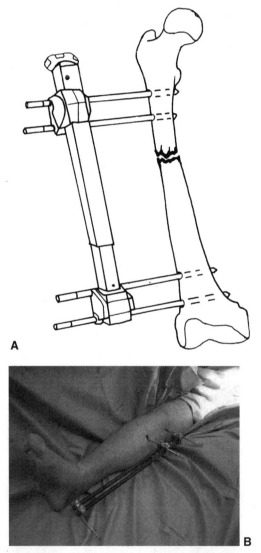

Figure 5–5. A: Drawing of fixator spanning femur fracture. (From Hoppenfeld S, Murthy V, eds. *Treatment and rehabilitation of fractures.* Philadelphia: Lippincott Williams & Wilkins; 2000, with permission.) **B:** Temporary external fixator for tibial pilon fracture spanning the ankle.

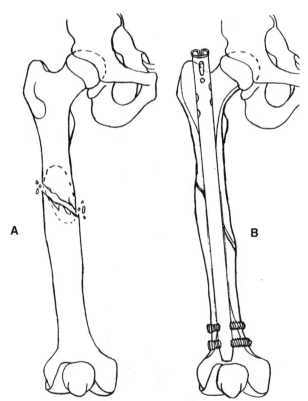

Figure 5–6. A,B: Midshaft femoral fracture before and after femoral nail insertion. (From Hoppenfeld S, Murthy V, eds. *Treatment and rehabilitation of fractures.* Philadelphia: Lippincott Williams & Wilkins; 2000, with permission.)

joints. Patients or family members are taught basic care of the pin sites, and their efforts will often significantly decrease the risk and severity of the pin infections. Occasionally pins will need to be changed to a different site or removed prematurely. Weight bearing is usually prohibited for temporary external fixators, but is often encouraged for treatment external fixators (if not immediately after placement then within a few weeks). Pelvic external fixators are an exception to this rule, as they are often used to stabilize anterior pelvic ring injuries and will allow for sitting and mobilization but not typically weight bearing (on the affected side).

INTRAMEDULLARY FIXATION

Also known as "rods" or "nails," intramedullary (IM) devices are placed down the shaft of long bones to stabilize fractures. They will typically be placed through small incisions around the hip or knee for femur and tibia and around the shoulder, elbow, or wrist for humerus and forearm fractures. By far the most common use is in the femur (Figs. 5–6 and 5–7) and tibia (Fig. 5–8). IM nails are load-sharing devices and typically allow at least limited weight bearing (depending on the fracture pattern) soon after surgery. Because they utilize small incisions,

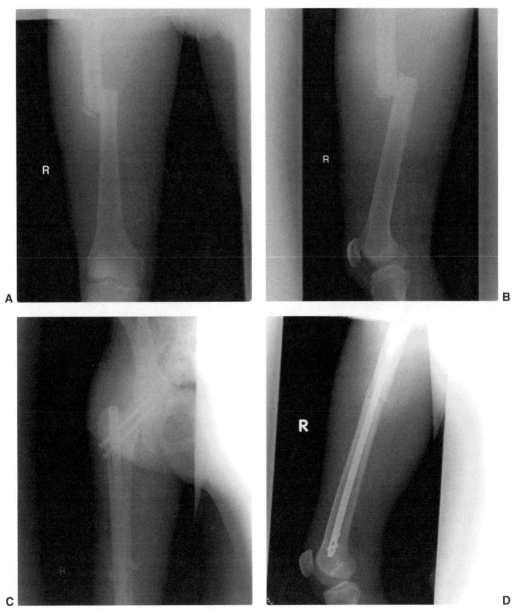

Figure 5–7. A–D: AP and lateral x-rays of midshaft segmental femur fracture before and after fixation with intramedullary nail.

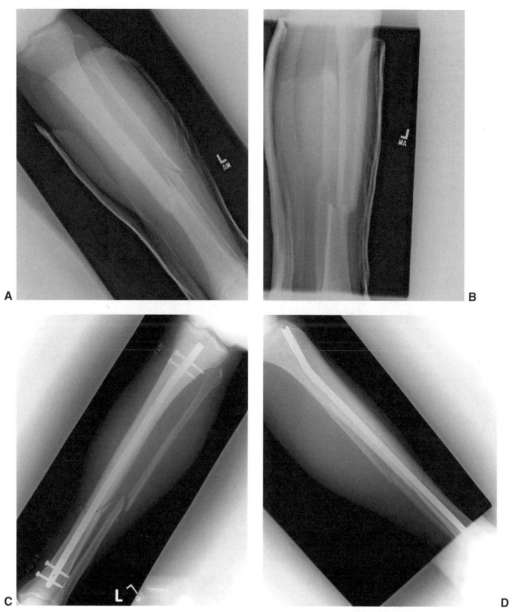

Figure 5–8. A–D: AP and lateral x-rays of tibial fracture before and after fixation with an intramedullary nail.

the more prolonged recovery period associated with large, extensive exposures is avoided and early rehabilitation is encouraged.

The most common complication of these devices is pain around the entry site, typically hip or knee pain. For tibial IM nails, studies have shown that between ~50% and 60% of patients complain of anterior knee pain regardless of the type of nail used or the surgical approach (9,10). This pain will typically subside by 1 year after surgery in many patients, but others will require nail removal for pain relief (10). With femoral nails, patients may complain of hip or knee pain. Femoral nails may

be inserted through the hip (antegrade) or the knee (retrograde); however, regardless of insertion site patients may complain of pain at the opposite end of the nail. The reason for this pain is unclear (assuming the nail is in good position and was inserted without complication). While many causes have been proposed, none have yet been confirmed (11).

IM nails typically have cross-locking screws at the top and bottom ends to provide rotational stability at the fracture site. These cross locks may be prominent or cause local irritation from the movement of tendons and muscles over their heads or tips. It is not uncommon to have to remove these cross locks once the fracture has healed because of local irritation. The nails themselves can usually stay in but on occasion patients who experience pain from them will request their removal. Removal typically requires a short period of protected weight bearing (2 to 6 weeks) postoperatively to allow the holes in the cortex to fill in and decrease the chance of refracture from minor trauma.

PLATE/SCREW CONSTRUCTS

Plate/screw constructs are one of the most common forms of operative treatment of fractures, particularly in periarticular regions. Recently, there has been an increase in the variety of specialized plates and screws designed specifically for a particular region and fracture type. There has also been an increase in interest in using smaller incisions to place these plates to avoid damaging the blood supply, which can disturb biologic healing at the fracture site. Depending on the fracture type and location, plates may be placed to provide rigid fixation by compressing the fracture fragments or be placed in a buttress or neutralization mode in which the plate may just hold the fragments in position but not provide rigid stabilization. Plates that provide rigid compression are commonly used in the forearm (Figs. 5–9 and 5–10) and humerus and may allow early range of motion and weight bearing. This approach can be particularly useful in polytrauma patients because it enables them to use their arms to walk with crutches and thus avoid being wheelchair-bound. Buttress-style plates are used in the periarticular regions and in the distal fibula for ankle fractures. Although these plates often do not allow immediate weight bearing, they are stable enough to permit a range of motion exercises to begin.

JOINT REPLACEMENTS (FOR TRAUMA)

On occasion, a fracture in a knee, hip, elbow, or shoulder region will be so severe that it is impossible to reconstruct and will necessitate a joint replacement. While these replacements are very successful and have an excellent track record when performed for arthritis, they can be problematic when performed for fracture. With fractures, associated soft tissue injuries or loss of bony landmarks make the replacement a more difficult surgery to perform, and outcomes are often less successful. These implants may be placed with additional fixation, such as cement or bone graft struts, and may have additional constraints built into them to make up for

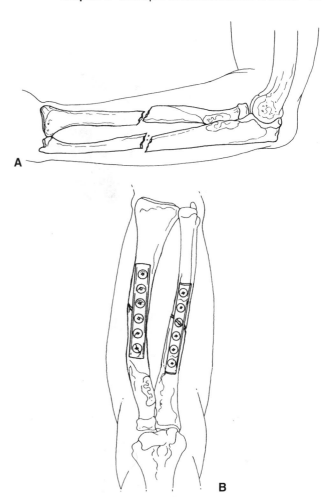

Figure 5–9. A,B: Drawing of radius fracture before and after plate and screw fixation. (From Hoppenfeld S, Murthy V, eds. *Treatment and rehabilitation of fractures.* Philadelphia: Lippincott Williams & Wilkins; 2000, with permission.)

the loss of normal surrounding bone or soft tissue. As such, the final range of motion may be less than otherwise anticipated and the rehabilitation associated with these surgeries may proceed at a slower pace than usual. Typically, range of motion exercises are encouraged as soon as possible after surgery; however, there may be limits on how aggressive the exercises should be. In the case of hip or knee replacement, there may be limited weight bearing to allow associated injuries to heal or for other fractures to consolidate before weight bearing. Regarding elbow and shoulder arthroplasty, motion is typically started immediately postoperatively, but weight bearing is limited for at least 6 weeks. These issues are usually handled on a case-by-case basis, and good communication between the physician and the rehabilitation team is essential.

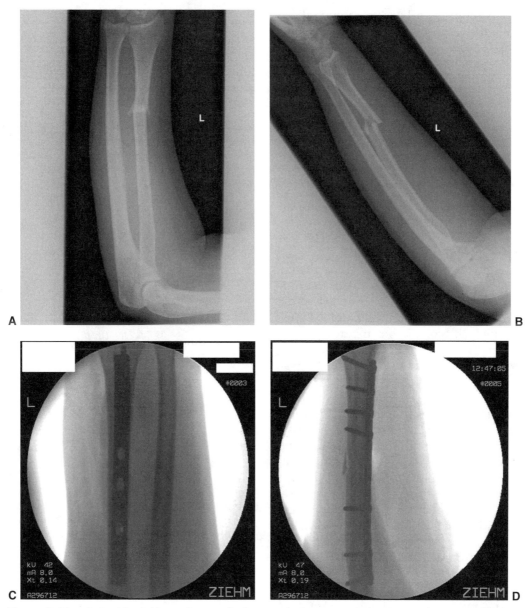

Figure 5–10. A–D: AP and lateral x-rays before and after open reduction and internal fixation of a radius fracture.

TRACTION

While traction used to be a mainstay of treatment for lower extremity (particularly femur) fractures, its use today is almost always temporary and serves to provide support to the surrounding soft tissue and prevent shortening and soft tissue contractures until more definitive surgery may be performed. Femoral and pelvic/acetabular fractures are the types that most commonly require temporary traction. However, if the patient has other comorbidities that might prevent surgery for an extended length of time, traction may be used for treatment for a period typically lasting approximately 6 weeks, after which a cast or brace may need to be applied for an additional 6 weeks.

There are significant downsides to traction. The patient is essentially bedridden during the 6-week period and at increased risk for developing pneumonia, deep venous thrombosis (DVT) and pressure sores, and requires a significant amount of nursing or family assistance. There must also be close follow-up during the first few weeks to ensure that the amount of traction is appropriate and that it is holding the fracture fragments in reasonable alignment. The traction pin sites must also be followed closely and kept clean. If a patient has an isolated injury and can follow commands, physical therapy can be initiated on their other extremities to try and prevent atrophy; however, the injured extremity often must be left alone (except for using ankle pumps and performing ROM exercises) until the traction is discontinued.

GERIATRIC PATIENTS— SPECIAL NEEDS

As the population ages but remains active, it is harder to define what constitutes a geriatric patient. Age >75 years is probably a reasonable indicator; however, there are certainly individuals >75 who are physiologically younger and can be treated as such. There are also 60-year-olds who are physiologically closer to 80-year-olds and should also be treated as such. For the most part, geriatric patients tend to have more medical comorbidities and have a greater risk of complications from surgical interventions, as well as increased risk of mortality from their injuries even many months later. Several studies have shown that a hip fracture in an elderly person leads to only a 50% chance of recovering pre-injury independent activities of daily living and is associated with a threefold increase in mortality if comorbidities are present (12–14). This result is less from the specific injury than from the associated complications that may develop. With less physiologic reserve, even minor postoperative or postinjury complications can have a major impact. As an example, geriatric patients may be less able to protect their weight bearing on an injured extremity because they cannot use crutches or a walker as a result of decreased upper extremity strength and/or balance problems. This situation may lead to their being bedridden or wheelchair-bound, increasing the risk of DVT or pulmonary embolism (PE) or pneumonia. They may also be more affected by postoperative pain medications that can cause temporary delirium and difficulties with balance and walking, which can delay mobilization and rehabilitation. They are also more likely to be osteopenic or have osteoporosis that can affect the overall stability of the repair and put them at risk for additional fractures from relatively minor trauma. Distal radius fractures, spinal compression fractures, and femoral neck fractures in the geriatric population are considered "sentinel events" and appropriate work-up for osteoporosis should be undertaken after these events if the patient has not had one already.

OTHER MEDICAL COMORBIDITIES

While the elderly are more at risk for medical comorbidities, younger patients may have them also, and these may affect the type of treatment for a particular injury, as well as the expected length of time for recovery and the appropriate rehabilitative plan. Diabetes is becoming more prevalent in the adult population and is thought to be linked to rising levels of obesity and increased sedentary behavior. Although a multitude of complications can occur with diabetes, the microvascular disease, which effectively reduces blood flow to healing fracture sites, and polyneuropathy, which causes decreased sensation in the hands and feet and thus decreases protective sensation, are the two biggest impediments to healing. Diabetic patients are often treated more conservatively, are at higher risk for perioperative complications, and need to have their weight bearing protected for significantly longer periods of time. These factors of course also significantly delay functional rehabilitation and return to pre-injury status.

Obesity itself can be a complicating factor in fracture care—particularly in the morbidly obese patient (defined as Body Mass Index [BMI] >40 kg per m^2). Operative treatment of these patients is often more difficult as a result of their obesity, and they are typically more difficult to mobilize after surgery, requiring longer periods in bed or a wheelchair versus ambulating. These factors put them at a higher risk of perioperative complications and also delay their functional recovery. Coronary artery disease and peripheral vascular disease are other commonly encountered comorbidities and can increase perioperative risk and delay functional recovery unless well controlled prior to surgery. Close communication between the orthopaedic surgeon and the appropriate consulting specialist is therefore required to maximize pre-operative function and minimize perioperative risk as well as allow earlier rehabilitation to begin.

POLYTRAUMA PATIENTS— SPECIAL NEEDS

The polytraumatized patient frequently has at least two long bone injuries (or long bone and pelvis/acetabulum) along with abdominal chest and/or head injuries. Because of the nature of their injuries, such patients often require a stay in the ICU and may require several surgical procedures over days or weeks to fully address their injuries in a timely but safe manner. While in the ICU, they may be intubated or unable to follow commands, and beginning appropriate rehabilitation may be difficult. At the same time, they are also at risk for atrophy in all muscle groups from a combination of inactivity and the increased catabolic rate as their body tries to heal all their injuries. Thus, proper nutritional support and appropriate positioning aids and range of motion exercises to prevent contractures can be very helpful in minimizing any long-term consequences from a prolonged ICU stay. Close communication with the physical and occupational therapists will allow early intervention to prevent these consequences.

Once polytrauma patients have recovered from their initial injury and subsequent surgeries, they may be very limited in their mobility and may have significant weight-bearing restrictions on multiple extremities or be immobilized so that not even range of motion exercises can begin. While there is often some form of physical therapy that can occur, these patients may need placement in a skilled nursing facility (SNF) to allow some healing to occur prior to being able to participate in a more aggressive rehabilitation program. They may also have significant atrophy and/or impaired nutritional status and thus initial rehabilitation goals may need to be scaled back to take this into account. Increased nutritional intake in the form of high-protein/high-calorie meals and nutritional supplements should also be considered.

Polytrauma patients who have suffered a traumatic brain injury (TBI) can be particularly challenging with respect to early rehabilitation. In the acute phase after their injury, they are likely to be intubated or very confused. Depending on the severity of the injury, they may then recover somewhat but still have difficulty with more complex tasks and especially with short-term memory. The situation can be particularly difficult when weight-bearing restrictions or precautions for range of motion have been imposed, because patients may attempt to get out of bed without assistance or quickly forget recently learned techniques such as walking with a walker or crutches or mastering posterior hip precautions. TBI has also been associated with the rapid formation of heterotopic ossification (HO), whereby injured muscle and soft tissue are ossified into bone as the body attempts to heal the damaged area with something stronger. This process can have a debilitating effect on range of motion when it occurs in periarticular areas and may require surgery to remove the ossified tissue, which in itself can cause trauma and stimulate more HO. Indomethacin and radiation therapy are two techniques to prophylax against HO, but they are not widely used. Close follow-up and observation is the current recommendation for detection of HO (15).

CONTINUOUS PASSIVE MOTION

Continuous Passive Motion (CPM) is a technique used after repair of some periarticular fractures, including those of the tibial plateau and acetabulum. A CPM machine is attached to the affected extremity and essentially provides passive range of motion over preset limits that can be increased over time. The theory is that the motion will help reshape damaged cartilage into a smooth, congruent configuration and help prevent contracture by stretching the surrounding soft tissue (16). Routine use is somewhat controversial, and it should not be initiated if there is any question of surgical wound or overlying soft tissue stability. Because of the increased risk of infection and/or wound breakdown in these situations, the extremity is typically immobilized until the wounds/soft tissues show signs of healing. Motion exercises are then initiated.

COMPARTMENT SYNDROME

Compartment syndrome can occur in both high- and low-energy trauma and is most commonly seen in tibia fractures, although it may occur in any extremity. Crush injuries with massive soft tissue damage or injuries with prolonged ischemia times from vascular damage are at particular risk for this syndrome. Areas within the various extremities are divided into muscular compartments (separated by functional muscle groups) that are enclosed by a tight fascial layer. Essentially, bleeding into the injured compartment causes pressure within the compartment to rise, eventually cutting off the incoming blood flow and causing local hypoxia. If prolonged for >6 to 8 hours, significant muscle and peripheral nerve damage can occur with devastating consequences. Treatment of compartment syndrome requires immediate surgery to release the tight overlying fascia and relieve the pressure. The incisions are left open for several days to allow the underlying swelling to decrease, and then the wounds are closed or skin grafted (17). Extremities treated for compartment syndrome are generally immobilized during the acute phase, and no rehabilitation is begun until after the wounds are closed and the underlying medical condition is stabilized.

GOALS OF REHABILITATION

As soon as the fractures, the associated injuries, and the patient's medical condition have been stabilized, functional rehabilitation should begin as soon as possible. As noted previously, even a patient intubated in the ICU may have early rehabilitation begun through the use of passive range of motion and positioning aids. The goal is to prevent or at least minimize contractures, adhesions, and atrophy and to preserve range of motion in the affected region. These actions will help minimize recovery time in the later stages. Once the patient's condition is improved and his or her fractures have shown evidence of healing, there will be a gradual increase in the allowed activity level and weight bearing.

A typical progression pattern is illustrated in a tibial plateau fracture. Typically for 1 to 2 weeks postoperatively, the patient's knee is immobilized in a cast or splint to allow the wounds to heal. Alternatively, if the soft tissue is not thought to pose a significant risk of breakdown, a CPM machine may be used. After the wounds show they are healing, range of motion and strengthening exercises are begun, as well as crutch/walker training, but the patient is allowed only toe-touch weight bearing. A range of motion brace may be used to help control varus/valgus stability; however, this is typically just for patient comfort and not necessary to support the surgical repair and should not require limitations in flexion/extension. Many fractures show signs of healing after 6 weeks; however, periarticular fractures (such as the tibial plateau) are typically not strong enough to support weight bearing yet, and so restricted weight bearing is maintained for another 6 weeks. Depending on the relative stability of the fracture pattern and repair, weight bearing may be slowly advanced at 6 weeks or it may be 12 weeks from injury before the patient is allowed to weight bear as tolerated. At this point, more aggressive strengthening exercises are begun, because hopefully the range of motion at the knee has been preserved and now strengthening and normal gait are the goals. By 6 to 9 months postinjury the patient should have achieved a return to pre-injury function (or as close as possible); however, benefits from continued exercising can continue for 1 or more years postinjury.

Obviously, patient compliance and motivation play a large role in the recovery timeline, and those with secondary gain issues (such as some workmen's compensation patients) may never return to pre-injury status and may require disability rating and/or vocational retraining. This issue is a subject that requires an entire textbook.

INPATIENT REHABILITATION

When a patient is medically stable, but is not able to be discharged home because of activity restrictions, lack of assistance, or lack of necessary assistive modifications at home, inpatient rehabilitation may be an option. The patient must meet insurance and ability admission criteria such as being able to tolerate 3 hours of therapy per day. Inpatient rehabilitation can often yield multiple benefits by keeping the patient in the hospital environment for consultation if questions arise and allows closer monitoring of

wounds. The patient must be medically stable, requiring only long-term intervention such as finishing a course of IV antibiotics or bladder and bowel function training in the case of spinal or sacral injury.

PRECAUTIONS

On occasion, patients sent to rehabilitation or SNFs or who have been discharged home may have a change in symptoms or the onset of new symptoms that require further evaluation. These symptoms may be initially evaluated by a therapist or other rehabilitation team member.

INCREASE IN PAIN/SWELLING OR ERYTHEMA

Although some pain during rehabilitation is to be expected, acute changes, especially if accompanied by swelling or erythema around the wound site, require further evaluation. These symptoms may be signs of fracture displacement, hardware failure, DVT, or infection. Work-up will typically involve wound evaluation, radiographic evaluation, and possibly blood work to look for infection.

WOUND BREAKDOWN/DRAINAGE/ CHILLS/FEVER/NIGHT SWEATS

These conditions are all hallmarks of possible infection and require wound evaluation, medical evaluation for other possible causes of fever such as pneumonia, and blood work consisting of complete blood count, erythrocyte sedimentation rate (ESR), and C-reactive protein (CRP).

DECREASE IN RANGE OF MOTION

Patients who have been progressing with therapy but who have a sudden decrease in their range of motion require further evaluation, typically with x-rays. This symptom may be evidence of fracture displacement or hardware failure or may be due to soft tissue contracture or development of HO.

SIGNS/SYMPTOMS OF DEEP VENOUS THROMBOSIS OR PULMONARY EMBOLISM

Patents who suffer lower extremity long bone or pelvic trauma are at high risk for developing acute DVT. They will typically be managed with mechanical and chemical prophylaxis while in the hospital, and chemical prophylaxis may be continued for several weeks postoperatively. In spite of this, DVT may develop either while the patient is in the hospital or in a subacute care setting. Acute swelling in a lower extremity, especially if accompanied by calf tenderness and/or erythema, requires further evaluation. This evaluation will typically involve clinical assessment and then duplex Doppler scan to look for presence of acute thrombosis. Signs or symptoms such as tachycardia, shortness of breath, and pleuritic chest pain may be indicative of a PE and require rapid further evaluation, because this may be fatal. Treatment of DVT or PE typically involves anticoagulation therapy for 3 to 6 months.

SIGNS/SYMPTOMS OF REGIONAL COMPLEX PAIN SYNDROME

Previously known as reflex sympathetic dystrophy (RSD), regional complex pain syndrome (RCPS) can occur with major or minor trauma and is thought to be an aberrant response from the sympathetic nervous system in combination with other psychological factors, to set up a "pain circuit" whereby the patient's complaints will be out of proportion to the physical findings or injury. Such patients may complain of significant pain (often described as burning or aching) from just light touch, a sheet, or even the wind blowing on them. In later stages, the skin may undergo trophic and thermal changes and there may be significant disuse atrophy and contractures of the affected extremity. Treatment is multifactorial and is directed at blocking the sympathetic nervous system (typically with injections) using oral agents, such as amitryptaline and gabapentin; psychotherapy; and physical therapy. Use of narcotics should be minimized, If narcotics are used, they should be prescribed by only one person to avoid multiple prescriptions from multiple providers. The therapy should be gentle but persistent, and the patient needs to be encouraged to expect recovery to occur. To prevent disuse atrophy and patterns of avoidance behavior, the patient should also be instructed not to avoid using the affected extremity (18).

CONCLUSIONS

Patients with orthopaedic injuries, particularly if polytraumatized, present difficult challenges in rehabilitation and recovery. This chapter has reviewed some basic orthopaedic injuries and discussed therapeutic options and treatment goals. In today's busy and complex health care environment, the most important issues when dealing with these injuries are communication and teamwork. Since no one individual member of the health care team can do everything necessary for these patients, coordination among all the elements is critical for minimizing time to recovery and producing the best outcomes.

REFERENCES

1. MacKenzie EJ, Fowler CJ. Epidemiology. In: Moore EE, Feliciano DV, Mattox KL, eds. *Trauma*. 5th ed. New York, NY: McGraw-Hill; 2004:22–23.
2. Buckwalter JA, Einhorn TA, Sheldon RS, eds. Form and function of bone. *Orthopaedic basic science*. 2nd ed. Rosemont, IL: AAOS; 2004:319–369.
3. Buckwalter JA, Einhorn TA, Sheldon RS, eds. Bone injury, regeneration and repair. *Orthopaedic basic science*. 2nd ed. Rosemont, IL: AAOS; 2004:371–399.
4. Colton CL. The history of fracture treatment. In: Browner BD, Jupiter JB, Levine AM, et al., eds. *Skeletal trauma*. Philadelphia, PA: WB Saunders;1992:3–9.
5. Sarmiento A, Latta LL. Functional fracture bracing. *J Am Acad Orthop Surg*. 1999;7(1):66–75.
6. Sarmiento A, Zagorski JB, Zych GA, et al. Functional bracing for the treatment of fractures of the humeral diaphysis. *J Bone Joint Surg Am*. 2000;82(4):478–486.
7. Pape HC, Hildebrand F, Pertschy S, et al. Changes in the management of femoral shaft fractures in polytrauma patients: From early total care to damage control orthopaedic surgery. *J Trauma*. 2002;53(3):452–461.
8. French B, Tornetta P III. Hybrid external fixation of tibial pilon fractures. *Foot Ankle Clin*. 2000;5(4):853–871.
9. Schmidt AH, Finkmeier CG, Tornetta P III. Treatment of closed tibial fractures. *Instr Course Lect*. 2003;52:607–622.
10. Court-Brown CM, Gustilo T, Shaw AD. Knee pain after intramedullary tibial nailing: Its incidence, etiology and outcome. *J Orthop Trauma*. 1997;11(2):103–105.
11. Winquist RA. Locked femoral nailing. *J Am Acad Orthop Surg*. 1993;1(2):95–105.
12. Richmond J, Aharonoff GB, Zuckerman JD, et al. Mortality risk after hip fracture. *J Orthop Trauma*. 2003;17(1):53–56.
13. Eisler J, Cornwall R, Strauss E, et al. Outcomes of elderly patients with nondisplaced femoral neck fractures. *J Orthop Trauma*. 2003;17(Suppl 8):S31–S37.
14. Koval KJ, Skovron ML, Aharonoff GB, et al. Predictors of functional recovery after hip fracture in the elderly. *Clin Orthop*. 1998;348:22–28.
15. Pape HC, Marsh S, Morley JR, et al. Current concepts in the development of heterotopic ossification. *J Bone Joint Surg Br*. 2004;86B:783–787.
16. Salter RB. The biologic concept of continuous passive motion of synovial joints. The first 18 years of basic research and its clinical application. *Clin Orthop*. 1989;242:12–25.
17. McQueen MM, Gaston P, Court-Brown CM. Acute compartment syndrome. Who is at risk? *J Bone Joint Surg Br*. 2000;82(2):200–203.
18. Hogan CJ, Hurwitz SR. Treatment of complex regional pain syndrome of the lower extremity. *J Acad Orthop Surg*. 2002;10(4):281–289.

6

Rehabilitation after Traumatic Brain Injury

Kathleen R. Bell, Mary Pepping, and Sureyya Dikmen

Traumatic brain injury (TBI) remains the most common type of central nervous system (CNS) trauma in the United States, estimated to be ten times more common than spinal cord injury (SCI). Although the true frequency of these types of injuries remains unknown because of the problems in identifying and diagnosing their milder forms, surveys indicate that each year >1 million people in the United States are seen in emergency departments with a traumatic brain injury (1). Despite an overall decrease in TBI fatalities, >50,000 people die each year from TBI-related causes (2). Data from a seven-state surveillance program indicate that 22.6% of persons brought to hospitals with TBI die before or during hospital admission (3). The most significant determinants of hospital deaths are related to severity of brain injury and age of the patient (4).

The number of TBI patients admitted to acute care hospitals each year in the United States who survive until discharge is 230,000 (5). Approximately 80,000 to 90,000 persons in the United States are left with long-term disability from these injuries each year (5). However, of those who survived a TBI, only 25% were hospitalized, and 35% were treated in emergency rooms; 14% were treated in clinics and physicians' offices, and 25% did not receive care, indicating they sustained a milder injury (6). The South Carolina TBI Surveillance Program indicated that 86% of all new cases identified from 1996 to 2000 were mild (7).

ESTIMATED COSTS OF TRAUMATIC BRAIN INJURY

The costs associated with TBI can be divided into three components. The estimated costs associated with acute care vary according to the severity of injury. A person with a moderate TBI has an average length of stay of 6.7 days and average hospital costs of $8,189. Persons with severe TBI have a stay of 17.5 days in an acute care medical setting with average associated costs of $33,537 (8). Second, costs for rehabilitation hospitalization have been estimated to be about $46,000 for a median 23-day stay, although not all those injured receive inpatient rehabilitation (9). Lastly, there are more difficult-to-measure long-term indirect costs associated with loss of income and productivity of the patient and lost income of the significant other who provides care to the patient.

DEMOGRAPHICS AND CAUSES OF INJURY

The highest incidence of TBI is for men in the 15- to 24-year-old age range (5). Two other smaller peaks of increased occurrence are seen in the ages 0 to 2 years and for ages ≥70 years. Based on data from a 14-state surveillance system, hospitalization rates for

Table 6-1	Sports Associated with Concussion

Boxing
Football
Soccer
Ice hockey
Equestrian sports
Skateboarding
Roller-skating/in-line skating
Bicycling
Downhill skiing
Snowboarding
Less frequent: baseball, rugby, basketball, mountaineering, race-car driving

Note: The sports are listed in descending order to show the frequency with which they cause concussions. From Bailes JE, Cantu RC. Head injury in athletes. *Neurosurgery.* 2001;48(1):26–45; discussion 45–46, with permission.

TBI were highest for young males, older adults, American Indians, and Alaskan natives and blacks (10).

The most common cause of TBI is motor vehicle crashes (MVCs) (48%); similarly, the most common cause of death from MVCs is TBI. Second comes falls (23%), followed by violence (firearm-related [10%] and non-firearm-related [9%]) and sports injuries (11,12) (Table 6-1). Black males and American Indian/Alaskan native males had the highest rate of TBI due to assault, almost four times that for white males (10). For the elderly, on the other hand, falls are the most frequent cause of brain injury (13). These percentages are from the Centers for Disease Control, and there may be some geographic variability.

TYPES AND MECHANISMS OF BRAIN INJURY

The primary mechanism of closed head injuries is either by direct blows to the head (as in a fall or assault) or by more indirect means such as acceleration-deceleration (AD) forces. Generally, direct blows to the skull will result in the classic "coup-contra-coup" injury with a focal tissue abnormality directly at the site of the blow, as well as opposite to the location of the blow; namely, where the brain contacts the skull as it is decelerating. Because the brain is only loosely connected to the surrounding cranium, the motion of the brain lags behind that of the skull. Thus, as the skull comes to rest, the brain strikes the calvarium on the opposite side and another injury results.

Injuries such as those sustained in a motor vehicle crash are associated with AD forces that result in anterior-posterior motion of the brain mass within the skull. Because of the bony prominences of the orbits and sphenoid ridge inside the skull, lesions often result in the frontal, inferior frontal, and temporal lobes. Rotational forces often coincide with AD forces, resulting in a twisting of the cerebral hemispheres on the core brain structures and numerous axonal disruptions at the white-gray borders. This kind of trauma is defined as diffuse axonal injury.

At an organ and molecular level, there are numerous changes in the physiology of cerebral blood flow and vasculature after severe TBI. Cerebral blood flow is commonly reduced and pressure autoregulation impaired, as are responses to partial pressure of carbon dioxide in arterial blood ($Paco_2$). Vascular injury stems from damage to endothelial cells, increased blood–brain barrier permeability, and impaired compensatory mechanisms. Free radicals, leukotrienes, and cytokines are among the mechanisms that contribute to brain damage after trauma as are the excitatory neurotransmitters (acetylcholine and glutamate) (14).

OUTCOME AND DETERMINANTS OF OUTCOME

Outcome following traumatic brain injury ranges from death to full recovery. Time to maximal recovery may range from days or weeks to years, depending on severity of the injury and the type of function in question. Outcome is determined by a host of factors including severity of the brain injury, the characteristics of the person injured, time since injury, and a number of factors after the injury that may facilitate or hinder recovery.

There are several measures of diffuse brain injury severity. Severity of initial brain injury is often measured by the Glasgow Coma Scale (GCS), an index of depth of coma at a specified time after injury (15) (Table 6-2). This scale assesses eye opening, verbal response, and motor response, with scores ranging

Table 6-2	Glasgow Coma Scale		
Eye opening	Spontaneous	4
	To voice	3
	To pain	2
	None	1
Verbal response	Oriented	5
	Confused	4
	Inappropriate	3
	Incomprehensible	2
	None	1
Motor response	Obeys command	6
	Localizes pain	5
	Withdraws from pain	4
	Flexion	3
	Extension to pain	2
	None	1
Total score		1–15

from 3 to 15. Severe injuries are considered to be a GCS of ≤8. Moderate TBI is considered when the GCS is between 9 and 12, and mild TBI when the GCS is ≥13. Generally the lowest score obtained in the first 24 hours after resuscitation is used for classification purposes.

Measures of duration of impaired consciousness typically are a better predictor of outcome than measures of depth of coma such as the GCS. These measures include posttraumatic amnesia (PTA) and time from injury to consistently follow commands. Posttraumatic amnesia is the period of time from injury to the time when regular memory for day-to-day events return. PTA can be determined retrospectively (16) or prospectively (17). Prospectively assessed PTA may be a better predictor but is much more difficult to obtain because it requires daily monitoring of the return of memory to more normal levels. Time to follow commands is the time from injury to when the individual is able to follow simple commands consistently as defined by the motor component of the GCS (18). This index can often be obtained from careful review of nursing notes during acute care hospitalization.

Early somatosensory evoked potentials (SEPs) may also prove useful for predicting prognosis in TBI. A recent review has shown that those with TBI who have bilaterally absent median nerve responses have only a 5% (95% confidence interval [CI] = 2% to 7%) chance of awakening; most of those who do awaken in this setting will have severe disability. On the other hand, normal median nerve SEPs suggest an 89% chance of awakening (95% CI = 85% to 92%) while present, but abnormal SEPs suggest a 69% (95% CI = 61% to 77%) chance of awakening (19).

A number of measures have been used to assess functional outcomes in traumatic brain injury. The most commonly used is the Glasgow Outcome Scale (GOS) (20) and its new revised version the Glasgow

Outcome Scale-Extended (GOS-E). The GOS-E was developed to improve the reliability and sensitivity of the GOS (21). The GOS and GOS-E are the most commonly used measures in the neurosurgical community and in large clinical trials. The GOS-E groups patient outcomes into eight categories, ranging from Dead to Upper Good Recovery. Other commonly used measures of functional status include the Disability Rating Scale (22), Functional Independence measure (23), Community Integration Questionnaire (24), and more recently, the Functional Status Examination (FSE) (25), the Mayo-Portland Scale (26), and the Rancho Los Amigos level of Cognitive Functioning (27).

PHYSICAL AND MEDICAL CONSEQUENCES

SPASTIC HYPERTONIA AND OTHER MOVEMENT DISORDERS

Because of the widespread nature of traumatic brain lesions, motor control can be affected at multiple levels, resulting in a mixed picture of movement disorders. Spasticity of cerebral origin tends to present with a more mixed picture than that seen after the more localized lesions of spinal cord injury. Although many of the classic signs (e.g., clasp-knife phenomenon and graded response to speed of joint displacement) are present, there are frequently features of muscle tone rigidity and dystonia that may alter the peripheral neurologic examination and effectiveness of treatment after TBI. The classic description of the upper motor neuron syndrome includes enhanced stretch reflexes, released flexor reflexes in the lower limbs, a loss of dexterity, and weakness (28).

The presence of hypertonia and other movement disorders is highly correlated to the severity of brain injury. For patients with severe enough injury to be admitted to inpatient rehabilitation units, the prevalence of spastic hypertonia may be as high as 84% (29). Some of these disorders may be transient. Tremors may occur in up to 10% of persons with severe TBI; persistent tremors may be seen in another 9% (30). Persistent dystonias may occur in 4% and, strikingly, are often delayed in their onset (mean latency of onset of movement disorders in adults was estimated at 2.5 +/− 4.9 years) (30,31). Other manifestations of movement disorders include ballism and chorea, paroxysmal dyskinesias, tics, and parkinsonism.

Treatment for these disorders depends on the functional impact of the disorder and the point in time of recovery from TBI that treatment is to occur. Spastic hypertonia and movement disorders that do not result in significant functional impairment or discomfort do not require treatment. The realization that disorders may be transient or may change in time will also direct the use of less invasive and "permanent" solutions early during recovery. Physical modalities such as serial casting and splints, ice, stretching, and functional mobilization are important first considerations (32,33). Pharmacologic treatments for spastic hypertonia, such as dantrolene, baclofen, tizanidine, and diazepam, are more useful for relief of hypertonia and spasms but have side effects including sedation and possible cognitive impairment (34). Other treatments for spastic hypertonia include alcohol and phenol injections, botulinum toxin injections, and the use of intrathecal baclofen via continuous pump (35–37).

Another frequent disorder that impairs volitional movement after TBI is apraxia, which is an impairment in the ability to perform skilled, purposive limb movements associated with left frontoparietal hemisphere damage in right-hand dominant persons. Apraxias may be classified as either ideational (lacking the concept of movement or of object use) or ideomotor/limb-kinetic (lacking in operationalizing motor sequences). There have been few studies on therapy to address apraxia despite its adverse effect on function (38).

ENDOCRINE DISORDERS

Significant hyponatremia is common following an insult to the brain and can be manifested by altered mental status, seizures, or dehydration, requiring routine monitoring of electrolytes after moderate to severe TBI. There are three main diagnoses to be considered: the syndrome of inappropriate antidiuretic hormone secretion (SIADH), the cerebral salt-wasting syndrome (CSW), and acute adrenocortical insufficiency. SIADH results from a primary dysregulation of water metabolism; increases in extracellular fluid osmolality results in the release of antidiuretic hormone, with subsequent water retention (39). CSW, on the other hand, is thought to be associated with volume depletion (40). Acute adrenal insufficiency can occur with trauma and results in both glucocorticoid and mineralocorticoid deficiency, including hyponatremia (41). Both SIADH and CSW tend to be transient in patients after TBI and can be treated conservatively. Too rapid replacement of sodium using hypertonic saline solutions can trigger central pontine myelinolysis. SIADH can be treated with free water restriction and sodium replacement; CSW, with salt and fluid replacement. Certain medications, such as

carbamazepine, can exacerbate hyponatremia and should be monitored.

Diabetes insipidus (DI) is a more uncommon disorder of sodium particularly associated with optic chiasm or pituitary injury characterized by excessive renal free water excretion because of a relative lack of ADH. Clinical signs include polydipsia and polyuria. Chronic DI is treated with intranasal administration of 1-desamino-D-arginine vasopressin (dDAVP).

Pituitary dysfunction is probably more common than realized by most clinicians, and the symptoms in adults are often nonspecific and may include anorexia, malaise, weight loss, lethargy, nausea, seizures, hypothermia, hypotension, and hypoglycemia (42). Patients at risk for hypopituitarism include those with basilar skull fractures, diabetes insipidus, unexplained hypotension, weight loss, fatigue, loss of libido, or nonresponsive depression (42). A recent study noted that the occurrence of pituitary dysfunction was between 57% and 59% in persons with moderate to severe TBI (43). However, no significant correlation has been demonstrated between growth hormone function and outcome after TBI. Diagnosis may occur years after the actual injury as well (43,44). The level of deficiency at which growth hormone replacement should be administered has not been established.

DISORDERS OF THE SPECIAL SENSES
Visual Dysfunction

Studies describing the effects of traumatic brain injury on the visual system are surprisingly limited considering the frequency of clinical complaints of visual dysfunction. Schlageter noted that 59% of patients admitted to an acute TBI rehabilitation unit (and able to comply with testing) had impairments in one or more areas including pursuits, saccades, ocular posturing, stereopsis, extra-ocular movements, and near/far eso-/exotropia (45). In another study, convergence insufficiency was noted in 38% of acute TBI inpatients and 42% of patients followed up at 3 years after injury (46). The most common extra-ocular deficiencies were fourth nerve palsies (36% to 39%), third nerve palsies (25% to 33%), sixth nerve palsies (14%), and combined palsies (10% to 25%) (47,48).

Consideration of these deficiencies alone understates how vision may be impaired after TBI. While sensory input and reception via the primary visual system is necessary, intact functioning of the visual processing areas in the cortex and the function of visual memory is also important to the overall concept of visual function.

Often, formal evaluation of the visual system is impossible early after TBI because the patient is unable to cooperate with testing. At this stage, functional observations of inattention to parts of the environment, past-reaching, and odd, sustained head postures may be clues to the need for eventual visual evaluation. The overall treatment of visual dysfunction continues to be somewhat controversial. Correction of visual acuity and the use of prisms to partly correct for convergence disorders are widely accepted. Surgery for persistent cranial nerve palsy is also well accepted. Less well studied is vision therapy that seeks to use practice and training in visual tasks to improve visual processes. (An excellent review of this can be found in the chapter by Suter [49]).

Dizziness and Balance

Dizziness and impaired balance are common complaints after TBI and may have a number of etiologies. The most common of these is benign positional paroxysmal vertigo (BPPV) (50). With BPPV, the sense of dizziness or vertigo follows changes in head position (rolling over in bed, bending over, or looking upward). BPPV results from free-floating debris in the vestibular labyrinth disturbing endolymphatic pressure and copular deflection. BPPV can be both diagnosed and treated at the bedside by using the Dix-Hallpike maneuver for diagnosis and Epley maneuver for treatment. (For details of these maneuvers, see Furman and Cass, 1999 [51].) Bilateral involvement is more common in BPPV of traumatic origin than the idiopathic type (52).

Taste and Smell

Olfactory dysfunction may be more common than realized after TBI. Forty percent of persons undergoing formal testing for olfactory function had no awareness of their decreased abilities (53). Actual incidence estimates vary widely, from 13.7% to 56%, depending on how they are identified (53–55). The severity of trauma does appear to be correlated with the presence of these disorders (53,55). While a third of patients who complained of dysosmia demonstrated some improvement over months to years, few regain normal smell. Parosmias improved more frequently than anosmias (55).

DYSAUTONOMIA

Dysautonomia (also called "storming") is usually an episodic disturbance in autonomic inhibition, resulting in any or all of the following symptoms: hyperthermia, tachycardia, hypertension, diaphoresis, pupillary

dilatation, dystonic posturing, increased metabolic rate, and impaired consciousness. Though the actual site of brain injury resulting in this syndrome has not been identified, the release of adrenergic compounds results in the clinical picture. Dysautonomia is correlated with severity of injury and persisting episodes portend a poor prognosis. No specific diagnostic test is useful in identifying this syndrome. However, a thorough work-up to find the source of a possible infection or other cause for fever is warranted. Treatment of dysautonomia concentrates on symptom control and identifying possible triggers. Severe episodes that require intravenous medication for treatment will likely result in transfer of a patient to an intensive care unit. Opioids can be used to dampen sympathetic activity. Propranolol has been used to manage cardiovascular symptoms, limiting the possibility of cardiac damage, and may be used routinely to decrease the severity or frequency of episodes. Hyperthermia can be treated with acetaminophen or, when severe, with chlorpromazine, which can be given intramuscularly as well. Dantrolene sodium can be used to control the often severe posturing that accompanies these episodes. Many other medications have been used to treat dysautonomia; however, many of these have significant sedative effects that are detrimental to cognitive recovery (56).

POST-TRAUMATIC SEIZURES

Seizures that occur after a severe TBI comprise 20% of all epilepsy cases. The incidence of seizure disorder after TBI ranges from 5% to 19% for closed head injuries to 32% to 50% for penetrating wounds (57–60). A distinction is made between early seizures (those occurring during the first week after TBI) and late seizures. While early seizures are a risk factor for later seizures, they are not as predictive of posttraumatic epilepsy as is the occurrence of a late seizure. There is evidence that the administration of phenytoin during the first week after TBI protects against seizures during that first week, but there is no good evidence to support the routine use of any antiepileptic drug for prophylaxis after that time (61,62).

There are certain factors that predispose patients to a higher risk of posttraumatic epilepsy. These risks include penetrating injuries, bilateral contusions with subdural hematoma, skull fracture with dural penetration of fragments, higher severity of injury, older age, multiple neurosurgic procedures, early seizures, and presence of apolipoprotein E ε 4 allele (60,63–65).

The risk of recurrence is high after a late seizure; over 2 years, the cumulative incidence of recurrent late seizures was 86%, and 37% will have had ten or more late seizures within 2 years of injury (66). Therefore, treatment of late seizures is generally indicated. Phenytoin, carbamazepine, sodium valproate, and phenobarbital have all been demonstrated to be effective (62,67). Other antiepileptic drugs are likely to be effective in individual cases, depending on the type of seizure. All medications used to treat seizures have potentially adverse cognitive effects.

MUSCULOSKELETAL DISORDERS

In cases of severe traumatic brain injury, peripheral nerve and limb or axial fractures may be diagnosed late because of the patient's inability to communicate or localize pain. It has been estimated that between 10% and 34% of persons hospitalized for TBI have peripheral nerve injuries. Risk factors for peripheral nerve injury include long-bone fractures, poor limb positioning, casts, surgery, and spasticity (68–70). Fractures may also remain undetected (71,72). In persons with risk factors, abnormal postures or atypical neurologic recovery in a limb may be cues to underlying nerve or bone damage.

Heterotopic ossification (HO), the formation of mature lamellar bone in soft tissue, may also occur with severe traumatic brain injury. Risk factors for developing heterotopic ossification include severity of TBI, spasticity, and trauma or surgery near the joint (73). There may be a link between disturbed hormonal function (specifically, prolactin) and enhanced osteogenesis in persons with TBI (74). Areas most commonly affected by HO after TBI are the hips, shoulders, elbows, and knees. Signs of HO may include local swelling, decreasing range of motion at a joint, and systemic signs such as fever. The diagnosis is best confirmed with a three-phase bone scan (73). There is some evidence that the use of nonsteroidal anti-inflammatory drugs inhibit mineralization of bone and thus may reduce the occurrence of HO (73). Surgical removal after the bone matures is the only decisive method of treatment; although there may be slight recurrence within the first few years after resection, functional improvement is usually maintained (75,76). Local irradiation has been used after arthroplasty surgery to prevent ectopic bone formation and appears to be safe and well tolerated (73).

NEUROBEHAVIORAL CONSEQUENCES

Emotional and behavioral difficulties occur frequently, even in the absence of physical problems, and are major barriers to resuming prior social roles and responsibilities. These neurologically-based personality and behavioral changes can include problems with awareness of deficit, lack of initiative, impulsivity, disinhibition, rage reactions, loss of empathy or concern for others, flat affect, inappropriate comments and behaviors, uncontrolled laughing or crying, or emotional lability.

Apathy occurs frequently after TBI and can be defined as reduced goal-directed behavior as a result of a lack of motivation that is neurologically correlated to frontal lobe damage (77). There are no randomized, controlled trials of any drug for this condition, but various case reports support the use of such drugs as amantadine, methylphenidate, amphetamine, selegiline, and selective serotonin reuptake inhibitors (78–80).

Another serious neurobehavioral sequela of TBI is depression. The incidence of depression in the first year after TBI is approximately 30%, with elevated rates of depression persisting years after injury (81,82). Frequent comorbid symptoms are anxiety (76.7%) and aggressive behavior or irritability (56.7%) (82). Depression not only results in the risk of suicide but also in diminished psychosocial functioning and quality of life (83). There have only been a few small studies of pharmacologic treatment of depression but those have demonstrated positive response to both tricyclic and selective serotonin reuptake inhibitors (84–86). Although there are no randomized controlled trials of psychotherapy after TBI, it seems reasonable to combine drug therapy with counseling as well. Adjunctive treatments such as exercise and light exposure have not been studied in persons with TBI but should be added to a treatment program when appropriate.

Other types of neurobehavioral disorders seen after TBI include alcohol and substance abuse; these disorders typically precede the injury. As compared to pre-injury, a decrease in alcohol and drug use is seen in the first year after injury with gradual increase to premorbid levels, especially in the less severely injured (87–89). Posttraumatic stress disorder (PTSD) does occur after traumatic brain injury. PTSD is characterized by intrusive thoughts related to the trauma, anxiety, and avoidance behavior, and a variety of somatic and cognitive symptoms of hyperarousal. There has been controversy regarding the existence of PTSD after brain injury because the usual criteria include intrusive and distressing memories of the trauma. Many people after TBI have significant posttraumatic amnesia and amnesia in regard to the trauma itself (90,91). PTSD is often comorbid with depressive disorders (92). There is some evidence that the early treatment of acute stress syndrome with cognitive behavioral therapy, in addition to typical therapies, helps to prevent the evolution of PTSD (93). Although the incidence rate is small, persons with TBI have a higher risk for psychotic disorder that is also delayed in onset (94).

NEUROPSYCHOLOGICAL IMPAIRMENTS

Neuropsychological impairments refer to acquired cognitive difficulties, such as trouble with concentrating, remembering new information, processing information quickly, thinking flexibly, abstract reasoning, or solving new problems. In the more severe cases and in those with attendant focal injuries, the deficits may also include very basic and specific alterations in key language capacities and in visual-perceptual and visual-spatial skills. Depending on the severity of the diffuse injury and size and location of anatomic lesions, impairments may be observed in any or all of these functions.

Severity of the brain injury clearly has a decisive influence on neuropsychological outcome. Severity indexes such as coma length, coma depth, post-traumatic amnesia, one or both nonreactive pupils, and presence and severity of mass lesions have significant impact on outcome. We examined the neuropsychological functioning of a large group of patients on a comprehensive battery of neuropsychological measures 1 year after injury (95). Unlike many studies that focus on patients who are seeking clinical help with complicated recoveries, this one enrolled patients on the basis of their injury type and its characteristics. Functions assessed ranged from motor to higher-level executive functions and included finger-tapping speed, sustained and divided attention, memory and learning, verbal and performance intelligence, reasoning, and overall neuropsychological competency. The performance of these subjects as a group, and also subdivided by various severity indices, was compared with that of a group of general trauma subjects who had sustained injury to parts of their body other than the head.

Table 6-3 shows the performance of the TBI cases divided by time from injury to follow simple commands (TFC) as defined by the motor subscale of GCS, an index of length of impaired consciousness. Overall, the TBI subjects as a group performed significantly more poorly than the general trauma group. The impairments were not restricted to attention, memory, or speed of information processing—abilities thought to be sensitive to traumatic brain injury. Rather, the impairments were diffuse and also involved motor skills, general intellectual functions, new problem solving, and overall impairments. The magnitude and the pervasiveness of impairments, however, depended on severity of the brain injury. There was clearly a dose-response relationship between TFC and level of cognitive impairments. As a group, the performance scores of the subgroup with TFC <1 hour were comparable to those of general trauma group. Selective impairments on measures of attention and memory start to emerge with longer TFC of 1 to 24 hours. With long TFC lengths such as 1 to 2 weeks, nearly all measures are impaired as seen in the table. Similar dose-response relationship can be observed on other measures of brain injury severity. Figure 6–1 shows the relationship between overall neuropsychological impairment (Halstead Impairment Index) and several brain injury severity indexes including GCS, neurosurgical intervention for evacuation of space-occupying lesions, and number of nonreactive pupils. It is important to add that this composite index of neuropsychological impairment ranges from 0 (none of the tests show impairment) to 1.0 (all test results are in the impaired range).

The degree of neuropsychological impairments is greater soon after injury with recovery occurring over days, weeks, months, and possibly years. Degree of improvement and degree of residuals depend on degree of original loss. Figure 6–2 shows recovery of Wechsler Adult Intelligence Scale Performance Intelligence Quotient (PIQ) from 1 to 12 months in subgroups of patients divided on the basis of time to follow commands. Those with more severe brain injury show greater loss at 1 month compared to trauma controls. However, the slopes of improvement appear to be proportional to the degree of loss. An exception is the most severe group (i.e., TFC >29 days). In spite of greater improvement, however, those with greater initial loss end up with greater impairments at 1 year. This is the reason for the findings that neuropsychological impairments are better predictors of long-term outcomes than neurological indices of severity (96).

FUNCTIONAL STATUS

Traumatic brain injuries can leave those that survive them with various limitations and disabilities in everyday life. These limitations may involve a range of areas from basic functions, such as personal care and ambulation, to higher-level activities, such as social relationships, work, and leisure. While the nature of the disabilities is known to be varied, it is important to know how often these problems occur and the predictors of who is likely to have them.

Table 6-3	Weighted Median Scores for Trauma Controls and Head-injured Subjects Divided by Time to Follow Commands

Measure	Trauma controls[a]	<1 h[b]	1–24 h[c]	25 h to 6 d[d]	7–13 d[e]	14–28 d[f]	≥29 d[g]	r[h]
Motor Functions								
Finger Tapping, dominant hand	53	51	52	47[k]	49[j]	42[k]	11[k]	−0.51
Finger Tapping, nondominant hand	50	48	48	44[k]	45[j]	38[k]	16[k]	−0.47
Namewriting, dominant hand	0.50	0.50	0.53	0.60	0.60[i]	0.69[k]	3.15[k]	0.49
Namewriting, nondominant hand	1.30	1.41	1.44	1.87[i]	1.64[i]	1.82[i]	3.60[k]	0.43
Attention and flexibility								
Seashore Rhythm Test	27	27	26	27	26	24[k]	16[k]	−0.42
Trail Making Test, Part A	23	22	25	27[j]	26[i]	40[k]	101[k]	0.57
Trail Making Test, Part B	56	57	72[i]	63	71	132[k]	301[k]	0.50
Stroop Color and Word Test, Part 1	42	42	46	44	48[k]	70[k]	151[k]	0.51
Stroop Color and Word Test, Part 2	96	98	108	107	122[k]	162[k]	300[k]	0.49
Memory								
WMS–LM	11	10.5	10	10	9	8[j]	0.50[k]	−0.39
WMS–VR	11	12	10	11	11	9[i]	4[k]	−0.38
SR–RCL	89	89	84[i]	86[i]	75[k]	69[k]	24[k]	−0.53
WMS–LM, delayed	9	9	8	7[i]	7[i]	6[k]	0[k]	−0.46
WMS–VR, delayed	10	11	10	9	10	6[k]	0[k]	−0.45
SR–RCL, 30-min delay	9	8	8[i]	8	7[k]	5[k]	0[k]	−0.45
SR–RCL, 4-h delay	8	8	7	8	5[k]	4[k]	0[k]	−0.46
Verbal								
WAIS–VIQ	106	106	101	101	98	92[k]	57[k]	−0.45
Performance skills								
WAIS–PIQ	112	110	106	102[k]	102[j]	90[k]	56[k]	−0.55
TPT–T	0.36	0.35	0.40	0.61[k]	0.51[k]	1.10[k]	5.75[k]	0.61
Reasoning								
Category Test	24	22	28	41	32	72[k]	112[k]	0.54
Overall								
Halstead Impairment Index	0.1	0.1	0.3	0.4[k]	0.4[j]	0.7[k]	1.0[k]	0.59

WMS–LM, Wechsler Memory Scale—Logical Memory; WMS–VR, Wechsler Memory Scale—Visual Reproduction; SR–RCL, Selective Reminding Test—Total Recall; TPT–T, Tactual Performance Test—time per block; WAIS–VIQ, Wechsler Adult Intelligence Scale—Verbal Intelligence Quotient; WAIS–PIQ, Wechsler Adult Intelligence Scale—Performance Intelligence Quotient.

[a] $n = 121$.
[b] $n = 161$.
[c] $n = 100$.
[d] $n = 52$.
[e] $n = 37$.
[f] $n = 32$.
[g] $n = 53$: median is untestable, lowest observed score recorded.
[h] All significant at $p < 0.001$.
[i] $p < 0.001$.
[j] $p < 0.01$.
[k] $p < 0.001$.
From Dikmen SS, Machamer JE, Winn HR, et al. Neuropsychological outcome at 1-year post head injury. *Neuropsychology.* 1995c;9(1):80–90, with permission.

As mentioned previously, the most commonly used index to describe overall outcome in TBI is the GOS and more recently its revised version, the GOS-E (21). The best data on overall outcome and its predictors in patients with severe head injury using the GOS are those contributed by three large multicenter studies: the International Coma Data Bank, the Pilot Phase of the National Coma Data Bank, and the Full Phase Coma Data Bank (97–99).

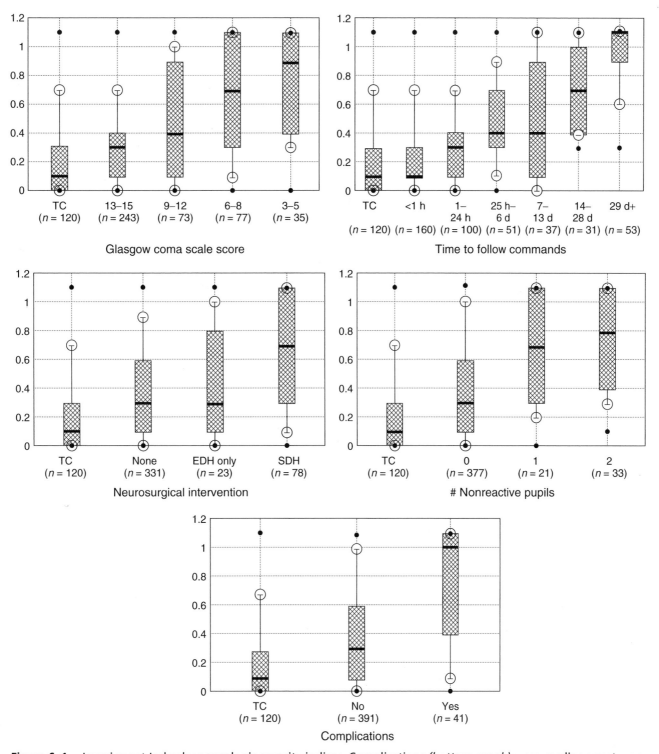

Figure 6–1. Impairment Index by neurologic severity indices. Complications *(bottom graph)* were cardiac arrest, ventriculitis, and meningitis. TC, trauma control; EDH, epidural hematoma; SDH, subdural or intracerebral hematoma or contusion. (From Dikmen SS, Machamer JE, Winn HR, et al. Neuropsychological outcome at 1-year post head injury. *Neuropsychology.* 1995c;9[1]:80–90, with permission.)

Severe head injury was defined as a GCS of ≤8 at 6 hours of injury. The GOS has five categories: death, persistent vegetative state, severe disability, moderate disability, and good recovery. The differentiation between the last two categories is based on the patient's dependence on others for self-care activities and the patient's ability to participate in normal social life. Based on large series of cases with severe TBI (defined as GCS ≤8 at 6 hours), approximately 45% of patients die early and half of those surviving

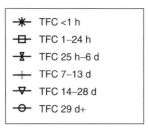

PIQ = 38 represents untestable

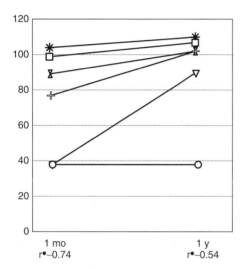

Figure 6–2. Median performance intelligence quotient (PIQ) scores by time to follow command (TFC) groups. (From Dikmen SS, Machamer JE, Winn HR, et al. Neuropsychological outcome at 1-year post head injury. *Neuropsychology.* 1995c;9[1]:80–90, with permission.)

sustain sufficiently severe impairments to make them totally or significantly dependent on others. Even the good recovery category of the GOS, which includes approximately 50% of the surviving patients, does not assure close to pre-injury level of functioning (100).

More detailed information on outcome for survivors of TBI with a broad spectrum of TBI severity is shown in Table 6-4 as assessed by the Sickness Impact Profile (SIP) (96). The subjects were 410 adults hospitalized for their brain injury and prospectively followed to 1 year. The results of this group at 1 year after injury were compared with a group of friends and a group of trauma controls (i.e., a group who had sustained an injury to body parts other than the head). Subjects reported how much dysfunction (in percentages) they experienced due to health or head injury in various areas of everyday life. As can be seen, friend controls in this age group do not report much health-related dysfunction. In contrast, TBI cases do report problems especially in the areas of employment, recreation, and cognitive functioning and to a lesser extent in almost all areas assessed, including sleep and rest, emotional behavior, and ambulation. Note, however, that trauma controls also report similar problems but not to the same extent, suggesting that some of the disabilities seen in TBI cases might be related to other injuries sustained in the same accident.

The effects of TBI can be long lasting and permanent in more severely injured persons. Longer-term

				TFC						
	FC	TC	HI	<1 h	1–24 h	25 h–6 d	7–13 d	14–28 d	≥29 d	r
No. tested/untested	88/0	124/0	410/27	166/0	103/0	50/2	36/2	29/1	26/22	
Sleep and rest	1	10	12	9	10	16	21[a]	20	19	0.20[c]
Emotional behavior	1	10	12	11	13	14	15	12	14	0.07
Body care and movement	0	3	4	3	3	3	7	7	12[b]	0.22[c]
Home management	0	8	8	6	8	7	10	18[a]	20[a]	0.21[c]
Mobility	0	2[a]	5	3	5	5	7	7	14[c]	0.23[c]
Social interaction	0	7[b]	10	10	11	10	14[a]	12	14	0.13[b]
Ambulation	0	6	6	5	5	4	8	8	16[a]	0.20[c]
Alertness behavior	0	9[c]	16	14	15	17	19	23[b]	20[a]	0.14[c]
Communication	0	5	7	6	5	14	10	12	18[b]	0.23[c]
Recreation and pastimes	1	12	16	13	16	20	22	23	28[a]	0.21[c]
Eating	0	1	1	1	1	2	2	3	4	0.14[b]
Work	0	14[c]	23	14	23	28[a]	31[b]	52[c]	47[c]	0.34[c]
Psychosocial	0	8[b]	11	10	11	13	15	14	16[a]	0.17[c]
Physical	0	4	5	4	4	4	7	7	14[a]	0.20[c]
Total	0	6[a]	9	7	8	10	12[a]	14[b]	17[c]	0.26[c]

Table 6-4 Sickness Impact Profile (SIP): Weighted Mean of Percentage of Dysfunction at 1 Year

FC, friend control group; TC, trauma control group; HI, head-injured group; TFC, time to follow commands.
Note: Superscripts in the TC column indicate the results of the comparison between trauma controls and the head-injured group as a whole. Superscripts in the TFC columns indicate the results of the comparisons between each TFC group and the trauma control group. Superscripts in the last column reflect the relationship between level of severity (TFC) and outcome.
[a]*p* <0.05.
[b]*p* <0.01.
[c]*p* <0.001.
From Dikmen SS, Ross BL, Machamer JE, et al. One year psychosocial outcome in head injury. *J Int Neuropsychol Soc.* 1995d;1(1):67–77, with permission.

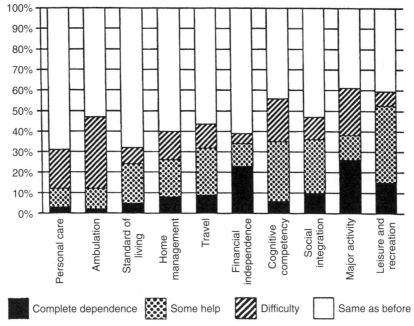

Figure 6–3. Functional Status Examination endorsements at 3 to 5 years after traumatic brain injury. The percentage of cases at different levels of functioning within each area of everyday life is shown. (From Dikmen SS, Machamer JE, Powell JM, et al. Outcome 3 to 5 years after moderate to severe traumatic brain injury. *Arch Phys Med Rehabil.* 2003;84[10]:1449–1457, with permission.)

outcome at 3 to 5 years after injury was examined in a group of adults with moderate to severe traumatic brain injury using the Functional Status Examination (FSE) (101,102). Significant limitations were reported by subjects in nearly all areas of activities of daily living. Recovery to pre-injury levels ranged from 65% in personal care to 40% in cognitive competency, major activity, and leisure and recreation, as seen in Figure 6–3. The degree of limitations, however, was related to the severity of injury (101).

A functional area that has probably received more attention than others is employment (103–105). Return to work is clearly compromised after the injury as a result of the various impairments and disabilities from the injury to the brain, as well as from injuries sustained to other body parts in the same accident. Overall statistics regarding return to work are not very meaningful, because whether the person returns to work, when he or she returns, and in what capacity relate to the characteristics of the person injured (e.g., education, gender, previous work history), the severity of the head injury and associated neuropsychological problems, and severity of other system injuries (105). Figure 6–4 shows survival curves representing rates of return to work over time as a function of severity of injury, pre-injury job stability, extremity injury, and neuropsychological status at 1 month after injury assessed by the Halstead Impairment Index.

APPROACH TO MANAGEMENT OF TRAUMATIC BRAIN INJURY: EARLY REHABILITATION INTERVENTIONS

EARLY MEDICAL MANAGEMENT

Potential complications that may result in later impaired function may begin very early in those with severe traumatic brain injuries. Therefore, early rehabilitation consultation is important to address prevention of complications and to assist in developing a plan of management in the critical care period and immediately afterwards.

In particular, the prevention of joint contractures and skin breakdown is most critical in the intensive care unit. Using proper positioning, splinting, and turning schedules should be part of a care plan in the intensive care unit for any patient with reduced consciousness. The presence of elevated muscle tone and spasticity in persons with severe TBI increases the importance of these measures. It is not possible to accurately predict the long-term functional outcome for any individual during the first week after TBI, so these precautions should be universal.

There is no literature supporting the implementation of sensory stimulation protocols in improving long-term outcome. However, using familiar sounds or music is not harmful and may be soothing for the family as well as the patient.

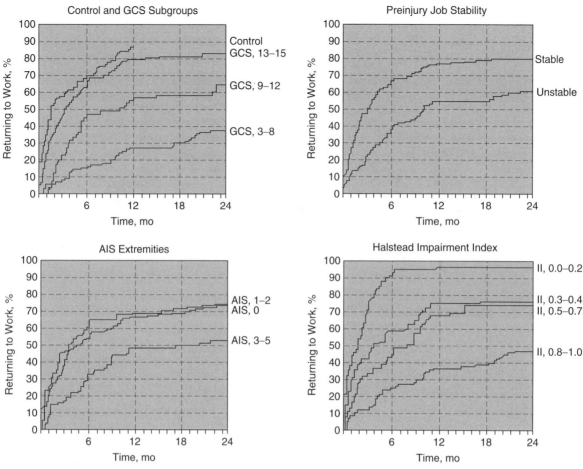

Figure 6–4. Estimated percentage first returning to work by subgroups defined on the basis of initial Glasgow Coma Scale (GCS) *(top left)*, job stability *(top right)*, Abbreviated Injury Scale (AIS) score for the extremities *(bottom left)*, and neuropsychological performance at 1 month after injury, using Halstead Impairment Index (II) *(bottom right)*. (From Dikmen SS, Temkin NR, Machamer JE, et al. Employment following traumatic head injuries. *Arch Neurol.* 1994;51[2]:177–186, with permission.)

THE ACUTELY AGITATED PATIENT

Posttraumatic agitation commonly accompanies recovery from severe TBI and is related to confusion and disinhibition. The features of agitation are not well defined; at one end, increased psychomotor activity is cited and, at the other, physical aggression and explosive anger (106). Early agitation co-varies with the degree of cognitive impairment, particularly attention (107,108). This type of agitation should be distinguished from episodic dyscontrol syndromes seen later during recovery. Medications used to treat agitation have included lithium, neuroleptics, antidepressants, psychostimulants, anticonvulsants, buspirone, dopaminergic drugs, beta blockers, and hormonal drugs. Treatments vary widely because there is little objective research supporting the use of any class of drug (109). Three points can be made in reference to the treatment of agitation in the acute care hospital or acute care rehabilitation unit. It is

important to monitor behavior response to interventions in a systematic fashion, using a modified single-subject research methodology. There are scales available to help track behavior, such as the Agitated Behavior Scale (110) and the Overt Aggression Scale (111). Certain drugs may have more effect on cognition than others. For instance, haloperidol significantly impaired problem solving in rats compared to olanzapine, which did not (112). Environmental controls should be included in any intervention plan to treat acute agitation. Agitation may be in response to environmental factors (e.g., noise, light) or to internal factors (e.g., need to urinate, pain). It is important to first analyze the situation to remove environmental and other easily addressed triggers and to use the environment to provide a calming influence (dimming the lights, music appropriate to the patient's tastes, fewer intrusions, treating pain). Allowing the patient movement with the use of enclosed beds or floor mats can be advantageous.

If these measures do not alleviate agitation or if there is a risk of injury to the patient or staff, then medications can be used to control the agitated state.

THE MINIMALLY RESPONSIVE PATIENT AND THE VEGETATIVE STATE

About 10% of persons hospitalized with TBI are in a minimally responsive or vegetative state during the first month after injury (113,114). At 6 months in the European Brain Injury Consortium survey, approximately 3% continued to be in a vegetative state (115). Minimally responsive state is defined as one in which the patient has generalized responses to the environment. The vegetative state is one in which no response to the environment can be detected, although the patient may have wake-sleep cycles, roving eye movements, tearing, and even occasional vocalizations (116). The diagnosis of vegetative state cannot be made until 12 months after injury; late recoveries are seen occasionally, although functional recovery is usually very limited (117). Survival in the vegetative state depends on the quality of external care but does not usually exceed 10 years. Positron emission tomography (PET) studies in individuals demonstrating isolated cognitive functions in an overall vegetative state have revealed islands of functioning brain tissue isolated from integrative centers (118). Present means of evaluation do not permit enough specificity to allow for definitive clinical decision making or decisions about resources (119).

Early after injury, it is most important to systematically evaluate the patient for responsiveness on a regular basis. Skin care, limb range of motion and positioning devices, mobilization into the sitting position with adequate trunk and head support, and good nutritional and respiratory support are important both for comfort and to allow for function if neurologic recovery occurs. There is little evidence to support the effectiveness of coma stimulation programs, although from an ethical standpoint, persons in minimally responsive or vegetative states deserve humane care, comfort, and human contact (120).

ACUTE REHABILITATION OF MODERATE AND SEVERE TBI

Much of the efforts during the acute rehabilitative phase of moderate and severe TBI are focused on optimizing mobility and independence in basic self-care activities and treating associated medical disorders. The emphasis in this phase for mobility is on regaining ambulation or at least independent use of a wheelchair. Recovery of independent ambulation skills occurs during the first 3 months after an injury; only 14% of those not ambulatory at 3 months

will become so later (121). Cognitive rehabilitation is directed at orientation and using simple memory strategies with cuing. Family members are involved to a large degree in training to compensate for the patient's cognitive problems in learning and memory. More and more aspects of TBI rehabilitation are being shunted to later treatment in the outpatient as inpatient stays grow progressively shorter (between 1990 and 1996, length of stay was reduced to an average of 2.25 days per year [122]).

LATER REHABILITATION INTERVENTIONS

COMMUNITY REINTEGRATION

The notion and practice of community reintegration as guiding therapeutic philosophy and treatment delivery paradigm was first embraced by the postacute brain injury rehabilitation field in the late 1970s (123) and early 1980s (124). With dramatic improvements in medical technology and early management of severe TBI, ever-increasing numbers of young adult survivors of severe TBI were leaving the acute care or inpatient rehabilitation setting still in need of comprehensive services to help them resume productive lives.

Programs need to address the TBI survivors' primary obstacles to better function, including significant problems with memory and new learning, poorly regulated behavior, reduced awareness of deficits and social impact, and trouble applying or generalizing what they learned in one setting to other, real-life situations. Ideally, comprehensive interdisciplinary treatment can provide for optimal functional improvement.

Early models for community reintegration programs were abstracted from those used in other clinical populations. Sources included the psychiatric community's milieu-based theory of treatment (125), appreciation for the value of a strong therapeutic alliance in helping people heal (126), and knowledge of psychotropic medications. Professionals in the area of developmental disabilities (127,128) brought expertise in sheltered or assisted employment, job coaching, and supported, independent living in group homes. Members of the psychology community brought their long-standing expertise in psychometric test development and neuropsychological evaluation (129), as well as the theories of learning (130) from which flowed principles of behavior management. The rise of rehabilitation medicine as a specialty area of practice for physicians, especially in the past 30 years, has also allowed further support and refinement of community reintegration models. When medical support is provided by a practitioner who looks at functional outcomes, and at the complex interface among physical, biochemical, cognitive, emotional, behavioral, vocational, leisure, interpersonal, and family concerns, a patient's chance to achieve better functioning in their real-life settings is maximized (131,132).

Community reintegration as a treatment paradigm is typically used now to describe particular types of intensive postacute brain injury rehabilitation programs (123,124,133–136). These programs are characterized by the use of an interdisciplinary staff with emphasis upon the successful real-life use of each patient's skills and abilities, whether the program occurs in a transitional residential setting, the patient's own home and community, or as part of outpatient programs in clinic settings. In each setting, successful outcome is measured by the patient's or client's ability to resume whatever levels of independence at home and at work that are possible, given their level of residual impairments.

This comprehensive level of intervention is necessary for many people who survive severe TBI simply because the range and degree of residual changes in function that persist are so profound in their impact on the person's function. In many instances, however, the injured person does not have obvious physical signs of brain damage once they are 6 to 12 months postinjury, thus the term "the silent epidemic." For most of these individuals, it will be the combination of cognitive and interpersonal deficits that make independent and successful community reintegration highly unlikely unless well-orchestrated treatment is provided.

When one follows large groups of young and working-age people with TBI over long periods of time (101,135), the actual degree of independent involvement in normal, community-based activities can vary considerably, as can levels of emotional and psychosocial adjustment (137). The community options range from the somewhat restrictive (24-hour onsite supervision in a residential facility) to the fully reintegrated.

In general, it appears that for patients who were able to return to some form of employment or productive activity outside the home after their injuries, there is good preservation of richness in life with opportunities for relationships with people at work, development of new friendships, travel and independence related to driving ability, and the use of community facilities, such as the local café, library, buses, shopping, movies, restaurants, and parks. For patients who are not able to work, the scope of their community involvement may be somewhat less expansive. Contact with peers may occur through community day programs that provide social and educational support or through activities

that are organized or accessed through family guidance. Memberships in church organizations, taking classes at the local community college, and participating in exercise programs at the local YMCA may all be additional outlets for either of the groups noted above.

When people with severe brain injury who are otherwise able to manage most of the basic activities of daily living are not able to live at home, they may benefit from living at a group home. Group homes are houses in regular neighborhoods, privately owned and operated, for four to six adults with similar needs and 24-hour oversight by trained caregivers.

Some patients remain so severely impaired that 24-hour institutional care is the only solution. There may be outings, and there may be room to gradually increase one's level of independence within the setting, but there are usually serious behavioral impairments or high levels of nursing care present that make successful placement outside a nursing facility unlikely or unsafe.

Many severely injured patients, who were unmarried young men or women at the time of their accidents, return to the care of their aging parents, and become a part of their parents' extended community. It is not clear where this group of patients will reside for the long term after the death of their parents—for example, with a sibling, in a group home, in an assisted living setting, or independently with some regular contact and support from a case manager, family, or friends. Increased risk for the development of dementia later in life has also been noted in the severely brain-injured population. In addition, those patients who were somewhat older at time of injury (i.e., age ≥60), have an additional major set of risk factors affecting their long-term recovery and return to functioning (138).

For the purposes of this chapter, we will focus our discussion to nonresidential community-based rehabilitation treatment models. Three broad models of such nonresidential care have evolved. Each of these models has its own unique set of strengths and weaknesses (Table 6-5). Each model also appears to work well with a particular subgroup of the postacute traumatic brain injury population.

The most common model is the clinic-based, outpatient interdisciplinary treatment program, with a dedicated core team, a comprehensive interdisciplinary evaluation phase that precedes treatment, well-defined individual and group interventions, and some form of job station or work trial, where the integration of strategies and real-world function can be fine-tuned. These programs can range from the exceptionally thorough and intense to a rather bare-bones framework, but they usually have a strong psychotherapeutic sensibility.

| Table 6-5 | Important Features of Three Community Reintegration Programs: Strengths and Weaknesses |

Key Features	NRP Clinic-based	RWW Model	Vocational Model
Behavioral (highly disruptive) management	−	+	−
Comprehensive treatment	+	+	−
Continuity of care	−/+	+	−/+
Cost	+	−	+
Daily informal staff contact	+	−/+	−/+
Ease of communication among staff	+	−/+	−/+
Family involvement	−/+	+	−
Group therapies	+	−	−
Local residency not required	+	−	−
Staff boundary problems not likely	−/+	−/+	+
Transportation not an issue	−	+	−
Treatment delivered in home	−	+	−
Treatment delivered at work station or job site	−/+	+	+
Wait time brief to access treatment	−	+	−/+

+, strength; −, weakness; −/+, features may vary by specific program or patient.

The most comprehensive programs of this genre tend to have two strong treatment tracks, one for return to work or school, and one for improving independence without a return to work goal. While the ultimate outcome goals are somewhat different for each of these subgroups of TBI survivors, both groups will receive an extensive set of individual and group therapies in a full-time, 4- to 5-day per week format. Family participation is encouraged through individual sessions with the patient and family group. Staff involvement may include daily meetings to plan and prioritize patient care issues and approaches. A daily milieu-based community meeting of patients and therapists to review each person's progress and issues for that day also occurs. There is also a well-developed work trial or job station component for those patients capable of return to work, and strong support from vocational rehabilitation counselors (VRCs) on the treatment team, who liaison with the patient's "outside" VRC in the community. The goal is to help the patient get ready for the next phase of community involvement, mostly by improving functioning in the clinic setting prior to passing the mantle to school personnel, to VRCs in the community, or to the patient, family, and nurse case managers who will continue with oversight of the case. Team members make themselves available to community personnel for consultation once active clinic treatment has come to an end.

A second model of community reintegration ("Rehabilitation Without Walls") is the comprehensive home rehabilitation format. In this model, all screening, evaluation, and treatment occur in the TBI survivor's home, neighborhood, community, and/or place of work. There is no clinic setting, and a flexible group of therapists is employed. Since 24-hour-a-day supervision in the home or community is available with this model, people can often transition to home from their acute care or brief inpatient rehabilitation stay, no matter how cognitively impaired they are, as long as they are medically stable and not physically violent. For some patients, this option also means they do not have to be discharged to a skilled nursing facility if they are still too impaired for more traditional outpatient treatment programs. (See Pace et al. for outcomes from a home- and community-based program [139].)

The third model of community reintegration (140–144) is primarily an expanded version of long-standing vocationally based models. In this model, selected patients are encouraged to engage with some kind of productive activity as soon as possible in their outpatient phase of treatment. While physical therapy (PT), occupational therapy (OT), or speech therapy may be provided to address specific deficits seen as obstacles to employment, the emphasis is on addressing behaviors and strategies having a primary adverse effect upon work. If depression, anxiety, or other psychological concerns are found to present obstacles to employment, those issues are then individually addressed.

The potential advantages and disadvantages of each model are summarized in Table 6-5. It is clear from the literature (145) that different models can work well for different subgroups of patients, and that each model may result in strong positive outcomes. Clinically, it appears that patients who are struggling with reduced awareness of their residual strengths and weaknesses, acceptance of their changes, exploring ways to forge a meaningful new life, and identifying and managing the interpersonal problems that will affect personal and work lives may benefit from the intense and comprehensive nature of the outpatient neurorehabilitation program (NRP) model. Clients who are too impaired initially to participate in outpatient rehabilitation, have significant behavioral disturbances (absent physical violence), or are likely to require seamless continuity of care to maximize new learning, may be likely to do best with the comprehensive home model. For patients for whom return to work is both a clear goal and a clear possibility, early transition to vocational activities may be the ideal circumstance. Re-establishing improved function in a work setting, with all the practical and psychological benefits that paid employment can bring, is a cost-effective approach for this subgroup of TBI patients.

Telemedicine support for community reintegration is being explored for those patients unable to access facility-based comprehensive programs or in-home programs because of geographic distance or a lack of funding. Telephone-based counseling and education is one means of providing limited rehabilitation services to TBI patients (146,147).

COGNITIVE REHABILITATION

While cognitive neuroscientists and cognitive rehabilitation therapists still have much work to do to forge a more heuristic, practical, and synergistic connection (148) between theories of brain function and ways to remediate cognitive deficits, the daily work of treating patients whose cognitive problems would otherwise preclude resumption of a normal life must go on. Controversies remain about the nature and usefulness of "cognitive retraining" (149,150); namely, what it is, what mechanisms are at play, and how one measures or demonstrates their efficacy.

Early controversy was understandable when practitioners were claiming that cognitive rehabilitation restored brain function or that plunking a patient down in front of a computer with very little therapist input or oversight would magically lead to recovery of function and generalization of skills. However, it has long been possible to teach people how to think more effectively. For instance, directed teaching has been demonstrated to improve problem solving in persons without brain injury (151). Cicerone's extensive review of studies in the cognitive rehabilitation literature for patients with brain injury (136) also provides ample evidence that specific kinds of cognitive rehabilitation interventions for specific kinds of cognitive problems can be effective.

A recent, well-controlled outcome study from Australia by Ponsford and her colleagues followed a large group of patients with TBI. One group of patients received extensive treatment in their homes and communities focused upon practical skills, while the other group received a comprehensive set of outpatient neurorehabilitation therapies in a more traditional clinic setting (152). The presence or absence of a formal cognitive retraining component made a significant difference to long-term functional outcome in this controlled study. The patients who received formal cognitive rehabilitation that targeted higher-level cognitive problems performed better in their homes and communities than those who did not receive the training. This finding ran contrary to expectations (152), given the emphasis in recent years on real-life activities in real-life settings as the only gold standard for gaining enduring improvements in cognitive or behavioral function.

The point of cognitive rehabilitation interventions is not to assume or suggest that altered brain functions can be restored or neurologically improved via the use of therapies. No one knows what role cognitive rehabilitation techniques may or may not play in the possible re-establishment of brain pathways or in neuronal sprouting. The goal of treatment is to improve the patient's attention, memory, problem solving, or other thinking and neurobehavioral issues (e.g., tangentiality, impulsivity) in their day-to-day life.

In effective and appropriate cognitive rehabilitation, the therapist develops and teaches useful strategies and compensatory techniques to improve the patient's performance across a range of tasks and settings. The therapist and team then monitor and refine those strategies and techniques to further improve the patient's performance. This process occurs directly in the therapy hour or home setting, and indirectly by reviewing homework assignments, from reports from family members, friends, and employers, and by obtaining feedback from other treating staff. Those staff observe whether or not the patient is generalizing use of the taught strategies in their treatment hours (e.g., in PT or OT) and also note any improvements in the targeted skills and behaviors. As a result, the patient has multiple opportunities to try out the new skills and multiple sources of professional feedback to gain increased ease and expertise with the use of the strategies.

It is good to be wary of claims that a particular computer program can "restore brain function," or that biofeedback leads to significant and permanent changes in "brain wave activity" or improved function, unless there is clear and strong scientific evidence to support the specific claim. In the meantime, sending patients to good postacute treatment programs, in any or all of the models described above, will maximize their chances of returning to work.

COGNITIVE ENHANCEMENT

The use of pharmacologic means to enhance cognition after TBI is in evolution. The neuroanatomic and neurochemical structures underpinning various aspects of cognition are still being mapped. There are only a few studies looking at the effects of medication on such functions as arousal and attention, initiation, organization and planning, and memory (153,154).

Of cognition-enhancing drugs, dextroamphetamine and methylphenidate, operating on the dopaminergic and noradrenergic systems, have been best studied. These drugs have been used to treat children with attention deficit hyperactivity disorder and have been demonstrated to increase on-task behavior and decrease hyperactivity. Amphetamines cause wakefulness, alertness, and improved concentration and physical performance. Most studies have found some benefit of these neurostimulants on vigilance, processing speed, and memory. It must be emphasized that there are few class I studies to support these findings (155). Amantadine is a dopaminergic agent that has also been studied to some degree in TBI. Again, positive effects have been seen in other disorders such as Parkinson disease, and there has been some promising pilot work performed with this drug (156,157). Cholinomimetic agents (such as citicoline, physostigmine, tacrine, donepezil, and rivastigmine) have been reported to be of benefit in case series in TBI with modest improvement in memory and overall energy levels (158). Treating depression in persons with TBI may result in improved cognitive function as well. A number of other drugs have been used and reported in case series to improve aspects of cognition such as bromocriptine, selegiline, and desipramine (159). Clearly, more research needs to be done to develop clear indications for using neurostimulants and for which populations or what specific cognitive conditions they may be helpful. In the meantime, there is much clinical, empirical use of these agents in persons with TBI. Using an assessment measure (standardized or individualized) to provide objective evidence of improvement in persons with TBI is extremely helpful when deciding whether any medication is useful for an individual.

MILD TBI AND CONCUSSION

Mild traumatic brain injury (MTBI, or concussion) constitutes an important public health problem because it occurs frequently. Probably 75% of all TBIs are mild in nature. It is difficult to accurately estimate the incidence of MTBI because many persons with MTBI are not seen in hospitals or emergency rooms and most statistics do not include persons who receive medical care in other facilities or not at all. Estimates based on a national survey are that 1.5 million people survive a TBI, with 35% of those treated and released from emergency departments, 14% receiving treatment in clinics and physicians' offices, and 25% never receiving medical care (6). Many sports-related injuries are mild in nature, with only 12% hospitalized (125,160). Many persons hospitalized with TBI only stay one night.

There is no universally accepted definition of mild traumatic brain injury. At this time, the recommended conceptual definition of MTBI by the Centers for Disease Control is an injury to the head as a result of blunt trauma or acceleration or deceleration forces that results in one or more of the following conditions: i) any period of observed or self-reported transient confusion, disorientation, or impaired consciousness; ii) dysfunction of memory around the time of injury; and iii) loss of consciousness lasting <30 minutes. In addition, there may be observed signs of neurological or neuropsychological dysfunction that when identified soon after injury can be used to support the diagnosis of MTBI, such as the following: i) seizures immediately following injury to the head; ii) for infants and young children, irritability, lethargy, or vomiting following head injury; and iii) symptoms among older children and adults such as headache, dizziness, irritability, fatigue, or poor concentration (7).

In addition to these criteria for the diagnosis of an MTBI, there should be a credible mechanism sufficient to generate injury (161). Unfortunately, the Glasgow Coma Scale was not originally formulated to describe and categorize milder injuries and is not sensitive to milder injuries. It is possible for an injury to be scored as mild on the GCS even in the presence of abnormalities on imaging studies. Currently these kinds of cases (GCS 13 to 15 with computed tomography [CT] or imaging abnormalities) are referred to as complicated mild or moderate head injuries based on the findings that outcomes are similar to those with GCS of 9 to 12 (162).

While for most clinical purposes MTBI are classified as such on the basis of the previously mentioned criteria and a GCS score of 13 to 15, there have been a number of gradation scales for sports-related concussion that relate to return-to-play criteria (Table 6-6). Recommendations about return to play are still being tested for validity. However, self-reported memory problems in athletes that persist hours after concussion are a good indicator of severity and should be a primary factor to consider in returning an athlete to play (163). Multiple

Table 6-6	Grading Systems for Concussion		
	Cantu (165)	**Colorado Medical Society (165)**	**AAN Practice Parameter (166)**
Grade 1	No LOC; PTA <30 min	Confusion without amnesia; no LOC	Transient confusion; no LOC; concussion symptoms or mental status abnormalities on examination resolve in ≤15 min
Grade 2	LOC ≤5 min in duration or PTA lasting ≥30 min but ≤24 h	Confusion with amnesia; no LOC	Transient confusion; no LOC; concussion symptoms or mental status abnormalities on examination last ≥15 min
Grade 3	LOC ≥5 min or PTA ≥24 h	LOC	Any LOC, either brief (s) or prolonged (min)

AAN, American Academy of Neurology; LOC, loss of consciousness; PTA, post-traumatic amnesia.

concussions predispose a player to more future concussions and result in slower recovery of neurologic function (163).

Generally, recovery from MTBI occurs rapidly. By one month, the effects are mild and selective in young persons with no prior compromising conditions (167–169). Based on the literature, by about three months, these problems resolve in most cases, although a fraction will continue to have problems (167,170–172). Although accurate statistics regarding the number of persons affected are not known, a small percentage have persisting symptoms (including fatigue, insomnia, headache, blurred vision, depressed mood, dizziness, and nausea), often referred to as postconcussion syndrome, that may last significantly longer. There have been no good predictors to indicate which individual may experience difficulty in recovery. Litigation has been implicated by some in slow recovery but studies have been conflicting and resolution of legal matters does not always result in resolution of symptoms.

Management of concussion or MTBI involves initial rest and treatment of associated symptoms. Patients should be instructed to simplify their responsibilities as much as possible at work and home for a few days up to a few weeks. Adequate sleep and avoidance of alcohol or other sedating drugs are recommended. After the first few days, remobilization, while avoiding activities that involve body contact or jarring, is also very important. Early education about the expected course of recovery has been demonstrated to be helpful in several limited studies (173–175).

Symptoms commonly noted in postconcussion syndrome include insomnia, memory difficulties, sensitivity to light and sound, fatigue, headaches, slow performance, poor concentration, anxiety, irritability, word-finding difficulties, distractibility, poor balance, and difficulty in thinking. Many of these symptoms can also be seen in a nonconcussed population and others may be derivative from the presence of pain or anxiety. For instance, insomnia, while present in many people with postconcussive symptoms, is very common in a general rehabilitation population (176). However, there is some evidence to support the notion that alterations to the physiologic stress pathways may in part be responsible for the persistence of some symptoms (161). Regardless, it is important to help the patient isolate symptoms and their treatment from whether or not they were caused by a brain injury. The following paragraphs discuss some general approaches to these common complaints.

Insomnia, particularly difficulty with sleep maintenance, occurs in 27% to 54% of persons with TBI (177,178). This symptom increases dramatically in the setting of pain complaints (179). Early after TBI, there is also an elevated occurrence of sleep apnea, more often central than obstructive (180). Environmental adaptations should be implemented early (such as adequate light exposure and exercise during the day, quiet activities before sleep, darkened room during sleep hours, and minimizing interruptions during the night on the rehabilitation unit). Sedative/hypnotic medications should be tailored to whether the problem is initiation of sleep (short-acting medications) or inability to maintain sleep (longer acting agents). Hypersomnia, on the other hand, can occur in persons with moderate to severe TBI in the absence of identifiable sleep disorders (181).

Although headache is commonly seen after mild TBI, it is misleading to use the singular term posttraumatic headache as a diagnosis. Headaches are likely due to biomechanical forces acting on the neck and muscles inserting onto the skull, but one may also see exacerbation of previous migraine symptoms or, less often, the onset of new migraine headaches. Sleeplessness, anxiety, and blurred vision may worsen headache symptoms so it is crucial to adequately address these co-existing issues. A good examination of the skull, neck, and shoulder girdle is essential. Cervicogenic pain radiating into skull is best treated with physical therapy, rather than with headache-specific medication. It is important to educate the patient in the proper use of medication to treat headaches, such as avoiding the use of regular analgesics, which can cause medication-rebound headaches.

PREVENTION OF TRAUMATIC BRAIN INJURY

While our focus has been on the rehabilitation management of traumatic brain injuries, it is obvious that the most effective way to improve outcomes is to prevent these injuries in the first place. There are a number of ways in which brain injury can be prevented or ameliorated by the use of proper equipment during certain activities. The use of bicycle helmets, for instance, reduced the risk for bicycle-related head injury in Seattle by 74% to 85% (182). The Centers for Disease Control recommend that bicycle helmets be worn by all ages in all places ridden (183). Although motorcycle helmets have been demonstrated to have equivalent efficacy, a number of states have repealed their laws requiring the use of helmets. The results: deaths of nonhelmeted persons at the scene increased from 40% to 75% and severity of injury increased dramatically in Arkansas with virtually identical results in Florida (184,185). There is also some evidence that the use of seat belts, and airbags combined with seat belts, results in a decrease in facial and head trauma in adults involved in motor vehicle crashes (186).

Sports with high incidences of concussion and head injury can be made somewhat safer with appropriate gear and behavior regulation. While professional boxing remains inexcusable with its ultimate goal of causing head injury, amateur boxing has used headguards and strict regulations about body contact and suspending the fight (187). Similarly, it is interesting to note that first concussions occur in Canadian youth hockey around the age of 15, when more aggressive play and body checking are allowed (188).

ACKNOWLEDGMENTS

The authors would like to acknowledge the support of grant award H133A020508, University of Washington Traumatic Brain Injury Model System, National Institute on Disability and Rehabilitation Research, Department of Education.

REFERENCES

1. Guerrero J, Thurman DJ, Sniezek JE. Emergency department visits associated with traumatic brain injury: United States, 1995-1996. *Brain Injury.* 2000; 14(2):181–186.
2. Adekoya N, Thurman DJ, White DD, et al. Surveillance for traumatic brain injury deaths—United States, 1989-1998. *MMWR Surveill Summ.* 2002;51(10):1–14.
3. Thurman DJ, Alverson C, Browne D, et al. *Traumatic brain injury in the United States: A report to congress.* Atlanta, GA: Centers for Disease Control; 1999c.
4. Kraus JF. Epidemiology of head injury. In: Cooper PR, ed. *Head injury.* 3rd ed. Baltimore, MD: Williams & Wilkins; 1993:1–25.
5. Thurman D, Alverson C, Dunn KA, et al. Traumatic brain injury in the United States: A public health perspective. *J Head Trauma Rehabil.* 1999a;14(6):602–615.
6. Sosin DM, Sniezek JE, Thurman DJ. Incidence of mild and moderate brain injury in the United States, 1991. *Brain Inj.* 1996;10(1):47–54.
7. National Center for Injury Prevention and Control. *Report to congress on mild traumatic brain injury in the United States: Steps to prevent a serious public health problem.* Atlanta, GA: Centers for Disease Control; 2003.
8. McGarry LJ, Thompson D, Millham FH, et al. Outcomes and costs of acute treatment of traumatic brain injury. *J Trauma.* 2002;53(6):1152–1159.
9. Mayer NH, Pelensky J, Whyte J, et al. Characterization and correlates of medical and rehabilitation charges for traumatic brain injury during acute rehabilitation hospitalization. *Arch Phys Med Rehabil.* 2003;82(2):242–248.
10. Langlois JA, Kegler SR, Butler JA, et al. Traumatic brain injury-related hospital discharges. Results from a 14-state surveillance system, 1997. *MMWR Surveill Summ.* 2003;52(4):1–20.
11. Centers for Disease Control. Traumatic brain injury— Colorado, Missouri, Oklahoma, and Utah, 1990-1993. *MMWR Morb Mortal Wkly Rep.* 1997a;46(1):8–11.
12. Centers for Disease Control. Sports-related recurrent brain injuries—United States. Centers for Disease Control and Prevention. *Int J Trauma Nurs.* 1997;3(3):88–90.
13. Cross J, Trent R, Adekoya N. Public health and aging: Nonfatal fall-related traumatic brain injury among older adults—California 1996-1999. *MMWR.* 2003;52(13):276–278.
14. DeWitt DS, Prough DS. Traumatic cerebral vascular injury: The effects of concussive brain injury on the cerebral vasculature. *J Neurotrauma.* 2003;20(9): 795–825.
15. Teasdale G, Jennett B. Assessment of coma and impaired consciousness: A practical scale. *Lancet.* 1974;2:81–84.
16. Levin HS. Neurobehavioral outcome of closed head injury: Implications for clinical trials. *J Neurotrauma.* 1995;12(4):601–610.
17. Russell WR, Smith A. Post-traumatic amnesia in closed head injury. *Arch Neurol.* 1961;5:4–17.

18. Dikmen SS, Ross BL, Machamer JE, et al. One year psychosocial outcome in head injury. *J Int Neuropsychol Soc.* 1995d;1(1):67–77.

19. Robinson LR, Micklesen PJ, Tirschwell DL, et al. Predictive value of somatosensory evoked potentials for awakening from coma. *Crit Care Med.* 2003;31: 960–967.

20. Jennett B, Snoek J, Bond MR, et al. Disability after severe head injury: Observations on the use of the Glasgow Outcome Scale. *J Neurol Neurosurg Psychiatry.* 1981a;44:285–293.

21. Wilson JT, Pettigrew LE, Teasdale GM. Structured interviews for the Glasgow Outcome Scale and the extended Glasgow Outcome Scale: Guidelines for their use. *J Neurotrauma.* 1998;15(8):573–585.

22. Rappaport M, Hall KM, Hopkins K, et al. Disability rating scale for severe head trauma: Coma to community. *Arch Phys Med Rehabil.* 1982;63:118–123.

23. Hamilton BB, Granger CV, Sherwin FS. Uniform national data system for medical rehabilitation. In: Fuhrer M, ed. *Rehabilitation outcomes: Analysis and measurement.* Baltimore, MD: Brookes; 1987.

24. Willer B, Kreutzer JS, Gordon WA. Assessment of community integration following rehabilitation for traumatic brain injury. *J Head Trauma Rehabil.* 1993; 8(2):75–85.

25. Dikmen SS, Machamer J, Miller B, et al. Functional status examination: A new instrument for assessing outcome in traumatic brain injury. *J Neurotrauma.* 2001;18(2):127–140.

26. Malec JF, Kragness M, Evans RW, et al. Further psychometric evaluation and revision of the Mayo-Portland Adaptability Inventory in a national sample. *J Head Trauma Rehabil.* 2003;18(6):479–492.

27. Malkmus D, Booth BJ, Kodimer C. *Rehabilitation of head injured adults: Comprehensive management.* Downey, CA: Professional Staff Association of Rancho Los Amigos Hospital; 1980.

28. Mayer N. Clinicophysiologic concepts of spasticity and motor dysfunction in adults with an upper motor neuron lesion. *Muscle Nerve Suppl.* 1997;6:S1–S13.

29. Yarkony G, Saghal V. A major complication of craniocerebral trauma. *Clin Orthop Rel Res.* 1987;219:93.

30. Krauss JK, Jankovic J. Head injury and posttraumatic movement disorders. *Neurosurgery.* 2002;50(5): 927–940.

31. Scott BL, Jankovic J. Delayed-onset progressive movement disorders after static brain lesions. *Neurology.* 1996;46(1):68–74.

32. Pohl M, Ruckriem S, Mehrholz J, et al. Effectiveness of serial casting in patients with severe cerebral spasticity: A comparison study. *Arch Phys Med Rehabil.* 2002;83(6):784–790.

33. Bell KR, Halar EM. Contractures: Prevention and management. *Crit Rev Phys Rehabil Med.* 1990;1(4): 231–246.

34. Gracies J-M, Elovic E, McGuire J, et al. Traditional pharmacological treatments for spasticity Part II: General and regional treatments. *Muscle Nerve Suppl.* 1997;6:S92–S120.

35. Chua KSG, Kong K-H. Alcohol neurolysis of the sciatic nerve in the treatment of hemiplegic knee flexor spasticity: Clinical outcomes. *Arch Phys Med Rehabil.* 2000;81(10):1432–1435.

36. Simpson DM. Clinical trials of botulinum toxin in the treatment of spasticity. *Muscle Nerve Suppl.* 1997;6:S169–S175.

37. Van Schaeybroeck P, Nuttin B, Lagae LES, et al. Intrathecal baclofen for intractable cerebral spasticity: A prospective placebo-controlled, double-blind study. *Neurosurgery.* 2000;46(3):603–612.

38. Smania N, Girardi F, Domenicali C, et al. The rehabilitation of limb apraxia: A study in left-brain-damaged patients. *Arch Phys Med Rehabil.* 2000;81(4):379–388.

39. Diringer MN. Management of sodium abnormalities in patients with CNS disease. *Clin Neuropharmacol.* 1992;15(6):427–447.

40. Palmer BF. Hyponatremia in patients with central nervous system disease: SIADH versus CSW. *Trends Endocrinol Metab.* 2003;14(4):182–187.

41. Webster JB, Bell KR. Primary adrenal insufficiency following traumatic brain injury: A case report and review of the literature. *Arch Phys Med Rehabil.* 1997;78(3):314–318.

42. Childers MK, Rupright J, Jones PS, et al. Assessment of neuroendocrine dysfunction following traumatic brain injury. *Brain Inj.* 1998;12(6):517–523.

43. Bondanelli M, De Marinis L, Ambrosio MR, et al. Occurrence of pituitary dysfunction following traumatic brain injury. *J Neurotrauma.* 2004;21(6):685–696.

44. Benvenga S, Campenni A, Ruggeri RM, et al. Clinical review 113: Hypopituitarism secondary to head trauma. *J Clin Endocrinol Metab.* 2000;85(4): 1353–1361.

45. Schlageter K, Gray B, Hall K, et al. Incidence and treatment of visual dysfunction in traumatic brain injury. *Brain Inj.* 1993;7(5):439–448.

46. Cohen M, Groswasser Z, Barchadski R, et al. Convergence insufficiency in brain-injured patients. *Brain Inj.* 1989;3(2):187–191.

47. Lepore FE. Disorders of ocular motility following head trauma. *Arch Neurol.* 1995;52:924.

48. Fitzsimons F, Fells P. Ocular motility problems following road traffic accidents. *Br Orthop J.* 1989;46:40.

49. Suter PS. Rehabilitation and management of visual dysfunction following traumatic brain injury. In: Ashley MA, ed. *Traumatic brain injury: Rehabilitative treatment and case management.* Boca Raton, FL: CRC Press; 2004:209–249.

50. Davies RA, Luxon LM. Dizziness following head injury: A neuro-otological study. *J Neurol.* 1995; 242(4):222–230.

51. Furman JM, Cass SP. Benign paroxysmal positional vertigo. *N Engl J Med.* 1999;341(21):1590–1596.

52. Katsarkas A. Benign paroxysmal positional vertigo (BPPV): Idiopathic versus post-traumatic. *Acta Otolaryngol.* 1999;119(7):745–749.

53. Callahan CD, Hinkebein JH. Assessment of anosmia after traumatic brain injury: Performance characteristics of the University of Pennsylvania smell identification test. *J Head Trauma Rehabil.* 2002; 17(3):251–256.

54. Ogawa T, Rutka J. Olfactory dysfunction in head injured workers. *Acta Otolaryngol Suppl.* 1999;540: 50–57.

55. Doty RL, Yousem DM, Pham LT, et al. Olfactory dysfunction in patients with head trauma. *Arch Neurol.* 1997;54(9):1131–1140.

56. Lemke DM. Riding out the storm: Sympathetic storming after traumatic brain injury. *J Neurosci. Nurs.* 2004;36(1):4–9.

57. Asikainen I, Kaste M, Sarna S. Early and late post-traumatic seizures in traumatic brain injury rehabilitation patients: Brain injury factors causing late

seizures and influence of seizures on long-term outcomes. *Epilepsia.* 1999;40:584–589.

58. Salazar AM, Jabbari B, Vance SC, et al. Epilepsy after penetrating head injury. I. Clinical correlates: A report of the Vietnam head injury study. *Neurology.* 1985a;35:1406–1414.
59. Bushnik T, Englander J, Duong TT. Medical and social issues related to posttraumatic seizures in persons with traumatic brain injury. *J Head Trauma Rehabil.* 2004;19(4):296–304.
60. Annegers JF, Hauser WA, Coan SP, et al. A population-based study of seizures after traumatic brain injuries. *N Engl J Med.* 1998;338(1):20–24.
61. Temkin NR, Dikmen SS, Wilensky AJ, et al. A randomized, double-blind study of phenytoin for the prevention of post-traumatic seizures. *N Engl J Med.* 1990;323(8):497–502.
62. Brain Injury Special Interest Group of the American Academy of Physical Medicine and Rehabilitation. Practice parameter: Antiepileptic drug treatment of posttraumatic seizures. *Arch Phys Med Rehabil.* 1998; 79(5):594–597.
63. Englander J, Bushnik T, Duong TT, et al. Analyzing risk factors for late posttraumatic seizures: A prospective, multicenter investigation. *Arch Phys Med Rehabil.* 2003;84(3):365–373.
64. Diaz-Arrastia R, Gong Y, Fair S, et al. Increased risk of late posttraumatic seizures associated with inheritance of APOE epsilon4 allele. *Arch Neurol.* 2003; 60(6):818–822.
65. Annegers JF, Coan SP. The risks of epilepsy after traumatic brain injury. *Seizure.* 2000;9(7):453–457.
66. Haltiner AM, Temkin NR, Dikmen SS. Risk of seizure recurrence after the first late posttraumatic seizure. *Arch Phys Med Rehabil.* 1997;78(8):835–840.
67. Yablon SA. Posttraumatic seizures. *Arch Phys Med Rehabil.* 1993;74(9):983–1001.
68. Cosgrove JL. A prospective study of peripheral nerve lesions occurring in traumatic brain-injured patients. *Am J Phys Med Rehabil.* 1989;68(1):15–17.
69. Stone L, Keenan MA. Peripheral nerve injuries in the adult with traumatic brain injury. *Clin Orthop.* 1988;233:136–144.
70. Shen J. Peripheral nerve injury following traumatic brain injury. *Phys Med Rehabil State Art Rev.* 1993; 7(3):503–518.
71. Kushwaha VP, Garland DG. Extremity fractures in the patient with a traumatic brain injury. *J Am Acad Orthop Surg.* 1998;6(5):298–307.
72. Sobus KM, Alexander MA, Harcke HT. Undetected musculoskeletal trauma in children with traumatic brain injury or spinal cord injury. *Arch Phys Med Rehabil.* 1993;74(9):902–904.
73. Buschbacher R. Heterotopic ossification: A review. *Crit Rev Phys Rehabil Med.* 1992;4(3,4):199–213.
74. Wildburger R, Zarkovic N, Tonkovic G, et al. Posttraumatic hormonal disturbances: Prolactin as a link between head injury and enhanced osteogenesis. *J Endocrinol Invest.* 1998;21(2):78–86.
75. Ebinger T, Roesch M, Kiefer H, et al. Influence of etiology in heterotopic bone formation of the hip. *J Trauma.* 2000;48(6):1058–1062.
76. Ippolito E, Formisano R, Farsetti P, et al. Excision for the treatment of periarticular ossification of the knee in patients who have a traumatic brain injury. *J Bone Joint Surg Am.* 1999;81(6):783–789.

77. Andersson S, Bergedalen AM. Cognitive correlates of apathy in traumatic brain injury. *Neuropsychiatry Neuropsychol Behav Neurol.* 2002;15(3):184–191.
78. Wroblewski BA, Glenn MB. Pharmacological treatment of arousal and cognitive deficits. *J Head Trauma Rehabil.* 1994;9(3):19–42.
79. Marin RS, Fogel BS, Hawkins J, et al. Apathy: A treatable syndrome. *J Neuropsychiatry Clin Neurosci.* 1995;7(1):23–30.
80. Roca RP, Santmyer K, Gloth FM, et al. Improvements in activity and appetite among long-term care patients treated with amantadine. A clinical report. *J Am Geriatr Soc.* 1990;38(6):675–677.
81. Dikmen SS, Bombardier CH, Machamer JE, et al. Natural history of depression in traumatic brain injury. *Arch Phys Med Rehabil.* 2004;85(9):1457–1464.
82. Jorge RE, Robinson RG, Moser D, et al. Major depression following traumatic brain injury. *Arch Gen Psychiatry.* 2004;61(1):42–50.
83. Hibbard MR, Ashman TA, Spielman LA, et al. Relationship between depression and psychosocial functioning after traumatic brain injury. *Arch Phys Med Rehabil.* 2004;85(4 Suppl 2):S43–S53.
84. Fann JR, Uomoto JM, Katon WJ. Sertraline in the treatment of major depression following mild traumatic brain injury. *J Neuropsychiatry Clin Neurosci.* 2000;12(2):226–232.
85. Perino C, Rago R, Cicolini A, et al. Mood and behavioural disorders following traumatic brain injury: Clinical evaluation and pharmacological management. *Brain Inj.* 2001;15(2):139–148.
86. Wroblewski BA, Joseph AB, Cornblatt RR. Antidepressant pharmacotherapy and the treatment of depression in patients with severe traumatic brain injury: A controlled, prospective study. *J Clin Psychiatry.* 1996;57(12):582–587.
87. Kreutzer JS, Witol AD, Marwitz JH. Alcohol and drug use among young persons with traumatic brain injury. *J Learn Disabil.* 1996;29(6):643–651.
88. Dikmen SS, Machamer JE, Donovan DM, et al. Alcohol use before and after traumatic head injury. *Ann Emerg Med.* 1995b;26(2):167–176.
89. Bombardier CH, Temkin NR, Machamer J, et al. The natural history of drinking and alcohol-related problems after traumatic brain injury. *Arch Phys Med Rehabil.* 2003;84(2):185–191.
90. Harvey AG, Brewin CR, Jones C, et al. Coexistence of posttraumatic stress disorder and traumatic brain injury: Towards a resolution of the paradox. *J Int Neuropsychol Soc.* 2003;9(4):663–676.
91. Bryant RA. Posttraumatic stress disorder and mild brain injury: Controversies, causes and consequences. *J Clin Exp Neuropsychol.* 2001;23(6):718–728.
92. Levin HS, Brown SA, Song JX, et al. Depression and posttraumatic stress disorder at three months after mild to moderate traumatic brain injury. *J Clin Exp Neuropsychol.* 2001;23(6):754–769.
93. Bryant RA, Moulds M, Guthrie R, et al. Treating acute stress disorder following mild traumatic brain injury. *Am J Psychiatry.* 2003;160(3):585–587.
94. Fann JR, Burington B, Leonetti A, et al. Psychiatric illness following traumatic brain injury in an adult health maintenance organization population. *Arch Gen Psychiatry.* 2004;61(1):53–61.
95. Dikmen SS, Machamer JE, Winn HR, et al. Neuropsychological outcome at 1-year post head injury. *Neuropsychology.* 1995c;9(1):80–90.

96. Dikmen S, Machamer JE. Neurobehavioral outcomes and their determinants. *J Head Trauma Rehabil.* 1995a;10(1):74–86.

97. Foulkes MA, Eisenberg HM, Jane JA, et al. Group at TCDBR. The Traumatic Coma Data Bank: Design, methods, and baseline characteristics. *J Neurosurg.* 1991;75:S8–S13.

98. Marshall LF, Gautille T, Klauber MR. The outcome of severe closed head injury. *J Neurosurg.* 1991;75: S28–S36.

99. Chesnut RM. Evolving models of neurotrauma critical care: An analysis and call to action. *Clin Neurosurg.* 2000;46:185–195.

100. Tate RL, Lulham JM, Broe GA, et al. Psychosocial outcome for survivors of severe blunt head injury: The results from a consecutive series of 100 patients. *J Neurol Neurosurg Psychiatry.* 1989;52:1128–1134.

101. Dikmen SS, Machamer JE, Powell JM, et al. Outcome 3 to 5 years after moderate to severe traumatic brain injury. *Arch Phys Med Rehabil.* 2003;84(10):1449–1457.

102. Temkin NR, Machamer JE, Dikmen SS. Correlates of functional status 3-5 years after traumatic brain injury with CT abnormalities. *J Neurotrauma.* 2003; 20(3):229–241.

103. Sherer M, Novack TA, Sander AM, et al. Neuropsychological assessment and employment outcome after traumatic brain injury: A review. *Clin Neuropsychol.* 2002a;16(2):157–178.

104. Sherer M, Sander AM, Nick TG, et al. Early cognitive status and productivity outcome after traumatic brain injury: Findings from the TBI model systems. *Arch Phys Med Rehabil.* 2002b;83(2):183–192.

105. Dikmen SS, Temkin NR, Machamer JE, et al. Employment following traumatic head injuries. *Arch Neurol.* 1994;51(2):177–186.

106. Fugate LP, Spacek LA, Kresty LA, et al. Definition of agitation following traumatic brain injury: I. A survey of the Brain Injury Special Interest Group of the American Academy of Physical Medicine and Rehabilitation. *Arch Phys Med Rehabil.* 1997;78(9):917–923.

107. Corrigan J, Mysiw WJ, Gribble MW, et al. Agitation, cognition, and attention during post-traumatic amnesia. *Brain Inj.* 1992;6(2):155–160.

108. Bogner JA, Corrigan JD, Fugate L, et al. Role of agitation in prediction of outcomes after traumatic brain injury. *Am J Phys Med Rehabil.* 2001;80(9):636–644.

109. Deb S, Crownshaw T. The role of pharmacotherapy in the management of behaviour disorders in traumatic brain injury patients. *Brain Inj.* 2004;18(1):1–31.

110. Corrigan JD. Development of a scale for assessment of agitation following traumatic brain injury. *J Clin Exp Neuropsychol* 1989;11(2):261–277.

111. Yudofsky SC, Silver JM, Jackson W, et al. The Overt Aggression Scale for the objective rating of verbal and physical aggression. *Am J Psychiatry.* 1986; 143(1):35–39.

112. Wilson MS, Gibson CJ, Hamm RJ. Haloperidol, but not olanzapine, impairs cognitive performance after traumatic brain injury in rats. *Am J Phys Med Rehabil.* 2003;82(11):871–879.

113. Levin HS, Saydjari C, Eisenberg HM, et al. Vegetative state after closed-head injury. A traumatic coma data bank report. *Arch Neurol.* 1991;48(6):580–585.

114. Rudehill A, Bellander BM, Weitzberg E, et al. Outcome of traumatic brain injuries in 1,508 patients: Impact of prehospital care. *J Neurotrauma.* 2002; 19(7):855–868.

115. Murray GD, Teasdale GM, Braakman R, et al. The European brain injury consortium survey of head injuries. *Acta Neurochir (Wien).* 1999;141(3):223–236.

116. The Multi-Society Task Force on PVS. Medical aspects of the persistent vegetative state (1). *N Engl J Med.* 1994a;330(21):1499–1508.

117. The Multi-Society Task Force on PVS. Medical aspects of the persistent vegetative state (2). *N Engl J Med.* 1994b;330(22):1572–1579.

118. Plum F, Schiff N, Ribary U, et al. Coordinated expression in chronically unconscious persons. *Philos Trans R Soc Lond B Biol Sci.* 1998;353(1377):1929–1933.

119. Andrews K. Prediction of recovery from post-traumatic vegetative state. *Lancet.* 1998;351(9118):1751.

120. Lombardi F, Taricco M, De Tanti A, et al. Sensory stimulation of brain-injured individuals in coma or vegetative state: Results of a Cochrane systematic review. *Clin Rehabil.* 2002;16(5):464–472.

121. Katz DI, White DK, Alexander MP, et al. Recovery of ambulation after traumatic brain injury. *Arch Phys Med Rehabil.* 2004;85(6):865–869.

122. Kreutzer JS, Kolakowsky-Hayner SA, Ripley D, et al. Charges and lengths of stay for acute and inpatient rehabilitation treatment of traumatic brain injury 1990–1996. *Brain Inj.* 2001;15(9):763–774.

123. Ben-Yishay Y, Diller L. Rehabilitation of cognitive and perceptual defects in people with traumatic brain damage. *Int J Rehabil Res.* 1981;4(2):208–210.

124. Prigatano GP, Fordyce DJ, Zeiner HK, et al. Neuropsychological rehabilitation after closed head injury in young adults. *J Neurol Neurosurg Psychiatry.* 1984;47(5):505–513.

125. Kutschinski WR. Milieu therapy under the primary caretaker system at the University of Michigan's Children's Psychiatric Hospital. *Child Psychiatry Hum Dev.* 1977;8(1):31–42.

126. Kahn EM, White EM. Adapting milieu approaches to acute inpatient care for schizophrenic patients. *Hosp Community Psychiatry.* 1989;40(6):609–614.

127. Bitter JA. Using employer job-sites in evaluation of the mentally retarded for employability. *Ment Retard.* 1967;5(3):21–22.

128. Krauss MW, MacEachron AE. Competitive employment training for mentally retarded adults: The supported work model. *Am J Ment Defic.* 1982;86(6): 650–653.

129. Lezak MD. *Neuropsychological assessment.* New York, NY: Oxford University Press; 1976.

130. Hilgard ER, Bower GH. *Theories of learning.* Englewood Cliffs, NJ: Prentice-Hall; 1975.

131. Stolov WC, Clowers MR. *Handbook of severe disability: A text for rehabilitation counselors, other vocational practitioners, and allied health professionals.* Washington, DC: US Department of Education, Rehabilitation Services Administration; 1981.

132. Kottke F, Lehmann JF. *Krusen's handbook of physical medicine and rehabilitation.* Philadelphia, PA: WB Saunders; 1990.

133. Pepping M, Roueche JR. Psychosocial consequences of severe brain injury. In: Tupper D, Cicerone K, eds. *The neuropsychology of everyday life: Issues in development and rehabilitation.* Vol. II. Boston, MA: Kluwer Academic Publishers; 1990.

134. Malec JF, Basford JS. Postacute brain injury rehabilitation. *Arch Phys Med Rehabil.* 1996;77(2):198–207.

135. Klonoff PS, Lamb DG, Henderson SW. Milieu-based neurorehabilitation in patients with traumatic brain

injury: Outcome at up to 11 years postdischarge. *Arch Phys Med Rehabil.* 2000;81(11):1535–1537.

136. Cicerone KD, Mott T, Azulay J, et al. Community integration and satisfaction with functioning after intensive cognitive rehabilitation for traumatic brain injury. *Arch Phys Med Rehabil.* 2004;85(6):943–950.

137. Hanks RA, Temkin N, Machamer J, et al. Emotional and behavioral adjustment after traumatic brain injury. *Arch Phys Med Rehabil.* 1999;80(9):991–997.

138. Rothweiler B, Temkin NR, Dikmen SS. Aging effect on psychosocial outcome in traumatic brain injury. *Arch Phys Med Rehabil.* 1998;79(8):881–887.

139. Pace GM, Schlund MW, Hazard-Haupt T, et al. Characteristics and outcomes of a home and community-based neurorehabilitation programme. *Brain Inj.* 1999;13(7):535–546.

140. Wehman PH, Kreutzer JS, West MD, et al. Return to work for persons with traumatic brain injury: A supported employment approach. *Arch Phys Med Rehabil.* 1990;71(13):1047–1052.

141. Wehman P, Sherron P, Kregel J, et al. Return to work for persons following severe traumatic brain injury. Supported employment outcomes after five years. *Am J Phys Med Rehabil.* 1993;72(6):355–363.

142. Yasuda S, Wehman P, Targett P, et al. Return to work for persons with traumatic brain injury. *Am J Phys Med Rehabil.* 2001;80(11):852–864.

143. Malec JF, Buffington AL, Moessner AM, et al. A medical/vocational case coordination system for persons with brain injury: An evaluation of employment outcomes. *Arch Phys Med Rehabil.* 2000;81(8):1007–1015.

144. Fraser RT, Clemmons D, Trejo W, et al. Program evaluation in epilepsy rehabilitation. *Epilepsia.* 1983;24(6):734–746.

145. Malec JF, Degiorgio L. Characteristics of successful and unsuccessful completers of 3 postacute brain injury rehabilitation pathways. *Arch Phys Med Rehabil.* 2002;83(12):1759–1764.

146. Bell KR, Hoffman JM, Doctor JN, et al. Development of a telephone follow up program for individuals following traumatic brain injury. *J Head Trauma Rehabil.* 2004;19(6):502–512.

147. Bell KR, Temkin NR, Esselman PC, et al. The effect of scheduled telephone counseling on outcome after moderate to severe traumatic brain injury: A randomized trial. *Arch Phys Med Rehabil.* 2005;86(5):851–856.

148. Powell JM, Hunt E, Pepping M. Collaboration between cognitive science and cognitive rehabilitation: A call for action. *J Head Trauma Rehabil.* 2004;9(3):266–276.

149. Jordan BD. Cognitive rehabilitation following traumatic brain injury. *JAMA.* 2000;283(23):3123–3124.

150. Prigatano GP. Rehabilitation for traumatic brain injury. *JAMA* 2000;284(14):1783; author reply 1784.

151. D'Zurilla T, Goldfried M. Problem solving and behavior modification. *J Abnorm Psychol.* 1971;78:107–126.

152. Ponsford J. Update on neuropsychological rehabilitation in Australia. Vipiteno, Australia: Second International Conference on Neuropsychological Rehabilitation; June 9–12, 2004.

153. Glenn MB. A differential diagnostic approach to the pharmacological treatment of cognitive, behavioral, and affective disorders after traumatic brain injury. *J Head Trauma Rehabil.* 2002;17(4):273–283.

154. Cope DN. An integration of psychopharmacological and rehabilitation approaches to traumatic brain injury rehabilitation. *J Head Trauma Rehabil.* 1994; 9(3):1–18.

155. Whyte J, Vaccaro M, Grieb-Neff P, et al. Psychostimulant use in the rehabilitation of individuals with traumatic brain injury. *J Head Trauma Rehabil.* 2002; 17(4):284–299.

156. Cowell LD, Cohen RF. Amantadine: A potential adjuvant therapy following traumatic brain injury. *J Head Trauma Rehabil.* 1995;10(6):91–94.

157. Meythaler JM, Brunner RC, Johnson A, et al. Amantadine to improve neurorecovery in traumatic brain injury-associated diffuse axonal injury: A pilot double-blind randomized trial. *J Head Trauma Rehabil.* 2002;17(4):300–313.

158. Blount PJ, Nguyen CD, McDeavitt JT. Clinical use of cholinomimetic agents: A review. *J Head Trauma Rehabil.* 2002;17(4):314–321.

159. Mysiw WJ, Clinchot DM. Medications to enhance cognitive functioning. *Phys Med Rehabil Clin N Am.* 1997;8(4):781–796.

160. Thurman DJ, Branche CM, Sniezek JE. The epidemiology of sports-related traumatic brain injuries in the United States: Recent developments. *J Head Trauma Rehabil.* 1998;13(2):1–8.

161. Rees PM. Comtemporary issues in mild traumatic brain injury. *Arch Phys Med Rehabil.* 2003;84(12): 1885–1894.

162. Williams DH, Levin HS, Eisenberg HM. Mild head injury classification. *Neurosurgery.* 1990;27(3): 422–428.

163. Guskiewicz KM, McCrea M, Marshall SW, et al. Cumulative effects associated with recurrent concussions in collegiate football players: The NCAA Concussion Study. *JAMA.* 2003;290(19):2549–2555.

164. Cantu RC. Cerebral concussion in sport. Management and prevention. *Sports Med.* 1992;14(1):64–74.

165. Kelly JP, Nichols JS, Filley CM, et al. Concussion in sports. Guidelines for the prevention of catastrophic outcome. *JAMA.* 1991;266(20):2867–2869.

166. Subcommittee QS. Practice parameter: The management of concussion in sports (summary statement). *Neurology.* 1997;48(3):581–585.

167. Levin HS, Amparo E, Eisenberg HM, et al. Magnetic resonance imaging and computerized tomography in relation to the neurobehavioral sequelae of mild and moderate head injuries. *J Neurosurg.* 1987;66: 706–713.

168. Dikmen SS, McLean A, Temkin N. Neuropsychological and psychosocial consequences of minor head injury. *J Neurol Neurosurg Psychiatr.* 1986;49: 1227–1232.

169. Paniak C, Reynolds S, Phillips K, et al. Patient complaints within 1 month of mild traumatic brain injury: A controlled study. *Arch Clin Neuropsychol.* 2002;17:319–334.

170. Alexander MP. Mild traumatic brain injury: Pathophysiology, natural history, and clinical management. *Neurology.* 1995;45:1253–1260.

171. Barth JT, Macciocchi SN, Giordani B, et al. Neuropsychological sequelae of minor head injury. *Neurosurgery.* 1983;13:529–533.

172. Levin HS, Grafman J, Eisenberg HM. *Neurobehavioral recovery from head injury.* New York, NY: Oxford University Press; 1987.

173. Paniak C, Toller-Lobe G, Durand A, et al. A randomized trial of two treatments for mild traumatic brain injury. *Brain Inj.* 1998;12(12):1011–1023.

174. Paniak C, Toller-Lobe G, Reynolds S, et al. A randomized trial of two treatments for mild traumatic brain injury: 1 year follow-up. *Brain Inj.* 2000;14(3):219–226.

175. Mittenberg W, Canyock EM, Condit C, et al. Treatment of post-concussion syndrome following mild head injury. *J Clin Exp Neuropsychol.* 2001;23(6):829–836.

176. Fichtenberg NL, Zafonte RD, Putnam S, et al. Insomnia in a post-acute brain injury sample. *Brain Inj.* 2002;16(3):197–206.

177. Thaxton L, Myers MA. Sleep disturbances and their management in patients with brain injury. *J Head Trauma Rehabil.* 2002;17(4):335–348.

178. Clinchot DM, Bogner J, Mysiw WJ, et al. Defining sleep disturbance after brain injury. *Am J Phys Med Rehabil.* 1998;77(4):291–295.

179. Beetar JD, Guilmette TJ, Sparadeo FR. Sleep and pain complaints in symptomatic traumatic brain injury and neurologic populations. *Arch Phys Med Rehabil.* 1996;77:1298–1302.

180. Webster JB, Bell KR, Hussey JD, et al. Sleep apnea in adults with traumatic brain injury: A preliminary investigation. *Arch Phys Med Rehabil.* 2001;82:316–321.

181. Masel BE, Scheibel RS, Kimbark T, et al. Excessive daytime sleepiness in adults with brain injuries. *Arch Phys Med Rehabil.* 2001;82(11):1526–1532.

182. Thompson RS, Rivara FP, Thompson DC. A case-control study of the effectiveness of bicycle safety helmets. *N Engl J Med.* 1989;320:1361–1367.

183. Centers for Disease Control and Prevention Injury-control recommendations: Bicycle helmets. *MMWR Surveill Summ.* 1995;44(RR-1):1–17.

184. Bledsoe GH, Schexnayder SM, Carey MJ, et al. The negative impact of the repeal of the Arkansas motorcycle helmet law. *J Trauma.* 2002;53:1078–1087.

185. Hotz GA, Cohn SM, Popkin C, et al. The impact of a repealed motorcycle helmet law in Miami-Dade County. *J Trauma.* 2002;52:469–474.

186. Mouzakes J, Koltai PJ, Kuhar S, et al. The impact of airbags and seat belts on the incidence and severity of maxillofacial injuries in automobile accidents in New York State. *Arch Otolaryngol Head Neck Surg.* 2001;127(10):1189–1193.

187. Jako P. Safety measures in amateur boxing. *Br J Sports Med.* 2002;36:394–395.

188. Goodman D, HGaetz M, Meichenbaum D. Concussions in hockey: There is cause for concern. *Med Sci Sports Exerc.* 2001;33:2004–2009.

7

Spinal Cord Injury

Diana D. Cardenas, Jeanne M. Hoffman, and Pam L. Stockman

EPIDEMIOLOGY OF TRAUMATIC SPINAL CORD INJURY

The incidence of spinal cord injury (SCI) in the United States is estimated to be about 40 cases per million population per year or approximately 11,000 new cases per year. Since there is no mandatory national surveillance system for such injuries in place, the true incidence is unknown. The estimated prevalence in the United States as of December 2003 is between 219,000 and 279,000 persons. Recent data suggest that the age at injury is correlated to survival, with a markedly decreased life expectancy in older persons, especially those with cervical injuries and complete injuries as compared to age-matched controls. The average age at injury for those injured after 2000 is 35.9 years, which is higher than in past decades. Another trend is an increase in the proportion of those who were at least 61 years of age at injury, which has increased from 4.7% in the 1970s to 11.4% since 2000. Male patients comprise about 80% of all those who are injured and the ratio of 4:1, male patients to female patients, has remained stable for the last three decades.

ETIOLOGY/PATHOPHYSIOLOGY

The most common etiology of SCI since 1990 is motor vehicle accidents (40.9%), followed by falls (22.4%), acts of violence (21.6%), and sports injuries (7.5%). The proportion of spinal cord injuries from acts of violence (primarily gunshot wounds) and falls has increased steadily since 1973. The most frequent neurologic category is incomplete tetraplegia (30.8%), followed by complete paraplegia (26.6%), incomplete paraplegia (19.7%), and complete tetraplegia (18.6%). Rarely is there a complete transection of the spinal cord; however, complete transection is not necessary for a complete lesion. Bleeding, infarction, and severe crush injuries can all produce clinically complete lesions. Serial examinations are important to determine if there has been any change in the patient's neurologic status. To date, there remains only one pharmacologic intervention, immediate intravenous administration of methlyprednisolone, which has been shown to have a beneficial effect on recovery after acute SCI. This steroid helps reduce free radical damage and lipid peroxidation when given within the first few hours of injury.

MODEL SPINAL CORD INJURY SYSTEMS

The Department of Education through the National Institute on Disability and Rehabilitation Research has funded a program since the mid-1970s to collect data from large SCI centers into a national data bank. The results of this Model Systems program provide useful information regarding the epidemiology, costs, and complications associated with SCI. The data collected includes the use of the standards for neurologic classification developed under the leadership of the American Spinal Injury Association (ASIA) (1). This standard classification system ensures that better information regarding outcomes across multiple centers is available. Those involved in SCI care should be familiar with this classification system.

NEUROLOGIC CLASSIFICATION

Determination of the neurologic level of injury is made based on the results of the motor and sensory examination. Classification of the injury is made by examination of the sensory and motor levels, as well as by the pattern of injury. Standard dermatome and myotome references have been established by ASIA. The level of injury is defined as the last caudal segment with intact motor and sensory innervation. The initial examination should occur within 72 hours of the injury and be conducted with the patient in the supine position. The injury is defined as incomplete if there is sparing of sensory or motor function below the neurologic level that includes the S4/5 segments. Comprehensive clinical examination of the SCI patient, with correct ASIA classification, is imperative not only for documenting clinical changes, but also for determining functional prognosis. Practitioners should refer to the *International Standards for Neurological and Functional Classification of Spinal Cord Injury*, published by ASIA, for comprehensive instructions (1). Examination and classification are facilitated by having the scoring chart (Fig. 7–1) available for marking during the exam.

ASIA scoring requires that the key muscles in the myotome have at least antigravity grade-3 muscle strength and be considered to have intact innervation if the segment above has grade 5 strength. A left and right motor and sensory level may be obtained. Refer to Figure 7–1 for the ten key muscles. It is also important to know the concept of upper motor neuron (UMN) and lower motor neuron (LMN) injury. Volitional, controlled muscle movement requires both UMN and LMN innervation. Assessment of UMN versus LMN injury must be made once the period of spinal shock resolves after the initial injury.

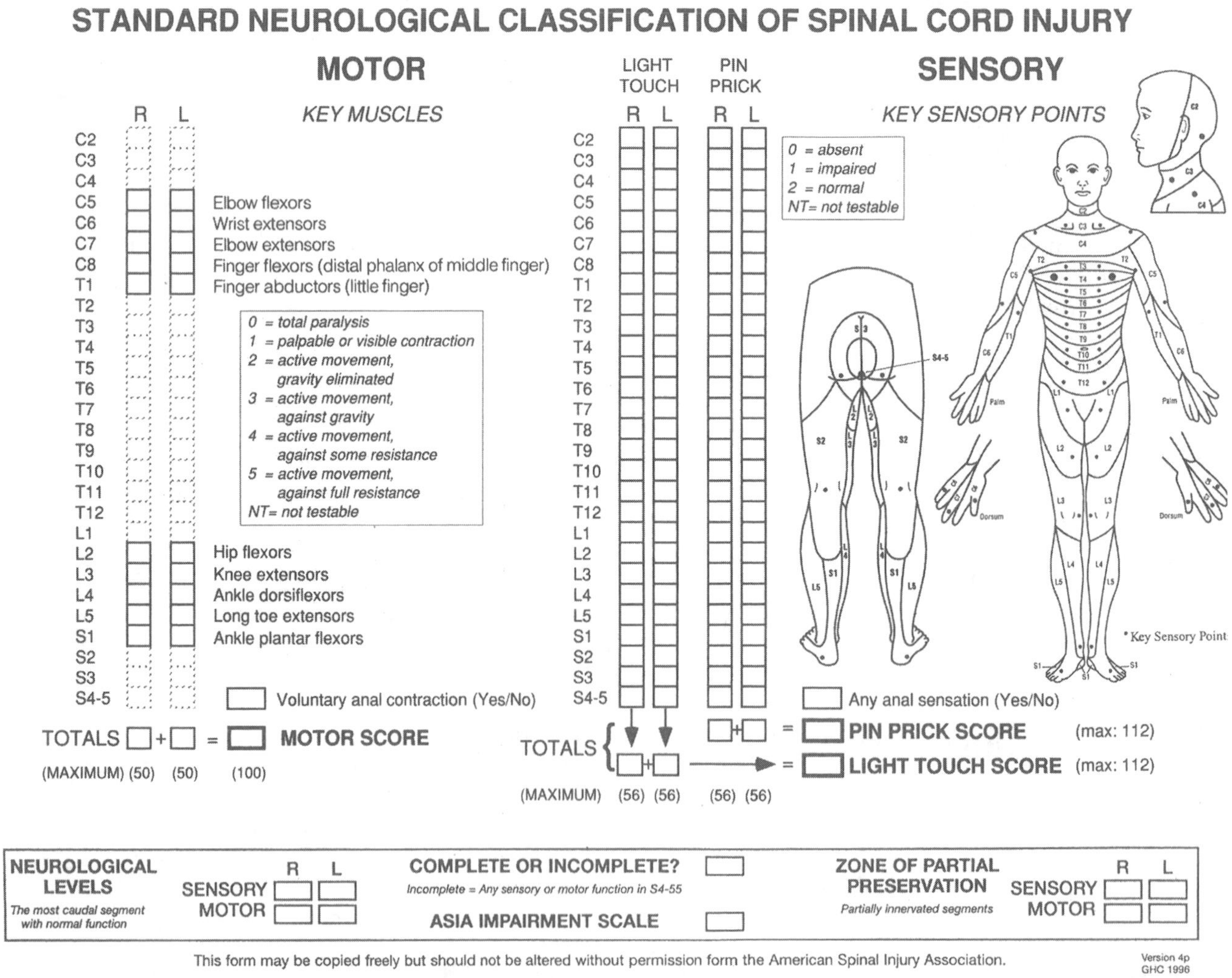

Figure 7–1. Standard neurologic classification of spinal cord injury, 2000. (From American Spinal Injury Association and the International Medical Society of Paraplegia. *International standards for neurological classification of spinal cord injury.* Chicago, IL: American Spinal Injury Association and the International Medical Society of Paraplegia; 2000, with permission.)

CLINICAL SYNDROMES THAT CAN RESULT FROM SCI

At least six different clinical syndromes can result from SCI. The characteristics of the injury determine which syndrome results. Four of these syndromes are depicted in Figure 7–2. Each one carries its own set of prognostic indications and impact on treatment. These syndromes are as follows:

Central Cord Syndrome

Central cord syndrome usually results from a cervical-level hyperextension injury with hematoma formation in the central cervical spinal cord, which results in weaker upper extremities compared to lower extremities (Fig. 7–2).

Brown Sequard Syndrome

Brown Sequard syndrome occurs from a lesion to half of the spinal cord in the axial plane, resulting in weakness, spasticity, and alteration of light touch on one side of the body, with decreased pain/temperature sensation on the opposite side (caused by the decussation of the anterolateral spinothalamic tract within the cord) (Fig. 7–2).

Cauda Equina Syndrome

Cauda equina syndrome occurs when lesions below the conus medullaris result in LMN type of symptoms, with flaccid lower extremities, bowel, and bladder.

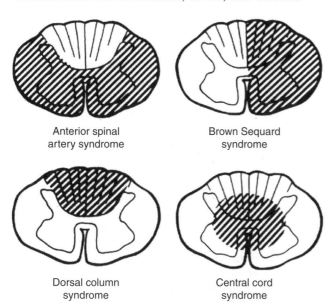

Anterior spinal artery syndrome

Brown Sequard syndrome

Dorsal column syndrome

Central cord syndrome

Figure 7–2. Incomplete clinical syndromes. (From Hays RM, Kraft GH, Stolov WC, eds. *Chronic disease and disability: A contemporary rehabilitation approach to medical practice*. New York, NY: Demos Publications; 1994:144, with permission.)

Conus Medullaris Syndrome

Conus medullaris syndrome occurs with lesions at the level of the conus and usually results in an areflexic bladder, bowel, and lower limbs.

Anterior Spinal Artery Syndrome

Anterior spinal artery syndrome (also known as the anterior cord syndrome) results from vascular injury to the anterior spinal artery, thus causing bilateral weakness, spasticity, and loss of pain/temperature sensation with sparing of bilateral proprioception and light touch sensation associated with the posterior columns (Fig. 7–2).

Dorsal Column Syndrome

Dorsal column syndrome (also known as the posterior cord syndrome) is a rare syndrome that occurs with a lesion to the posterior third of the spinal cord, causing loss of posterior column sensory function and motor weakness (Fig. 7–2).

ACUTE MANAGEMENT ISSUES

The acutely injured patient requires a comprehensive systematic assessment. This includes evaluation of spinal stability, as well as assessment of neurologic, musculoskeletal, pulmonary, cardiovascular, gastrointestinal, genitourinary, and integumentary systems. The role of the physiatrist is to assist in early consultative care of the patient, to lead the team that works with the patient during initial inpatient rehabilitation, and to bring a systematic and coordinated team approach to all the patient's bodily functions. The initial rehabilitation is critical to the patient to prevent complications and for his or her future health and well-being.

EVALUATION OF SPINAL STABILITY

Skeletal spinal stability evaluation is based on a division of upper cervical, lower cervical, and thoracolumbar injuries. Radiographic studies must visualize all components of the spine. A cervical spine x-ray series must include an open-mouth odontoid view, swimmer's view (to visualize C7), and anterior-posterior, lateral, and bilateral oblique views. A computerized tomography (CT) scan is also often needed to identify fractures and the extent of compromise, and magnetic resonance imaging (MRI) is needed to determine ligamentous injury affecting stability. Based on the type and extent of injury, it is determined if the injury requires surgery versus external orthotic intervention. Postoperatively the injury will require an additional 10 to 12 weeks for complete healing; therefore, an external orthotic device must often be used to reduce motion across the surgical construct. The choice of orthotic device depends on the degree and type of stabilizing force required. There are many different types of cervical orthoses, including the Minerva, halo vest, Miami J, and Philadelphia collar. Thoracolumbar sacral orthoses (TLSO) are also available in a variety of brands; however, a custom-molded TLSO is usually the best choice for optimal stability. After the appropriate period of time, flexion/extension films in an upright position with external support removed must be obtained in order to determine stability. When stability is achieved, the individual is usually weaned away from use of a brace, as the underlying muscles will be initially deconditioned and weakened.

INITIAL REHABILITATION

MUSCULOSKELETAL ASSESSMENT

Following the period of spinal shock, patients with UMN lesions will begin developing spasticity. Spasticity is a velocity-dependent increase in tone and may be elicited by using a reflex hammer on tendons or by giving quick-stretch to the muscle. Most SCI patients develop a primarily extensor pattern of lower-extremity spasticity. Spasticity can also be exacerbated or set off by a variety of medical complications, such as urinary tract infections (UTIs), heterotopic ossification (HO), pressure ulcers, or a noxious stimulus such as an ingrown toenail. Assessment of spasticity should be performed with the patient in different positions, since an extended posture will usually enhance spasticity, and components of postural flexion will tend to diminish spasticity. The patient may complain of increased spasticity at night when in a recumbent extended position.

The Ashworth scale or the modified Ashworth scale is a simple bedside measure that is easy to administer and is often used along with tendon taps and testing for clonus to evaluate spasticity (2,3). In the Ashworth scale, 0 = no increase in tone and 4 = limb rigid in flexion extension with lesser degrees of tone between these endpoints.

Assessment of musculoskeletal pain after SCI is complex. Musculoskeletal pain must be distinguished from neuropathic pain caused from abnormal neural signals initiated by the spinal cord damage. This distinction is important because both the pharmacologic and nonpharmacologic treatment is dependent upon the etiology of the pain. Musculoskeletal pain is more likely to be related to activity and, unlike neuropathic spinal cord injury pain, is affected by change of position (4). Treatment will be discussed in the next section. Clinicians should perform a comprehensive pain assessment, using an objective scale when possible. The visual analog scale is frequently and easily used. The patient is requested to rate the degree of pain on a 10-point scale of intensity, with a score of 0 as no pain and a score of 10 as the worst pain one can imagine. Pain assessment should include questions about traumatic versus nontraumatic sources of the pain, and situations that cause the pain to be better or worse. SCI patients will usually describe neuropathic pain as burning, tingling, radiating, hypersensitive, or as a pressure sensation, but no term is pathognomonic. Discrete skeletal pain following trauma should be radiographically studied, as fractures are sometimes missed on initial examination. SCI patients are prone to developing overuse syndromes, entrapment neuropathies such as carpal tunnel syndrome or ulnar neuropathies and radiculopathies. These may develop acutely or after chronic injury and should be evaluated by electrodiagnostic testing based on clinical presentation.

PULMONARY ASSESSMENT

The most frequent pulmonary complications after SCI are atelectasis and pneumonia caused by impairment of both ventilation and the coughing mechanism. The higher the level of SCI, the more severe the impairment. Injuries caudal to T12 generally spare pulmonary dysfunction. T12 to T5 lesion levels show progressive loss of abdominal and intercostal muscle function that impairs the force of coughing as well as expiration. Complete lesions above T5 basically eliminate coughing, and patients with C5 or higher lesions also have weakness of inspiration. Initially, patients with C4 neurologic level commonly require mechanical ventilation but can typically be weaned off the ventilator. At and above the C3 level, diaphragmatic innervation is disrupted, necessitating mechanical ventilation. Those with high incomplete lesions, however, may eventually be weaned from mechanical ventilation. Initial assessment of ventilatory compromise should include possible trauma-associated injuries such as hemothorax or lung contusions. Concomitant head injury increases the chance of aspiration or the development of neurogenic pulmonary edema. Initial assessment should include bedside pulmonary function testing (PFT) with forced vital capacity, tidal volume, negative inspiratory pressure, and arterial blood gases. Restrictive changes are seen on PFT, and mid-to low-cervical-level lesions typically result in vital capacities of 1,000 to 1,500 mL. In addition, patients with cervical lesions, particularly those with a tracheotomy, are at risk for dysphagia and should be evaluated for swallowing dysfunction since dysphagia can lead to aspiration of food or secretions and pneumonia.

CARDIOVASCULAR EVALUATION

Early detection of deep venous thrombosis (DVT) and the associated risk of pulmonary embolism (PE) should be given careful consideration, even in light of prophylaxis. In the acute phase of SCI, PE is a common cause of death. Assessment for DVT is usually by a venous Doppler (duplex scan), and a laboratory D-dimer study may be of value. A negative D-dimer test essentially rules out DVT or PE; however, many other conditions may produce a positive test result. A ventilation-perfusion scan is usually the preliminary study used to rule out PE; however, a pulmonary arteriogram or spiral computerized tomography may be more definitive.

Orthostatic hypotension is a common occurrence immediately after SCI because of the loss of the sympathetic peripheral vasoconstriction. Sympathetically mediated hypotension should be distinguished from a lack of hydration or intravascular volume. Treatment of neurogenic orthostatic hypotension is addressed in the treatment section. Brachycardia is also common after cervical SCI as the heart loses its sympathetic input but maintains its parasympathetic supply via the vagus nerve. When severe, brachycardia may require use of an on-demand pacemaker.

GENITOURINARY EVALUATION

During the period of spinal shock, the bladder is usually areflexic, and an indwelling catheter should be placed to allow drainage. Assessment of the genitourinary (GU) system after spinal shock has resolved will help determine whether the individual has sustained a UMN versus an LMN injury and the presence of detrusor sphincter dysynergia (DSD). Baseline evaluation of the function of the GU system during the first weeks postinjury should include a renal ultrasound and x-ray of the kidneys, ureters, and bladder (KUB) or CT. The choice and timing of urodynamic studies will depend on the level and type of SCI, pattern of neurologic return, and degree of spasticity. Urodynamic studies evaluate bladder sensation and compliance, resting and voiding intravesicular pressures, detrusor activity, and voiding flow rates. These studies are best delayed until after spinal shock has resolved. Urodynamic studies will help determine the functional classification of neurogenic bladder, as well as suggest the type of bladder management to be prescribed.

Patients with spastic tetraplegia and insufficient hand function (even with splints) may wish to continue with an indwelling Foley catheter, rather than depend on an attendant to perform an intermittent catheterization procedure (ICP) every 4 to 6 hours. Even if a condom catheter bladder management method is chosen, SCI males with DSD may not be able to adequately drain the bladder without the placement of a sphincterotomy or sphincter stent. The many considerations that are weighed to determine the optimal bladder management for an individual include prognosis for bladder recovery, prognosis for recovery of hand function, type of neurogenic bladder, control of incontinence, presence of DSD, ability to transfer, sexual activity, and lifestyle. The goals of bladder management are to maintain continence, allow adequate emptying of the bladder, prevent accumulation of postvoid residual volumes above 150 to 200 cc, and enable the individual to be as functionally independent as possible.

Sexual functioning is often affected by SCI, since neural function is important for the production of erection and ejaculation. In men with a UMN lesion, 60% to 90% will have reflex erections, but these erections may be inconsistent and fleeting. Very few men with UMN lesions will have consistent emission, ejaculations, or orgasm unless the injury is incomplete. Ejaculations in those with complete UMN lesions have been reported to range from only 1% to 3% with no interventions such as electrical stimulation. Vaginal lubrication for women with UMN lesions will also be inconsistent and reflex in nature. Men with injuries from T10 through T12 with a UMN lesion may have more psychic erections and increased emission and ejaculations compared to those with higher lesions.

Men with a complete LMN lesion below T10 usually are not expected to produce reflex erections, but about 20% may have psychic erections, which are generally somewhat fleeting. Ejaculations are more likely in men with LMN lesions, since the sympathetic fibers are relatively spared. About 5% of men report ejaculations occurring without the use of electrical stimulation. When electrical stimulation is used, the percentage of men reporting ejaculation greatly increases (5–7). Women with complete SCI have been reported to achieve reflex genital vasocongestion but not psychogenic genital vasocongestion (8). The reader is referred to reviews for a discussion of pregnancy and menopause in women with SCI (9–11).

GASTROINTESTINAL EVALUATION

During the period of spinal shock immediately post-SCI, a paralytic ileus is common but should resolve within a week as the bowel regains intrinsic activity. Gastrointestinal bleeding is an uncommon occurrence, perhaps owing to the routine use of ulcer prophylaxis (12). During the first 3 weeks of hospitalization, the most common gastrointestinal complications are ileus, peptic ulcer disease, and gastritis (13). Pancreatitis is a potentially serious complication that can occur from three mechanisms in those without a history of alcoholism or gallbladder disease: (i) spasm of the sphincter of Oddi; (ii) activation of trypsinogen by hypercalcemia; and (iii) increased viscosity of pancreatic secretions caused by steroids (14). During the transitional and chronic phases, assessment of neurogenic bowel is similar to that of the neurogenic bladder. A scheduled bowel program should be established as soon as possible and will depend on the type of injury. If the individual has spasticity, and a spastic external anal sphincter, it is likely that a UMN-type of bowel exists. The UMN bowel program consists of judicious use of stool softener medications and insertion of a suppository, followed by digital stimulation of the rectum until the bowels reflexively evacuate stool. This routine should be performed daily or every other day. Lack of limb spasticity and a flaccid external anal sphincter after spinal shock has resolved indicate an LMN-type of bowel. The LMN bowel program consists of judicious use of stool-bulking agents, Valsalva maneuver, and/or manual disimpaction of stool. Individuals may require daily or twice-daily disimpaction in order to maintain continence, due to the flaccid characteristic of the bowel and sphincter. The LMN-type of bowel is more difficult to manage than the UMN bowel.

INTEGUMENT EVALUATION

Neurogenic skin is at significant risk for pressure and shear injury, especially over bony prominences. SCI patients must immediately be placed on a special mattress that allows for enhanced equal distribution of pressure and turned at least every 2 hours. Prior to seating the individual in a wheelchair, the wheelchair must be fitted with a special cushion, and the individual's weight must be shifted every 15 to 20 minutes. The transition of responsibility for maintaining skin integrity and prevention of pressure/shear injury from caregivers to the patient is an interdisciplinary rehabilitation team effort. Prevention and comprehensive management of pressure ulcers is a multifaceted effort and will be addressed in the treatment section.

DUAL DIAGNOSIS: SPINAL CORD INJURY WITH TRAUMATIC BRAIN INJURY

SCI adaptation requires the ability to attend to, concentrate on, understand, process, retrieve, integrate, and use information. In addition, there are a large number of tasks that an individual with SCI needs to learn in order to become as independent in their function as possible. When an individual with SCI has also suffered a traumatic brain injury (TBI), the rehabilitation process can become more complicated and make learning essential information more difficult.

TBI is often underidentified because the initial medical effort focuses on addressing the SCI. Often the potential diagnosis of a TBI, especially a mild brain injury, is not even considered until a patient is found unable to learn in rehabilitation. Mild head injury is defined as having an initial Glasgow Coma Scale (GCS) score between 13 and 15, no loss of consciousness or only brief loss of consciousness (<20 minutes), and a normal CT scan. Risk factors for TBI in the setting of SCI include younger age (15 to 35), male gender, alcohol or drug use, risk-taking behavior, and cause of injury, including motor vehicle accident, act of violence, or fall. Motor-free cognitive assessments are recommended in order to identify deficits in memory, attention, and problem-solving skills.

In addition, cognitive difficulties can exist prior to a SCI and can affect an individual's success in rehabilitation. Individuals may have a history of brain injury or may have a significant alcohol or substance abuse history, which can contribute to decreased cognition.

It has been suggested that from 40% to 50% of SCI patients exhibit cognitive difficulties (15). When individuals with SCI present with learning difficulties, an effort should be made to determine the cause. Potential causes include a co-occurring TBI, which, as mentioned previously, may not have been identified, a prior history of cognitive difficulties, current medications that may lead to impaired cognition, a history of learning disability, limited education, depression, pain, fatigue, and even adjustment issues.

Brain injury affects an individual's ability to learn, attend, and process information, but it also can have behavioral and emotional consequences that can interfere with rehabilitation. Individuals with brain injury can have impaired judgment and safety awareness, as well as difficulty with impulse control, which may require added supervision. Consultation of speech therapists to assist with cognitive rehabilitation and the development of a behavioral management plan may be useful for those patients with dual diagnoses of SCI and brain injury.

PROGNOSIS/OUTCOME/FOLLOW-UP

The prognosis of improvement and functional outcome following SCI is complex and multifaceted, extending beyond the scope of this chapter. The most accurate way to predict recovery is the standardized physical examination as endorsed by the *International Standards for Neurological and Functional Classification of Spinal Cord Injury Patients* (16). This comprehensive examination will determine the initial level and classification of the injury. Other diagnostic tests such as MRI may be helpful in further determination of prognosis. The presence of extensive cord edema and hemorrhage indicates a poor prognosis. Electrophysiologic tests, such as somatosensory evoked potentials, have not proven more useful than the clinical examination for predicting motor recovery. The presence of initial strength in a muscle caudal to the injury is a significant predictor, at any level of injury, of achieving functional antigravity strength later. Individuals with SCI will often gain significant strength at the root level just caudal to the injury. Other factors, such as preservation of pinprick sacral sensation or volitional anal contraction, also portend an improved prognosis. Rate of improvement is another important factor, with most motor recovery occurring in the first 3 to 6 months. Incomplete injuries have a better prognosis overall for ambulation and functional outcome than do complete injuries.

Charts have been published that correlate the neurologic level of injury with functional outcome, delineating expected independence with activities of daily living, as well as mobility. These charts are useful; however, each injury is different, and factors such as associated injuries, age, patient motivation, and family support must be considered. A thorough understanding of the pathophysiology of the injury and factors affecting neurologic recovery will assist in predicting ultimate functional capability. Patients should receive optimal pharmacologic and therapeutic interventions to enhance recovery. Patient education about recovery mechanisms, as well as about the methods used to determine prognosis, is an essential component of the rehabilitation process.

FUNCTIONAL OUTCOMES IN SCI

The question of whether a patient will walk again is often posed following a spinal cord injury. The ability to communicate predictable functional outcomes is vital in planning the course of rehabilitation, communicating with the rehabilitation team, and determining disposition setting, equipment needs, and caregiver support. In general, the neurologic (motor) level and severity (ASIA impairment scale) of the SCI predicts functional outcomes. Other factors involved in functional outcomes must be considered. Factors such as comorbidities (e.g., TBI), obesity, age, motivation, psychosocial and socioeconomic factors, disposition setting, access to health care and rehabilitation services in post acute rehabilitation, and shortened lengths of stay (LOS) in acute care rehabilitation facilities may affect functional outcomes.

Shortened LOS are occurring throughout all of the health care delivery system and have been especially hard-hitting in the field of rehabilitation medicine. Comparisons within the Model SCI Systems from the 1973 to 1977 period to the 1995 to 2002 period demonstrate that average LOS in an acute care setting decreased from 25 to 19 days while rehabilitation LOS decreased from 122 days to 46 days (17,18).

Countless studies have cited recovery and functional improvement within the first few months after a traumatic SCI. Functional improvement occurs faster with incomplete SCI. For those with incomplete injuries, one half to two thirds of the 1-year motor recovery occurs within the first 2 months after injury (19). Ongoing recovery continues but slows after 3 to 6 months (20,21). Recovery of motor function continues past 1 year and has been documented up to 2 years postinjury (22).

SCI patients with higher ASIA impairment levels have varying degrees of recovery. Research on complete tetraplegia has provided the most predictable source of information on functional outcomes. Most of this information is about muscles at or near the level of injury. Recovery in muscles graded trace to fair minus (1 to 3) indicates a better prognosis than muscles with a muscle grade of absent (0). For muscles with initial muscle strength of trace to poor (1 to 2), 90% achieve antigravity strength (3) by 1 year (22). Of those with an initial strength of 0, 64% achieve antigravity strength (3) by 2 years (22).

There is great discrepancy between the amount of time an individual with SCI rehabilitates in an acute care setting (1 to 2 months) and the time in which functional recovery occurs (3 to 6 months). The long-term impact of shortened LOS *and* the fact that this stay does not overlap with the period in which motor recovery is greatest has not been fully realized. Often rehabilitation must continue after discharge from the acute care rehabilitation unit in different venues: in skilled nursing facilities, at home, or in outpatient rehabilitation centers. Therefore, efforts should be made to educate patients and families and ensure continued rehabilitation follow-up for optimal functional outcomes.

Functional outcome-based guidelines provide estimates of the effect of rehabilitation on functional abilities. These guidelines have implications for the level of care required, as well as for estimating the cost of care, for an individual with SCI. The Consortium of Spinal Cord Medicine has used extensive data from research conducted by the National Spinal Cord Injury Statistical Center on the functional independence measure (FIM), and expert clinical observation and judgment, to develop outcome-based guidelines.

EXAMPLES OF FUNCTIONAL OUTCOMES IN SCI

C1 through C4 Tetraplegia

C1 through C3 Motor Impairment

Total paralysis of trunk, upper extremities, lower extremities, ventilator dependent.

C4 Motor Impairment

Paralysis of trunk, upper extremities, lower extremities; inability to cough, low endurance, and respiratory reserve secondary to paralysis of intercostals.

The individual with tetraplegia at C1 through C4 has neck movement—flexion, extension, and rotation. They are dependent on caregivers for self-care, transfers, and bed mobility. Those with complete C1 through C3 SCI will require some form of mechanical ventilation. These individuals may be candidates for phrenic nerve stimulators and diaphragmatic pacing. Individuals with C4 tetraplegia generally do not require chronic mechanical ventilation but may need continuous positive airway pressure (CPAP) or bilevel positive airway pressure (BiPAP) at night to assist with hypoventilation. An individual with this high-level SCI can be independent in drinking fluids with setup of a secured container or sport hydration system and straw positioned near the mouth. Power wheelchair independence including tilt backs is possible with the use of controls activated by the head, mouth, tongue, voice, infrared devices, or breath. Environmental control units (ECUs) with operational inputs similar to those that control wheelchairs increase independence by providing computer/telephone access and operation of lights, fans, TV, doors, security systems, and other devices in the home setting. Mouthsticks may be used if the individual demonstrates sufficient head control/neck strength. Individuals with C1 through C4 tetraplegia are not candidates for independent driving, because they must have functional use of one upper limb to operate a specialized driving system. Although some independence can be achieved via ECUs, a 24-hour attendant is required for personal care and homemaking tasks. Tables 7-1 and 7-2 provide a summary of functional outcomes and equipment for individuals with C1 through C3 and C4 tetraplegia, respectively.

C5 Tetraplegia

C5 Motor Impairment

Paralysis of trunk and lower extremities, absence of elbow extension, pronation, all wrist and hand movement.

The individual with C5 tetraplegia has added antigravity strength (3/5) in the biceps as well as in the deltoids and rhomboids, and partial innervations of the brachialis, brachioradialis, supraspinatus, infraspinatus, and serratus anterior. Movements gained include shoulder flexion, extension, and abduction; elbow flexion; forearm supination; and weak scapular adduction and abduction. It is essential to monitor the ongoing risk of elbow flexion and forearm supination contractures as a result of unopposed active biceps movement. These individuals remain at risk for respiratory complications because of impaired accessory muscles of respiration. They usually do not have sufficient upper extremity strength to execute independent transfers but can operate power wheelchairs, including tilt backs with appropriately placed controls/switches. Partial biceps innervation allows for possible independence with self-feeding and grooming skills using splints, overhead slings, or mobile arm supports and assistive devices. Use of a tenodesis splint requires the ability to abduct and internally rotate at the shoulder in order to orient the hand and splint to the object appropriately. A ratchet tenodesis splint allows for function without the use of wrist extensors. The ratchet mechanism allows the individual to externally activate the splint. C5 tetraplegia is the highest level of SCI that an individual can have and retain the potential to return to driving with specialized equipment and a wheelchair-accessible vehicle. A formal driver evaluation is necessary but should not be performed until the individual has reached their full potential strength, at least 8 months postinjury. Since most functional activities will require assistive devices, consideration may be given to tendon transfers for gross hand function once neurologic recovery is considered complete. Individuals will require approximately 16 hours of attendant care daily to assist with self-care and homemaking tasks. See Table 7-3 for functional outcomes and potential equipment for individuals with C5 tetraplegia.

Table 7-1	Expected Functional Outcomes for Levels C1 through C3

	Expected Functional Outcome	Equipment
Respiratory	Ventilator dependent Inability to clear secretions	2 ventilators (bedside, portable) Suction equipment Generator/battery backup
Bowel	Total assist	Padded reclining shower/commode chair
Bladder	Total assist	
Bed mobility	Total assist	Full electric hospital bed with Trendelenburg feature and side rails
Bed/wheelchair transfers	Total assist	Transfer board Power or mechanical lift with sling
Pressure relief/ positioning	Total assist; may be independent with equipment	Power recline and/or tilt wheelchair Wheelchair pressure-relief cushion Postural support and head control devices as indicated Hand splints if indicated Specialty bed or pressure-relief mattress if indicated
Eating	Total assist	
Dressing	Total assist	
Grooming	Total assist	
Bathing	Total assist	Handheld shower Shampoo tray Padded reclining shower/commode chair (if roll-in shower available)
Wheelchair propulsion	Manual: total assist Power: independent with equipment	Power recline and/or tilt wheelchair with head, chin, or breath control and manual recliner Vent tray
Standing/ ambulating	Standing: total assist Ambulation: not indicated	
Communication	Total assist to independent depending on work station setup and equipment	Mouthstick, high-tech computer access, environmental control unit Adaptive devices everywhere as indicated
Transportation	Total assist	Attendant-operated van or accessible public transportation
Homemaking	Total assist	
Assist required	24-hour attendant care Able to instruct in all aspects of care	

Adapted from Paralyzed Veterans of America. *Outcomes following traumatic spinal cord injury: A clinical practice guideline for health care professionals.* Washington, DC: Paralyzed Veterans of America; 1999.

C6 Tetraplegia

C6 Motor Impairment

Paralysis of trunk and lower extremities; absence of wrist flexion, elbow extension, and hand movement.

The individual with C6 tetraplegia has added at least antigravity strength (3/5) in the radial wrist extensors (extensor carpi radialis longus and brevis). Additional muscles partially innervated include supinator, pronator teres, clavicular head of pectoralis major, and latissimus dorsi. Movements gained also include scapular abduction and radial wrist extension. Paralysis of the intercostals compromises the respiratory system, causing low endurance and vital capacity. Individuals with this condition may require assistance to clear secretions.

With the addition of active wrist extension, tenodesis grasp, which allows the fingers to pinch, is possible (23).

The C6 tetraplegic who has at least 3+/5 wrist extension may benefit from a wrist-driven flexor hinge splint (WDFH splint) to improve the strength of tenodesis pinch, which is shown in Figures 7–3 and 7–4. These splints are very costly and may not be covered by insurers unless medically justified (e.g., for use in self-catheterizing), and the user often finds them cumbersome. In follow-up studies with those who have been fitted and trained with the tenodesis splints, there is inconsistent long-term use. Careful consideration must be given to whether to allow for contractures or muscle shortening to develop in the finger flexors to create a tenodesis grasp.

Table 7-2	Expected Functional Outcomes for Level C4

	Expected Functional Outcome	Equipment
Respiratory	May be able to breathe without a ventilator	If not ventilator free, see C1–C3 for equipment
Bowel	Total assist	Padded reclining shower/commode chair
Bladder	Total assist	
Bed mobility	Total assist	Full electric hospital bed with Trendelenburg feature and side rails
Bed/wheelchair transfers	Total assist	Transfer board Power or mechanical lift with sling
Pressure relief/ positioning	Total assist; may be independent with equipment	Power recline and/or tilt wheelchair Wheelchair pressure-relief cushion Postural support and head control devices as indicated Hand splints if indicated Specialty bed or pressure-relief mattress if indicated
Eating	Total assist	
Dressing	Total assist	
Grooming	Total assist	
Bathing	Total assist	Handheld shower Shampoo tray Padded reclining shower/commode chair (if roll-in shower available)
Wheelchair propulsion	Manual: total assist Power: independent	Power recline and/or tilt wheelchair with head, chin, or breath control and manual recliner Vent tray
Standing/ ambulating	Standing: total assist Ambulation: not indicated	Tilt table Hydraulic standing table
Communication	Total assist to independent depending on work station setup and equipment	Mouthstick, high-tech computer access, environmental control unit
Transportation	Total assist	Attendant-operated van or accessible public transportation
Homemaking	Total assist	
Assist required	24-hour attendant care to include homemaking Able to instruct in all aspects of care	

Adapted from Paralyzed Veterans of America. *Outcomes following traumatic spinal cord injury: A clinical practice guideline for health care professionals.* Washington, DC: Paralyzed Veterans of America; 1999.

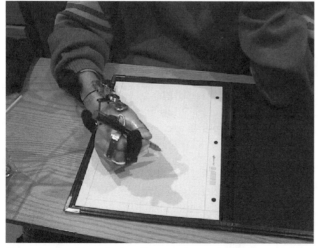

Figure 7–3. Tenodesis splint used to assist with pen grasp.

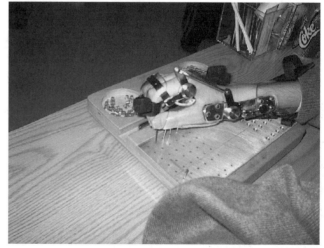

Figure 7–4. Tenodesis splint used to promote pinch.

Table 7-3	Expected Functional Outcomes for Level C5	
	Expected Functional Outcome	**Equipment**
Respiratory	Low endurance and vital capacity secondary to paralysis of intercostals; may require assist to clear secretions	
Bowel	Total assist	Padded shower/commode chair or padded transfer tub bench with commode cutout
Bladder	Total assist	Adaptive devices may be indicated (electric leg bag emptier)
Bed mobility	Some assist	Full electric hospital bed with Trendelenburg feature with patient's control and side rails
Bed/wheelchair transfers	Total assist	Transfer board Power or mechanical lift with sling
Pressure relief/ positioning	Independent with equipment	Power recline and/or tilt wheelchair Wheelchair pressure-relief cushion Hand splints Specialty bed or pressure-relief mattress if indicated Postural support devices
Eating	Total assist for setup, then independent eating with equipment	Long opponens splint Adaptive devices as indicated
Dressing	Lower extremity: total assist Upper extremity: some assist	Long opponens splint Adaptive devices as indicated
Grooming	Some to total assist	Long opponens splint Adaptive devices as indicated
Bathing	Total assist	Handheld shower Padded tub transfer bench or shower/commode chair
Wheelchair propulsion	Manual: independent to some assist indoors on noncarpeted surface, level surface; some to total assist outdoors Power: independent	Power: power recline and/or tilt with arm drive control Manual: lightweight rigid or folding frame with hand rim modifications
Standing/ ambulating	Standing: total assist Ambulation: not indicated	Hydraulic standing frame
Communication	Independent to some assist after setup with equipment	Long opponens splint Adaptive devices as indicated
Transportation	Independent with highly specialized equipment; some assist with accessible public transportation; total assist for attendant-operated vehicle	Highly specialized modified van with lift
Homemaking	Total assist	
Assist required	Personal care: 10 h/d Home care: 6 h/d Able to instruct in all aspects of care	

Adapted from Paralyzed Veterans of America. *Outcomes following traumatic spinal cord injury: A clinical practice guideline for health care professionals.* Washington, DC: Paralyzed Veterans of America; 1999.

Individuals with C6 tetraplegia can usually achieve independence with feeding, grooming with assistive devices, and use of a tenodesis splint. Upper-body dressing independence can be achieved, but individuals will likely require some assistance with lower-body dressing. Clothing fasteners or fastener devices such as loops or self-fastening closures on shirts, shoes, and pants are necessary for optimal independence.

Extensive training is needed for an individual with C6 tetraplegia to achieve independence with functional transfers. A sliding board and a trapeze over the bed may be necessary for this. Some men are able to perform self-catheterization using a clean catheter with a tenodesis splint, but not using the condom catheter. Women will likely require continued assistance with self-catheterization. Independent bowel management is not likely, even with assistive devices (Digistim, suppository inserter). Independent manual wheelchair propulsion is possible, but the wheelchair may require plastic-coated rims or knobs. A power wheelchair may be an appropriate option for community mobility, especially if the individual is to return to work. Return to driving at this level requires significant evaluation of the individual's strength, active range of motion, and functional skills to determine the most appropriate equipment (seating, steering, hand controls) and van modifications. Individuals with C6 tetraplegia will continue to require an attendant approximately 10 hours daily for personal care and homemaking. See Table 7-4 for a summary of functional outcomes and equipment.

Careful consideration may be given to tendon transfers for gross hand function. These procedures can improve function. The criteria for tendon transfer intervention include complete neurologic recovery and maximized existing function; no or negligible spasticity in the hand; full range of motion; at least 4/5 strength in muscles transferred; and the individual's motivation and commitment to extensive postoperative rehabilitation. Tendon transfers of the pronator teres to the flexor digitorum profundus, the brachioradialis to the flexor pollicis longus, and the posterior deltoid to the triceps can provide active finger and thumb movement, as well as elbow extension (24).

C7 through C8 Tetraplegia

C7 through C8 Motor Impairment

Paralysis of trunk and lower extremities; partial hand intrinsics with limited grasp and release/dexterity.

The individual with C7 through C8 tetraplegia has added triceps, serratus anterior, pronator quadratus, extensor carpi ulnaris, flexor carpi radialis, flexor digitorum profundus and superficialis, interrossei/lumbricals, and abductor pollicis. Movements gained at C7 include elbow extension, scapulae stabilization protraction and elevation, ulnar wrist extension, and wrist flexion. At C8, digit flexion and extension and thumb flexion, extension abduction, and circumduction allow for improved hand and finger function. The respiratory system is compromised because of the lack of intercostals, causing low endurance and vital capacity. Individuals with this condition may require assistance to clear secretions.

Individuals with C7 tetraplegia will likely have enough upper-extremity motor return to become independent with eating, grooming, dressing, and bathing with appropriate assistive devices and durable medical equipment. Men are likely to achieve independence with self-catheterization, but women may still require assistance, especially if lower-limb spasticity is present. Bowel management independence is possible with assistive devices, although it is likely that most individuals will continue to require assistance. Independent transfers, weight shifts, pressure reliefs, and manual wheelchair use are feasible with extensive training. Most individuals with C7 through C8 SCI have enough shoulder strength to operate a modified van with a standard steering wheel and to be able to operate a car with hand controls. They may require a wheelchair-accessible van if they are unable to load/unload their wheelchair independently. Individuals will require approximately 8 hours of attendant care daily to assist with self-care and homemaking tasks. Table 7-5 summarizes the functional outcomes and equipment for individuals with C7 through C8 tetraplegia.

T1 through T9 Paraplegia

T1 through T9 Motor Impairment

Partial paralysis of lower trunk, paralysis of lower extremities.

The individual with T1 tetraplegia has added hand intrinsics and the thumb, which are fully innervated at T1. With T2 through T9 paraplegia, there is also added intercostal and erector spinae muscle. The movements gained at T1 are fully functioning upper limbs. The movement gained at T2 through T9 is an improved but compromised respiratory system, resulting in a less impaired vital capacity and endurance. Abdominal and thoracic back muscle strength improves at T6. Independence is achieved in all self-care tasks including bowel and bladder management and functional mobility. In the lower thoracic levels with bracing, standing is possible as well as ambulation, but it is not likely a long-term functional goal due to very high requirements for energy expedition. Standing is a prerequisite for walking. There must be adequate tolerance to vertical positioning prior to ambulation. The use of a standing frame or standing frame/parallel bars and bilateral lower-extremity orthoses may be appropriate to achieve vertical tolerance prior to formal gait training. Bilateral lower-extremity orthoses, such as hip-knee-ankle-foot orthoses (HKAFOs), reciprocating gait orthosis (RGOs) (T5 through T7), knee-ankle-foot othoses (KAFOs) (T8 through T12) with knee lockouts, and fixed or hinged ankle-foot orthoses (AFOs) with floor reaction modifications, may be indicated for the individual with SCI depending upon completeness and

Table 7-4	Expected Functional Outcomes for Level C6	
	Expected Functional Outcome	**Equipment**
Respiratory	Low endurance and vital capacity secondary to paralysis of intercostals; may require assist to clear secretions	
Bowel	Some to total assist	Padded shower/commode chair or padded transfer tub bench with commode cutout
Bladder	Some to total assist with equipment; may be independent with leg bag emptying	Adaptive devices if indicated
Bed mobility	Some assist	Full electric hospital bed Side rails Full to king standard bed may be indicated
Bed/wheelchair transfers	Level: some assist to independent Uneven: some to total assist	Transfer board Mechanical lift
Pressure relief/ positioning	Independent with equipment and/or adapted techniques	Power recline wheelchair Wheelchair pressure-relief cushion Pressure-relief mattress or overlay if indicated Postural support devices
Eating	Independent with or without equipment, except cutting which is total assist	Adaptive devices as indicated (e.g., U-cuff, tendenosis splint, adapted utensils, plate guard)
Dressing	Lower extremity: some to total assist Upper extremity: independent	Adaptive devices as indicated (e.g., button, hook, loops on zippers, pants; socks, self-fasteners on shoes)
Grooming	Some assist to independent with equipment	Adaptive devices as indicated (e.g., U-cuff, adapted handles)
Bathing	Upper body: independent Lower body: some to total assist	Handheld shower Padded tub transfer bench or shower/commode chair
Wheelchair propulsion	Manual: independent indoors, some to total assist outdoors Power: independent with standard arm drive on all surfaces	Power: may require power recline or standard upright power wheelchair Manual: lightweight rigid or folding frame with modified rims
Standing/ ambulating	Standing: total assist Ambulation: not indicated	Hydraulic standing frame
Communication	Independent with or without equipment	Adaptive devices as indicated (e.g., tendenosis splint; writing splint for keyboard use, button pushing, page turning, object manipulation)
Transportation	Independent driving from wheelchair	Modified van with lift Sensitized hand controls Tie-downs
Homemaking	Some assist with light meal preparation; total assist for all other homemaking	Adaptive devices as indicated
Assist required	Personal care: 6 h/d Home care: 4 h/d	

Adapted from Paralyzed Veterans of America. *Outcomes following traumatic spinal cord injury: A clinical practice guideline for health care professionals.* Washington, DC: Paralyzed Veterans of America; 1999.

return of function, ambulation goals, and personal preference. The Parastep System, a functional electrical stimulation (FES) device, is an option for ambulation training. The FES requires the presence of an intact reflex arc, so only individuals with UMN lesions are candidates. Individuals with T1 through T9 paraplegia will require approximately 2 hours of attendant care daily to assist with homemaking tasks. See Table 7-6 for a summary of expected functional outcomes and equipment.

Table 7-5	Expected Functional Outcomes for Levels C7 through C8	
	Expected Functional Outcome	**Equipment**
Respiratory	Low endurance and vital capacity secondary to paralysis of intercostals; may require assist to clear secretions	
Bowel	Some to total assist	Padded shower/commode chair or padded transfer tub bench with commode cutout
Bladder	Independent to some assist	Adaptive devices if indicated
Bed mobility	Independent to some assist	Full electric hospital bed or full to king standard bed
Bed/wheelchair transfers	Level: independent Uneven: independent to some assist	With or without transfer board
Pressure relief/ positioning	Independent	Wheelchair pressure-relief cushion Pressure-relief mattress or overlay if indicated Postural support devices
Eating	Independent	Adaptive devices as indicated
Dressing	Lower extremity: independent to some assist Upper extremity: independent	Adaptive devices as indicated
Grooming	Independent	Adaptive devices as indicated
Bathing	Upper body: independent Lower body: independent to some assist	Handheld shower Padded tub transfer bench or shower/commode chair
Wheelchair propulsion	Manual: independent on all indoors surfaces and level outdoor terrain, some assist with uneven terrain	Manual: lightweight rigid or folding frame with modified rims
Standing/ ambulating	Standing: independent to some assist Ambulation: not indicated	Hydraulic or standard standing frame
Communication	Independent	Adaptive devices as indicated
Transportation	Independent car if independent with transfer and wheelchair loading/unloading; independent driving modified van from captain's seat	Modified vehicle Transfer board
Homemaking	Independent with light meal preparation and homemaking; some to total assist for complex meal prep and heavy housecleaning	Adaptive devices as indicated
Assist required	Personal care: 6 h/d Home care: 2 h/d	

Adapted from Paralyzed Veterans of America. *Outcomes following traumatic spinal cord injury: A clinical practice guideline for health care professionals.* Washington, DC: Paralyzed Veterans of America; 1999.

T10 through L1 Paraplegia

T10 through L1 Motor Impairment

Paralysis of lower extremities.

The individual with T10 through L1 paraplegia has fully innervated intercostals, external obliques, and rectus abdominus. With L1 paraplegia, there is also partial innervation of hip flexors, such as iliopsoas. The movements gained at T10 through L1 include good trunk stability and improved potential for ambulation with orthoses. At L1, individuals will likely achieve household ambulation with bilateral KAFOs using a four-point gait with crutches. The respiratory system is fully intact. Independence is achieved in all self-care tasks, including bowel and bladder management, and functional mobility in a

Table 7-6	Expected Functional Outcomes for Levels T1 through T9

	Expected Functional Outcome	Equipment
Respiratory	Compromised vital capacity and endurance	
Bowel	Independent	Elevated padded toilet seat or padded tub bench with commode cutout
Bladder	Independent	
Bed mobility	Independent	Full to king standard bed
Bed/wheelchair transfers	Independent	May or may not require transfer board
Pressure relief/ positioning	Independent	Wheelchair pressure-relief cushion Pressure-relief mattress or overlay if indicated Postural support devices
Eating	Independent	
Dressing	Independent	
Grooming	Independent	
Bathing	Independent	Handheld shower Padded tub transfer bench or shower/commode chair
Wheelchair propulsion	Independent	Manual: lightweight rigid or folding frame
Standing/ ambulating	Standing: independent Ambulation: typically not functional	Standing frame
Communication	Independent	
Transportation	Independent in car with transfer and wheelchair loading/unloading	Hand controls
Homemaking	Independent with complex meal preparation and light housekeeping; some to total assist for heavy housecleaning	
Assist required	Home care: 3 h/d	

Adapted from Paralyzed Veterans of America. *Outcomes following traumatic spinal cord injury: A clinical practice guideline for health care professionals.* Washington, DC: Paralyzed Veterans of America; 1999.

wheelchair. Individuals will require approximately 2 hours of attendant care daily to assist with homemaking tasks. Table 7-7 lists expected functional outcomes and equipment.

L2 through S5 Paraplegia

L2 through S5 Motor Impairments

Partial paralysis of lower extremities.

The individual with L2 through S5 paraplegia has fully intact abdominal muscles, most trunk muscles, partially to fully innervated hip flexors, extensors, abductors, knee flexors and extensors, and ankle dorsiflexors and plantar flexors. With L3 paraplegia, quadriceps and iliopsoas are fully innervated. Movements gained include hip flexion, extension, abduction and adduction, internal and external rotation, and knee extension. Ankle dorsiflexion is partially innervated at L4. Ankle plantar flexors are gained at S1. The individual at these levels is fully independent in all self-care and functional mobility. Bowel and bladder management methods are dependent upon whether there is a UMN lesion or LMN lesion. Regardless, bowel and bladder management should be performed independently. At the L3 level, community ambulation using a four-point gait usually requires AFOs with crutches or canes. At this level they will likely be able to operate a standard vehicle and may or may not require use of hand controls. Individuals may require minimal (0 to 1 hour) attendant care daily to assist with homemaking tasks. Expected functional outcomes and equipment are similar to those for individuals with T10 through L1 paraplegia and are summarized in Table 7-7.

Table 7-7	Expected Functional Outcomes for Levels T10 through S5	
	Expected Functional Outcome	**Equipment**
Respiratory	Intact respiratory function	
Bowel	Independent	Padded standard or raised toilet seat
Bladder	Independent	
Bed mobility	Independent	Full to king standard bed
Bed/wheelchair transfers	Independent	May or may not require transfer board
Pressure relief/ positioning	Independent	Wheelchair pressure-relief cushion Pressure-relief mattress or overlay if indicated Postural support devices
Eating	Independent	
Dressing	Independent	
Grooming	Independent	
Bathing	Independent	Handheld shower Padded tub transfer bench
Wheelchair propulsion	Independent	Manual: lightweight rigid or folding frame
Standing/ ambulating	Standing: independent Ambulation: functional, some assist to independent	Standing frame Forearm crutches or walker Knee, ankle, foot orthosis (KAFO)
Communication	Independent	
Transportation	Independent in car with transfer and wheelchair loading/unloading	Hand controls
Homemaking	Independent with complex meal preparation and light housekeeping; some assist for heavy housecleaning	
Assist required	Home care: 0–2 h/d	

Adapted from Paralyzed Veterans of America. *Outcomes following traumatic spinal cord injury: A clinical practice guideline for health care professionals.* Washington, DC: Paralyzed Veterans of America; 1999.

ADDITIONAL THERAPEUTIC CONSIDERATIONS

STANDING/AMBULATION

The physiologic and psychological benefits of standing and ambulation are significant and include the possible decrease in spasticity and bone loss. Enhancement of the function of the internal organs, specifically the bowel and bladder, respiratory capacity, and positional pressure relief, are also important. In addition, decreased depression and improved self-concept have been widely reported with standing and ambulation. Repeated standing may improve the recovery of lower extremity venous return and improved overall cardiovascular

system function. Standing is a prerequisite for walking. Standing is possible with the use of a standing frame or a tilt table. Tilt tables are especially useful in the early stages to monitor and immediately reposition in the event of orthostatic hypotension. There must be adequate tolerance to vertical positioning prior to ambulation. Given the neurologic presentation of the individual, adequate strength, joint integrity of the hips, knees, ankles, and spine stability, the lack of lower-extremity contractures, and the individual's motivation, consideration may be given to ambulation retraining. The physiatrist in consultation with the orthopaedic surgeon needs to determine guidelines for standing mobilization with or without the spinal stabilization orthoses such as a TLSO brace. Once the individual is able to tolerate static standing, standing balance (including free standing) in parallel bars must be achieved. Additional components that need to be mastered are weight shifts, core or trunk control, and gait sequencing. Re-evaluation of bracing throughout gait retraining will optimize the individual's potential.

The body weight support system (BWSS) is a good alternative to parallel bars for individuals who wish to start ambulation but who have questionable proximal strength and fear of falling. One such system is shown in Figure 7–5. A combination of BWSS and parallel bar gait training may best suit the individual. Once individuals have mastered the techniques in the parallel bars, ambulation with assistive devices such as a reciprocating walker, crutches, or canes may be considered. Some drawbacks to ambulation that need to be considered and discussed with the individual throughout the entire process include whether the amount of energy expended is worth the mode of locomotion and whether the strain of additional weight bearing on the upper extremities will lead to overuse syndromes and/or orthopaedic injuries.

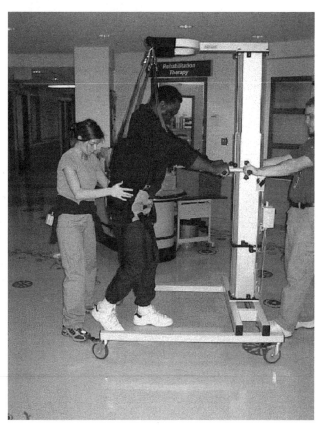

Figure 7–5. Body weight support system.

RECREATION AND SPORTS ACTIVITIES

The majority of people who sustain spinal cord injuries are young, active individuals who not only grieve the loss of their capacity to participate in sports but also everyday leisure activities. Recreational therapy, along with the Americans with Disabilities Act and a multitude of organizations, has made many sports and therapeutic activities accessible to individuals with SCI.

During the initial rehabilitation stay, recreational therapists provide an essential part of treatment by initiating and assessing community mobility. Identifying possible leisure activities and attending community outings prepare individuals with SCI for community re-entry. Recreational therapists assess an individual's values and recreational interests and provide education and counseling related to skills and opportunities for leisure pursuits. Community outings allow for practice with activities, such as shopping, attending sporting events, and other enjoyable activities, that allow for maximal independence at discharge.

In the long term, individuals for SCI often develop sedentary lifestyles. Repetitive motion injuries, cumulative joint trauma, pain, joint contractures, and deconditioning can result from that same sedentary lifestyle. SCI and subsequent physiological decline can also lead to depression and other psychosocial consequences.

For individuals with SCI, exercise is effective in improving endurance and maintaining muscle mass. Strength, flexibility, increased bone density, improved postural tolerance, and cardiopulmonary function are also enhanced with exercise. The function and type of exercise of the individual with SCI must be balanced to reduce the risk of injury.

An exercise program for individuals with SCI requires special considerations because of potential complications and injuries. Factors to be considered include (i) thermal regulation, (ii) fractures and re-injury, (iii) overuse injuries, (iv) pain, and (v) autonomic dysreflexia. Exercise, equipment selection, appropriate retraining, nutritional status, and monitoring of skin and joint integrity will maximize the benefit for individuals with SCI.

Advanced technology and equipment have improved access and reduced injuries while providing greater opportunity to participate in more diverse sports and leisure activities. Anyone with SCI can lead an active lifestyle, whether it involves a leisure activity or amateur/professional competition. Information on recreational sports can be found on the

Internet at sites including Disabled Sports USA (www.dsusa.org), Wheelchair Sports (www.wsusa. org), International Wheelchair Tennis Federation (www.itfwheelchairtennis.com), and U.S. Quad Rugby Association (www.quadrugby.com).

ASSISTIVE TECHNOLOGY DEVICES/ ENVIRONMENTAL CONTROL UNITS

An important means of enhancing strengths and compensating for limitations is technology. Technology plays an important role in every aspect of daily life with or without a disability. Assistive technology devices include any piece of equipment that is used to maintain or increase independence with functional capabilities. Assistive technology devices designed to increase an individual's level of function and independence can be instrumental in providing a person with SCI the highest level of function possible after injury. Assistive technology devices not only can be incorporated for daily self-care activities but also can be valuable tools for improving recreational, vocational, and communication skills. However, it is important to note that more than 50% of assistive technology devices prescribed are abandoned within 6 months (25). This result has been attributed to the following causes: (i) a change (improvement or deterioration) in the needs of the person with SCI; (ii) a mismatch between the technology and the disability; (iii) the user's limited interest in or anxiety with use of the technology; (iv) inadequate training; and (v) failure of the device(s) to meet the needs of the person with SCI in his or her environment or community. In order to determine the most appropriate assistive technology devices a comprehensive evaluation is necessary for the best possible match between technology and the person with SCI. An ecologic approach that is a client-centered evaluation may yield the best results for matching technology with disability.

The evaluation should include the following: (i) an overview of the work or living environment to determine existing and potential modifications (including job/task, behavioral, and environmental modifications); (ii) identification of the person's goals; (iii) determination of the person's learning style and preferences, and cognitive and functional skills deficits or limitations; (iv) evaluation of the activity to determine physical, cognitive, and social demands; and (v) identification of appropriate assistive technology (26).

Low-technologic intervention is recommended initially. Often low-tech modifications without great cost can minimize previously existing barriers. If these modifications do not facilitate the goals of the person or overcome the barriers, then higher-tech options may be prudent. The matching of technology with the person can be very time consuming and the course of action may change given the environment and the nature of the person's deficits. Ultimately, assistive technology can have a great impact on individuals with a spinal cord injury and their quality of life.

HOME MODIFICATIONS

The functional level of individuals with SCI can have significant implications in their ability to access their home. During initial rehabilitation after SCI the establishment of a safe and appropriate disposition setting is essential. A home evaluation provides the rehabilitation team with the necessary information to determine modifications and/or appropriateness of the home. When evaluating the home setting, it is important to keep the goals of the individual, the level and severity of injury, prognosis for functional recovery, social support, income, and financial resources in mind.

During an initial home evaluation, the focus is typically on essential modifications that must be made to allow an individual to have a safe discharge, and it will include evaluation of entrances and how activities of daily living can be conducted in the current space. Recommendations may also be made for future reconstruction. Evaluation of entrances and doorways includes all areas the individual will enter from, or egress to, such as the sidewalk, driveway, and garage or carport. The pathways from these key areas should be relatively smooth, passable, and flat. Often the entry requires modifications such as a ramp (www.abledata.com). Careful thought and planning should be given for a secondary exit should an emergency occur. In addition to the rehabilitation team, an emergency preparedness organization may be a useful resource in assisting with developing an emergency plan.

Interior and exterior doorway specifications vary. Adequate space at the entry is needed to allow the individual in the wheelchair to clear the door while opening it. Removal of screen doors is recommended to reduce barriers. A wedge of durable material may be installed for ease in passing a wheelchair over the threshold if it is >1 in. Intermediate solutions can be found to access the interior rooms where doorways are often smaller, including removing doors or changing the swing of the door to allow access to bedrooms and bathrooms.

The accessible bathroom should ideally be adjacent to the accessible bedroom. The bathroom almost always requires the greatest modifications and is related to the level of impairment of the individual with SCI. Equipment can be evaluated during the inpatient stay to determine temporary solutions. Bedrooms should be cleared of any unnecessary furniture and have a minimum of 5-ft-by-5-ft clearance for wheelchair maneuverability. A minimum clearance of 3 feet on one side of the bed is needed for accessibility. Dressers can be adapted with accessible handles to accommodate impaired coordination.

In the kitchen, commonly used appliances should be placed within reach. It is recommended that during the rehabilitation stay the individual with SCI be evaluated and retrained on kitchen safety and independence.

In addition to accessing the home, a variety of safety issues need to be considered when the individual with SCI returns home. Safety recommendations can include the following:

- Maintaining a backup power source;
- Having an accessible telephone and/or medical alert system;
- Maintaining a temperature of 70° F at all times;
- Making sure that house numbers are visible from the street for emergency service response;
- Notifying the police, fire, and utility companies that an individual with a disability lives in the dwelling. Discounts on utility rates may be available. In addition, emergency services may request additional information on the layout of the home to keep on record;
- Installing and maintaining working smoke and carbon monoxide detectors;
- Ensuring that rugs are low pile and that throw rugs are removed;
- Ensuring that light switches, thermostats, and all essential environmental control units are within reach.

When reconstruction can begin, there are many contractors who specialize in universal or accessible design. With reduced lengths of stay, follow-up therapies are imperative for successful transition to the home. Additional problems may arise that were previously unforeseen, and therapeutic intervention in the home can address these issues in a timely manner. When individuals are forced to give up their home because of architectural barriers or lack of social and community support, renting may be possible. In that event, or if an individual is already renting, extensive civil rights legislation—such as the Americans with Disabilities Act, the

Fair Housing Amendments of 1988 (FHAA), the American National Standards Institute (ANSI) Standards A117.1-1986, and the Uniform Federal Accessibility Standards (UFAS) (www.usdoj.gov/crt/ada/stdspdf.htm)—protects the disabled individual's housing rights. Included in these laws are standard dimensions and characteristics for door widths, wheelchair mobility clearance, grab bars, heights for environmental controls, and signals to accommodate for sensory loss. Additional codes, laws, and guidelines may be imposed at the state, county, or city level.

TREATMENT OF POTENTIAL MEDICAL COMPLICATIONS

There are a number of potential medical complications that may occur as result of a spinal cord injury. These include pulmonary complications, deep venous thrombosis, pulmonary embolism, autonomic dysreflexia, pressure ulcers, heterotopic ossification, urinary tract infections, spasticity, chronic pain, gastrointestinal complications, overuse syndromes, posttraumatic syringomyelia. Some of these complications, for example, deep venous thrombosis and pulmonary embolism, are much more common during the acute stage after SCI. Others may occur anytime after SCI, for example, UTI or pain, and they may become life long problems. Still other complications such as autonomic dysreflexia and spasticity do not occur until after the period of spinal shock ends. The following is a discussion of some of these more common complications and suggested treatment.

PULMONARY COMPLICATIONS

Patients with complete SCI, especially those with tetraplegia, are at a greater risk for atelectasis and pneumonia than those with incomplete injuries or paraplegia. Atelectasis and pneumonia are more common during the first 3 weeks after injury (27). Prevention includes deep breathing exercises, regular changes in bed position, incentive spirometry, and "quad" coughing for those who do not have adequate abdominal strength. Vigorous pulmonary toilet can decrease the incidence of pulmonary complications. A useful alternative to tracheal suctioning is the intervention provided by mechanical exsufflation, which creates deep insufflation followed by an immediate decrease in pressure to create a forced exsufflation. Mechanical exsufflation can produce a peak cough expiratory force that is comparable to a normal cough and greater than that produced by a manually assisted cough, and thus is appropriate for management of pulmonary secretions (28). It may be applied via endotracheal or tracheostomy tubes, or via oral-nasal interfaces.

Weaning from a ventilator in the SCI patient may proceed more slowly than in patients with strictly pulmonary problems alone, since SCI may impair the function of intercostal and abdominal muscles. Often, the patient who is weaned during the day has more difficulties at night and may benefit from continued ventilation at night or the use of BiPAP. The patient with a complete C1 or C2 tetraplegia may be an appropriate candidate for phrenic nerve stimulators, also called diaphragm pacing. Individuals with SCI at the C3 and C4 levels usually are not candidates for phrenic pacing since the LMNs supplying the phrenic nerve (i.e., the anterior horn cells) usually are not intact. If the patient is incomplete, even if only by sensory examination, weaning may still be possible many months postinjury. Implanting phrenic nerve stimulators has the potential to damage the phrenic nerves and should therefore be avoided in sensory incomplete patients in the first year or two postinjury. Damage to the nerves in the incomplete patients would risk needing to use a ventilator on a permanent basis when weaning might have been possible otherwise.

DEEP VENOUS THROMBOSIS AND PULMONARY EMBOLISM

The risk for DVT is highest in the first few weeks after injury. The reported incidence of DVT has ranged from 47% to 100%. One study reported that 62% of patients had a positive venogram 6 to 8 days after injury (29). Patients with acute SCI are predisposed to the development of DVT based on the presence of all three components of the Virchow triad for the development of thrombosis (30). The incidence of clinically noted PE is much lower, ranging from 3% to 15% (31,32). The true incidence of PE after acute SCI is unknown since >50% of PEs in patients with DVT are asymptomatic (33).

Current published *Clinical Practice Guidelines* recommend DVT prophylaxis for 8 to 12 weeks after acute SCI depending on risk factors (34). It is important to attempt to prevent lower-extremity DVTs with compression stockings, sequential compression devices (SCDs) or pumps, and either adjusted-dose heparin or low–molecular weight heparin. The SCDs usually lose value quickly once the patient becomes wheelchair mobile and can be discontinued. In our experience, a single DVT confined to the calf often becomes multiple DVTs or may extend above the knee; thus, it may be better for the patient with SCI who develops a DVT in the calf to institute full anticoagulation. Even patients with the ability to ambulate in a few days after SCI appear at significant risk for DVT and require the same degree of prophylaxis and vigilance. Duplex ultrasonography is a useful noninvasive tool for the detection of DVT. Since DVT may lead to PE, it is important to ask the patient with or without DVT regarding chest or shoulder pain or discomfort, cough, or shortness of breath, and to report any such symptoms anytime during the course of treatment. A high index of suspicion is needed for diagnosis when symptoms are minimal. Treatment of DVT and PE in the patient with SCI is essentially the same as that for a neurologically intact patient.

AUTONOMIC DYSREFLEXIA

The signs and symptoms of autonomic dysreflexia (AD) include an acute elevation of blood pressure associated with headache, sweating, flushing above the lesion, nasal congestion, piloerection, and, sometimes, bradycardia. AD may occur in the patient with a spinal cord injury at or above the T6 level after the period of spinal shock. The most common causative agent is bladder distention followed by bowel distention. However, any noxious stimulus below the level of the lesion may lead to AD. The treatment is directed at removing the stimulus, for example, checking the urinary catheter for kinks if indwelling, or catheterizing the bladder if on intermittent catheterization. Sometimes the blood pressure requires immediate treatment, often using nitro-paste, nitroglycerin 1/150 sublingually, or an agent such as hydralazine. At times the patient may need chronic prophylaxis with an alpha blocker. *Clinical Practice Guidelines* for detection and treatment of AD have been published by the Consortium for Spinal Cord Medicine (35). The patient and family should be educated in the signs and symptoms of AD and initial management and prevention.

PRESSURE ULCERS

Pressure ulcers, which are one of the costliest complications that can occur, may develop anytime after SCI. Prevention of pressure ulcers is critical during the acute phase, as care of even small wounds can prevent mobilization of the patient. Grade I pressure ulcers may be present on the sacrum by the time the patient is taken off of the backboard, and the length of time spent on a backboard is significantly correlated with the development of pressure ulcers (36). Ulcers develop in dependent areas of the body, usually over bony prominences. Sacral ulcers are the most common type during initial hospitalization and ischial ulcers in chronic SCI (37). Unrelieved pressure and shear injury are the usual etiologies of skin breakdown and require multidisciplinary team assessment and intervention, as well as patient vigilance, for short- and long-term management. Patients who use a manual wheelchair are instructed in methods of relieving pressure by lifting the body or by leaning from side to side. Patients with tetraplegia who do not have enough upper-body function to perform an adequate pressure relief require a power tilting mechanism to enable weight shifting. Pressure-support surfaces such as mattresses and wheelchair cushions must be carefully assessed, based on the individual's body habitus and functional level. Once a pressure ulcer develops, the pressure must be alleviated in order to heal the wound, which may entail bed rest on a dynamic mattress. In cases with deep ulcers, myocutaneous flap surgery may be required for healing.

The major risk factors for pressure ulcers in persons with SCI include immobility, completeness of SCI, urinary incontinence, older age, cognitive impairment, anemia, and hypoalbuminemia. The majority of studies have found an increased risk for skin breakdown in patients with paraplegia versus tetraplegia (38). There are other comorbid medical complications that predispose a patient to poor skin integrity and the development of pressure ulcers or make healing difficult. These conditions can include low levels of testosterone (endogenous anabolic protein synthesis stimulus), poorly controlled diabetes, poor nutrition, and peripheral vascular disease. The patient with multiple medical complications during the acute stage is at risk unless caloric needs are met. There is a tendency for physicians to accept great loss of body mass as part of the paralysis without regard for the nutritional status of the patient. Once an individual develops an open wound, the body develops a state of catabolism, which causes lean body weight loss and perpetuates healing difficulty. Many studies show a direct correlation between low albumin levels and the presence, severity, and duration of pressure ulcers. Studies also show that SCI patients with pressure ulcers may have almost twice as much nutritional intake as control-matched individuals without ulcers and still be unable to take in enough substrate for protein synthesis that is required to heal a wound. Patients with open wounds, weight loss, and low albumin should be considered for short-term treatment with an anabolic medication, such as oxandrolone, in order to attenuate the catabolic state. Comprehensive assessment and management of pressure ulcers is beyond the scope of this chapter.

HETEROTOPIC OSSIFICATION

The etiology of HO is unknown but is likely related to a combination of immobility and neurogenic and traumatic factors since it also may be seen after TBI, burns, and total hip replacement. HO is the abnormal development of bone in the soft tissues surrounding a joint and occurs in about 16% to 53% of patients with SCI. A triple-bone scan is abnormal before calcification appears on x-rays. Elevation of alkaline phosphatase is helpful in diagnosis and monitoring response to treatment, which may consist of disodium etidronate or indomethacin. In refractory cases, surgery and radiation therapy may be necessary. The most common location for HO to develop is at the hips, but HO has been found in many different locations. HO develops only below the level of the lesion in persons with SCI.

SPASTICITY

Spasticity may interfere with function or self-care or lead to contractures and pain. The most basic form of treatment is stretching, but this may provide only temporary relief of spasms. Several medications are available including baclofen, tizanidine, and dantrolene sodium. Diazepam may provide quick relief of spasticity but is addicting and therefore not a first-line drug. Common antispasticity medications are shown in Table 7-8. Blocks using

Table 7-8	Common Medications Used for Spasticity	
Name	**Mechanism of Action**	**Dosage**
Baclofen	Agonist of GABA-$_B$ receptor	5–10 mg qd increased to as much as 150 mg in divided doses
Tizanidine	Agonist of α_2-adrenergic receptors in CNS	Start 2–4 mg qhs; gradual increase to maximum of 12 mg PO t.i.d.
Dantrolene sodium	Blocks calcium release from the sarcoplasmic reticulum	25 mg qd for 1 week, then gradually increase to 300–400 mg daily in divided doses
Diazepam	Facilitates GABA$_A$-mediated inhibition in CNS	2–10 mg PO, 2–4 times daily

qd, every day; qhs, every night at bedtime; t.i.d., 3 times a day; PO, by mouth.

phenol or botulinum toxin may be beneficial in those resistant to oral medications. Some patients may not obtain enough relief of spasticity with medications or blocks and may benefit from the use of intrathecal baclofen. The choice of treatment should proceed from the least invasive to the more invasive treatments. Common infections such as UTIs may aggravate spasticity. Of note the newer selective serotonin reuptake inhibitors used for depression may increase spasticity (39).

URINARY TRACT INFECTIONS

UTIs are quite common in patients with SCI during the initial hospitalization and in many persons throughout the remainder of life. The signs and symptoms of UTI may include increased spasticity, cloudy and odorous urine, urinary incontinence, autonomic dysreflexia, general malaise, fever, and chills. Patients with complete injuries do not sense dysuria. Intermittent catheterization (IC) is less likely to lead to recurrent UTIs; however, this applies only to those who perform self-catheterization, since having caregivers perform IC is more likely to be associated with febrile episodes of UTI (40). Indwelling catheters increase the risk of UTIs and are also associated with an increased risk of renal and bladder calculi, epididymitis, fistula formation, and the development of bladder carcinoma (41). Prophylaxis with low dose of an antibiotic may be useful in reducing the incidence of UTI, but causes of recurrent UTIs should be sought before instituting antibiotic prophylaxis. Antibiotic prophylaxis is not recommended for hospitalized SCI patients.

CHRONIC PAIN

Another common complication is the development of chronic pain. This may be sensed above, at, or below the level of the injury. The incidence of chronic pain has been estimated to be about 79% (42). Two major categories of pain after SCI are neuropathic and musculoskeletal. Neuropathic pain includes four types of pain: (i) pain produced by the spinal cord injury and sometimes referred to as central pain or spinal cord injury pain, which occurs below the level of the injury; (ii) transitional zone pain, which occurs at the level of the injury and is sometimes called segmental pain; (iii) radicular pain, which may occur at any dermatomal level and is usually unilateral; and (iv) visceral pain, which is perceived in the abdomen.

Treatment of neuropathic pain in SCI is largely empirical. Drugs that have been used include narcotics, antidepressants, anticonvulsants, and others. Of the antidepressants, amitriptyline, a tricyclic

antidepressant, was not found effective in pain relief in a recent double-blind, placebo-controlled trial of persons with SCI and chronic pain (43). Trazodone, a heterocyclic antidepressant that, unlike tricyclic antidepressants, selectively inhibits serotonin and norepinephrine reuptake in a ratio of 25:1, also failed to show significant pain relief in patients with SCI pain (44). The newer selective-serotonin reuptake inhibitors may produce an increase in spasticity and do not seem clinically effective for treatment of chronic SCI pain. Gabapentin has been found beneficial in SCI pain and has a better side effect profile than tegretol, a similar but older drug used for chronic neuropathic pain. The dose of gabapentin needs to be started low, 100 to 300 mg each night, to avoid unpleasant side effects but then should be gradually increased to a maximum of 2,700 mg per day in divided doses or until complete pain relief has occurred.

Although narcotics are addicting, there are patients with SCI pain who will need to be maintained for the long term on narcotics. It is important to establish a strict agreement with the patient regarding dosing because tolerance may develop and the patient may seek more medication over time. Generally combining types of drugs is helpful in reducing the need for higher doses of narcotics whenever pain is exacerbated. Any increased stress or illness may increase neuropathic pain, and efforts should be made to reduce the stressors that occur in the life of the patient as well as nociceptive stimuli such as calculi and UTIs. Nonpharmacologic modalities such as acupuncture, relaxation techniques, exercise, and self-hypnosis are useful to varying degrees.

POST-TRAUMATIC SYRINGOMYELIA

The development of a syrinx, a fluid-filled cavity within the spinal cord, can be a devastating late complication of SCI. Symtomatic post-traumatic syringomyelia (PTS) is estimated to occur in 3% to 6% of SCI patients, and the pathogenesis is unclear. The cavity typically develops within the initial injury site, followed by enlargement and extension above and below the level of injury. The cavity usually develops in the relatively hypovascular area of the cord in the gray matter between the dorsal horns and posterior columns, and it may progressively expand with resulting loss of sensory and/or motor function. Extension may occur from pressure pulses within the epidural venous system, exacerbated by certain activities that cause valsalva (e.g., coughing, sneezing, straining at stool, exercising). Ascending sensory level or change in neurologic exam consistent with ascending neurologic level should alert the clinician to the possibility of PTS.

Diagnosis is ascertained by a comprehensive history and physical exam followed by MRI. Signs and symptoms may include ascending sensory and/or motor loss, new onset of pain or worsening of chronic neuropathic pain, and autonomic changes such as orthostatic hypotension, sweating, AD, or increased spasticity. The sensory loss is dissociated with greater loss of pain and temperature but relative preservation of light touch sensation and proprioception. A cyst at the level of injury only is not considered PTS. There is no definitive correlation between the size of the syrinx and severity of deficit. Once PTS is diagnosed, each patient must be individually considered regarding treatment. Surgical treatments include shunts and duraplasty, but recurrence is common.

CARDIOVASCULAR COMPLICATIONS

Because of loss of function below the level of the lesion and resulting difficulty in exercising, SCI patients have difficulty maintaining cardiovascular fitness. This relatively sedentary lifestyle promotes obesity, glucose intolerance, elevated cholesterol, and low levels of high-density lipoprotein (HDL). Cardiac etiologies are second only to pulmonary etiologies as causes of death in chronic SCI. Studies show a 16.9% incidence of ischemic heart disease in the SCI population, compared to 6.9% in age-matched controls. Silent ischemia may occur with higher-level lesions. Prior to initiating treatment of hypertension, secondary causes such as autonomic dysreflexia, renal artery stenosis, and renal insufficiency should be ruled out.

Hypotension is also a complex complication in acute and chronic SCI. Many factors are responsible for chronically lower baseline blood pressure, including reduced venous return, venous pooling in lower extremities, and loss of sympathetic peripheral vasoconstriction. Decreased stroke volume and left ventricular atrophy also contribute to a lower baseline blood pressure. In addition to low baseline blood pressure, individuals with acute SCI are particularly prone to significant orthostatic hypotension. Multiple approaches may be used to compensate for loss of sympathetic reflex peripheral vasoconstriction upon arising. Nonpharmacologic methods include compression stockings, abdominal binders, and the use of tilt-in-space or recliner wheelchairs. Pharmacologic interventions may include administering sympathomimetic agents prior to arising, giving salt tablets, or giving a mineralcorticoid. Midodrine is a selective α-1 agonist and is the preferred sympathomimetic agent over ephedrine, which has alpha- as well as beta-adrenergic properties. Small doses of fludrocortisone acetate, a mineralocorticoid, may enhance blood pressure through volume expansion.

ENDOCRINE COMPLICATIONS

Studies have shown that the SCI population has significantly increased risk for developing type II diabetes mellitus, likely due to insulin resistance. The etiology of insulin resistance includes muscle wasting, adiposity, and relative inactivity. Prompt diagnosis and treatment is important in order to prevent both microvascular and macrovascular complications.

Male SCI patients may develop acute or chronic low endogenous testosterone levels from suppression of gonadotropins as well as from impairment in thermoregulation. Hypogonadal men may develop further muscle wasting, osteoporosis, decreased skin integrity (increasing the risk for developing pressure ulcers), and depression. Prior to initiation of androgen replacement therapy, prostate cancer should be ruled out. Women with SCI have also been reported to develop transient amenorrhea and galactorrhea with hyperprolactinemia (45).

Antidiuretic hormone (ADH) is secreted in response to hypovolemia and increased serum osmolality. In normal individuals, it is secreted in diurnal surges with highest levels at night, thus preventing nocturnal diuresis. In some SCI patients, the diurnal rhythm may be impaired, and exogenous ADH therapy may be beneficial at night. This is especially important if large nocturnal urine volumes are precluding a successful intermittent catheterization program for bladder management.

SCI patients with concomitant brain injury may develop adrenal insufficiency, resulting in hyperkalemia, hyponatremia, and hypotension. Acute glucocorticoid treatment immediately after SCI may exacerbate this tendency, and it may be difficult to distinguish orthostatic hypotension from impaired sympathetic tone from that of adrenal insufficiency. Patients with dual diagnoses of SCI and brain injury may also develop the syndrome of inappropriate antidiuretic hormone (SIADH).

Osteoporosis below the level of the lesion develops immediately after SCI and may result in impaired calcium metabolism. Acutely injured individuals should receive increased fluids to deter the development of immobilization hypercalcemia. Nausea, abdominal pain, and elevated ionized calcium should alert the clinician to this diagnosis. Patients generally respond well to biphosphanate medication, such as intravenous pamidronate disodium (46).

Neurogenic factors affect hypothalamic temperature regulation, and individuals with higher lesion levels may be poikilothermic. The body takes on the temperature of the environment and places the SCI patient at risk for hyperthermia in warm weather and hypothermia in cold weather.

PSYCHOSOCIAL ADJUSTMENT FOLLOWING SCI

INITIAL ADJUSTMENT

Spinal cord injury typically leads to a change in function that requires adjustment to learning a new method of mobility prior to discharge from the hospital. This change in mobility also often results in a change in economic status because of lengthy hospitalization and an extended rehabilitation period, which can be an additional source of stress.

While grief often plays a role in adjustment to a new level of disability, this is not always the case. It is important to recognize individual adjustment, as the expectations of staff for a patient to be grieving or depressed following injury can lead to increased suffering for individuals who may have different methods of coping. Research suggests that staff often have beliefs about how patients should react to spinal cord injury, especially with cervical-level injuries, that differ significantly from those of injured patients themselves (47).

While differences in expectations of how patients cope with spinal cord injury are evident, the rates of diagnosable depression are higher than in the general population. Research suggests that rates of depression range between 25% to 40% in individuals with spinal cord injury, compared to approximately 5% in the general population (48). Given this significantly higher rate, it is important to assess for depression and provide treatment, both psychotherapy and medication if appropriate, throughout the rehabilitation stay. Depressive behavior has been found to be associated with longer hospital stays, less improvement during rehabilitation, and the occurrence of complications such as pressure sores and UTIs (49). Depression may be suspected if a significant change in behavior occurs, such as refusal to participate in therapies, or if patients stop making progress without any other medical barriers existing.

Anxiety may also play a significant role in acute adjustment. Several factors can lead to increased anxiety in patients, including the uncertainty of prognosis, a heightened sense of vulnerability, decreased mobility, lack of control of their environment, and an increased amount of time to focus on themselves. In addition, anxiety can be increased by sleep difficulties and a lack of routine. Individuals with increased anxiety often benefit from development of a regular schedule, increased control by making choices about their care and/or schedule, and addressing barriers to reduced sleep, such as decreasing noise or decreasing stimuli when staff turn the individual at night or check vitals.

It is not uncommon for patients to report that they plan to "walk out of here" during their initial rehabilitation, and concerns are often raised about "denial" or an individual's inability to face reality. While it is often very difficult to determine an individual's eventual outcome soon after injury, some estimates of long-term function can be estimated, and concerns are often raised about how to move patients from denial of their condition to a more "realistic" viewpoint. It is important to balance the need for reality with a patient's and family's need for hope. Often, focusing on adaptation to current disability rather than adjustment to the possible future reality is most useful. If injured patients can participate with therapy and work with staff on appropriate and safe discharge plans, then maintaining denial should not be considered a barrier to treatment, and successful long-term adjustment to decreased function is likely. If patients refuse to participate until they are able to walk, then further psychological intervention is necessary.

Families may also have significant difficulty coping with the patient's new level of dependence. They too may maintain a sense of denial and unrealistic hope for future function. However, as with the patient's adaptation, if families are working with staff to ensure an appropriate and safe discharge, adjustment to the long-term reality is likely to occur over time. Families may need significant assistance with obtaining information about how to access and/or provide the increased care that their injured family member may need as well as how to cope with the often significant financial impact that can occur with a new disability.

In order to maximize adjustment postdischarge, gradual re-entry into the community is recommended during the inpatient rehabilitation stay. Working with therapeutic recreation staff and patients' families to engage in community passes to practice outdoor mobility and become familiar with transportation issues and access can be useful. When possible, encouraging an overnight pass before discharge is recommended to assist patients and their family with overcoming any barriers to returning home.

LONG-TERM ADJUSTMENT

As mentioned previously, rates of depression are higher in those with SCI compared to the general population, and continued monitoring of depression and anxiety is essential. Depression in nonhospitalized individuals has been associated with spending more time in bed, fewer days outside of the home, and higher medical expenses (49). Increased suicide risk is an important outcome of depression that must be monitored. Research suggests that rates of suicide are approximately five to ten times higher in individuals with SCI than in the general population (approximately 1% of all deaths) and that risk for suicide is highest in the first 5 years postinjury (50). Suicide can occur through overt action, self-neglect, and refusal to get required health care (49). Risk factors for suicide following SCI are similar to those in the general population and include alcohol and drug abuse, psychiatric history, family problems, and a history of suicide attempts prior to injury (49). If people learn to successfully cope with their injury early, the rate of suicide decreases to that of the general population.

Anxiety has also been found to occur more frequently following SCI than in the general population. In addition, social anxiety and social phobia have been found to develop in people with SCI (49).

Even if patients have coped successfully with their initial adjustment after injury, coping skills may be taxed after discharge home as individuals face the reality of the impact of their injury. Individuals may encounter significant barriers to returning to their own homes and often face reduced social support as their mobility is restricted.

Developing a sense of purpose and engaging in social roles are important for individuals following SCI. Such roles can include educational, vocational, and/or avocational activities. For those individuals previously in the workforce, the new injury may require a career change. Vocational counseling during inpatient rehabilitation will assist individuals in transitioning to a return to school or work, or in beginning to determine interests and discuss options for acquiring new skills. While more than 50% of individuals with SCI are typically employed prior to their injury, fewer than 25% are employed after injury. Research also suggests that those who return to paid employment are more likely to be paraplegic versus tetraplegic, younger at time of injury, further from time of injury, and have a higher level of education prior to injury (51).

Engaging in exercise and recreational activities is important following SCI, not only to increase participation in social activities, but also to maintain health and wellness. Individuals with SCI are prone to obesity, given the potentially sedentary lifestyle that can follow restricted mobility. Modes of exercise and access to recreational activities are frequently very different from the activities that individuals engaged in pre-injury, and a willingness to try new activities should be encouraged.

While many individuals with SCI return to competitive employment and engage in healthy lifestyles, some do not. Unhealthy lifestyles can result from continued denial of their situation or a return to previously unhealthy behaviors. Behavioral noncompliance with medical recommendations or self-neglect can result in skin breakdown, UTIs, and autonomic dysreflexia.

Substance abuse, of both alcohol and drugs, is often an ongoing issue after SCI. Often individuals will be reluctant to address these issues initially after injury. Often, they will report that they do not need treatment because they no longer use any drugs or alcohol, other than those medications prescribed. However, return to these behaviors after discharge is often rapid (52). This rapid return to alcohol and/or drug use may impair their recovery and/or willingness to participate in therapies. Alcohol abuse after SCI has been related to decreased self-care, judgment, and involvement in productive activities. Increased incidence of secondary complications, including pressure sores, has also been found (53). Motivational interviewing has been used with some success as an early intervention (54).

A return to smoking cigarettes is also of concern. While most people who smoke understand the potential negative impact to their lungs, including the possibility of lung cancer, emphysema, and shorter life expectancy, most do not know about the increased risk of pulmonary complications following SCI. With higher-level injuries, reduced ability to breathe normally can be complicated by smoking where the capacity is reduced and the ability to cough and move secretions from the lungs is impaired, and it leads to a higher risk of infection. In addition, smoking has been found to increase pressure sores, decrease wound healing after surgery, and increase the risk of bladder cancer (www.craighospital.org/sci/mets/smoking.asp).

Despite the difficulties with adjustment following SCI, research has consistently found subjective rating of quality of life for those with all levels of SCI to be comparable to individuals without SCI over time. In fact, it is not uncommon for individuals to state benefits of the change in their function, including an increase in their sense of patience, better relationships with family and friends, and pride in their ability to adapt (55).

Peer mentoring or counseling can be helpful through both modeling and emotional support. Contact with peers can be formally arranged by rehabilitation staff or can occur informally by individuals interacting during their physical or occupational therapy visits or involvement in SCI educational programs. More formal interaction with peers is often integrated with inpatient rehabilitation programs. However, with shorter lengths of stay, such interaction may be difficult to coordinate. In addition, timing of such visits needs to be considered as newly injured individuals may not be emotionally ready to meet someone living with an SCI. Psychologists and other rehabilitation staff should be involved in the decision about the best timing for introducing a peer mentor.

SEXUALITY AND INTIMATE RELATIONSHIPS

Sexual desire typically is unchanged after SCI; however, sexual satisfaction tends to be diminished. It is essential to provide information on sexuality to both patients and their partner (if they have a current partner at the time of injury). While individuals may not be thinking about sexual function/sexuality during the initial period after injury, introduction of the topic is important as outpatient visits may be very limited and focused. In addition, individuals can be uncomfortable raising the issue; therefore, inpatient and outpatient providers need to offer information or ask about this issue rather than waiting for it to come up.

Information should describe not only devices and medical intervention to deal with such issues as erection and ejaculation for men and lubrication, menses, and pregnancy for women, but also how to communicate about sex and sexuality. Individuals often have fears about bowel and bladder accidents, which can be addressed, and partners may have fears about hurting the individual with SCI during sex. While physicians and psychologists can provide medical information and discuss communication and intimacy, it may also be useful for peers to share their own experiences. An important message to convey is that there are many approaches to improving sexual function and sexuality, but successful sexual adjustment may require new patterns and methods that individuals had not considered before their injury.

Individuals' body image and self-esteem can be affected after SCI, making a return to sexual relationship with their partner or developing new intimate relationships more difficult. Change in body image and self-esteem can result from change in function as well as the beliefs that an individual has about individuals with disabilities. It is not uncommon for people to hold beliefs about disability prior to

injury that can negatively affect their own adjustment, including feeling pity or sympathy, avoiding individuals with disability due to discomfort, assuming cognitive impairment and/or dependence with physical disability, and not treating those with disabilities as equals. These beliefs may need to be addressed directly with patients and/or their partner to increase self-esteem and improve their body image after SCI.

SUMMARY

Spinal cord injury remains a cause of significant disability to hundreds of thousands of Americans, and trauma is its number one cause. Prevention efforts are important to help reduce the incidence of this disability. Rehabilitation has improved the functional outcomes following an SCI, and new technologic advances continue to improve the quality of life of many. The functional outcomes that may be expected are related primarily to the neurologic level of injury, but outcomes are influenced by such factors as age, body habitus, comorbidities, social support, and funding sources. The person with an SCI may face many possible complications; however, the future appears brighter with the increased research effort to improve recovery.

REFERENCES

1. Marino RJ, ed. *International standards for neurological classification of spinal cord injury*. Atlanta, GA: ASIA; 2000.
2. Ashworth B. Preliminary trial of carisoprodol in multiple sclerosis. *Practitioner*. 1964;192:540–542.
3. Bohannon RW, Smith MB. Interrater reliability of a modified Ashworth scale of muscle spasticity. *Phys Ther*. 1986;67:206–207.
4. Cardenas DD. Current concepts of rehabilitation of spinal cord injury patients. *Spine State Art Rev*. 1999; 13:575–585.
5. Griffith ER, Tomko MA, Timms RJ. Sexual function in spinal cord injured patients: A review. *Arch Phys Med Rehabil*. 1973;54:539–543.
6. Brindley GS. Electroejaculation: Its technique, neurological implication and uses. *J Neurol Neurosurg Psychiat*. 1981;44:9.
7. Bennett CJ, Seager SW, Vasher EA, et al. Sexual dysfunction and electroejaculation in men with spinal cord injury: Review. *J Urol*. 1988;139:453–457.
8. Sipski ML, Alexander CJ, Rosen RC. Physiological parameters associated with psychogenic sexual arousal in women with complete spinal cord injuries. *Arch Phys Med Rehabil*. 1995;76:811–818.

9. Baker ER, Cardenas DD. Pregnancy in spinal cord injured women: A review of the literature. *Arch Phys Med Rehabil.* 1996;77:501–507.

10. Baker ER, Cardenas DD, Benedetti TJ. Risks associated with pregnancy in spinal cord injured women. *Obstet Gynecol.* 1992;80:425–428.

11. Jackson AB. Menopausal issues after spinal cord injury. *Top Spinal Cord Inj Rehabil.* 2001;7:64–71.

12. Cardenas DD, Farrell-Roberts L, Sipski ML, et al. Management of gastrointestinal, genitourinary, and sexual function. In: Stover SL, Delisa JA, Whiteneck GG, eds. *Spinal cord injury: Clinical outcomes from the model systems.* Gaithersburg, MD: Aspen; 1995:120–144.

13. Albert TJ, Levine MJ, Balderston RA, et al. Gastrointestinal complications in spinal cord injury. *Spine.* 1991;16:S522–S525.

14. Berczeller PH, Bezkor MF. Gastrointestinal complication. In: Berczeller PH, Bezkor MF, eds. *Medical complications of quadriplegia.* Chicago, IL: Year Book; 1986:95–107.

15. Macciocchi SN, Bowman B, Coker J, et al. Effect of co-morbid traumatic brain injury on functional outcome of persons with spinal cord injuries. *Am J Phys Med Rehabil.* 2004;83:22–26.

16. ASIA, IMSOP. International standards for neurological classification of spinal cord injury, revised 2000. Atlanta, GA: American Spinal Injury Association and the International Society of Paraplegia; 2000.

17. Stover SL, Hall KM, Delisa JA. System benefits. In: Stover SL, Whiteneck GG, Delisa JA, et al. eds. *Spinal cord injury: Clinical outcomes from the model systems.* Gaithersburg, MD: Aspen; 1995:317–326.

18. Cardenas DD, Hoffman JM, Kirshblum S, et al. Etiology and incidence of rehospitlization after traumatic spinal cord injury: A multicenter analysis [abstract]. *Arch Phys Med Rehabil.* 2004;85:1757–1763.

19. Bracken M, Holford TR. Neurological and functional status 1 year after acute spinal cord injury. *J Neurosurg.* 2002;96:259–266.

20. Waters RL, Adkins RH, Yakura JS, et al. Motor and sensory recovery following incomplete tetraplegia. *Arch Phys Med Rehabil.* 1994a;75:67–72.

21. Waters RL, Adkins RH, Yakura JS, et al. Motor and sensory recovery following incomplete tetraplegia. *Arch Phys Med Rehabil.* 1994b;75:306–311.

22. Ditunno JF Jr, Stover SK, Freed MM, et al. Motor recovery of the upper extremities in traumatic quadriplegia: A multicenter study. *Arch Phys Med Rehabil.* 1992;73:431–436.

23. Hollar LD. Spinal Cord Injury. In: Trombly C, ed. *Occupational therapy for physical dysfunction.* Baltimore, MD: Williams & Wilkins; 1995:795–813.

24. Waters RL, Sie IH, Gellman H, et al. Functional hand surgery following tetraplegia. *Arch Phys Med Rehabil.* 1996;77:86–94.

25. Phillips B, Zhao H. Predictors of assistive technology abandonment. *Assist Technol.* 1993;5:36–45.

26. Johnson K, Dudgeon B, Amtmann D. Assistive technology in rehabilitation. *J Voc Rehabil.* 1997;8:389–403.

27. Goetter WE, Stover SL, Kuhlemeier KV, et al. Respiratory complications following spinal cord injury: A prospective study. *Arch Phys Med Rehabil.* 1986;67:628.

28. Bach JR. Mechanical exsufflation, noninvasive ventilation, and new strategies for pulmonary rehabilitation and sleep disordered breathing. *Bull N Y Acad Med.* 1992;68:321–340.

29. Rossi E, Green D, Rosen J, et al. Sequential changes in factor VIII and platelets preceding deep vein thrombosis in patients with spinal cord injury. *Br J Haematol.* 1980;45:143–151.

30. Virchow R. Neuer fall vontodlichen. Embuli der lungernarterie. *Arch Pathol Anat.* 1856;10:225–228.

31. Walsh J, Tribe C. Phlebothrombosis and pulmonary embolism in paraplegia. *Paraplegia.* 1965;3:209–213.

32. Naso F. Pulmonary embolism in acute spinal cord injury. *Arch Phys Med Rehabil.* 1974;55:275–278.

33. Huisman MV, Buller HR, ten Cate JW, et al. Unexpected high prevalence of silent pulmonary embolism in patients with deep venous thrombosis. *Chest.* 1989; 95:498–502.

34. CSCM. Prevention of thromboembolism in spinal cord injury. In: *Spinal cord medicine clinical practice guidelines.* Washington, DC: Consortium of Spinal Cord Medicine; 1997:9–10.

35. CSCM. Acute management of autonomic dysreflexia: Individuals with spinal cord injury presenting to health-care facilities. *J Spinal Cord Med.* 2002; 25:S67–S88.

36. Mawson AR, Biundo JJ, Neville P, et al. Risk factors for early occurring pressure ulcers following spinal cord injury. *Am J Phys Med Rehabil.* 1988;67:123–127.

37. Yarkony GM, Heinemann AW. Pressure ulcers. In: Delisa JA, Whiteneck GG, eds. *Spinal cord injury: Clinical outcomes from the model systems.* Gaithersburg, MD: Aspen; 1995:100–119.

38. Byrne DW, Salzberg CA. Major risk factors for pressure ulcers in the spinal cord disabled: A literature review. *Spinal Cord.* 1996;34:255–263.

39. Stolp-Smith KA, Wainberg MC. Antidepressant exacerbation of spasticity. *Arch Phys Med Rehabil.* 1999; 80:339–342.

40. Cardenas DD, Mayo ME. Bacteriuria with fever after spinal cord injury. *Arch Phys Med Rehabil.* 1987;68: 291–293.

41. Cardenas DD, Hooton TM. Urinary tract infection in persons with spinal cord injury. *Arch Phys Med Rehabil.* 1995;75:272–280.

42. Turner JA, Cardenas DD, Warms CA, et al. Chronic pain associated with spinal cord injuries: A community survey. *Arch Phys Med Rehabil.* 2001;82:501–508.

43. Cardenas DD, Warms CA, Turner JA, et al. Efficacy of amitriptyline for relief of pain in spinal cord injury: Results of a randomized controlled trial. *Pain.* 2002; 96:365–373.

44. Davidoff G, Guarracini M, Roth E, et al. Trazodone hydrochloride in the treatment of dysesthetic pain in traumatic myelopathy: A randomized, double-blind, placebo-controlled study. *Pain.* 1987;29:151–161.

45. Berezin M, Ohry A, Shemesh Y, et al. Hyperprolactinemia, galactorrhea and amenorrhea in women with a spinal cord injury. *Gynecol Endocrinol.* 1989;3:159–163.

46. Massagli TL, Cardenas DD. Immobilization hypercalcemia treatment with pamidronate disodium after spinal cord injury. *Arch Phys Med Rehabil.* 1999;9: 998–1000.

47. Bach JR, Tilton MC. Life satisfaction and well-being measures in ventilator assisted individuals with traumatic tetraplegia. *Arch Phys Med Rehabil.* 1994;75: 626–632.

48. Kennedy P, Rogers BA. Anxiety and depression after spinal cord injury: A longitudinal analysis. *Arch Phys Med Rehabil.* 2000;81:932–937.

49. Richards JS, Kewman DG, Pierce CA. Spinal cord injury. In: Frank RG, Elliott TR, eds. *Handbook of rehabilitation psychology*. Washington, DC: American Psychological Association; 2000:11–27.

50. DeVivo MJ, Black KJ, Richards JS, et al. Suicide following spinal cord injury. *Paraplegia*. 1991;29:620–627.

51. Chapin MH, Kewman DG. Factors affecting employment following spinal cord injury: A qualitative study. *Rehabil Psychol*. 2001;46:400–416.

52. Heinemann AW, Keen M, Donohue R, et al. Alcohol use by persons with recent spinal cord injury. *Arch Phys Med Rehabil*. 1988;69:619–624.

53. Elliott TR, Kurylo M, Chen Y, et al. Alcohol abuse history and adjustment following spinal cord injury. *Rehabil Psychol*. 2002;47:278–290.

54. Bombardier C, Rimmele C. Alcohol use and readiness to change after spinal cord injury. *Arch Phys Med Rehabil*. 1998;79:1110–1115.

55. Patterson DR, Miller-Perrin C, McCormick TR, et al. When life support is questioned early in the care of patients with cervical-level quadriplegia. *N Engl J Med*. 1993;328:506–509.

8

Rehabilitation after Traumatic Lower Extremity Amputation

Joseph M. Czerniecki

EPIDEMIOLOGY OF TRAUMATIC AMPUTATION

The epidemiological characteristics of extremity amputation vary considerably depending upon geographical factors, the relative frequency of diabetes and atherosclerosis, the presence of or residual effects of military conflict, the predominance of farming or heavy industry, and the use of different types of motor vehicles. These factors make it difficult to compare published data and interpret differences in the prevalence of amputation between studies. There are regional variations in the United States that may be related to the population characteristics, such as age and ethnic origin (1). Similarly, there is even greater variation when the epidemiology of amputation is considered from a more global perspective. In Burma (2), for example, 87% of upper-extremity amputations are related to trauma and 47% of lower-extremity amputations are trauma related. Similarly, in Saudi Arabia during the 1980s (3), it was reported that 87% of upper-extremity and 53% of lower-extremity amputations were trauma related. In Europe and North America, current data suggest that only 3% to 4% of amputations are trauma related and a similar proportion are related to tumors, while >90% are related to a combination of peripheral vascular disease or diabetes (4–6). While the incidence of traumatic amputation is relatively low in North America, the prevalence is proportionately higher because individuals with trauma-related amputations live longer after injury than those with amputations due to vascular disease or diabetes.

Dillingham (7), in his retrospective survey, provides the greatest insights into the epidemiology of lower-extremity traumatic amputation in large United States metropolitan areas. He studied the epidemiologic factors and outcomes of 78 individuals with amputations treated during a 10-year period at a major urban trauma center. These data reinforce the notion that traumatic amputation is largely a problem experienced by young men. More than 85% of the population were male and a comparable proportion were younger than 40 years of age. The use of motor vehicles accounted for 75% of the trauma-related lower-extremity amputations. Occupants of motor vehicles incurred 11% of the amputations; pedestrians, 23%; riders of motorcycle crashes had the most amputations at 42%. It is important to note from a rehabilitation perspective that although the majority of these patients will have isolated extremity injury, a significant proportion will have major injuries to other body parts that will complicate both their acute care and long-term outcome (head and neck injury, 14%; thoracic injury, 13%; abdominal injury, 9%).

The distribution of amputation levels related to trauma in a major university hospital in Seoul, South Korea (8), is remarkably similar to the distribution in the previously mentioned study by Dillingham (7). The most common amputation level is the transtibial level, accounting for slightly more than 50%, with transfemoral (including knee disarticulation) being approximately 40%. Partial foot amputations and hip disarticulations account for the remaining 10%. In Dillingham (7), the frequency of amputation at the knee disarticulation was remarkably high, at 16%.

143

AMPUTATION DECISION MAKING IN THE "MANGLED LIMB"

One of the most challenging decisions to make in the evaluation of the patient with severe injury to the distal lower extremity is whether to embark on a plan to salvage the lower extremity or to have the patient undergo primary amputation. In some ways, an even more difficult decision is when to discontinue the plan to attempt salvage. The patient, the patient's family, and the surgeon may have, at this point, invested significant time and energy, with the accompanying financial and emotional toll, and therefore may have a difficult time considering amputation.

Because of the difficulties associated with these decisions, extensive efforts have been made to quantify the severity of injury and determine a threshold at which the salvage of the extremity is not possible and amputation is the treatment of choice. Some of these measures include the Mangled Extremity Score (MESS); the Limb Salvage Index (LSI); the Predictive Salvage Index (PSI); the Nerve Injury, Soft-Tissue Injury, Skeletal Injury, Shock, and Age of Patient Score (NISSA); and the Hannover Fracture Scale-97 (HFS-97). To varying degrees each of these measures attempts to quantify factors that might predict failure of limb salvage and therefore the need for amputation. The local extremity factors include a quantification of the extent of soft tissue injury or defect; the presence, absence, and severity of vascular injury; the presence and extent of nerve injury; and the location and extent of osseous injury. Some of these measures assess the patient in a more global way, but only in the limited dimensions of age and the presence or absence of systemic manifestations of injury, as determined by the presence or absence of shock. Initial studies of the predictive utility of these measures were encouraging. Johansen (9), for example, initially showed in a retrospective analysis that a MESS score above threshold was 100% predictive of need for amputation. Similarly, Russel (10) showed that the LSI had a 100% correlation with limb amputation and salvage. More recently, other investigators using retrospective research designs have been less enthusiastic about the utility of these measures. Dagum et al. (11) showed sensitivities of between 0.4 and 0.6 in three of these measures. Similarly, Bonanni et al. (12) showed sensitivities of between 0.2 and 0.6 for these measures. That is, scores above the threshold predicted need for amputation only about 50% of the time. In the only prospective multicenter evaluation (13) of these indexes in different subpopulations of

lower-extremity injury (those with differing severity of fractures with and without vascular injuries), these measures had sensitivities that varied with the different subpopulations, but overall the sensitivities mirrored those of the previously mentioned retrospective studies. Of value, however, is that these indexes generally had specificities of >0.9. Bosse (13) summarized the utility of these measures by saying that "the indices are incapable of identifying patients who will eventually require an amputation, [but] they might be useful as a screening test to support the entry of an extremity into the limb salvage pathway." That is, a score below threshold has a high probability of leading to a successfully salvaged extremity, but there is a moderate probability that limbs of patients with a score above the threshold value can also be salvaged.

The previously mentioned research provides insights into a "first layer" approach to decision making in the mangled extremity. That is, it addresses the question, can it be determined at the time of injury and presentation to the emergency room which extremity can be salvaged and which will require amputation? An additional and critical layer in the decision making is related to the prediction of functional outcome. In an ideal world, it would be advantageous to predict at the time of injury not only if a limb can be salvaged but also if the functional outcome of the individual with a salvaged extremity would be better than if an amputation were performed. To date there are no outcome measurement tools available that address this question. One is therefore left to rely on the clinical expertise of the surgeon and physical medicine and rehabilitation (PM&R) specialist to try to anticipate the functional outcome of either amputation or limb salvage.

REHABILITATION MANAGEMENT IN THE PERIOPERATIVE PERIOD

THE PREOPERATIVE PERIOD

The primary role of the rehabilitation specialist in the preoperative period is to assist the orthopaedic surgeon in the informed consent process, amputation decision making, and patient education.

The Informed Consent Process

Historically, informed consent was used as a process of legal protection for the physician and hospital. Generally, it included statements only of risk of death or specific complications. The informed consent process has evolved considerably so that it should now be used as a tool to facilitate quality patient-physician interaction and to enable shared decision making in terms of health care interventions. To quote James Bernat (14), "Reasonable people need to know their treatment options, the general risks, benefits, and probable outcomes of each option, and the reasons that the physician has recommended a specific treatment." In the context of the patient who presents to the emergency room with extensive lower-extremity trauma, it is critical that the patient be informed of his or her treatment options and potential outcomes. In the following section, the role of physiatrists in this process will be described. Their expertise in understanding the outcome of amputation and the interaction of premorbid and concurrent disease processes, as well as the interaction of prosthetic provision, enables them to provide a key component in the informed consent process.

THE DECISION TO AMPUTATE OR ATTEMPT LIMB SALVAGE

LIMB SALVAGE

At the outset, it is important to consider not only whether the limb can be salvaged from a technical perspective, but whether its salvage will more likely return the patient to his or her premorbid level of function than if an amputation were performed. It is the functional status of the patient that is the key issue, not the salvage of the extremity.

The first step in patient evaluation, therefore, is to determine the patient's premorbid level of function. This includes not only their vocational status, but also their avocational interests. Their premorbid functional status must be established in sufficient detail to know what their mobility requirements are, including periods of time standing, walking, and stair climbing; ambulation over complex terrain; and sports participation, including frequency and intensity. The second step is to try to determine the relative importance to the patient of preserving each of these various functional tasks and also the relative importance of the psychological aspects of preserving the cosmetic and body image aspects of a "normal" compared with a prosthetic extremity. With this background, the clinical team is setting the stage to establish the goals of the patient's health care intervention.

The first key question for the health care team is whether or not the limb can be salvaged from a technical perspective. This question itself may require

input from the orthopaedic surgeon, the vascular surgeon, if there has been vascular injury, and/or the plastic surgeon if there is a significant soft tissue defect that might require free flap or other skin grafts. In many situations, it is difficult to answer this question definitively. Oftentimes, the surgeon must approximate the percentage probability that the limb can be successfully salvaged.

Of equal importance to whether or not the limb can be salvaged is to define what would be involved in the salvage process. The factors to be considered include the number of surgical procedures, the time course of future reconstruction, and the extent of function during the time course of salvage. For example, the salvage of the extremity might take six to eight surgical procedures over the course of 18 months with the need for casts and crutch walking during this time. This course might require the patient to take considerable analgesic medication, undergo intensive physical therapy, and miss work during the salvage and reconstructive efforts.

The final consideration is what functional outcome the patient might expect at the conclusion of the salvage attempt. How closely will the patient's functional status approximate his or her premorbid level of function? For example, will salvage necessitate an extensive split thickness skin graft that may be prone to skin breakdown in the long term, with intermittent reductions in mobility to heal the skin breakdown? Will there be a significant risk for residual contracture, pain, or sensory motor impairment that will limit the function of the extremity for higher levels of mobility?

AMPUTATION

Once the details of salvage have been defined, it is important to define the details of the amputation branch of the decision tree. Although some orthopaedic specialists have extensive expertise in amputation rehabilitation and amputation outcome prediction, the physiatrist with expertise in the rehabilitation of the amputee is in an ideal position to play an important role in this area.

There is little research to guide the clinician in the prediction of functional outcome in the traumatic amputation patient. Attempts have been made in the dysvascular population (15) with some success. One is therefore left to use clinical experience and expertise in this process. The data set that should be used in addition to the patient's premorbid vocational and avocational status includes preamputation comorbid medical surgical disorders, social support system, psychological status, and current comorbid medical and surgical disorders. In addition to assessing these historical features, it is essential to perform a detailed physical examination, including mental, neurologic, musculoskeletal, and functional status. With this information and with a base of clinical experience in the care of many patients with a wide spectrum of amputation levels, one can reasonably predict what that individual's probable level of function will be at a number of relevant amputation levels. The typical time course of recovery and rehabilitation can also be determined.

This information is provided to the orthopaedic surgeon and the patient so that together they can weigh the potential impact of either branch of the decision tree in terms of its time course, frequency, and intensity of medical/surgical intervention, as well as the functional endpoint and long-term course, as they make their decision.

PATIENT EDUCATION

If the decision is made that amputation is necessary, the patient and family may experience a wide variety of psychological reactions. It is relatively uncommon for a patient facing this decision to have experience with the potential outcome after amputation. There are often extensive concerns about future mobility, sexuality, and ability to function as a spouse and/or parent, as well as potential concerns about being a burden to family members. The potential psychological reactions may include despair, depression, and anxiety.

One of the important goals of patient education is instilling a sense of hope. Although there has not been specific research into aspects of hope and hopelessness in the context of the amputee, research into other patient populations suggests that a sense of hopelessness is associated with adverse health outcomes. In the case of the amputee, it is important to instill a sense of "realistic optimism." This goal can be accomplished by the physician through direct patient-physician interaction, as well as in conjunction with an appropriately selected peer support person.

Although there has been limited research into the types of educational strategies and their effects, a study by Mortimer et al. (16) has shown that generally amputation patients are not happy with the amount of information they receive and how they receive it. The important elements to include in the educational process are information about where the amputation will take place, the typical postoperative management strategy, how much pain patients will typically experience and how long will it last, phantom limb pain, the typical time course to prosthetic fitting, what the rehabilitation process will be

and how long will it last, and, most vital, what their probable functional outcome will be.

EARLY POSTAMPUTATION MANAGEMENT

The key issues in the early rehabilitation of the amputee are to enhance wound healing, shape the residual limb in preparation for prosthetic fitting, prevent joint contracture, reduce pain, prevent secondary injury to the healing residual limb, and prevent the secondary complications associated with bed rest and immobility.

Early Postoperative Residual Limb Management

The most important goals of residual limb management in the early postoperative period are to prevent proximal joint contracture, protect the healing incision line, enhance healing, reduce edema, and shape the residual limb in preparation for future prosthetic fitting.

There has been considerable debate regarding the optimal strategy for managing the postamputation residual limb. There have been many advocated wound management strategies, including soft dressings, rigid dressings, immediate postoperative prostheses, removable rigid dressings, pneumatic dressings, and Unna dressings. Some have been advocated for specific amputation levels, while others have been more universally recommended for all lower-extremity amputation levels. Unfortunately there have been few well-designed studies that have adequately weighed the risks, benefits, cost-effectiveness, and functional outcome of the different postoperative management strategies. This topic was recently critically reviewed by Smith (17).

Soft dressings, which include a gauze dressing with an elasticized wrap bandage for compression, have been used at all major lower extremity amputation levels. They have been used to a greater extent by nonorthopaedic surgeons (18). The advantages of the procedure may include ease of application and the ability to observe the healing incision line in cases where there is a wound complication that may require debridement or frequent dressing changes. Potential disadvantages of this technique include a lack of protection of the residual limb from external trauma if the patient should happen to injure it during a transfer. There is no immobilization of the proximal joint so that flexion contractures may develop, which can have a significant adverse effect on the outcome. The use of physical therapy, patient/ nursing staff education and/or a posterior splint may decrease the likelihood of contracture of proximal joints. The proper application of the elasticized wrap requires a significant amount of skill, so that excessive proximal pressure and residual limb choking do not occur. There is also a significant staff time requirement because the position of the wrap constantly shifts and loosens, especially when patients are in bed. This necessitates frequent reapplication.

Rigid dressings have been used at all major lower-extremity amputation levels distal to and including the hip disarticulation level. Their use has largely been abandoned except for the transtibial, Symes, and, to a lesser extent, the transmetatarsal amputation levels. The rigid dressing typically includes a light gauze dressing at the incision line with an open cell foam distal pad, with padding over key boney landmarks, covered by layers of elastic and conventional plaster. At the transtibial amputation level, which is the most common amputation level where the rigid dressing is used, the key boney landmarks include the anterior border of the tibia, the distal anterior tibia, the fibular head, and the patella. It is suspended on the leg either through a waist belt or by compression of the cast as it hardens, over the medial and lateral femoral condyles. The advantages of this dressing are that it immobilizes the knee in extension, thus avoiding knee flexion contracture; immobilizes the soft tissues of the healing incision line; protects the residual limb from external trauma; and helps to compress and shape the residual limb in preparation for prosthetic fitting. At the transtibial amputation level, compared with the soft dressing, this approach may result in earlier prosthetic fitting and gait training (19) and may result in fewer surgical revisions (20).

The immediate postoperative prosthesis (IPOP) technique has been used at all levels from hip disarticulation through Symes but has been largely abandoned at all levels except the transtibial and, to a lesser extent, at the Symes amputation level. This technique uses a rigid dressing as described previously except with the distal attachment of a prosthetic pylon and foot. This approach therefore has the purported advantages of the rigid dressing but in addition allows either immediate or early postoperative progressive weight bearing. Early weight bearing may further enhance shaping of the residual limb and may have psychological and physiological benefits because of the earlier return to ambulation. Unfortunately, there are few well-done comparative trials that have evaluated the effect of the IPOP dressing against other management strategies. General cautionary statements have been made about the possible adverse effects of early weight bearing on patients with amputation secondary to vascular disease or diabetes (21).

The removable rigid dressing has been used exclusively at the transtibial amputation level (22). It includes a distal soft dressing over the wound with a rigid plaster cast that extends only to the level of the patella. This device simulates a conventional below-the-knee prosthetic socket except it is made of plaster. No pylon or prosthetic foot is attached. Weight bearing is begun through the distal end of the plaster cast against a padded pommel. The wound can be inspected to allow the effect of early weight bearing to be evaluated, prosthetic socks can be added to accommodate shrinkage of the residual limb, and the residual limb is protected by the rigid cast. Potential disadvantages include the lack of effective suspension systems other than the waist belt with an anterior strap; also the knee is not immobilized in extension so there may be greater risk of knee flexion contracture. The only comparative study done suggests that this device may be more effective at reducing edema and shaping the residual limb than a soft dressing (23).

A variety of pneumatic compressive devices have been developed to protect shape and immobilize the residual limb. Generally these devices have been developed to function similarly to the rigid dressing, or the IPOP, but they are lighter in weight and have more adjustable control over the amount of tissue compression and therefore allow more edema reduction and shaping than the rigid dressing. They also are removable to allow wound inspection and dressing changes to occur. Some of these are nonweight-bearing devices and some allow partial weight bearing during ambulation. In one comparative study, Schon (24) found a reduced risk of wound healing complications and need for surgical revision using these devices compared with a soft dressing.

The Unna dressing is a bandage that has typically been used in the management of venous stasis ulcers. It is a bandage that is embedded with a number of medications that, when applied to the postamputation residual limb, forms a semirigid dressing. It has been used at both the transtibial and transfemoral amputation levels (25). Wong and Edelstein (25) showed that the use of the Unna semirigid dressing resulted in enhanced wound healing and a greater frequency of prosthetic fitting with successful ambulation.

Overall, although there is data that suggest wound management strategies that create external compression result in enhanced wound healing and earlier and more likely prosthetic fitting, there is an acute need for better prospective randomized study designs with more well-defined endpoints, using more established outcome measures (17). In the absence of these studies and based upon the consensus in the data that postoperative management strategies with external compression seem to be effective, there is little to separate the relative effectiveness of different forms of external compression. It is recommended therefore that each amputation center develop knowledge and expertise with a given type of wound management strategy and to use it consistently to avoid possible complications.

THE OUTCOME AFTER SEVERE LOWER-EXTREMITY TRAUMA

OUTCOME AFTER AMPUTATION

Our understanding of the outcome of traumatic lower-extremity amputation has been enhanced significantly by the work of Dillingham (7) and Pezzin (26). Their epidemiologic study of a population of urban trauma center–managed patients best reflects the typical outcomes that one might expect in this country. The 78 amputation patients in this group included 51% with transtibial, 20% with transfemoral, and 16% with knee disarticulation amputations. This population had a mean age of 32 years at the time of injury with the mean follow-up time of >7 years. It is interesting to note that the mental health component of the SF-36 Health Survey revealed no significant differences compared with age- and gender-matched norms. The physical dimensions of the SF-36 do, however, reveal significant differences. The extent of bodily pain, ability to maintain physical roles, and overall physical functioning are significantly reduced compared to individuals without amputations.

Pain is primarily related to the amputation, but pain is also important in the contralateral limb. Phantom limb pain is a very common sequela of lower-extremity amputation and has been reported to occur to varying degrees in almost all individuals with lower-extremity amputations. In Dillingham's (7) population of individuals with traumatic lower-extremity amputations, severe phantom limb pain was present in 25% of patients. These results mirror those of a mixed population of patients with dysvascular and traumatic amputations. Using the Chronic Pain Grade, Ehde et al. (27) showed that 25% of amputation patients had a pain of grade III or IV, which indicates moderate to severe disability related to pain, and using the Numerical Pain Rating scale, 40% will have pain rated as >5/10. These results also mirror those of Steinbach, who showed that 27% of combat-injured individuals with lower-extremity amputations had either continuous or frequent phantom limb pain (28).

Residual limb pain is also an important cause of disability. Dillingham (7) found that 36% of his population rated their residual pain as either severe, continuous, or intermittent. The extent of residual limb pain, although seemingly very high, has been confirmed in other studies. Once again, Ehde et al. (27) showed that 60% of individuals with lower-extremity amputations in her study reported either moderately or severely bothersome residual limb pain. Smith et al. (29) similarly showed that 39% of patients reported that residual limb pain interfered with activity either "moderately or a lot." In addition to residual limb pain, persons with amputations experience disability related to mechanical skin injury, heat, and perspiration. Mechanical skin injury occurs in approximately 24% of subjects, and difficulties with skin irritation and perspiration occur in an additional 24% of subjects. In spite of problems with pain and mechanical skin injury, prosthetic use is very high overall, averaging 80 hours per week (7). From a more global perspective, there is only a moderate probability that those who incur a traumatic lower-extremity amputation will return to work. The return-to-work rate was very poor overall, with only 58% returning to work, and those who returned to work typically returned to less physically demanding jobs (7). These results parallel those seen in other studies (11,30).

It is becoming increasingly apparent that in addition to experiencing pain and limitation of function related to the primary disability of amputation, individuals with amputations will incur secondary musculoskeletal disability. It is particularly important to consider these factors when evaluating the global disabling effects of amputation across the life span of the individual with lower-extremity amputation. Only recently have studies begun to quantify the extent of secondary musculoskeletal pain and disability in such individuals. In the control population, low back pain has an approximate point prevalence of 30%, whereas in individuals with amputations, it is between 52% and 76% (27,29). Individuals with transfemoral amputations may have a greater incidence of back pain than persons with transtibial amputations (29). The precise underlying mechanisms that predispose to low back pain in individuals with amputations have not been established; however, it appears that leg length discrepancy may be a contributing factor (31). In addition to low back pain, individuals with lower-extremity amputations seem to be at increased risk of pain and degenerative arthritis of the lower-extremity joints, in particular the knee on the intact side. Recent epidemiological evidence (32) has shown that individuals with transtibial amputations have a twofold increased incidence of knee pain and those with transfemoral amputations have a threefold increased incidence of knee pain, compared with age-matched controls. Hungerford and Cockin (33) have also shown accelerated degenerative arthritis on radiologic studies of the intact knee of patients with amputations. This investigation reinforces the notion that accelerated degenerative changes occur in individuals with amputations and that it is influenced by amputation level. Interestingly, knee pain is actually reduced on the prosthetic side of transtibial amputation patients compared to the same control group. It may be that the gait pattern is modified on the amputated side to minimize lower-extremity loading.

In summary, traumatic amputation of the lower extremity exacts a significant toll on survivors, with 48% reporting their health to be somewhat or much worse than prior to their amputation. Only 58% returned to employment, and pain and physical limitation are much greater than in an age-matched control group. Prosthetic use is very high, but generally there is substantial dissatisfaction with the function of the prosthesis, with only 43% of patients reporting satisfaction with the comfort. In the long term, there is a significant risk of low back pain and contralateral limb articular pain that may further limit function.

OUTCOME AFTER SALVAGE

In the context of the compromised outcome after amputation, it is important to determine if the outcome of patients who have undergone successful limb salvage is any different from that of those who did not. Karladani et al. (34) evaluated a small sample of patients with Gustilo type IIIB and IIIC fractures. Type III open fractures of the tibia are those that are created by high energy and are associated with extensive soft tissue damage. Type IIIA are those that have adequate soft tissue coverage of bone, type IIIB are those that have exposure of bone and massive contamination, and type IIIC are those that have associated vascular injury. The majority, approximately 90%, were satisfied overall with their results. However, depression was evident in 28% and only 64% returned to work. In terms of mobility, 15% of patients walked with crutches, and an additional 28% could only walk <1 km. Pain at rest ranged from 0 to 40/100 on a 100 mm visual analogue scale, while pain during walking ranged from 0 to 71/100 with a mean of 36. These results confirm the significant adverse effects these extensive lower-extremity injuries have on ultimate function and mobility.

In contrast to the work of Karladani (34), which focused primarily on quantifying the outcome of individuals with salvaged severely injured lower-extremity injuries, some studies have compared the outcome of those with primary amputation after traumatic injury with those that have undergone limb salvage (35). Some studies have included the additional population of those that have undergone transtibial amputation as a delayed procedure after prolonged attempts at limb salvage (11,30). Unfortunately, all of these studies are retrospective studies. Generally, there do not appear to be striking differences in the outcomes of these groups in terms of the state of well-being (30) or mental health. Dagum (11) used the SF-36, and in the mental component, which includes subscales such as vitality, mental health, and social functioning, there was no difference, and in fact, there were no differences from a normal control population of similar age. Similarly, Georgiadis (35), using the Nottingham Health Profile, showed no significant differences in energy, emotional reactions, or sense of social isolation. Regarding physical functioning and mobility, there is some controversy. Dagum's (11) results suggest improved physical functioning scores on the SF-36 in the limb salvage group, while others (35) have found there were no differences in reported ability to walk, run, jump, or climb stairs. Georgiadis (35) did find, however, that those with limb salvage had greater reported adverse effects on health status and ability to work or engage in recreational activities. Although long-term pain is a frequent issue in both individuals with amputations and those with limb salvage, there is little to no difference between the two populations (11,35). An important aspect of functional outcome assessment in the individual with severe lower-extremity trauma is return to work. These individuals tend to be young and male; therefore, the economic impact and effect on overall financial status, as well as disability costs throughout their lifetime, are significant. The return to work rate and the time to return to work are surprisingly consistent across studies. Dagum (11) found a return to work rate of approximately 65% in both the amputation and salvage groups, which is similar to the results of Karladani (34) in his study of those with type IIIB or IIIC lower-extremity injuries that were salvaged. Those with primary amputation return to work significantly earlier than those with salvage, and in those with secondary amputation, the return to work is most delayed. The average time to return to work in the primary amputation group in Dagum's study (11) was 9 months compared to 17 months in the salvage group and 36 months in the late amputation group. These times to return to work are almost identical to those in Fairhurst's (30) retrospective review of type III fractures: 6 months in the primary amputation group, 18 months in the salvage group, and 36 months in the late or secondary amputation group. In a number of studies, investigators have tried to assess from a more global perspective what patients' perceptions are about their decisions to pursue either a salvage or amputation pathway. The conclusions of course are limited, because there is a reductive bias built into the answer by the patients' previous decisions about their treatment, but they may offer some general insights into whether people would have chosen their choice of treatment if faced with the same problem again. Those who chose salvage would choose the same course again between 60% (30) and 88% (34) of the time. It is interesting to note, however, that of those patients who had delayed amputation, 75% wished that they had their amputation performed as a primary procedure. This result suggests that those who had pursued a course of salvage, albeit one that was not successful, and ultimately experienced their functional status as an individual with an amputation, would have made a different decision. As discussed earlier, it is indeed a challenge to determine who should have primary amputation and who should embark on a pathway of limb salvage. Of equal importance, however, is the difficulty in determining when to abandon attempts at limb salvage. Once beginning this course of treatment with its investment of time, psychological energy, pain, and money, it is easy for both the patient and surgeon to continue.

In summary, based upon limited data and research involving less than optimal study designs, there are few differences between those with salvage of a severely injured lower extremity compared to those that have undergone amputation. Pain, ultimate sense of well-being, psychological status, probability of employment, and so on, are very similar. There is controversy about individuals' level of physical functioning and perception of ability to pursue vocational and recreational interests. Some data suggest that those with salvaged extremities perform to a higher level of mobility while other data suggest that those with transtibial amputations do. There are two clear differences. First, the time to reach optimal mobility and return to work is much less after amputation, and second, the health care costs incurred in this process are much lower. Further prospective studies, using validated outcome measures to further help us understand which patients should have amputation and which should have limbs salvaged, are necessary. Additionally, it would be useful to know whether or not over the life span of the individual there are differences in each population's ability to maintain mobility with fewer additional secondary disabilities.

PROSTHETIC FITTING AFTER LOWER EXTREMITY AMPUTATION

TRANSMETATARSAL AMPUTATION

A transmetatarsal amputation is an amputation across all of the metatarsals, removing all of the toes and the distal portions of the metatarsals. This amputation level typically uses a long plantar flap with a distal dorsal closure and plantar soft tissue covering the distal cut ends of the metatarsals. This amputation level is preferred when there is good general perfusion to the foot and there is adequate soft tissue on the plantar surface to construct the plantar flap, as well as adequate sensation on the plantar surface. The pathology or tissue defect is typically limited to a number of toes up to the level of the metatarsal heads. This amputation level is preferred if there is a need for more than two rays to be amputated.

The prosthetic and orthotic management is variable depending on the length of the transmetatarsal amputation. Generally, provided the surgeon is able to preserve robust soft tissue coverage, the greater the length of the metatarsal that can be preserved the better. In fact, if possible, a metatarsophalangeal disarticulation is the best choice because it preserves the weight-bearing characteristics and the specialized soft tissues under the metatarsal heads. With the long transmetatarsal amputation, the key functional problems that need to be addressed are a tendency to develop an equinus contracture; a reduction in the effective lever arm length of the foot with its effect on gait characteristics; reduced surface area for dissipation of tissue pressures associated with ambulation; and, to a lesser extent, stabilization of the shoe on the residual foot. To remedy the tendency towards an equinus contracture, an Achilles tendon lengthening or, less commonly, a Gastroc-slide or Strayer procedure (36) is often performed at the time of the amputation. The remaining problems are dealt with through prosthetic/orthotic fitting and foot-wear modifications. To increase the effective toe lever to normal, it is common to insert a spring steel or carbon fiber insert between the outsole and the midsole of the shoe that extends only to the level of the metatarsal heads before amputation. To increase the surface area for distribution of forces on the plantar surface, a custom-molded in-shoe orthotic is provided; to stabilize the shoe on the foot, a toe filler is provided. This filler prevents the residual limb from sliding within the shoe. It is important that the toe filler have a dorsal V-notch across it at the location of the metatarsal heads. The notch ensures a normal "toe break" or point of flexion of the shoe during the second half of stance phase. If there are continued problems with the shoe being unstable on the foot, a high-top lace-up or self-fastening closure shoe will provide additional stability.

For the patient with a short transmetatarsal amputation the previously mentioned problems associated with the transmetatarsal amputation are the same, only exaggerated. One of the primary issues is that it is virtually impossible to stabilize the shoe on the residual limb, which results in excessive motion and "pistoning" of the residual limb in the shoe, which not only causes risk of mechanical skin breakdown, but prevents normal biomechanical function of the foot/shoe complex. In this case, a custom-molded thermoplastic ankle foot orthosis (AFO) with a toe filler is necessary. The custom contouring of the sole portion optimizes pressure distribution under the residual foot. Extending the sole portion to the area of the metatarsal heads restores the toe lever, and the toe filler assists in forming the toe lever as well as preventing distal migration of the residual limb in the shoe. The posterior, or leg portion, assists in stabilizing the shoe on the residuum and also transmits the forces of the toe lever to the leg. For patients with a relative contraindication to a thermoplastic AFO, a double metal upright AFO may be required. This is commonly rejected, however, because of weight, cosmesis, and a tendency for it to make abnormal noises during gait.

THE SYMES AMPUTATION

The Symes is a controversial amputation level. In the literature there are some strong advocates for amputation at this anatomic level because of the potential benefits of improved balance and stability, reduced metabolic cost of ambulation, and the potential for limited weight bearing and ambulation in the home environment without a prosthesis. Those that view this amputation level less favorably suggest that there are problems with maintaining stability of the distal heel pad, with associated difficulties of maintaining a comfortable prosthetic fit.

This surgical procedure involves removal of all of the osseus structures of the foot, as well as the malleoli to the level of the distal articular surface of the tibia. Subsequently, a long plantar flap is constructed using the soft tissues of the plantar surface of the calcaneus. This results in preservation of the architectural and structural characteristics of these specially adapted tissues to allow end bearing either

in a prosthesis, or for very limited ambulation outside of the prosthesis. Excessive mobility of the heel pad is attributed to inadequate healing at the time of initiation of weight bearing and the dynamic pull of tendons such as the Achilles tendon or the tibialis posterior tendon that attach to the heel pad by scar formation. It is therefore recommended that weight bearing after Symes amputation be delayed for 6 weeks, whether or not the skin and subcutaneous tissues appear to be healed adequately, to ensure optimal stabilization of the heel pad. Recently, Smith (37) described the direct suturing of the Achilles tendon to the posterior aspect of the tibia so that dynamic muscle tension does not tend to displace the position of the heel pad away from the distal end of the tibia.

The principal challenge of prosthetic provision after Symes amputation is the bulbous shape of the distal portion of the residual limb. Special prosthetic socket designs are necessary to ensure that there is total contact of the socket wall with the residual limb while still allowing ingress of the residual limb into the prosthesis. The two typical prosthetic socket solutions are the closed Symes prosthesis and the windowed Symes prosthesis. The closed Symes prosthesis has an inner pelite or other closed celled foam layer that covers the residual limb but is built up to an additional thickness at the narrowest supramalleolar level, so that its external dimension is equal to that at the distal bulbous end. The liner is then slit on the medial aspect over a length of approximately 15 cm so that when the patient dons the liner, the bulbous portion will cause the slit to open and allow ingress of the bulbous end. Subsequently, the slit will close when it is completely donned. After donning the liner, the patient dons the rigid prosthetic socket. The windowed Symes prosthesis differs in that it typically does not have an inner liner. It consists of an epoxy or polyester resin socket with an oval medial window that is approximately 15 cm long and 7 cm wide at the level of the medial supramalleolar area. The presence of the window allows the patient to don the prosthesis without difficulty because with the window removed the bulbous distal end is allowed to pass easily into the socket. Once the residual limb is in place, the hard cover to the window is replaced and held in place by a circumferential self-fastening strap.

Each of these prosthetic socket types has advantages and disadvantages. The closed Symes does provide for an inner foam liner, which may enhance comfort, but the cosmetic contour of the prosthesis has been described as "stovepipe" in appearance as it lacks any normal external ankle contour. The external contour of the windowed Symes has a normal ankle conformation, although there is a self-fastening closure. Soft tissue cushioning is typically provided by prosthetic socks.

An additional challenge of fitting a Symes prosthesis is to achieve equal and symmetrical leg lengths. With the distal heel pad on the residual limb plus the additional length associated with the use of a liner and the external socket, there is very little space left for the prosthetic foot. This problem has been solved by the development of low-profile Symes feet by a number of prosthetic manufacturers. Because of limitations in the effective mechanical spring function, these prosthetic feet are less dynamic than designs that are used at higher amputation levels.

THE TRANSTIBIAL AMPUTATION LEVEL

There are a number of surgical approaches that may be used to perform an amputation at the transtibial level. These approaches include an anterior-posterior fish mouth closure, the skew flap, the sagittal flap, and the long posterior flap techniques. The fish mouth closure should be avoided especially in the dysvascular patient, because of problems with flap perfusion and less than adequate soft tissue coverage, especially on the distal anterior tibia. The sagittal flap uses an anterolateral musculocutaneous flap and a posteromedial gastrocnemius musculocutaneous flap. The Skew flap consists of anteromedial and posterolateral fasciocutaneous flaps with a superficial posterior muscle flap to be contoured over the distal boney tibia (38). The posterior flap technique uses a long posterior myocutaneous flap that is brought up around the distal end of the residual limb and is sutured across the anterodistal portion of the residual limb. There is greater agreement about the way the osseus structures should be handled. The tibial is sectioned transversely with the distal anterior portion beveled to minimize its prominence, and the fibula is sectioned approximately 1.5 cm shorter than the tibia. A procedure that has been advocated by some is the Ertl procedure (38). This procedure results in a portion of the amputated fibula that is oriented horizontally between the distal fibula and tibia and kept in place with a screw. Ultimately a fusion will result. Advocates of this procedure note a greater potential to have a partially end-bearing residual limb because of the improved surface area for loading, as well as potential advantages of rigidly stabilizing the fibula. Unfortunately, there is little scientific investigation that supports its utility. It has been argued that in individuals with dysvascular amputations, the long posterior flap provides better soft tissue coverage at the distal end of the residual limb. It is also thought

by some that the long posterior myocutaneous flap may have greater healing potential because of the presence of perforating myocutaneous vessels from the underlying gastrocnemius that may enhance perfusion to the distal portion of the flap. Others have disagreed with this assertion and, based upon vascular anatomy, feel that the skew flap has the greatest probability of healing and provides adequate distal soft tissue coverage (39).

In the case of individuals with traumatic amputations, one of the most important surgical considerations is to preserve the length of the residual limb. Preservation will optimize the effective lever arm length for transmission of muscular forces, and it also enhances the overall surface area for distribution of the forces applied to the soft tissues of the residual limb during standing and walking. The preservation of length sometimes requires the surgeon to use creative flaps and soft tissue approaches. In the young traumatic amputation patients, limitations of perfusion are a less important consideration, therefore allowing a greater flexibility in the surgical technique. A common question in amputation surgery and rehabilitation is the extent to which residual limb length should be preserved, when preserving length results in a limb with compromised soft tissue coverage. That is, should a short or very short transtibial amputation be performed to obtain a residual limb with good soft tissue coverage, or should the surgeon perform an amputation that results in a long residual limb but with soft tissue coverage that may require split thickness skin graft or free flap? This is a complicated issue. Of greatest importance is probably not whether there is split thickness skin graft but where it is located and whether or not there is adequate subcutaneous tissue separating it from underlying bone. With currently available interface systems, long-term successful function can be obtained in the presence of split thickness skin graft, especially if it is not overlying an area of boney prominence or, at least, it is not adherent to underlying bone. The preservation of length does of course have reasonable limits. Some have advocated an optimal length of 19 cm distal to the knee joint or just proximal to the myocutaneous junction of the gastrocnemius soleus. These limits have been established to allow adequate muscle and subcutaneous tissue at the distal end of the residual limb.

There are many options available when formulating a prosthetic prescription at the transtibial amputation level. The primary goals are to have a prosthesis that is comfortable, minimizes applied forces to the residual limb, is well suspended, allows for effective stabilization of the residual limb in the prosthetic socket, and has optimum biomechanical function for the functional priorities of the individual patient. Before arriving at a prosthetic prescription, it is important to define the patient's expected level of function. This will be based largely upon the premorbid level of function and the current status. The current status includes an evaluation of cognitive function, neuromuscular function, and musculoskeletal function, as well as a detailed evaluation of the residual limb. The residual limb evaluation should include an assessment of residual limb length, shape, soft tissue characteristics, extent of healing, and presence of pain/hypersensitivity. It would be impossible to arrive at a prosthetic prescription for all possible clinical contexts, so only a limited number will be discussed. These prescriptions will be based on the assumption that no other significant cognitive, musculoskeletal, or neurological injury exists, and because the traumatic amputee is typically relatively young and active, on the assumption that the patient has at least moderately active functional goals.

For the patient with the very short residual limb, the surface area available for distributing the loads associated with body weight, as well as the muscular forces associated with standing and walking, is very small. In addition, there is difficulty in maintaining stability of the residual limb in the prosthetic socket. As a result, careful attention must be paid to the socket design and the characteristics of the interface material between the socket and the residual limb. There are three socket design characteristics that can effectively increase the surface area for distribution of forces and increase the stability of the residual limb in the prosthetic socket. These include the patellar tendon-bearing supracondylar (PTS) socket, the patellar tendon-bearing supracondylar suprapatellar (PTSS) socket, and the side joint and thigh lacer (SJTL). The PTS socket extends the medial lateral brim of the socket further proximally and commonly uses a pelite liner that has been built up over the medial femoral condyle. The PTSS socket is the same as a PTS socket in the medial-lateral plane but also has a proximal extension over the patella. Both of these designs extend the proximal contours to provide additional stability of the socket on the residual limb, and they use a foam interface material to provide cushioning. The SJTL is attached to a typical patellar tendon-bearing socket. It includes a medial and a lateral metal upright that extends one-half to two-thirds of the way up the thigh with a single axis joint at the level of the functional center of rotation of the knee joint. The uprights have a leather thigh corset attached to the uprights with an anterior lace-up or self-fastening closure. The use of the SJTL allows a portion of the body weight to be carried by the musculature and

soft tissues of the thigh instead of on the very short residual limb. The choice between the PTS or PTSS and the SJTL rests primarily with patient tolerance to the added weight, the cosmetic consequences, and the bulk of the side joint and thigh lacer. For the patient with higher activity goals, especially if involved in vocational or avocational goals that require extensive walking, carrying of heavy loads, or walking over complex terrain, the SJTL is advisable.

For the patient with an average length residual limb or longer, the typical prosthetic socket design involves a combination of traditional patellar tendon bearing plus total surface bearing, for even distribution of loads across the whole surface of the residual limb. The most commonly used interface system for the active transtibial amputee is a silicone or urethane roll on a suspension sleeve with a distal locking pin. These systems are rolled onto the residual limb directly against the skin and extend to approximately 5 cm above the brim of the socket. Typically they have a distal pin that engages in a shuttle lock at the distal end of the prosthetic socket. There are many different manufacturers of these systems. In fact, each manufacturer often makes a number of different designs, each with unique thicknesses, stiffnesses, and distributions of silicone or urethane. They also vary in whether they are manufactured as a straight tube or whether they are in a preflexed position. Although there is little research to guide our choice of interface, they all work in a similar manner. The silicone or urethane interface is designed to enhance the distribution of normally oriented forces and also to reduce applied shear forces to the residual limb, and the presence of the distal locking pin prevents pistoning of the residual limb in the prosthetic socket, further minimizing applied shear stresses to the soft tissues. These systems allow for the adjustment of socket fit when there is a reduction in residual limb volume, through the addition of prosthetic socks. The ability to adjust the socket fit is a very important issue, especially early after amputation when there are often very significant and rapid reductions in residual limb volume.

In all transtibial amputation patients, there are a myriad of choices of prosthetic pylon and foot/ankle components. The two primary choices in pylon type are endoskeletal or exoskeletal. The endoskeletal system is essentially a lightweight tubular pylon that is attached to the distal end of the socket proximally and the prosthetic foot distally. An advantage of this system is that prosthetic realignment can be easily accomplished at any time after prosthetic fitting. This ability is particularly important in the new amputation patient during the early stages of gait training when there can be considerable variability in gait characteristics, which requires concomitantly more frequent readjustments of alignment. The cosmetic characteristics of the endoskeletal system rely on a foam cover to be applied on the outside of the endoskeletal pylon, which is cosmetically contoured and pigmented to match the remaining intact limb. The principal disadvantage of the endoskeletal system is that it is more difficult to keep clean and tears more easily when exposed to environments that may be damaging. The exoskeletal system is indicated for the patient who would like a more durable and more easily cleaned prosthetic limb. One relatively new component that has been added to the therapeutic armamentarium for individuals with transtibial amputations is the vertical impact-absorbing pylon. This is a component that is typically added to the endoskeletal system. It is designed much like an automotive or mountain bike shock absorber to minimize impact loads that are transmitted from the ground to the residual limb. The indications for this system are unclear because it has received only limited study. It may be beneficial for amputation patients with higher activity levels who subject their residual limb to increased loading conditions during avocational or vocational pursuits. The only reported disadvantages of these systems are that they do add weight to the prosthesis and, as with most mechanical systems, that they may require more frequent repair and maintenance.

Finally, one must consider the type of prosthetic foot ankle mechanism that should be incorporated into the prosthetic limb. One of the primary philosophical questions that physiatrists and prosthetists consider is whether or not the first prosthetic foot/ankle mechanism provided should be the one that you envision will best meet the patients' long-term functional needs, or whether it should be the one that would best meet their immediate functional needs. In part, this decision must be made on pragmatic considerations such as whether the insurer will pay for sophisticated components and how often they will allow replacement of components. Generally it is my belief that patients early in their prosthetic rehabilitation should be fit with components that meet their immediate functional needs. These goals often are simply to return to safe bipedal ambulation in household and community environments. At the outset, this may only involve ambulation with upper-extremity assistive devices. These functional activities do not require a sophisticated energy-storing device or a device that allows multidimensional motion. In fact, many of the energy-storing components that are currently available are manufactured with a number of different spring stiffnesses that must be "tuned" to the patient's body

weight and activity level. Consequently, if, for example, you are prescribing an energy-storing component for someone who you think will jog in the future, you will be prescribing a foot that is excessively stiff for conditions of day-to-day ambulation. This type of foot may in fact have a detrimental effect on the individual's gait. Ultimately, the majority of traumatic amputation patients will benefit from more sophisticated foot/ankle mechanisms. Their use and function have been reviewed elsewhere (40).

THE TRANSFEMORAL AMPUTATION

Amputation at the transfemoral level leads to a significant decrement in function compared to the transtibial amputation level. The optimal length residual limb is one that is approximately 10 to 12 cm proximal to the knee joint line (41). The residual limb will then have adequate length to optimize tissue loading, as well as an optimal lever arm length for transmitting muscular forces. This length also allows for adequate space for the prosthetic knee unit, so that the prosthetic knee center is at the same position as the anatomic knee center on the remaining limb. The amputation surgical procedure should include a myodesis or a myoplasty. A myodesis is the surgical suture of the anterior muscles to the posterior muscles over the distal end of the femur. This technique results in improved soft tissue coverage over the distal end of the femur. Furthermore, fixing of the distal ends of the hamstrings to the rectus femoris enables these muscles to function as accessory hip extensors and flexors, respectively. In the case of the myoplasty, the distal ends of the quadriceps and hamstrings are attached to the femur by passing sutures through drill holes at the distal end of the femur. The biomechanical effect of this procedure is very similar to that of the myodesis. There has been considerable controversy about the role of the adductors and what should be done with them at the time of amputation surgery. Gottshalk (41) has been a strong advocate of placing the residual femur in a position of physiological adduction during the surgical procedure and passing the adductor magnus over the distal end of the femur and suturing it to the lateral aspect of the femur with it under tension. The hypothetical benefit of this modification of transfemoral amputation technique is to improve the biomechanical function of the hip abductors during prosthetic limb stance phase, therefore reducing the commonly observed compensated gluteus medius gait with its exaggerated lateral trunk shift, observed during prosthetic stance phase. The details of the biomechanical principles underlying this gait abnormality are beyond the scope of this work but can be reviewed in more detail (42).

There are many different kinds of prosthetic options for the transfemoral amputation patient. Although there are similarities in the kinds of components that are prescribed for both dysvascular and traumatic transfemoral amputation patients, there are also distinct differences. The choices and types of appropriate prosthetic sockets are essentially the same in the two populations as are the suspension systems. There is a different class of prosthetic knee units and prosthetic feet that is available, and more appropriate, for the younger active amputation patient.

In individuals with traumatic transfemoral amputations, the most common socket prescription is a total contact narrow mediolateral prosthetic socket (narrow M/L) with a flexible brim, flexible wall design. The narrow M/L socket is conceptually analogous to the ischial containment socket but differs radically from the quadrilateral socket, which was the only socket design available 10 to 15 years ago (43). The narrow M/L socket design has become the standard of prosthetic care for the amputation patient. It was developed on an empirical basis with the goals of enhancing comfort, biomechanical function, and ultimately the metabolic costs of ambulation. Research has shown that compared with the quadrilateral socket, it results in a reduced lateral trunk shift to the prosthetic side during prosthetic stance phase (44), as well as a reduced metabolic cost of ambulation, especially at faster walking speeds (45).

The narrow M/L prosthetic socket can be fabricated out of rigid materials throughout its length and contour or it can be fabricated out of a flexible inner plastic socket with a rigid outer socket that has been cut away in key areas. The outer rigid socket can be trimmed at the proximal brim to allow only the flexible inner socket to contact the soft tissues, providing a more compliant and comfortable material that reduces shear stresses at the margins of the socket. This would be described as a narrow M/L flexible brim design. The rigid outer socket can also be extensively windowed anteriorly and posteriorly at the midlength of the socket, exposing the inner flexible socket. This design theoretically allows for improved heat transfer and a more compliant socket wall to allow expansion of the residual limb musculature as they are activated during gait. The windows in the external hard socket are referred to as the flexible wall design. There is little available data to support the benefits of a flexible brim, flexible wall design over the hard socket; however, it may be considered if there is difficulty in achieving a comfortable socket fit with a hard socket.

Specialized interface materials are not typically necessary in the residual limb with adequate soft tissue integrity. The soft tissue envelope of the normal transfemoral residual limb usually provides a very adequate interface. In the case where there are compromised soft tissues, a silicone roll-on suspension system may reduce mechanical skin injury.

Suspension of the transfemoral prosthesis may be achieved through a number of systems. The two most common are a suction suspension system and a silicone roll-on suspension system with a distal locking pin. The suction suspension system uses a valve at the distal end of the prosthetic socket. Typically, the patient would apply a stockinette to the residual limb, place the end of the stockinette through the valve opening, and gradually "pull" the soft tissues of the residual limb into the prosthetic socket. The valve is then replaced into the valve opening to prevent the ingress of air. This is a very positive suspension system. The primary disadvantage is that it requires a stable residual limb volume. It is not possible to adjust residual limb volume through the application or subtraction of prosthetic socks. The silicone roll-on suspension system with a distal locking pin uses a silicone or urethane sleeve that is everted and subsequently rolled on to the residual limb. This has a distal locking pin that fits into a shuttle lock at the distal end of the prosthetic socket. Removing the prosthesis is easily performed by pressing a button on the outside of the shuttle lock, which releases the locking mechanism. This system is also a very positive suspension system and has advantages over the suction suspension in that changes in residual limb volume can be made by the addition or subtraction of prosthetic socks. Other suspension systems include the hip joint and pelvic band and the Silesian bandage suspension. The hip joint and pelvic band are used exclusively when there is hip abductor weakness or there is a very short transfemoral residual limb. The Silesian bandage suspension is an external strap that is attached anteriorly and posteriorly to the prosthetic socket and wraps around the pelvis. It is rarely used in contemporary transfemoral prosthetic provision.

There are a multitude of prosthetic knee joints available. Their functional characteristics can be broadly divided into their stance phase and swing phase control mechanisms. Details of their function are beyond the scope of this work (46). Generally the young individual with a traumatic transfemoral amputation without concomitant neuromuscular injury and a reasonable length residual limb would be prescribed a knee that has a hydraulic swing phase control mechanism. The chief advantage of the hydraulic swing phase control mechanism is that it allows improved timing and control of the swing phase dynamics of the prosthetic knee across a broad spectrum of walking speeds. Recent advances in prosthetics have led to the development of microprocessor-controlled knees. These knees have sensors in the pylon and in the knee joint itself that determine the current ambulatory speed and conditions and automatically adjust the damping of the prosthetic knee so that it is optimized under these conditions. At this time there are microprocessor-controlled knees that control only swing phase and some that control both swing and stance phase. The microprocessor-controlled knees that can control stance can allow controlled flexion of the prosthetic knee going down stairs and ramps, which is impossible with conventional prosthetic knee mechanisms. These components significantly increase the price of prosthetic limbs that may cost up to US $40,000 and therefore are not being allowed by some insurers. Although there are a number of research studies that are ongoing at this time, current data has only shown that these components can reduce the metabolic costs of ambulation at walking speeds outside of the typical self-selected walking speed (47).

REFERENCES

1. Ephraim PL, Dillingham TR, Sector M, et al. Epidemiology of limb loss and congenital limb deficiency: A review of the literature. *Arch Phys Med Rehabil.* 2003; 84(5):747–761.
2. Hla P. A 15-year survey of Burmese amputees. *Prosthet Orthot Int.* 1988;12:65–72.
3. Al-Turaiki HS, Al-Falahi LA. Amputee population in the kingdom of Saudi Arabia. *Prosthet Orthot Int.* 1993; 17:147–156.
4. Rommers GM, Vos LD, Groothoff JW, et al. Epidemiology of lower limb amputees in the north of the Netherlands: Aetiology, discharge destination and prosthetic use. *Prosthet Orthot Int.* 1997;21(2):92–99.
5. Ebskov LB, Schroeder TV, Holstein PE. Epidemiology of leg amputation: The influence of vascular surgery. *Br J Surg.* 1994;81(11):1600–1603.
6. Pohjolainen T, Alaranta H. Epidemiology of lower limb amputees in southern Finland in 1995 and trends since 1984. *Prosthet Orthot Int.* 1999;23(2):88–92.
7. Dillingham TR, Pezzin LE, MacKenzie EJ, et al. Use and satisfaction with prosthetic devices among persons with trauma-related amputations: A long-term outcome study. *Am J Phys Med Rehabil.* 2001;80(8): 563–571.
8. Kim YC, Park CI, Kim DY, et al. Statistical analysis of amputations and trends in Korea. *Prosthet Orthot Int.* 1996;20(2):88–95.
9. Johansen K, Daines M, Howey T, et al. Objective criteria accurately predict amputation following lower extremity trauma. *J Trauma.* 1990;30(5):568–572; discussion 572–573.
10. Russel WL, Sailors DM, Whittle TB, et al. Limb salvage versus traumatic amputation. A decision based on a seven-part predictive index. *Ann Surg.* 1991;213: 473–481.
11. Dagum AB, Best AK, Schemitsch EH, et al. Salvage after severe lower-extremity trauma: Are the outcomes

worth the means? *Plast Reconstr Surg.* 1999;103(4): 1212–1220.
12. Bonanni F, Rhodes M, Lucke JF. The futility of predictive scoring of mangled lower extremities. *J Trauma.* 1993;34(1):99–104.
13. Bosse MJ, MacKenzie EJ, Kellam JF, et al. A prospective evaluation of the clinical utility of the lower-extremity injury-severity scores. *J Bone Joint Surg Am.* 2001;83A(1):3–14.
14. Bernat JL. Informed consent. *Muscle Nerve.* 2001; 24(5):614–621.
15. Campbell WB, Ridler BM. Predicting the use of prostheses by vascular amputees. *Eur J Vasc Endovasc Surg.* 1996;12(3):342–345.
16. Mortimer CM, Steedman WM, McMillan IR, et al. Patient information on phantom limb pain: A focus group study of patient experiences, perceptions and opinions. *Health Educ Res.* 2002;17(3):291–304.
17. Smith DG, McFarland LV, Sangeorzan BJ, et al. Postoperative dressing and management strategies for transtibial amputations: A critical review. *J Rehabil Res Dev.* 2003;40(3):213–224.
18. Choudhury SR, Reiber GE, Pecoraro JA, et al. Postoperative management of transtibial amputations in VA hospitals. *J Rehabil Res Dev.* 2001;38(3):293–298.
19. Baker WH, Barnes RW, Shurr DG. The healing of below-knee amputations: A comparison of soft and plaster dressing. *Am J Surg.* 1977;133(6):716–718.
20. Mooney V, Harvey JP Jr, McBride E, et al. Comparison of postoperative stump management: Plaster vs. soft dressings. *J Bone Joint Surg Am.* 1971;53(2):241–249.
21. Boucher HR, Schon LC, Parks B, et al. A biomechanical study of two postoperative prostheses for transtibial amputees: A custom-molded and a prefabricated adjustable pneumatic prosthesis. *Foot Ankle Int.* 2002; 23(5):452–456.
22. Wu Y, Keagy RD, Krick HJ, et al. An innovative removable rigid dressing technique for below-the-knee amputation. *J Bone Joint Surg Am.* 1979;61(5):724–729.
23. Mueller MJ. Comparison of removable rigid dressings and elastic bandages in preprosthetic management of patients with below-knee amputations. *Phys Ther.* 1982;62(10):1438–1441.
24. Schon LC, Short KW, Soupiou O, et al. Benefits of early prosthetic management of transtibial amputees: A prospective clinical study of a prefabricated prosthesis. *Foot Ankle Int.* 2002;23(6):509–514.
25. Wong CK, Edelstein JE. Unna and elastic postoperative dressings: Comparison of their effects on function of adults with amputation and vascular disease. *Arch Phys Med Rehabil.* 2000;81(9):1191–1198.
26. Pezzin LE, Dillingham TR, MacKenzie EJ. Rehabilitation and the long-term outcomes of persons with trauma-related amputations. *Arch Phys Med Rehabil.* 2000;81(3):292–300.
27. Ehde DM, Czerniecki JM, Smith DG, et al. Chronic phantom sensations, phantom pain, residual limb pain, and other regional pain after lower limb amputation. *Arch Phys Med Rehabil.* 2000;81(8):1039–1044.
28. Steinbach TV, Nadvorna H, Arazi D. A five-year follow-up study of phantom limb pain in post traumatic amputees. *Scamd J Rehabil Med.* 1982;14:203–207.
29. Smith DG, Ehde DM, Legro MW, et al. Phantom limb, residual limb, and back pain after lower extremity amputations. *Clin Orthop.* 1999;361:29–38.
30. Fairhurst MJ. The function of below-knee amputee versus the patient with salvaged grade III tibial fracture. *Clin Orthop.* 1994;301:227–232.

31. Friberg O. Biomechanical significance of the correct length of lower limb prostheses: A clinical and radiological study. *Prosthet Orthot Int.* 1984;8(3):124–129.
32. Norvell DC, Czerniecki JM, Reiber GE, et al. The prevalence of knee pain and symptomatic knee osteoarthritis among veteran traumatic amputees and nonamputees. *Arch Phys Med Rehabil.* 2005;86:487–493.
33. Hungerford DS, Cockin J. Fate of retained limb joints in Second World War amputees. *J Bone Joint Surg Br.* 1975;57-B(1):111.
34. Karladani AH, Granhed H, Fogdestam I, et al. Salvaged limbs after tibial shaft fractures with extensive soft-tissue injury: A biopsychosocial function analysis. *J Trauma.* 2001;50(1):60–64.
35. Georgiadis GM, Behrens FF, Joyce MJ, et al. Open tibial fractures with severe soft-tissue loss. Limb salvage compared with below-the-knee amputation. *J Bone Joint Surg Am.* 1993;75(10):1431–1441.
36. Pinney SJ, Hansen ST Jr, Sangeorzan BJ. The effect on ankle dorsiflexion of gastrocnemius recession. *Foot Ankle Int.* 2002;23(1):26–29.
37. Smith DG. Amputation: Preoperative assessment and lower extremity surgical techniques. *Foot Ankle Clin.* 2001;6(2):271–296.
38. Smith DG, Fergason JR. Transtibial amputations. *Clin Orthop.* 1999;361:108–115.
39. Johnson WC, Watkins MT, Hamilton J, et al. Transcutaneous partial oxygen pressure changes following

40. skew flap and Burgess-type below-knee amputations. *Arch Surg.* 1997;132(3):261–263.
40. Nassan S. The latest designs in prosthetic feet. *Phys Med Rehabil Clin N Am.* 2000;11(3):609–625.
41. Gottschalk F. Transfemoral amputation. Biomechanics and surgery. *Clin Orthop.* 1999;361:15–22.
42. Czerniecki JM. Rehabilitation in limb deficiency. 1. Gait and motion analysis. *Arch Phys Med Rehabil.* 1996;77(Suppl. 3):S3–S8.
43. Pritham CH. Biomechanics and shape of the above-knee socket considered in light of the ischial containment concept. *Prosthet Orthot Int.* 1990;14(1):9–21.
44. Flandry F, Beskin J, Chambers RB, et al. The effect of the CAT-CAM above-knee prosthesis on functional rehabilitation. *Clin Orthop.* 1989;239:249–262.
45. Gailey RS, Lawrence D, Burditt C, et al. The CAT-CAM socket and quadrilateral socket: A comparison of energy cost during ambulation. *Prosthet Orthot Int.* 1993;17(2):95–100.
46. Michael JW. Modern prosthetic knee mechanisms. *Clin Orthop.* 1999;361:39–47.
47. Schmalz T, Blumentritt S, Jarasch R. Energy expenditure and biomechanical characteristics of lower limb amputee gait: The influence of prosthetic alignment and different prosthetic components. *Gait Posture.* 2002;16(3):255–263.

9

Diagnosis and Rehabilitation of Peripheral Nerve Injuries

Lawrence R. Robinson and Elizabeth L. Spencer Steffa

EPIDEMIOLOGY OF PERIPHERAL NERVE TRAUMA

Traumatic injury to peripheral nerves results in considerable disability across the world. In peacetime, peripheral nerve injuries most commonly result from trauma caused by motor vehicle accidents and, less commonly, from penetrating trauma, falls, and industrial accidents. Out of all patients admitted to level I trauma centers, it is estimated that roughly 2% to 3% have peripheral nerve injuries (1,2). If plexus and root injuries are also included, the incidence is about 5% (1).

In the upper limb, the nerve most commonly reported injured is the radial nerve, usually due to its proximity to the spiral groove of the humerus and its frequent injury by humeral fractures. The ulnar nerve is injured next most commonly, usually at the elbow, where it runs superficially but over the bony ulnar groove. The median nerve is injured less commonly than the radial or ulnar and is usually injured distally in the forearm (1,2). Lower limb peripheral nerve injuries are less common, with the sciatic most frequently injured, typically associated with hip or pelvic fractures. This is followed by peroneal and rarely tibial or femoral nerve injuries.

In wartime, peripheral nerve trauma is much more common, and much of our knowledge about peripheral nerve injury, repair, and recovery comes from experience derived in World Wars I and II, and subsequent wars (3–5).

In peacetime, as in wartime, peripheral nerve trauma is primarily an injury occurring in young males (1) with a peak between 20 and 25 years of age (90% males). The specific cause of injury varies according to geographic setting, in particular with respect to the frequency of gunshot wounds and motorcycle crashes. In recent studies from North America, the most frequent causes of injury were motor vehicle crash (46%) and motorcycle crash (10%), followed by pedestrian versus motor vehicle (8%) and gunshot wound (7%) (1). Looking at the statistics another way, however, the risk of peripheral nerve injury once one is admitted to a trauma center is higher with motorcycle crashes (5%), industrial accidents (6%), and gunshot wounds (6%) than with pedestrian accidents or motor vehicle crashes (2% each).

Brachial plexus injuries are also most frequently caused by motor vehicle crash (29%) and motorcycle crash (22%), followed by pedestrian versus motor vehicle (13%) and industrial injuries (7%).

Peripheral nerve injuries may be seen as an isolated nervous system injury but may also often accompany central nervous system (CNS) trauma, not only compounding the disability, but also making recognition of the peripheral nerve lesion problematic. Of patients with peripheral nerve injuries, about 60% have a traumatic brain injury (TBI) (1). Conversely, of those with TBI admitted to rehabilitation units, 10% to 34% have associated peripheral nerve injuries (6–8). It is often easy to miss peripheral nerve injuries in the setting of CNS trauma. Since the neurologic history and examination is limited, early hints to a superimposed peripheral nerve lesion might be only flaccidity, areflexia, and reduced movement of a limb.

Peripheral nerve injuries are of significant import as they impede recovery of function and return to work, and carry risk of secondary disabilities from falls, fractures, or other secondary injuries. An understanding of the classification, pathophysiology, and electrodiagnosis of these lesions is critical to the appropriate diagnosis, localization, and management of peripheral nerve trauma.

CLASSIFICATION OF NERVE INJURIES

For the purposes of this article, trauma is defined as injury resulting from kinetic energy applied to the nerve or limb. Examples include the kinetic energy of the patient moving at high speed into a car or wall, a bullet moving through tissue with a high velocity, or a sudden stretch of a limb. Kinetic energy (KE) is proportional to the mass of the object (m) and the square of the velocity (v):

$$KE = \tfrac{1}{2}mv^2$$

Thus, a doubling of the velocity (e.g., bullet velocity or motor vehicle speed) results in a fourfold increase in kinetic energy applied to the body or body part. Knife or wounds from other sharp objects are also included in this review, though the amount of kinetic energy necessary for a significant peripheral nerve injury is probably lower. While burns and electrical injuries also derive from high amounts of energy (thermal or electrical) applied to tissue, these injuries will not be considered here since the pathophysiology of these injuries is significantly different from those wounds resulting from kinetic energy.

There are two predominant schemes that have been proposed for classification of peripheral nerve traumatic injuries: that of Seddon (4) and that of Sunderland (5) (Table 9-1). The former is more commonly used in the literature. Seddon has used the terms *neurapraxia*, *axonotmesis*, and *neurotmesis* to describe peripheral nerve injuries (4). Neurapraxia is a comparatively mild injury with motor and sensory loss but no evidence of Wallerian degeneration. The nerve distally conducts normally. Focal demyelination and/or ischemia are thought to be the etiologies of the conduction block. Recovery may occur within hours, days, weeks, or up to a few months. Axonotmesis is commonly seen in crush injuries. The axons and their myelin sheaths are broken, yet the surrounding stromas (i.e., the endoneurium, perineurium, and epineurium) remain partially or fully intact. Wallerian degeneration occurs, but subsequent axonal regrowth may proceed along the intact endoneurial tubes. Recovery ultimately depends upon the degree of internal disorganization in the nerve, as well as the distance to the end organ. Sunderland's classification (in the following paragraph) further divides this category. Neurotmesis describes a nerve that has been either completely severed or is so markedly disorganized by scar tissue that axonal

| Table 9-1 | Classification Systems for Nerve Injury |

Seddon Classification	Sunderland Classification	Pathology	Prognosis
Neurapraxia	First degree	Myelin injury or ischemia Axons Disrupted	Excellent recovery in weeks to months Good to poor, depending upon integrity of supporting structures and distance to muscle
Axonotmesis	Second degree	Variable stromal disruption Axons disrupted Endoneurial tubes intact Perineurium intact Epineurium intact	Good, depending upon distance to muscle
	Third degree	Axons disrupted Endoneurial tubes disrupted Perineurium intact Epineurium intact	Poor Axonal misdirection Surgery may be required
	Fourth degree	Axons disrupted Endoneurial tubes disrupted Perineurium disrupted Epineurium intact	Poor Axonal misdirection Surgery usually required
Neurotmesis	Fifth degree	Axon disrupted Endoneurial tubes disrupted Perineurium disrupted Epineurium disrupted	No spontaneous recovery Surgery required Prognosis after surgery guarded

regrowth is impossible. Examples are sharp injury, some traction injuries, or injection of noxious drugs. Prognosis for spontaneous recovery is extremely poor without surgical intervention.

Sunderland (5) uses a more subdivided scheme to describe peripheral nerve injuries, with five groups instead of three. *First-degree injury* represents conduction block with completely intact stroma and corresponds to Seddon's classification of neuropraxia. Prognosis is good. *Second-degree injury* involves transection of the axon but with intact stroma. Recovery can occur by axonal regrowth along endoneurial tubes. *Third-degree injury* represents transection of the axon and endoneurial tubes, but the surrounding perineurium is intact. Recovery depends upon how well the axons can cross the site of the lesion and find endoneurial tubes. *Fourth-degree injury* involves loss of continuity of axons, endoneurial tubes, and perineurium. Individual nerve fascicles are transected and the continuity of the nerve trunk is maintained only by the surrounding epineurium. Traction injuries commonly produce these types of lesions. Prognosis is usually poor absent surgical intervention because of the marked internal disorganization of guiding connective tissue elements and associated scarring. *Fifth-degree injury* describes transection of the entire nerve trunk and is similar to Seddon's neurotmesis.

Some authors have described another "degree" of injury, known as *sixth-degree injury* (9). This is a mixed lesion with both axon loss and conduction block, each occurring in some fibers. This type of lesion is probably quite common and requires skillful electrodiagnostic data collection and analysis to separate it from pure axon loss lesions.

EFFECTS OF NEURAPRAXIA ON NERVE AND MUSCLE

As noted previously, neurapraxic injuries to peripheral nerves may be caused by ischemia or focal demyelination. When ischemia for a brief period (i.e., up to 6 hours) is the underlying cause, there are usually no structural changes in the nerve (10), though there may be edema in other nearby tissues.

On the other hand, in neurapraxic lesions caused by focal demyelination, there are anatomic changes predominantly affecting the myelin sheath but sparing the axon. Tourniquet paralysis has been used to produce an animal model of a neurapraxic lesion (11), though it is recognized that acute crush injuries may be different in mechanism from prolonged application of a tourniquet. In this model,

anatomic changes along the nerve are most marked at the edge of the tourniquet, where a significant pressure gradient exists between the tourniquet and nontourniquet areas. The pressure gradient essentially "squeezes" out the myelin with resulting invagination of one paranodal region into the next. As a result, there is an area of focal demyelination at the edge of the tourniquet (11). Larger fibers are more affected than smaller fibers.

In this area of focal demyelination, impulse conduction from one node of Ranvier to the next is slowed as current leakage occurs and the time for impulses to reach threshold at successive nodes of Ranvier is prolonged. Slowing of conduction velocity along this nerve segment ensues. More severe demyelination results in complete conduction block. This result has been reported to occur when internodal conduction times exceed 500 to 600 μsec (12). Since there are very few sodium channels in internodal segments of myelinated nerves, conduction in demyelinated nerves cannot simply proceed slowly as it would for normally unmyelinated nerves. Thus sufficient demyelination results in block of conduction rather than in simply more severe slowing.

There are relatively few changes in muscle as a result of neurapraxic lesions. Disuse atrophy can occur when neurapraxia is more than transient. There remains debate as to whether muscle fibrillates after a purely neurapraxic lesion (see below).

EFFECTS OF AXONOTMESIS ON NERVE AND MUSCLE

Soon after an axonal lesion, the process of Wallerian degeneration starts to occur in nerve fibers. This process is well described elsewhere (13,14) and will be only briefly reviewed here. There are changes in both the axon and the nerve cell body. In the axon, a number of changes occur in the first 2 days, including leakage of axoplasm from the severed nerve, swelling of the distal nerve segment, and subsequent disappearance of neurofibrils in the distal segment. By day 3, there is fragmentation of both axon and myelin with start of digestion of myelin components. By day 8, the axon has been digested and Schwann cells are attempting to bridge the gap between the two nerve segments. Nerve fibers may also degenerate for a variable distance proximally; depending upon the severity of the lesion, this retrograde degeneration may extend for several centimeters.

If the lesion is sufficiently proximal, there are also a number of changes at the nerve cell body level occurring after nerve trauma. Initially, within the first 48 hours, the Nissl bodies (the cell's rough endoplasmic reticulum) break apart into fine particles. By 2 to 3 weeks after injury, the cell's nucleus becomes displaced eccentrically and the nucleolus is also eccentrically placed within the nucleus. These changes may reverse as recovery occurs.

ELECTRODIAGNOSIS: TIMING OF CHANGES AND DETERMINING DEGREE OF INJURY

Optimal timing of electrodiagnostic studies will vary according to clinical circumstances. For circumstances in which it is important to define a lesion very early, initial studies at 7 to 10 days may be useful at localization and separating conduction block from axonotmesis. On the other hand, when clinical circumstances permit waiting, studies at 3 to 4 weeks postinjury will provide much more diagnostic information, since fibrillations will be apparent on needle EMG. Finally, in cases where a nerve lesion is surgically confirmed and EMG is used to only document recovery, initial studies at a few months postinjury may be most useful.

Changes may be seen in the compound motor action potential (CMAP), late responses (F and H waves), sensory nerve action potential (SNAP), and needle electromyography (EMG). Each of these studies has a somewhat different time course, which should be understood in order to evaluate peripheral nerve injury; they will also vary according to the severity of nerve injury.

THE COMPOUND MOTOR ACTION POTENTIAL

Neurapraxia

In purely neurapraxic lesions, the compound muscle action potential will change immediately after injury, assuming one can stimulate both above and below the site of the lesion (Fig. 9–1). When recording from distal muscles and stimulating distal to the site of the lesion, the CMAP should always be normal, since no axonal loss and no Wallerian degeneration has occurred. Moving stimulation proximal to the lesion will produce a smaller or absent CMAP, as conduction in some or all fibers is blocked. It should be remembered that amplitudes normally fall with increasing distance between stimulation and recording; hence there is some debate about how much of a drop in amplitude is sufficient to demonstrate conduction block. Amplitude drops exceeding 20% over a 25-cm distance or less are

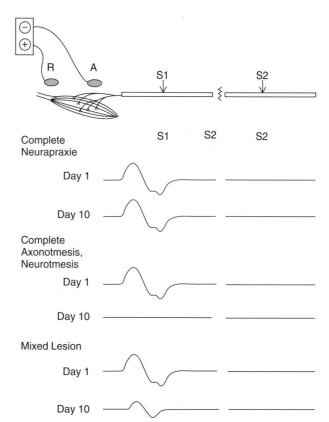

Figure 9–1. Schematic of changes on nerve conduction studies after neurapraxia, axonotmesis, and neurotmesis.

clearly abnormal; smaller changes over smaller distances are likely also suggestive of an abnormality. In addition to conduction block, partial lesions also often demonstrate concomitant slowing across the lesion. This slowing may be due to either loss of faster conducting fibers or demyelination of surviving fibers. All these changes in the CMAP will generally persist until recovery takes place, typically by no more than a few months postinjury. Most important, the distal CMAP will never drop in amplitude in purely neurapraxic injuries, since no axon loss or Wallerian degeneration occurs and the distal nerve segment remains normally excitable.

Axonotmesis and Neurotmesis

Electrodiagnostically, complete axonotmesis (equivalent to Sunderland grades 2, 3, and 4) and complete neurotmesis look the same, since the difference between these types of lesions is in the integrity of the supporting structures, which have no electrophysiologic function. Thus these lesions can be grouped together as axonotmesis for the purpose of this discussion.

Immediately after axonotmesis and for a "few days" thereafter, the CMAP and motor conduction studies look the same as those seen in a neurapraxic lesion. Nerve segments distal to the lesion remain excitable and demonstrate normal conduction while proximal stimulation results in an absent or small response from distal muscles. Early on, this picture looks the same as conduction block and can be confused with neurapraxia. Hence neurapraxia and axontomesis cannot be distinguished until sufficient time for Wallerian degeneration in all motor fibers has occurred, typically about 9 days postinjury (15).

As Wallerian degeneration occurs, the amplitude of the CMAP elicited with distal stimulation will fall. This effect starts at about day 3 and is complete by about day 9 (15). Neuromuscular junction transmission fails before nerve excitability (16,17). Thus in complete axonotmesis at day 9, one has a very different picture from neurapraxia. There are absent responses both above and below the lesion. Partial axon loss lesions will produce small amplitude motor responses, with the amplitude of the CMAP roughly proportional to the number of surviving axons. One can compare side-to-side CMAP amplitudes to estimate the degree of axon loss, though inherent side-to-side variability of up to 30% to 50% limits the accuracy of the estimate. Using the CMAP amplitude to estimate the degree of surviving axons is also most reliable only early after injury, before axonal sprouting has occurred. Use of this technique later after injury will tend to underestimate the degree of axon loss.

Mixed Lesions

Lesions that have a mixture of axon loss and conduction block provide a unique challenge. These lesions can usually be sorted out by carefully examining amplitudes of the CMAP elicited from stimulation both above and below the lesion and by comparing the amplitude with distal stimulation to that obtained from the other side. The percentage of axon loss is best estimated by comparing the CMAP amplitude from distal stimulation with that obtained contralaterally. Of the remaining axons, the percentage with conduction block is best estimated by comparing amplitudes or areas obtained with stimulation distal and proximal to the lesion. Thus, if a 1 mV response is obtained with proximal stimulation, a 2 mV response is obtained distally, and a 10 mV response is obtained with distal stimulation contralaterally, one can deduce that probably about 80% of the axons are lost, and of the remaining 20%, half are blocked (neurapraxic) at the lesion site. As mentioned previously, this analysis is most useful only in the acute phase, before re-innervation by axonal sprouting occurs.

F-WAVES

F-waves may change immediately after the onset of a neurapraxic lesion. In complete block, responses will be absent. However, in partial lesions, changes can be more subtle since F-waves are dependent upon only 3% to 5% of the axon population to elicit a response (18). Thus, partial lesions may have normal minimal F-wave latencies, and mean latencies, with reduced or possibly normal penetrance. While F-waves are conceptually appealing for detecting proximal lesions (e.g., brachial plexopathies), it is in few instances that they truly provide useful additional or unique information. They are sometimes useful in very early proximal lesions when conventional studies are normal, since stimulation does not occur proximal to the lesion, but they are not very good at distinguishing axon loss lesions from conduction block.

COMPOUND OR SENSORY NERVE ACTION POTENTIALS

Neurapraxia

The SNAP and compound nerve action potential (CNAP) will show changes similar to the CMAP after focal nerve injury. In the setting of neurapraxia, there is a focal conduction block at the site of the lesion, with preserved distal amplitude. However, the criteria for establishing conduction block in sensory nerve fibers are substantially different from those for the CMAP. When recording nerve action potentials, there is normally a greater drop in amplitude over increasing distance between stimulating and recording electrodes, caused by temporal dispersion and phase cancellation (19). Amplitude drops of 50% to 70% over a 25-cm distance are not unexpected, and it is less clear just what change in amplitude is abnormal. A large focal change over a small distance is probably significant. Slowing may also accompany partial conduction blocks, as for the CMAP. Responses elicited with stimulation and recording distal to the lesion are normal in pure neurapraxic injuries.

Axonotmesis and Neurotmesis

Immediately after axonotmesis, the SNAP looks the same as seen in a neurapraxic lesion. Nerve segments distal to the lesion remain excitable and demonstrate normal conduction while proximal stimulation results in an absent or small response. Hence neurapraxia and axontomeis cannot be distinguished until sufficient time for Wallerian degeneration in all sensory fibers has occurred, typically about 11 days postinjury (15). It takes slightly longer for sensory nerve studies to demonstrate loss of amplitude than for motor studies, namely, 11 days versus 9 days, because of the earlier failure of neuromuscular junction transmission compared to nerve conduction.

NEEDLE ELECTROMYOGRAPHY

Neurapraxia

The needle EMG examination in purely neurapraxic lesions will show neurogenic changes in recruitment with debatable abnormalities in spontaneous activity. As mentioned earlier, there is debate as to whether fibrillation potentials are recorded after a purely neurapraxic lesion. One study of peripheral nerve lesions in baboons has failed to demonstrate fibrillations in purely neurapraxic lesions (20). On the other hand, study of purely neurapraxic lesions in rats (21) has suggested fibrillations occur in blocked, but not denervated, muscle fibers. There are limited reports of fibrillations in humans with apparently predominantly neurapraxic nerve lesions (22,23), but it is difficult to know whether or not *any* axon loss had occurred in these patients, since nerve conduction studies are not sensitive for detecting minimal axon loss. Needle EMG is more sensitive for detecting motor axon loss than nerve conduction studies, and hence it is easy to imagine situations in which nerve conduction studies are within normal limits, but needle EMG detects minimal or mild axon loss.

Independent of whether or not needle EMG demonstrates fibrillation potentials in neurapraxia, the most apparent change on needle EMG will be changes in recruitment. These occur immediately after injury. In complete lesions (i.e., complete conduction block), there will be no motor unit action potentials. In incomplete neurapraxic lesions, there will be reduced numbers of motor unit action potentials firing more rapidly than normal (i.e., reduced or discrete recruitment). Recruitment changes alone are not specific for neurapraxia or axon loss.

Since no axon loss occurs in neurapraxic injuries, there will be no axonal sprouting and no changes in motor unit action potential (MUAP) morphology (e.g., duration, amplitude, or phasicity) anytime after injury.

Axonotmesis and Neurotmesis

A number of days after an axon loss lesion, needle EMG will demonstrate fibrillation potentials and positive sharp waves. The time between injury and onset of fibrillation potentials will be dependent in part upon the length of distal nerve stump. When the lesion is distal and the distal stump is short, it takes only 10 to 14 days for fibrillations to develop. With a proximal lesion and a longer distal stump (e.g., ulnar innervated hand muscles in a brachial plexopathy), 21 to 30 days are required for full development of fibrillation potentials and positive sharp waves (24). Thus, the electromyographer needs to be acutely aware of the time since injury, so that severity is not underestimated when a study is performed early after injury, and also so that development of increased fibrillation potentials over time is not misinterpreted as a worsening of the injury.

Fibrillation and positive sharp wave density are usually graded on a scale of 1 to 4. This is an ordinal scale, meaning that as numbers increase findings are worse. However, it is not an interval or ratio scale; that is, 4+ is not twice as bad as 2+ or 4 times as bad as 1+. Moreover, 4+ fibrillation potentials do not reflect complete axon loss and in fact may represent only a minority of axons lost (25,26). Evaluation of recruitment and particularly of distally elicited CMAP amplitude is necessary before one can decide on whether or not complete axon loss has occurred.

Fibrillation potential size will decrease over time since injury. Kraft (27) has demonstrated that fibrillations initially are several hundred microvolts in the first few months after injury. However, when lesions are more than 1 year old, they are unlikely to be over 100 μV in size. Fibrillations will also decrease in number as re-innervation occurs; however this finding is not usually clinically useful for two reasons. First, since a qualitative or ordinal scale of fibrillation density is typically used and an accurate quantitative measurement of fibrillation density is not available, comparison of fibrillation numbers from one examination to the other is not reliable (26). Second, even in complete lesions, fibrillation density will eventually reduce since the muscle becomes fibrotic and the number of viable muscle fibers falls; in this case, reduction in fibrillation numbers predicts not recovery, but rather muscle fibrosis.

Fibrillations may also occur after direct muscle injury, as well as nerve injury. Partanen and Danner (28) have demonstrated that after muscle biopsy patients have persistent fibrillation potentials starting after 6 to 7 days and extending for up to 11 months. In patients who have undergone multiple trauma, coexisting direct muscle injury is common and can be potentially misleading when trying to localize a lesion.

When there are surviving axons after an incomplete axonal injury, remaining MUAPs are initially normal in morphology but demonstrate reduced or discrete recruitment. Axonal sprouting will be manifested by changes in morphology of existing motor units. Amplitude will increase, duration will become prolonged, and the percentage of polyphasic MUAPs will increase as motor unit territory increases (26,29). This process occurs soon after injury. Microscopic studies demonstrate outgrowth of these nerve sprouts starting at 4 days after partial denervation (14,30). Electrophysiologic studies using single fiber EMG demonstrate an increase in fiber density starting at 3 weeks postinjury (31).

In complete lesions, the only possible mechanism of recovery is axonal regrowth. The earliest needle EMG finding in this case is the presence of small, polyphasic, often unstable motor unit potentials previously referred to as "nascent potentials." Observation of these potentials is dependent upon establishing axon regrowth as well as new neuromuscular junctions, and this observation represents the earliest evidence of re-innervation, usually preceding the onset of clinically evident voluntary movement (26). These potentials represent the earliest definitive evidence of axonal re-innervation in complete lesions. When performing the examination looking for new motor unit potentials, one must be sure to accept only "crisp," nearby motor unit potentials with a short rise-time, since distant potentials recorded from other muscles can be deceptive and could erroneously suggest intact innervation.

Mixed Lesions

When there is a lesion with both axon loss and conduction block, needle EMG examination can be potentially misleading if interpreted in isolation. If, for example, a lesion results in destruction of 50% of the original axons and conduction block of the other 50%, then needle EMG will demonstrate abundant (e.g., 4+) fibrillation potentials and no voluntary MUAPs. The electromyographer should ***not*** then conclude that there is a complete axonal lesion but should instead carefully evaluate the motor nerve conduction studies to figure out how much of the lesion is neurapraxic and how much axonotmetic. The important point here is to not take the presence of abundant fibrillations and absent voluntary MUAPs as evidence of complete denervation.

LOCALIZATION OF TRAUMATIC NERVE INJURIES

The localization of peripheral nerve injuries is sometimes straightforward but is potentially complicated by a variety of possible pitfalls. Localization is usually performed by two methods: (i) detecting focal slowing or conduction block on nerve conduction studies, or (ii) assessing the pattern of denervation on needle EMG.

Localizing peripheral nerve lesions by nerve conduction studies usually requires that there be a focal slowing or conduction block as one stimulates above and below the lesion. To see such a change, there must either be focal demyelination or ischemia, or the lesion should be so acute that degeneration of the distal stump has not yet occurred. Thus, lesions with partial or complete neurapraxia (caused by either demyelination or ischemia) can be well localized with motor nerve conduction studies, as can very acute axonal injuries.

In pure axonotmetic or neurotmetic lesions, it is more difficult if not impossible to localize the lesion using nerve conduction studies. In such a case, there will be mild and diffuse slowing in the entire nerve due to loss of the fastest fibers, or there will be no response at all. Conduction across the lesion site will be no slower than across other segments. In addition, provided enough time for Wallerian degeneration has elapsed (i.e., at least 9 days for motor fibers or 11 days for sensory fibers), there will be no change in amplitude as one traverses the site of the lesion. Thus, pure axon loss lesions are not well localized along nerve-by-nerve conduction studies.

There are some cases in which indirect inferences can be made about the location of purely axonal lesions. For instance, if the ulnar motor response is very small or absent and the median motor response is normal, this implies an ulnar neuropathy rather than a lower brachial plexus lesion. However, in such an instance, the site of pathology along the ulnar nerve may not be well defined.

Another indirect inference that can be made based upon sensory nerve conduction studies is placement of the lesion at a pre- versus postganglionic location. Lesions that are proximal to the dorsal root ganglion—namely, at the preganglionic level (proximal root, cauda equina, spinal cord)—tend to have normal sensory nerve action potential amplitudes, even in the setting of reduced or absent sensation (32,33). The finding of normal sensory nerve action potentials is a particularly bad prognostic sign when seen in the setting of possible root avulsion. On the other hand, lesions occurring distal to the dorsal root ganglion have small or absent SNAPs (when these are recorded in the appropriate distribution). Thus, SNAPs may be useful to differentiate root versus plexus or other pre- versus postganglionic locations. A limitation, particularly in partial lesions, is the wide variability in SNAP amplitudes seen in normal individuals. Mixed pre- and postganglionic lesions are also potentially difficult to interpret.

The other major electrodiagnostic method of determining the site of nerve injury is by needle

EMG. Conceptually, if one knows the branching order to various muscles under study, one can determine that the nerve injury is between the branches to the most distal normal muscle and the most proximal abnormal muscle. There are, however, a number of potential problems with this approach. First, the branching and innervation for muscles is not necessarily consistent from one person to another. Sunderland (5) has demonstrated a great deal of variability in branching order to muscles in the limbs, variability in the number of branches going to each muscle, and variability in which nerve or nerves supply each muscle. Thus, the typical branching scheme may not apply to the patient being studied, and consequently the lesion site can be misconstrued.

Second, the problem of muscle trauma and associated needle EMG findings can be misleading. As mentioned earlier, direct muscle trauma can result in positive sharp waves and fibrillations for months or longer after injury (28). Practically speaking, this effect can result in erroneously proximal lesion sites, or error in diagnosing more than one lesion. For example, in the setting of humeral fracture with radial neuropathy, the triceps not infrequently demonstrates fibrillation potentials from direct muscle trauma. However, one could be misled to localize the lesion to the axilla or higher rather than spiral groove if the triceps findings are not recognized as coming from direct muscle rather than from nerve injury.

Third, the problem of partial lesions can make for misdiagnosis to more distal sites. In partial ulnar nerve lesions at the elbow, for example, the forearm ulnar innervated muscles are often spared (34). Their preservation is thought to result at least partially from sparing of the fascicles in the nerve that are preparing to branch to the flexor digitorum profundus and the flexor carpi ulnaris; in other words they are in a relatively protected position. This finding could lead one to inadvertently localize the lesion distally to the distal forearm or wrist. Similarly, a lesion involving the median nerve in the arm (above the elbow) has been reported to cause findings only in the anterior interosseous distribution (35). Intraneural topography needs to be considered when making a diagnosis based on branching (36).

MECHANISMS OF RECOVERY

There are several possible mechanisms of recovery after traumatic nerve injury; knowledge of these mechanisms, along with the type of nerve injury, allows estimation of the probable course of recovery.

For motor fibers, resolution of conduction block (in neurapraxic lesions), muscle fiber hypertrophy (in partial lesions), distal axonal sprouting of spared axons, and axonal regeneration from the site of injury may contribute to recovery of strength.

Resolution of conduction block, whether based upon ischemia or demyelination, is probably the first mechanism to promote recovery of strength after nerve injury. Improvement after a solely ischemic lesion is relatively quick. Demyelinating injuries take longer as remyelination over an injured segment may take up to several months (37), depending upon the severity of demyelination and the length of the demyelinated segment.

In normal adults performing strengthening exercises, there are generally two mechanisms of increasing force production: initial neural mechanisms followed by later muscle fiber hypertrophy. The initial neural mechanisms are thought to involve improved synchronization of motor unit firing (38,39), and they result in increased efficiency (defined as muscle force per unit of electrical activity) in the absence of muscle fiber changes. After several weeks, there is muscle fiber hypertrophy, which results in further increases in strength. In patients with partial nerve lesions, it is unclear how much neural changes alone (namely, increased efficiency of firing) can contribute to increased strength, since there is loss of nerve fibers. However, it is likely that working the existing muscle fibers to fatigue in the setting of partial nerve injuries does produce enlargement of muscle fibers and consequent increases in force production.

Partial axonotmesis of motor nerves also produces distal sprouting of motor fibers from intact axons. It has been observed that within 4 days after nerve injury, sprouts are starting to form from intact axons, typically from distal nodes of Ranvier (nodal sprouts) or from nerve terminals (terminal sprouts) near denervated muscle fibers (30). Partial recovery in twitch tension has been reported as early as 7 to 10 days postinjury (40), though electrophysiologic correlates (e.g., polyphasic long duration motor units) usually take longer. Sometimes, when axonal regeneration occurs, those muscle fibers re-innervated by distal sprouting become dually innervated; namely, by both the sprout and the newly regenerated fiber (30,41). It is not well understood how multiple synapses are reduced.

Axonal regeneration contributes to recovery in both partial and complete axonotmesis and, with surgical approximation, neurotmesis. In complete axon loss lesions, this is the only mechanism for muscle recovery. It is noted that in the 24 to 36 hours after injury, the proximal nerve stump has started to sprout regenerating axons, and these have started to penetrate the area of injury. The recovery that results from this process depends upon the degree of injury, presence of scar formation, approximation of the two nerve ends, and age of the subject.

In relatively more minor axonotmetic lesions, in which the endoneurial tubes are preserved (i.e., Sunderland second-degree injuries), the axons can traverse the segment of injury in 8 to 15 days and then regenerate along the distal nerve segment at a rate of 1 to 5 mm per day (5), slightly faster for crush injuries than for sharp laceration, slightly faster for proximal than distal injuries, and slightly faster for younger individuals.

In more severe axonotmetic lesions in which there is distortion of endoneurial tubes with or without perineurial disruption (Sunderland third and fourth degrees), prognosis for spontaneous regrowth is worse. Extensive scarring reduces the speed at which regenerating axons can traverse the lesion and, more important, reduces the likelihood that they will ever reach their end organs. When regrowth occurs, it may also be misdirected to the wrong end organ. In some of these cases, particularly when a large neuroma is present, surgical intervention is required.

In complete neurotmesis (Sunderland fifth degree), axonal regrowth will usually not occur unless the nerve ends are freed from scar and surgically re-approximated. After surgical intervention, using either direct approximation or cable grafting, nerve growth will often occur along the endoneurial tubes of the distal segments. Use of cable grafts (e.g., sural nerve graft) does not provide axons directly, since these die after harvesting; the graft simply provides a pathway for axonal regrowth to occur (42,43).

In complete lesions, recovery of motor function will also depend upon integrity of the muscle when the axon reaches it. Most muscles remain viable for re-innervation for 18 to 24 months postinjury, though hand intrinsic muscles may not remain viable for as long, possibly only 6 months. However, past this time, because of fibrosis and atrophy, motor axon regrowth makes little difference, since muscle fibers—that is, the end organ—are no longer viable. For example, in complete lower trunk brachial plexus lesions, recovery of hand function is usually not expected no matter how good the surgical grafting might be; it simply takes too long for axons to reach the muscle.

Recovery of sensory function is dependent upon different mechanisms than is motor recovery. There may be redistribution of sensory fibers after an axonal injury, such that intact fibers provide cutaneous sensation to a larger area than previously (23,44). The mechanisms of axonal regeneration are similar to those mentioned earlier for motor axons. An important difference, however, is that one does not have end organs that may degenerate after 18 to 24 months as muscle does; hence sensory recovery may continue for a longer period of time than motor recovery does.

ELECTRODIAGNOSTIC EVALUATION OF PROGNOSIS

Determining the pathophysiology of a peripheral nerve traumatic injury can help with estimating prognosis. Those injuries that are completely or largely neurapraxic have a good prognosis for recovery within a few months (usually up to 3 months postinjury). Resolution of ischemia and remyelination should be complete by this time.

Mixed injuries typically have two or more phases of recovery (Fig. 9–2). The neurapraxic component resolves quickly as above and muscle fiber hypertrophy can provide additional recovery, but the axonal component is slower, since it depends upon distal axonal sprouting and on axonal regeneration from the site of the lesion. Thus patients usually experience a relatively rapid partial but incomplete recovery followed a slower further recovery. Sensory recovery may proceed for a longer time than motor (Fig. 9–3).

Partial axon loss lesions usually represent axonotmesis, though a partial neurotmesis (e.g., a laceration through part of the nerve) cannot always be excluded in such cases. In axonotmesis, recovery will depend upon axonal sprouting and regeneration. Thus, there will be some early recovery followed possibly by a later recovery if or when regenerating axons reach their end organs. The amplitude of the CMAP provides some guide to prognosis. In facial nerve lesions, it has been demonstrated that patients with CMAP amplitudes >30% of the other side have

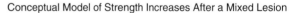

Conceptual Model of Strength Increases After a Mixed Lesion

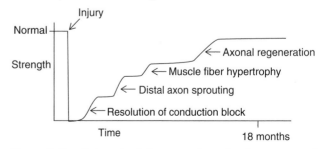

Figure 9–2. Conceptual diagram of mechanisms responsible for motor recovery after traumatic nerve injury.

Conceptual Model of Sensory Improvement After a Mixed Lesion

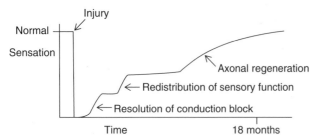

Figure 9–3. Conceptual diagram of mechanisms responsible for sensory recovery after traumatic nerve injury.

an excellent outcome; those with 10% to 30% have good but not always complete recovery; and those with <10% have a poor outcome (45).

Complete axonotmesis and neurotmesis have the worst prognosis. Recovery depends solely upon axonal regeneration that may or may not occur, depending upon the degree of injury to the nerve. In many cases of complete axon loss, it is not possible to know the degree of nerve injury except by surgical exploration with or without intraoperative recording, or looking for evidence of early re-innervation after the lesion. As a consequence, it is often recommended to wait 2 to 4 months and look for evidence of re-innervation in previously completely denervated muscles near the site of the lesion (43,46). Those lesions that have some spontaneous recovery are usually treated conservatively, since operative repair is unlikely to improve upon natural recovery. Those with no evidence of axonal regrowth usually have operative exploration with possible grafting.

SURGICAL INTERVENTIONS

Most surgical interventions can be conceptually separated into immediate reconstruction, early surgery, and delayed reconstruction. Immediate surgery—that is, within a few days of injury—occurs in a few very specific instances. Such treatment is reserved for sharp nerve lacerations, such as a wound from a knife or glass. If the nerve is completely severed, but the ends can be approximated with minimal tension, then an immediate re-anastamosis may be performed. However, immediate surgery is usually only attempted when the need for surgery is certain; in other words, it is clear that the nerve has been severed or that surgery is indicated for other reasons (e.g., fracture repair). Moreover, other local tissue trauma should be minimal. If nerve grafting is

required for approximation, then surgery is usually delayed for at least several weeks.

Early reconstruction is usually performed at roughly 3 to 4 weeks post-trauma. Typically, the need for surgery is already certain; that is, it is known that neurotmesis has occurred. The trauma may have consisted of blunt trauma or nerve traction. Or there may have been sharp laceration, but immediate reconstruction was not indicated. By 3 to 4 weeks postinjury, nerve retraction has typically occurred, or neuroma development has started. Thus, in these cases, some resection of the nerve ends is required and a nerve graft is interposed to provide an avenue in which the proximal axons can grow to their end organs. Early surgery is usually reserved for complete lesions in which there is little or no hope of spontaneous recovery.

Many times one is uncertain about the condition of the nerve at the site of injury. As stated previously, electrodiagnostic studies can document neurapraxic injuries and indicate when the prognosis is favorable. However, one cannot differentiate between axonotmesis and neurotmesis. If much of the supporting nerve structure is intact and internal disorganization is minimal, then spontaneous recovery will likely be much better than if surgical exploration and grafting are performed. On the other hand, if the lesion is complete neurotmesis, or scarring is so extensive that regrowth cannot proceed, then surgery would produce a better outcome. In these cases, a surgical decision is usually delayed by several months to see if re-innervation spontaneously occurs in muscles just distal to the lesion.

There are, however, some trade-offs to consider when deciding how long to wait to perform a surgical intervention. One would like to wait long enough for re-innervation to reach the most proximal muscles distal to the lesion. On the other hand, if one waits too long, there will be insufficient time to allow axons to grow through the graft and reach muscle within the 18- to 24-month window in which re-innervation is possible. The literature indicates, for example, that brachial plexus repair before 6 months has a significantly better outcome than those performed after 12 months (47), possibly due to earlier re-innervation of the intrinsic muscles.

Thus, most clinicians will wait up to 4 to 6 months to see if there is any clinical or EMG evidence of re-innervation before performing exploration and grafting. There have been, however, instances in our own experience in which evidence of new re-innervation was found only on the morning of surgery, and none had been seen only 1 to 2 weeks beforehand. Delayed reconstruction usually consists of nerve exploration, neurolysis, resection of any neuromas that may have formed, and interposition of grafts from the sural or other nerves. Delayed nerve reconstruction is typically reserved for proximal muscles. Since the muscle cannot be re-innervated after 18 to 24 months, there is little point in attempting cable grafting to resupply distal muscles.

Tendon transfers are another option for surgical reconstruction. This surgery is commonly performed after radial nerve injury instead of or in addition to radial nerve repair because it generally provides a good level of function in this setting (48–50). Of interest, the muscles after transfer change their firing pattern in accordance with their new mechanical function, indicating some retraining; some patients will even have individual finger movements but using a combination of finger flexor and extensor firing (51). Other nerve injuries that impair fine hand movements (e.g., ulnar and median) are less successfully treated by tendon transfer techniques.

Outcomes after surgery vary according to the nerve injured and the technique applied. In low-velocity missile injuries to the upper limb, for example, Taha has shown that radial nerve injuries have the best outcome (100% return to work), followed by median or ulnar nerve injuries (55% return to work); combined ulnar and median nerve injuries resulted in no patients returning to work (52). Kim et al. (53) have also shown in 260 patients with radial nerve injuries that outcomes are very good after surgical intervention with the majority regaining at least grade 3/5 strength. The same group found that repair of ulnar and median nerve injuries produced less favorable results (54). It is hypothesized that radial nerve injuries may have a better outcome both because they produce less sensory loss and less impairment of fine motor control of the digits. Moreover, unlike the radial nerve, the median and ulnar nerves are responsible for innervation of hand intrinsics.

REHABILITATION OF TRAUMATIC PERIPHERAL NERVE INJURIES

Rehabilitation of peripheral nerve injuries should include a focus on avoiding complications and further disability, improving function, and enhancing recovery after surgical interventions.

Although contractures are more likely to develop after spastic paralysis, they can also occur after flaccid paralysis associated with peripheral nerve lesions. If allowed to develop, contractures can prevent or reduce meaningful function in the event of re-innervation of involved muscles. Patients,

caregivers, and/or families need to be educated on how to perform passive range of motion (PROM) exercises daily. Positioning of the affected limb to avoid contractures is also important to enhance full range of motion.

Use of the limb should be encouraged for daily functional activities whenever possible and not contraindicated. There are several benefits of early activity in the limb. First, it will help to prevent disuse atrophy in muscles not affected by the peripheral nerve injury. Second, it will help to prevent contractures by having the limb used within the functional range of motion. Additionally there is some evidence from the study of rats that suggests it may improve recovery in other ways. van Meeteren et al. (55), for example, studied rats after sciatic nerve injury. Those required to use their hind limbs for 24 days after injury had better function and faster nerve conduction velocity (NCV) than sedentary animals from 50 to 150 days postinjury, suggesting that use of the limb could improve nerve function.

There are a number of modalities that have been applied to the limb in an effort to improve recovery after nerve injury. There have been many trials of electrical stimulation to the muscle to prevent muscle atrophy and possibly enhance recovery. The results of these trials have provided mixed results without providing convincing evidence that such stimulation will lead to improved outcomes. There are a vast number of paradigms that can be used for stimulation in terms of stimulation frequency, intensity, pulse duration, and the number of days and hours over which stimulation is given. Moreover, outcomes are likely influenced more by the degree of nerve injury than by what modality is applied to the muscle pending re-innervation. Thus, it is difficult to say that *no* form of electrical stimulation will be proven helpful. While there is some recent evidence that very low intensity (1 μA) stimulation of nerves in the rat after sciatic nerve injury may improve recovery (56), there is not yet enough evidence to support electrical stimulation to make this a standard of practice.

Ultrasound is another physical modality that may show some promise for enhancing recovery after peripheral nerve injury. There are studies showing efficacy for treatment of carpal tunnel syndrome (57) that may indicate promise for encouraging peripheral nerve regeneration, although other studies have failed to find an effect (58). There is also one study in rabbits in which ultrasound enhanced resolution of acute nerve conduction block (59). As yet, however, ultrasound still remains experimental and is not a standard of care. Further research in this area may be promising.

PERIPHERAL NERVE INJURY REHABILITATION SPLINTING

Splinting is an important part of rehabilitation care after peripheral nerve injury (60). The goals of splinting should be to prevent or minimize harmful contractures and other deformities, to substitute for lost motor control when possible, to enhance recovery after surgery, and to encourage early use of the limb for functional activities. When considering the best position for splinting, it is important to also consider the position of function.

Splint design and construction will depend greatly on the specific nerve injury. In the paralyzed hand for example, one wishes to both keep the appropriate ligaments stretched and also maintain a position of function. One will want about 30-degree wrist extension to enhance grip strength. At the metacarpal-phalangeal (MCP) joints, 90 degrees of flexion will both keep the collateral ligaments stretched and maintain a position of function. The interphalangeal (IP) joints are usually maintained in extension or only slight flexion in order to keep the finger flexors stretched. The thumb is usually kept in moderate abduction and opposition to provide a stable base for two- or three-point grasp. James described the "safe position" in 1970, stating, "The metacarpophalangeal joints are safe in flexion and most unsafe in extension; the PIP joints, conversely, are safe in extension and exceedingly unsafe if immobilized in flexion" (61,62) (Fig. 9–4).

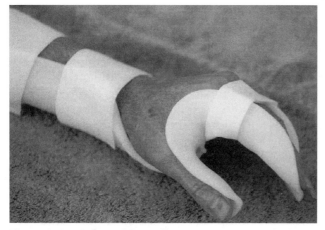

Figure 9–4. Safe position splint.

Special attention, for splinting as well as for other activities, needs to be directed toward preserving sites of surgical repair. Both tendon and peripheral nerve repairs have more successful outcomes if tension can be avoided for several weeks after repair (63). Thus, when planning a PROM program, constructing a splint, or having the patient participate in functional activities, tension must be avoided at all times for the first few weeks after surgical repair, and coordination between therapists and surgeon is essential.

Splints generally function as a first-class lever system using three points of pressure. Fess has described the splint forces generated and calculated that a forearm splint be two-thirds the length of the forearm and two-thirds the circumference (64). Four types of splints are used specific to the nerve injury and rehabilitation goals. The static splint has no moving parts and is used to protect and maintain correct joint alignment, motion, or functional position; prevent contractures; and support laxity. The dynamic splint uses moving parts and resistance and may be used to substitute for lost function. The static progressive splint has moving parts that use adjustable nonelastic traction, low load, and prolonged stress to scar tissue holding the joint at end range (65). Serial splints are static splints using progressive changes at end range to reduce contractures. Bell-Krotoski (66) states, "Tissue will lengthen and grow under constant stress because it is already a dynamic biologic system with constant change and remodeling." It is imperative that the therapist understand the mechanics of splinting forces as described by Fess and Brand. They documented critical soft tissue tolerance and had great understanding of splinting biomechanics and transfer of forces to unsplinted joints (61).

RADIAL NERVE SPLINTING PRINCIPLES

The high-level radial nerve injury creates loss of active wrist, finger, and thumb extension and weakness of supination and thumb radial abduction. Functional splints are worn during the day and a static "safe splint" at night. The wrist is functionally splinted in extension using either a static or dynamic splint (Fig. 9–5). Finger and thumb extension assistance may be needed to allow optimal hand function. The wrist splinted in extension will prevent overstretching extensor muscle groups. Wrist stabilization allows functional grasp and improved coordination (67) (Figs. 9–6, 9–7).

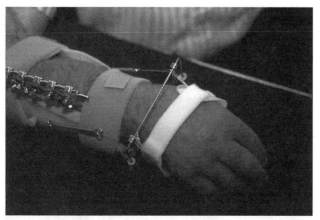

Figure 9–5. Radial nerve injury with fracture external fixator splinted in functional dynamic wrist extension splint to maintain muscle balance. Early motion also assisted in edema reduction.

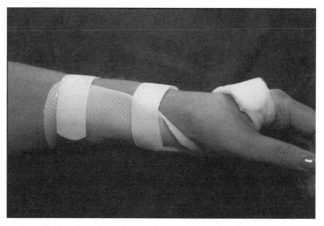

Figure 9–6. Static volar wrist extension splint.

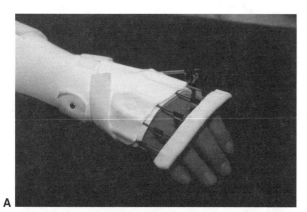

A

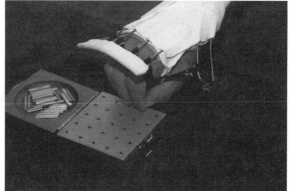

B

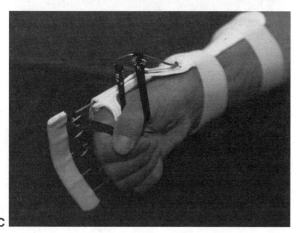

C

Figure 9–7. A–C: Dorsal static wrist extension splint with elastic digit extension loops as first described by James Sellers in the March 1980 *American Journal of Occupational Therapy*. The splint enhances prehension and does not limit full composite digit flexion.

■ Case Study

Radial Nerve Injury

A 21-year-old female student injured in a motor vehicle accident with high-level radial nerve lesion, post repair, was fit with a dynamic wrist extension, dynamic digit extension splint for daytime wear for her right dominant hand to allow continued classroom participation and note taking (Fig. 9–8). She did not drop any classes as a result of her injury. As the radial nerve function returned, the Phoenix wrist extension unit was removed and the Phoenix digit dynamic extension portion was customized as a hand-based splint (Fig. 9–9). The patient had good functional return with functional grasp strength and full active digit extension with wrist neutral but lacked full digit extension with wrist extension (Figs. 9–10—9–13).

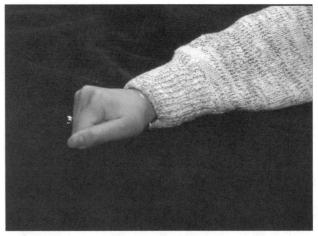

Figure 9–10. Functional full fist grasp.

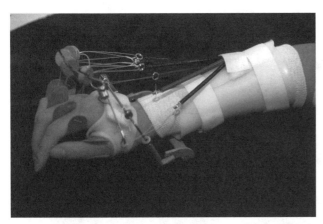

Figure 9–8. Dynamic wrist extension, dynamic digit extension splint.

ULNAR NERVE SPLINTING PRINCIPLES

Intrinsic muscle function of the ring and small fingers, wrist ulnar deviation, and flexion and ulnar digit sensation are compromised with ulnar nerve injury. A claw deformity with ring and small metacarpophalangeal joint hyperextension and phalangeal flexion may develop. Functional grip strength and full tight fist are not possible with the little finger metacarpophalangeal joint held in extension. Loss of thumb opposition and adduction and loss of the first dorsal interosseus muscle for index finger abduction produces a weak pinch. Splinting the ulnar metacarpophalangeal joints in slight flexion permits phalangeal extension, enabling hand function, and prevents proximal interphalangeal (PIP) joint flexion contracture formation. Anticlaw splinting works on the supple hand or when full passive motion is present but is not effective when contractures have formed. Proximal interphalangeal flexion contractures may be reduced by

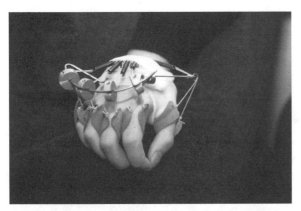

Figure 9–9. Customized hand-based digit extension splint.

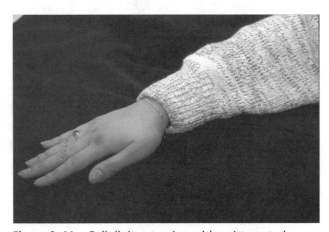

Figure 9–11. Full digit extension with wrist neutral.

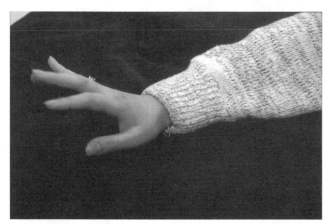

Figure 9–12. Decreased digit extension with wrist extension.

remodeling tissue using serial plaster of Paris individual digit casts as described by Bell-Krotoski (66,67) (Figs. 9–14, 9–15).

MEDIAN NERVE SPLINTING PRINCIPLES

The high-level median nerve creates loss of the extrinsic pronator muscles, radial wrist flexor, superficial digit flexors, index and long finger profundus flexors, and long thumb flexor. Distally, the median nerve innervates thenar abduction and opposition. Sensation for the entire palmar area of the hand and digits with the exception of the small and half

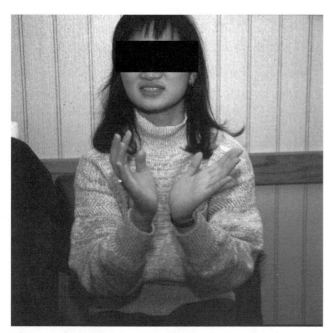

Figure 9–13. Injured right-hand motion compared to left normal extension.

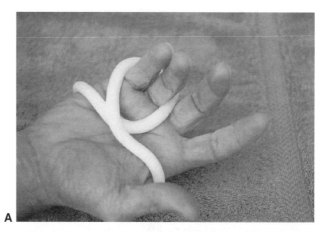

A

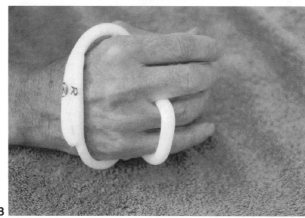

B

Figure 9–14. **A–B:** A figure-eight splint fabricated from low-temperature thermoplastic rod provides passive metacarpophalangeal flexion, permitting active proximal interphalangeal joint extension.

the ring fingers is lost. With sensory loss, functional hand and digit tasks must be performed within the visual field. The high-level median nerve injury splint provides radial digit metacarpophalangeal flexion of the radial fingers and thumb positioned in

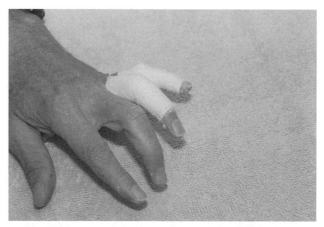

Figure 9–15. Serial digit casts as used to reduce proximal interphalangeal (PIP) flexion contractures.

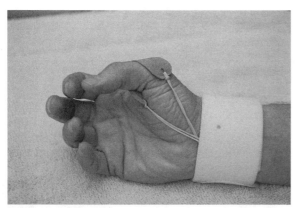

Figure 9–16. Wrist cuff with dynamic thumb palmar abduction sling assists palmar abduction.

palmar abduction opposition. A lower-level median nerve injury splint may be used to maintain the thumb web space and place the thumb in palmar abduction (67) (Figs. 9–16, 9–17).

BRACHIAL PLEXUS AND COMBINED PERIPHERAL NERVE INJURY SPLINTING PRINCIPLES

Splinting a brachial plexus or combined peripheral nerve injury requires understanding of each individual nerve function and deficits present. Ongoing treatment goals are customized as the different injured or repaired nerves recover at different rates or possibly have no recovery. Framptom (68) describes the therapist's role in the rehabilitation of brachial plexus lesions as a "prolonged process." A preganglionic lesion has no possible recovery as the nerve root has been torn from the spinal cord. A postganglionic traction lesion may have a good recovery depending on the severity of the injury.

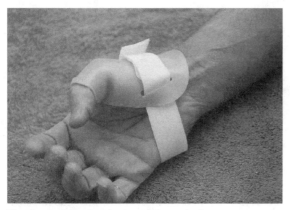

Figure 9–17. Static hand-based short opponens splint used to prevent thumb web space contracture.

Table 9-2	Passive Range of Motion and Splint Selection
PROM Increase	**Splinting**
About 20 degrees or more	No Splint
About 15 degrees	Static Splint
About 10 degrees	Dynamic Splint
About 0–5 degrees	Static Progressive Splint

From Flowers KR. A proposed decision hierarchy for splinting the stiff joint, with an emphasis on force application parameters. *J Hand Ther.* 2002;15(2):158–162, with permission.

The patient may be referred to therapy after loss of motion or with developed contractures. Determining the best splint and therapy approach for the stiff joint has been described by Flowers (69) using the Modified Weeks Test. The patient does not exercise or wear a splint on the day to be tested. Passive joint measurements are taken before using any modality or exercise. The patient then performs 20 minutes of a thermal modality with motion. The patient manually places the joint at end range for 10 minutes followed by immediate joint remeasurement. Change in passive range of motion (before modality/exercise to after modality/exercise) is used to determine the splint selection (Table 9-2).

■ Case Studies

Brachial Plexopathy
Case Number 1

A 39-year-old woman sustained a left nondominant brachial plexus traction shoulder dislocation injury when she fell into a snow hole while skiing. She had a completely flaccid hand and upper extremity. The day of injury, her upper arm was stabilized against her body and her forearm supported in a sling. She was fitted with a custom volar pan resting hand splint in the "safe position." She faithfully followed through with a passive motion home exercise program. The median and ulnar nerves began to recover at 3 months, and she was placed in a dynamic wrist extension and dynamic finger and thumb extension splint. Therapy focused on early use of the intrinsic hand muscles to decrease atrophy and contracture formation. The Phoenix wrist extension unit was selected because it allowed the patient to go into wrist flexion, which was essential to perform some of her daily living tasks. As the radial nerve function returned at 6 months, the forearm-based splint was converted to a hand-based splint for digit extension. As she continued to progress, the three ulnar digits were

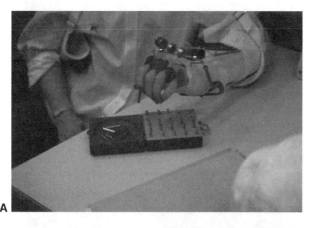

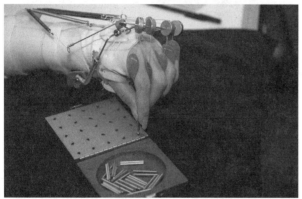

Figure 9–18. A–B: Dynamic wrist, finger, and thumb extension splint.

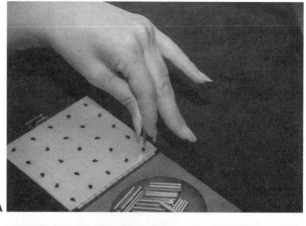

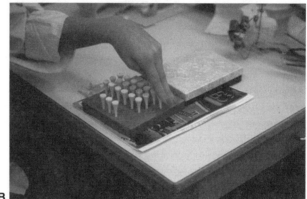

Figure 9–19. A–B: Early prehension without splint.

assisted in extension and the small finger in extension and adduction. At 1-year postinjury, she had full active wrist and digit flexion and extension with the exception of the middle finger distal interphalangeal joint lacking 15 degrees full extension. She stated she noticed intrinsic hand muscle fatigue with strenuous and prolonged use. She resumed her pre-injury, part-time office work using a keyboard (Figs. 9–18—9–22).

Case Number 2

A 56-year-old male with cerebral palsy due to birth trauma worked as an industrial machinist throughout his adult life. He performed most tasks with his less involved left dominant hand. As an adult, he sustained an iatrogenic brachial plexus injury during a left shoulder manipulation under anesthesia for frozen shoulder. He received therapy for his wrist, forearm, and shoulder. He received no preventative splinting or digit passive exercises until 6 months following injury when referred for hand therapy. By this time, he had already developed median and ulnar nerve claw deformities. His metacarpophalangeal extension and proximal interphalangeal flexion contractures were not successfully reduced with surgery or splinting. Dynamic splinting did not improve his dominant hand function. He was not able to return to work and retired on disability (Fig. 9–23).

Case Number 3

A 43-year-old male sustained a left dominant forearm crush injury with permanent radial nerve damage while working in forestry and struck by a burning falling tree. His forearm and wrist injury resulted in a proximal row carpectomy. He had significant loss of extension and had developed digit flexion contractures. He had no functional

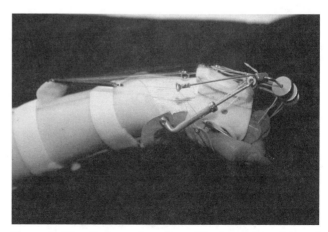

Figure 9–20. Early prehension with dynamic wrist and digit extension splint.

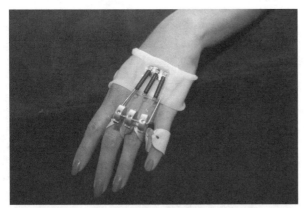

Figure 9–21. Wrist flexion while using dynamic extension splint.

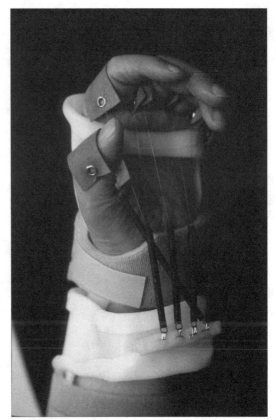

Figure 9–23. Dynamic splinting did not achieve return to functional hand use.

individual digit motion. Function was not improved with dynamic splinting. Before his injury, he worked in the office using a keyboard for 6 months in the winter and spring, and in the summer and fall, he fought forest fires. He was very motivated to return to his pre-injury occupation and had an accepting employer. He retrained hand dominance to the right, attended a community college for one quarter for keyboard training using one-handed techniques, and returned to the forestry department working inside. He noted that his keyboard speed was equal or better than that of fellow workers who used the hunt-and-peck technique (Fig. 9–24).

Case Number 4

A 26-year-old male involved in a farming accident sustained a right dominant humeral fracture, radial nerve laceration, and median and ulnar traction injury with flaccid upper extremity and unstable fracture. He was referred to therapy for a full arm splint with the hand and wrist placed in the "safe position" at 6 weeks post-injury. Passive motion was maintained for the wrist, hand, and digits while the fracture was surgically plated and the radial nerve repaired. The median and ulnar

nerve function returned before the radial nerve. He was treated with dynamic wrist and digit extension splinting (Figs. 9–25—9–27). At the end of 12 months, he had full return of all upper extremity and hand flexion and extension with the exception of the thumb interphalangeal joint lacking 15 degrees full extension. He was pleased with his outcome and returned to farming.

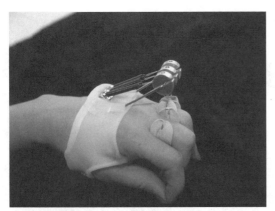

Figure 9–22. Hand-based dynamic digit extension.

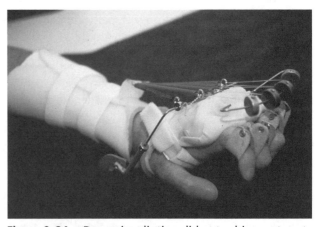

Figure 9–24. Dynamic splinting did not achieve return to functional hand use.

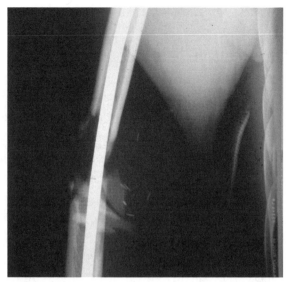

Figure 9–25. Humeral fracture separation with weight of arm and cast.

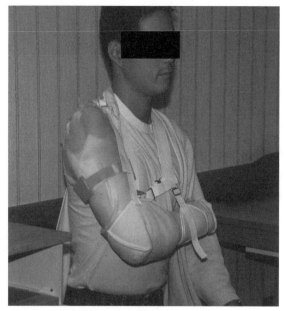

Figure 9–27. Full arm 36-inch-long splint with wrist and digits in "safe position" and sling.

OUTCOMES AFTER PERIPHERAL NERVE INJURIES

There is limited data on functional or vocational outcomes after specific nerve injuries, but further research in this area may be fruitful in predicting prognosis for return to functional activities. A problem with outcomes prediction is the wide variability in site and severity of nerve injury. One recent study, for example, has reported on the outcomes after median and ulnar nerve injury (70). Of those with median nerve injury, 80% returned to work, while 59% of those with ulnar nerve injury reported return to work. Individuals who had both nerves injured had only a 24% chance of returning to work. Factors associated with poor prognosis for return to work included: lower educational level, more physically demanding vocation, low compliance with therapy, weaker grip strength, and less sensory recovery.

REFERENCES

1. Noble J, Munro CA, Prasad VS, et al. Analysis of upper and lower extremity peripheral nerve injuries in a population of patients with multiple injuries. *J Trauma.* 1998;45(1):116–122.
2. Selecki BR, Ring IT, Simpson DA, et al. Trauma to the central and peripheral nervous systems. Part II: A statistical profile of surgical treatment new South Wales 1977. *Aust N Z J Surg.* 1982;52(2):111–116.
3. Haymaker W, Woodhill B. *Peripheral nerve injuries: Principles of diagnosis.* Philadelphia, PA: WB Saunders; 1953.
4. Seddon HJ. *Surgical disorders of the peripheral nerves.* 2nd ed. New York, NY: Churchill Livingstone; 1975.
5. Sunderland S. *Nerves and nerve injuries.* 2nd ed. New York, NY: Churchill Livingstone; 1978.
6. Cosgrove JL, Vargo M, Reidy ME. A prospective study of peripheral nerve lesions occurring in traumatic brain-injured patients. *Am J Phys Med Rehabil.* 1989; 68(1):15–17.
7. Garland DE, Bailey S. Undetected injuries in head-injured adults. *Clin Orthop.* 1981;155:162–165.
8. Stone L, Keenan MA. Peripheral nerve injuries in the adult with traumatic brain injury. *Clin Orthop.* 1988; 233:136–144.
9. Mackinnon S, Dellon AL. *Surgery of the peripheral nerve.* New York, NY: Thieme Medical Publishers; 1988.

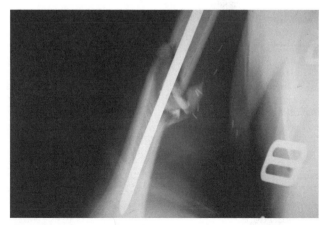

Figure 9–26. Weight of arm splinted and supported in sling.

10. Gilliatt RW. Acute compression block. In: Sumner AJ, ed. *The physiology of peripheral nerve disease*. Philadelphia, PA: WB Saunders; 1980:287–315.

11. Ochoa J, Fowler TJ, Gilliatt RW. Anatomical changes in peripheral nerves compressed by a pneumatic tourniquet. *J Anat*. 1972;113(3):433–455.

12. Rasminsky M, Sears TA. Internodal conduction in undissected demyelinated nerve fibres. *J Physiol*. 1972;227(2):323–350.

13. Dumitru D. *Electrodiagnostic medicine*. Philadelphia, PA: Hanley & Belfus; 1995.

14. Miller RG. AAEE minimonograph #28: Injury to peripheral motor nerves. *Muscle Nerve*. 1987;10(8):698–710.

15. Chaudhry V, Cornblath DR. Wallerian degeneration in human nerves: Serial electrophysiological studies. *Muscle Nerve*. 1992;15(6):687–693.

16. Gilliatt RW, Hjorth RJ. Nerve conduction during Wallerian degeneration in the baboon. *J Neurol Neurosurg Psychiatry*. 1972;35(3):335–341.

17. Gilliatt RW, Taylor JC. Electrical changes following section of the facial nerve. *Proc R Soc Med*. 1959;52:1080–1083.

18. Fisher MA. AAEM minimonograph #13: H reflexes and F waves: Physiology and clinical indications. *Muscle Nerve*. 1992;15(11):1223–1233.

19. Kimura J, Machida M, Ishida T, et al. Relation between size of compound sensory or muscle action potentials and length of nerve segment. *Neurology*. 1986;36(5):647–652.

20. Gilliatt RW, Westgaard RH, Williams IR. Extrajunctional acetylcholine sensitivity of inactive muscle fibres in the baboon during prolonged nerve pressure block. *J Physiol*. 1978;280:499–514.

21. Cangiano A, Lutzemberger L, Nicotra L. Non-equivalence of impulse blockade and denervation in the production of membrane changes in rat skeletal muscle. *J Physiol*. 1977;273(3):691–706.

22. Trojaborg W. Early electrophysiologic changes in conduction block. *Muscle Nerve*. 1978;1(5):400–403.

23. Weddell G, Glees P. The early stages in the degeneration of cutaneous nerve fibers. *J Anat*. 1941;76:65–93.

24. Thesleff S. Trophic functions of the neuron. II. Denervation and regulation of muscle. Physiological effects of denervation of muscle. *Ann N Y Acad Sci*. 1974;228:89–104.

25. Buchthal F. Fibrillations: Clinical electrophysiology. In: Culp WJ, Ochoa J, eds. *Abnormal nerves and muscle generators*. New York, NY: Oxford University Press; 1982:632–662.

26. Dorfman LJ. Quantitative clinical electrophysiology in the evaluation of nerve injury and regeneration. *Muscle Nerve*. 1990;13(9):822–828.

27. Kraft GH. Fibrillation potential amplitude and muscle atrophy following peripheral nerve injury. *Muscle Nerve*. 1990;13(9):814–821.

28. Partanen JV, Danner R. Fibrillation potentials after muscle injury in humans. *Muscle Nerve*. 1982;5(9S):S70–S73.

29. Erminio F, Buchthal F, Rosenfalck P. Motor unit territory and muscle fiber concentration in paresis due to peripheral nerve injury and anterior horn cell involvement. *Neurology*. 1959;9:657–671.

30. Hoffman H. Local re-innervation in partially denervated muscle: A histophysiological study. *Aust J Exp Biol Med Sci*. 1950;28:383.

31. Massey JM, Sanders DB. Single-fiber EMG demonstrates re-innervation dynamics after nerve injury. *Neurology*. 1991;41(7):1150–1151.

32. Brandstater ME, Fullerton M. Sensory nerve conduction studies in cervical root lesions. *Can J Neurol Sci*. 1983;10:152.

33. Tackmann W, Radu EW. Observations on the application of electrophysiological methods in the diagnosis of cervical root compressions. *Eur Neurol*. 1983;22(6):397–404.

34. Campbell WW, Pridgeon RM, Riaz G, et al. Sparing of the flexor carpi ulnaris in ulnar neuropathy at the elbow. *Muscle Nerve*. 1989;12(12):965–967.

35. Wertsch JJ, Sanger JR, Matloub HS. Pseudo-anterior interosseous nerve syndrome. *Muscle Nerve*. 1985;8(1):68–70.

36. Wertsch JJ, Oswald TA, Roberts MM. Role of intraneural topography in diagnosis and localization in electrodiagnostic medicine. *Phys Med Rehabil Clin N Am*. 1994;5:465–475.

37. Fowler TJ, Danta G, Gilliatt RW. Recovery of nerve conduction after a pneumatic tourniquet: Observations on the hind-limb of the baboon. *J Neurol Neurosurg Psychiatry*. 1972;35(5):638–647.

38. Milner-Brown HS, Stein RB, Lee RG. Synchronization of human motor units: Possible roles of exercise and supraspinal reflexes. *Electroencephalogr Clin Neurophysiol*. 1975;38(3):245–254.

39. Moritani T, deVries HA. Neural factors versus hypertrophy in the time course of muscle strength gain. *Am J Phys Med*. 1979;58(3):115–130.

40. Brown MC, Holland RL, Hopkins WG. Motor nerve sprouting. *Annu Rev Neurosci*. 1981;4:17–42.

41. Guth L. Neuromuscular function after regeneration of interrupted nerve fibers into partially denervated muscle. *Exp Neurol*. 1962;6:129–141.

42. Seddon HJ. Nerve grafting. *J Bone Joint Surg [Br]*. 1963;45:447–455.

43. Wood MB. Surgical approach to peripheral nervous system trauma. In: *AAEM Course C: Electrodiagnosis in traumatic conditions*. Rochester, NY: American Association of Electrodiagnostic Medicine; 1998:27–36.

44. Speidel CC. Studies of living nerves: Growth adjustments of cutaneous terminal arborization. *J Comp Neurol*. 1942;76:57–73.

45. Sillman JS, Niparko JK, Lee SS, et al. Prognostic value of evoked and standard electromyography in acute facial paralysis. *Otolaryngol Head Neck Surg*. 1992;107(3):377–381.

46. Kline DG. Surgical repair of peripheral nerve injury. *Muscle Nerve*. 1990;13(9):843–852.

47. Penkert G, Carvalho GA, Nikkhah G, et al. Diagnosis and surgery of brachial plexus injuries. *J Reconstr Microsurg*. 1999;15(1):3–8.

48. Dunnet WJ, Housden PL, Birch R. Flexor to extensor tendon transfers in the hand. *J Hand Surg [Br]*. 1995;20(1):26–28.

49. Skoll PJ, Hudson DA, de Jager W, et al. Long-term results of tendon transfers for radial nerve palsy in patients with limited rehabilitation. *Ann Plast Surg*. 2000;45(2):122–126.

50. Kruft S, von Heimburg D, Reill P. Treatment of irreversible lesion of the radial nerve by tendon transfer: Indication and long-term results of the Merle d'Aubigne procedure. *Plast Reconstr Surg*. 1997;100(3):610–616; discussion 617–618.

51. Illert M, Trauner M, Weller E, et al. Forearm muscles of man can reverse their function after tendon transfers: An electromyographic study. *Neurosci Lett.* 1986;67(2):129–134.

52. Taha A, Taha J. Results of suture of the radial, median, and ulnar nerves after missile injury below the axilla. *J Trauma.* 1998;45(2):335–339.

53. Kim DH, Kam AC, Chandika P, et al. Surgical management and outcome in patients with radial nerve lesions. *J Neurosurg.* 2001;95(4):573–583.

54. Kim DH, Han K, Tiel RL, et al. Surgical outcomes of 654 ulnar nerve lesions. *J Neurosurg.* 2003;98(5):993–1004.

55. van Meeteren NL, Brakkee JH, Hamers FP, et al. Exercise training improves functional recovery and motor nerve conduction velocity after sciatic nerve crush lesion in the rat. *Arch Phys Med Rehabil.* 1997;78(1):70–77.

56. Mendonca AC, Barbieri CH, Mazzer N. Directly applied low intensity direct electric current enhances peripheral nerve regeneration in rats. *J Neurosci Methods.* 2003;129(2):183–190.

57. Ebenbichler GR, Resch KL, Nicolakis P, et al. Ultrasound treatment for treating the carpal tunnel syndrome: Randomised "sham" controlled trial. *BMJ.* 1998;316(7133):731–735.

58. Oztas O, Turan B, Bora I, et al. Ultrasound therapy effect in carpal tunnel syndrome. *Arch Phys Med Rehabil.* 1998;79(12):1540–1544.

59. Paik NJ, Cho SH, Han TR. Ultrasound therapy facilitates the recovery of acute pressure-induced conduction block of the median nerve in rabbits. *Muscle Nerve.* 2002;26(3):356–361.

60. Chan RK. Splinting for peripheral nerve injury in upper limb. *Hand Surg.* 2002;7(2):251–259.

61. Fess EE. A history of splinting: To understand the present, view the past. *J Hand Ther.* 2002;15(2):97–132.

62. James JI. Common, simple errors in the management of hand injuries. *Proc R Soc Med.* 1970;63(1):69–72.

63. Schmidhammer R, Zandieh S, Hopf R, et al. Alleviated tension at the repair site enhances functional regeneration: The effect of full range of motion mobilization on the regeneration of peripheral nerves—histologic, electrophysiologic, and functional results in a rat model. *J Trauma.* 2004;56(3):571–584.

64. Duncan RM. Basic principles of splinting the hand. *Phys Ther.* 1989;69(12):1104–1116.

65. King JW. Practice forum static-progressive splints. *J Hand Ther.* 1992;5(1):36.

66. Bell-Krotoski JA. Biomechanics of soft-tissue growth and remodeling with plaster casting. *J Hand Ther.* 1995;8(2):131–137.

67. Fess EE, Phillips CA. *Hand splinting: Principles and methods.* 2nd ed. St. Louis, MO: Mosby; 1987:346.

68. Frampton VM. Management of brachial plexus lesions. *J Hand Ther.* 1988;1(3):115.

69. Flowers KR. A proposed decision hierarchy for splinting the stiff joint, with an emphasis on force application parameters. *J Hand Ther.* 2002;15(2):158–162.

70. Bruyns CN, Jaquet JB, Schreuders TA, et al. Predictors for return to work in patients with median and ulnar nerve injuries. *J Hand Surg [Am].* 2003;28(1):28–34.

10

Burns

Peter C. Esselman, Dana Y. Nakamura, and David R. Patterson

The rehabilitation of burn injuries presents unique challenges because of the prolonged acute care management and significant long-term physical and psychological impairments involved. It is estimated that more than 1 million individuals sustain burn injuries in the United States every year, resulting in approximately 50,000 hospital admissions per year (1). In 1995, there were 4,345 deaths caused by fire/burn injuries (2). The overall incidence of burn injuries requiring medical attention has declined over time from estimates of 1,000 per population of 100,000 in the 1950s and 1960s to an incidence of 420 per 100,000 in the early 1990s (1).

Mortality has decreased over time due to increased prevention of burns and improved medical treatment techniques. The Centers for Disease Control (CDC) reported that from 1985 to 1995 the age-adjusted death rate from fire/burns decreased 33% from 2.1 per 100,000 to 1.4 per 100,000 (2). The incidence of mortality in individuals with burn injuries is influenced by the size of the burn, the patient's age, and associated injuries such as inhalation injury. In data collected from 1991 to 1993 in patients admitted to burn centers, the overall mortality rate was 2.2% and the mortality in patients with inhalation injury was 29.4%. At that time, the burn size that was lethal to 50% of young adults (LD_{50}) was 81% total body surface area (TBSA). Mortality increased with age, and a burn of 29.5% TBSA was lethal to 50% of adults over the age of 70 (3). Improved acute care treatment techniques have decreased the mortality after severe burn injuries. Pruitt compared mortality between patients in 1950 to 1963 and 1987 to 1991 and found that the decrease in mortality was not uniform across all ages or size of burns. Small burns have never resulted in significant mortality,

and large burns in the elderly continue to present a high risk of death. The largest decrease in mortality is in the burn that resulted in about an 80% mortality rate in the 1950s (4). The increased survival rates for individuals with larger burn injuries has resulted in a greater need for burn rehabilitation treatment to maximize independence and restore lost function.

PROPERTIES OF NORMAL SKIN

To provide appropriate rehabilitation care to individuals with burn injuries, it is important to understand the properties of normal skin and how burns injure the skin. The primary function of the skin is to provide a protective barrier; prevent infection and fluid loss; regulate temperature; and provide sensory function. The skin is composed of the epidermis, dermis, and the hypodermis (Fig. 10–1). The epidermis or the outer layer of the skin is about 1 to 2 mm in thickness and provides a protective barrier. The inner layer of the epidermis is composed of the basal cells that divide to form the keratinocytes. The keratinocytes mature and migrate to the outer layer (stratum corneum) that is primarily composed of cellular debris and keratin. The process of cells moving from the basal layer to the surface takes 2 to 4 weeks. The epidermis is penetrated by the dermal appendages (hair follicles, sweat, and sebaceous glands) that come from the dermis. In addition to cells related to their primary function, these epidermal appendages contain epidermal cells. These epidermal cells can divide to regenerate the epidermis in superficial partial-thickness burns (5).

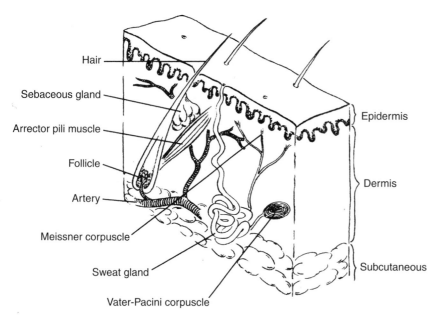

Figure 10–1. Cross section of normal skin illustrating the epidermis, dermis, and the epidermal appendages (hair follicles, sweat, and sebaceous glands). (From Achauer BM, Eriksson E. *Plastic surgery indications, operations and outcomes.* St. Louis: Mosby; 2000:24, with permission.)

The dermis is up to 5 mm thick. It has a vascular structure that provides nutrition to the epidermis and a collagen matrix to support the epidermis. The fibroblasts of the dermis synthesize the collagen and elastin, providing the strength and elasticity of the skin. The dermis also supports the dermal appendages and sensory nerve endings. The hypodermis consists of the subcutaneous fat layer (5).

CLASSIFICATION OF BURN INJURIES

Burn injuries are classified by etiology of injury, the size of the burn, depth of the burn, and the area burned. An estimate of burn size can be quickly determined by the rule of nines, providing easy calculation of burn size in adults (Fig. 10–2). A more

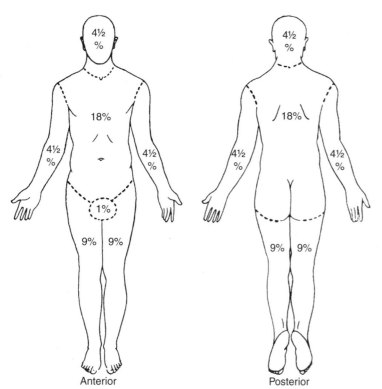

Figure 10–2. The rule of nines is a quick method for the calculation of the percentage of body surface area burned. (From Artz CP, Moncrief JA, Pruitt BA. *Burns: A team approach.* Philadelphia: W.B. Saunders; 1979:153, with permission.)

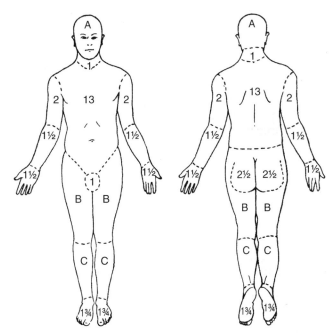

Relative Percentage of Areas Affected by Growth

Figure 10–3. The Lund and Browder method for calculation of burn size accounts for differences in body proportions in children. (From Artz CP, Moncrief JA, Pruitt BA. *Burns: A team approach.* Philadelphia: W.B. Saunders; 1979:160, with permission.)

	Age in Years					
	0	1	5	10	15	Adult
A—½ of head	9½	8½	6½	5½	4½	3½
B—½ of one thigh	2¾	3¼	4	4¼	4½	4¾
C—½ of one leg	2½	2½	2¾	3	3¼	3½

accurate method that will account for the differences in body area proportions in children is the Lund and Browder method for calculation of burn size (6) (Fig. 10–3).

Burns are described as superficial (first degree), partial thickness (second degree) or full thickness (third degree) (Fig. 10–4). A superficial burn involves only the epidermis and is usually minor except in the very young or elderly. Sunburn is an example of a superficial burn injury, and this usually heals in 3 to 7 days. Partial-thickness burns include the epidermis and dermis and are characterized as superficial

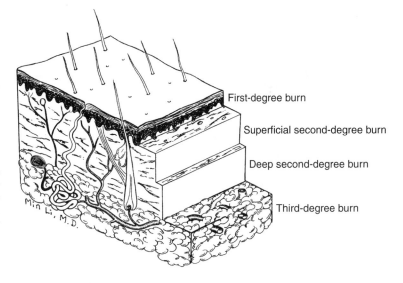

First-degree burn

Superficial second-degree burn

Deep second-degree burn

Third-degree burn

Figure 10–4. In determining depth of burn injury, a superficial (first-degree) burn involves only the epidermis. A partial-thickness (second-degree) burn involves the superficial or deep dermis, and a full-thickness burn (third-degree) extends to subdermal tissues. (From Achauer BM, Eriksson E. *Plastic surgery indications, operations and outcomes.* St. Louis: Mosby; 2000:361, with permission.)

or deep. In superficial partial-thickness burns the superficial portion of the dermis is destroyed. These wounds are painful due to the preserved nerves and appear red, blister, and will blanch with pressure. A superficial partial-thickness burn will heal in 7 to 21 days. The epidermal cells in the epidermal appendages are a primary source of epidermal regeneration and healing in superficial partial-thickness burns. A deep partial-thickness burn involves almost all the dermis and may take >14 days to heal with hypertrophic scarring or may need grafting. A full-thickness burn includes the entire epidermis and dermis extending to the hypodermis. These burns are not painful because the sensory nerves are destroyed and the wound is dry with an eschar. Full-thickness burns require excision and grafting (7).

The American Burn Association defines a burn injury that should be referred to an established burn center as a burn that includes any of the following criteria (8):

1. Partial-thickness burn of >10% TBSA.
2. Burn that involves the face, hands, feet, genitalia, perineum, or major joints.
3. Full-thickness burn in any age group.
4. Electrical injury, including lightning injury.
5. Chemical burn.
6. Inhalation injury.
7. Burn injury in patients with pre-existing medical conditions that could complicate treatment.
8. Burn injury in patients with concomitant trauma in which the burn injury poses the greatest risk of morbidity or mortality.
9. Burn injury in children in hospitals without qualified personnel or equipment for the care of children.
10. Burn injury in patients who will require special social, emotional, or long-term rehabilitative treatment.

INITIAL MANAGEMENT OF BURN WOUNDS

Debridement and prevention of infection are important in the initial management of burn wounds. Debridement removes the eschar, which is avascular nonviable necrotic tissue. This is routinely completed during daily wound care on the burn unit and promotes wound healing and minimizes the risk of infection. Topical agents can be used to prevent infection. Silver nitrate solution was used in the past and found to be effective in reducing infection.

Unfortunately silver nitrate permanently stains all surfaces brown and is not currently used routinely. Silver can be applied to the wound in the form of silver sulfadiazine (Silvadene) as a water-soluble cream, or mafenide acetate (Sulfamylon) in a cream or solution can be used. These agents have broad antibacterial properties and can penetrate into the eschar.

Full-thickness wounds or deep partial-thickness wounds that will take longer than 2 to 3 weeks to heal are treated with early excision of the necrotic tissue and autografting using skin from a donor site on the patient. Tangential excision of deep partial-thickness burns is the sequential removal of eschar until reaching the deeper intact dermal tissue. In full-thickness burns the excision is made down to subcutaneous fat or other underlying intact tissue. Split-thickness skins grafts (STSG) are taken from a donor site and include the epidermis and part of the dermis and can vary in thickness. The tissue can be applied without any alteration as a sheet graft to a small area or when grafting the face, hands, or neck or over joints. This method provides an improved cosmetic and functional result in these locations. In larger burns the split-thickness skin graft is meshed, expanding to cover a wound several times the original size. Meshed grafts are avoided in exposed areas since they heal with a characteristic mesh pattern (9).

Full-thickness skin grafts (FTSG) include the entire dermis and provide a thicker skin covering and less wound contraction. These grafts are small and sutured closed since large FTSG donor sites will not heal spontaneously. FTSG can be used to graft small areas such as the eyelid, lip, and tip of the nose, where a good cosmetic result is very important (9).

Patients with large burns often benefit from temporary wound coverage with a biologic dressing such as a xenograft or allograft. A xenograft is skin from a pig and can be placed over a burn wound to provide a temporary covering and prevent infection. Allograft skin from organ donors can also be used to provide temporary wound coverage. It can prevent infection and allow time for further wound vascularization and healing in preparation for an autograft. An allograft will be rejected by the patient's immune system within 2 to 3 weeks (9).

There is increasing use of dermal replacement products in the management of large burns when there are limited graft donor sites. Integra is a product that has been shown to be safe and effective in the treatment of burn wounds and is associated with a decrease in hospital length of stay (10,11). Integra is composed of a dermal replacement layer of bovine collagen in a matrix of shark cartilage chondroitin-6-sulfate covered by a silicone layer. The collagen layer serves as a matrix for infiltration of fibroblasts and other cell types from the wound bed and is vascularized forming a neodermis in 2 to 3 weeks. At that time the silicone layer is removed and a thin autograft is placed on the wound for final closure and healing.

Donor sites from split-thickness skin grafts can be managed as partial thickness injuries to the skin and will heal with epithelialization from the deeper dermis within 2 to 3 weeks. It is important to decrease pain caused by the donor site and promote healing. Acticoat can be used to cover the donor site. Acticoat is composed of a rayon/polyester sheet with a polyethylene mesh coated with silver. The silver is released from the material and prevents wound infection while providing a covering to the wound. In addition, with the Acticoat there is no need for frequent dressing changes, decreasing the pain from the donor site.

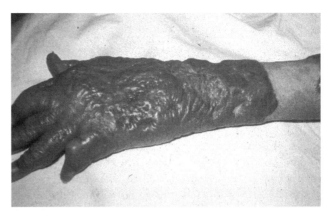

Figure 10–5. Hypertrophic scarring is characterized by a red, raised, and rigid scar that can cause distortion of surrounding tissue and contractures.

COMPLICATIONS OF BURN INJURIES

HYPERTROPHIC SCARRING

While scar formation is a normal part of the wound healing process, hypertrophic scarring can cause contractures and deformities. The cause of hypertrophic scarring is unknown, but the adverse effects can be minimized by decreasing the time to healing and reducing the amount and intensity of inflammation and edema (12,13). In addition, the prevalence of hypertrophic scarring is poorly documented (14).

Clinical Presentation

Burn hypertrophic scarring presents clinically with a red, raised, and rigid mass that contracts relentlessly and distorts surrounding skin (Fig. 10–5). The histological picture of scar tissue is one of highly vascularized tissue with collagen and myofibril elements oriented in whorls and nodules separated by edematous spaces.

The contractile forces of hypertrophic scar progress as collagen fibers are randomly laid down, with peak scarring at 4 to 6 months from the time of injury. The time to maturation varies from 6 months to 2 years with an average of 1 year. The scar is assessed as mature when it is pale, flat, and pliable.

The risk of developing hypertrophic scar is related to the size, depth, and location of burn, time to healing, and patient race and age. Hypertrophic scar formation is more prevalent in children (15). The prevalence in people with darker skin may be due to an increased reactivity of melanocytes to

melanocyte-stimulating hormone. It is also known that hypertrophic scars commonly develop in areas of motion, such as the joints, because tension promotes collagen deposits while lessening collagen lysis (16). The time to obtain healing of the wound is also a factor in hypertrophic scarring. Wounds that heal within 21 days have a 33% incidence of hypertrophic scarring, and wounds that take longer than 21 days to heal have a 78% incidence (15).

Pressure Therapy

Pressure therapy is routinely used to prevent or treat hypertrophic scarring, but further research is needed to clarify the effectiveness of pressure therapy (17–19). The basic premise of pressure therapy is that it decreases circulation to an area, and thus retards scar development (20). Patients who are at high risk of developing hypertrophic scar are fit with pressure garments and devices (Fig. 10–6). In general, patients with wounds that heal in less than

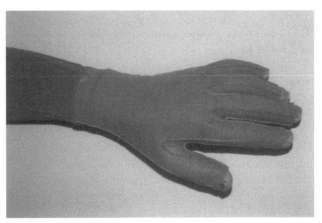

Figure 10–6. Pressure garments are worn to prevent and treat hypertrophic scarring.

10 days require no pressure, and patients with wounds that heal in 10 to 21 days may benefit from pressure. Patients with wounds that take longer than 21 days to heal will definitely require pressure therapy. In addition, children and people with darker skin are at increased risk of scarring and are routinely fit with pressure garments. The elderly typically do not require pressure therapy because they rarely develop hypertrophic scars.

The recommended amount of pressure is 20 to 40 mm Hg, and despite precise fitting techniques, pressure garments do not provide a consistent amount of pressure at the scar/garment interface (21). A computer-based method such as the I-scan system (Tekscan, Inc.) is an accurate and reliable measure of pressure under garments (19,21) and face masks (18) and can be used for standardization of pressure application.

Patient education regarding the purpose and benefits of pressure garments is important to successful outcome. Pressure garments are worn continuously, except for daily hygiene. Patient noncompliance with wearing pressure garments may be due to difficulty donning the garment, pain, heat intolerance, and differences in patient and clinician perceptions (22). Knowledge and education about the benefits of wearing garments has been shown to have the greatest positive effect on patient compliance (23). Comfort measures such as easier donning and doffing, better sizing, cooler fabric, more custom options such as pockets for silicone and pressure inserts, and zippers also increase adherence with wearing pressure garments.

In addition to custom-measured and fabricated pressure garments, other pressure techniques include wraps (Ace bandages, cohesive bandages, Silipos Gel-E-Roll), tubular pressure bandages (Tubigrip, digit sleeves), commercially available garments (Isotoner gloves, Jobst interims), and inserts. Topical silicone products are now widely used for pressure therapy. It is still unclear how topical silicone works; however, clinicians report improvement in the appearance of burn scars, as well as a beneficial effect on pruritus and pain.

CONTRACTURE/JOINT DEFORMITIES

The aggressive treatment of contractures and joint deformities is important to maximize the functional outcome after a severe burn injury. The techniques available for treatment include positioning, splinting, range of motion (ROM) exercises with stretching, and serial casting.

Positioning

The purposes of positioning are to minimize edema, prevent tissue destruction, and maintain the soft tissues in an elongated state to facilitate functional recovery (24). Positioning methods must prevent contracture but not compromise the patient's mobility and function. Individualized positioning programs are based on the medical status, ROM, location of burn, depth of burn, and level of patient cooperation.

A general principle is that the position of patient comfort will equal the position of contracture. This position of comfort is characterized by neck flexion, shoulder adduction, elbow flexion, hip/knee flexion, and ankle plantarflexion. Individualized plans and programs are developed to prevent these common contractures.

When a patient demonstrates cooperation and compliance with the therapy program, basic positioning techniques and principles apply. When a patient is unable to comply with the positioning plan, increased attention and detail are necessary for successful outcomes. Positioning devices may be made more secure or alternative measures such as plaster and fiberglass casts and external fixation can be employed. Special considerations apply to positioning pediatric patients, as they may be fearful of the hospital environment, anxious due to previous painful treatments, uncooperative, and unable to understand the reasons for specific therapeutic interventions.

Postoperative positioning is important for graft healing and requires 24-hour attention of all team members. It is important to communicate the positioning plan so that it is understandable to all team members, even those with limited experience caring for burn patients. Communication of positioning needs can occur by a number of means such as written information, diagrammed instructions, and photos or videos.

Splinting

Splinting techniques and methods have changed over the years, but the overall goals are the same: to prevent loss of motion and deformity, promote functional independence, protect anatomic structures, preserve skin graft integrity, and restore function (25–29).

To provide appropriate splinting, it is important to have a good understanding of the process and mechanism of wound healing and to recognize the phases of wound healing. Burn injuries that take

>21 days to heal have an increased risk of scarring, and these wounds are often treated with grafting. In burn injuries that heal without grafting, the indications for splints vary during the phases of healing. In the initial inflammatory phase of the burn injury, lasting several days, the healing tissue needs support. Static splinting is used with some period of controlled exercises out of the splint. This is followed by a proliferative healing phase that can last several weeks with increased cellular activity and collagen production. Dynamic or static splinting is used to provide gentle prolonged stretch that influences the direction and alignment of collagen tissue. The maturation healing phase can last as long as 1 to 2 years as the scar matures with increased tissue resistance to stretching forces. The best method to apply force in this phase is with serial static, static progressive, or dynamic splinting. Serial casting may also be indicated during this period of healing. These methods maintain stretch for prolonged periods of time to allow tissue accommodation and lengthening.

In splint design, it is important to consider biomechanical principles of design, simplicity to ensure compliance, and practicality to allow function while wearing the splints. Correct fit ensures alignment and orientation of underlying structures to prevent joint compression and ligamentous stretch, conformity to surface areas to avoid friction that can alter skin integrity, and contouring to avoid causing pressure sores over body prominences. Efficiency of splint construction and fit are important considerations. Prefabricated splints may save time and expense but should be used only if they meet the criteria for good fit. Splint design, construction, and fit also take into consideration individual patient factors, the planned length of time of splint use, function, and ease of use.

Individual factors include the reliability, cognition, and lifestyle of the patient, and ability to follow through with the splinting plan. With pediatric patients, for example, a special splint or fastening techniques may need to be designed to keep the child from moving in the splint or removing it completely. Cohesive wraps work well for holding a splint in place and can easily be managed by parents. The use of self-riveting silicone in pediatric hand splints helps with correct positioning of the hand, enhances the palmar arch, prevents skin breakdown, and has the added benefit of scar management for finger flexion contractures (30).

The length of time the splint is to be used will also affect the splint design. If the splint will be used for only a short time, the splint can be simple and cost-effective. If it is to be used for long term, long-lasting materials will hold up over time and rivet straps will hold components in place.

Splint design should optimize function of the extremity. Splint only the joint that needs to be immobilized and allow continued ROM of other joints. It is also important to allow for optimum sensation with hand splints to maximize hand function.

The ease of splint application and removal will influence splint compliance. Modifications for easy donning and doffing will allow the patient increased independence—for example, riveting an elastic abdominal binder to the front edge of an axillary splint to increase patient independence with application and removal (31).

Exercise

Exercise is an essential part of burn rehabilitation, and programs are developed on the basis of the unique characteristics of the individual patient and burn wound. The purpose of exercise is to preserve mobility and function, preserve strength and conditioning, and counteract contracting forces of scar tissue. Patients are taken through dependent or guided exercise programs, which transition into independent programs and increased functional activities. Over time, patients assume responsibility for their therapy programs and are empowered to achieve their goals, thus increasing self-esteem, motivation, and sense of accomplishment (32).

The extent of the burn and the location and the level of pain experienced by the patient dictate the intensity of exercises. A general guideline is to do frequent exercises throughout the day with shorter sessions versus fewer sessions of longer duration. Gains made with ROM and stretching may need to be maintained with splints and positioning and additional exercises. Continuous passive motion (CPM) is beneficial for positioning of an extremity while providing continued movement. It is important to remember, however, that CPM should be used as an adjunct to hands-on therapy and not as a replacement.

The burn patient's exercise program may include passive, active-assist, and active ROM; resistive exercises; strengthening and conditioning; functional activities; and joint mobilization. Other soft tissue management techniques such as massage and myofascial release, and physical agent modalities such as paraffin, fluidotherapy, hot packs, ultrasound, and electrical stimulation may be used.

Soft tissue mobilization or massage is recommended for its direct mechanical effect to elongate, soften, and increase pliability of immature scars (33) and increase ROM. Edema reduction is another possible benefit. Massage has the added benefit of relaxing a patient and decreasing resistance to exercise, and it aids in decreasing pruritus (34,35). Friction massage is not recommended due to possible development of epidermal lesions and blisters from friction on inelastic and thin tissue (34).

Many traditional contracture prevention techniques limit dynamic motion. It becomes critical to decide when and where to compromise on scar contracture prevention and to promote function. It is important to put an emphasis on functional activities to increase independence and control. Patients are taught that the performance of basic activities of daily living (ADL) and functional activities are all considered exercise. Many normal functional tasks may actually promote the development of contractures (29). For example, few ADL require flexion and abduction of the shoulder past 90 degrees, which may increase the risk of an axillary contracture. The incorporation of play activities when working with children improves outcome compared to rote exercise (36).

Serial Casting

Serial casting has been shown to be effective for the management of soft tissue contractures (37,38). Richard et al. compared multimodal (exercise, pressure, massage) to progressive (serial casting, dynamic splints, static progressive splints) treatment techniques for the correction of burn scar contractures. They found that with ROM deficits being equal, the progressive group required less than half the time to correct contracture than did the multimodal group (38).

Serial casting is based on Dr. Paul Brand's concept of "inevitable gradualness," which maintains that holding tissue at the end of its elastic limit will make the tissue relax (39). The repeated process of resetting the resting length and tissue's elastic limit is effective in increasing ROM and stretching skin contractures. A long duration stretch with low force enhances the permanent plastic deformation of contracted tissue.

Serial casting is indicated in patients with contractures 18 to 24 months postburn that have not responded to traditional methods (40). Casting is also indicated in the noncompliant or pediatric patient. Innovative ideas such as reusable prefabricated foot plates (41), metacarpal-phalangeal joint blocks (42), and bubbling out heels (43), have contributed to a resurgence of serial casting.

AMPUTATIONS

In extremities with severe burns, an aggressive approach with early decision for limb salvage and intense inpatient and outpatient therapy can result in >90% of patients achieving satisfactory functional outcome (44). However, when the extremity is devoid of all sensation or the soft tissue damage is so extensive that it precludes salvage of a functional limb, amputation is the only option.

Overall functional goals must be considered in the decision to amputate and plan for level of and type of amputation. Stable, durable skin is desired at the amputation site, but this is often not available in individuals with large burns (45). It is important to evaluate the ability of the patient to use a prosthetic device and become functionally independent. This evaluation includes factors that are present in all patients with amputations such as the ability to tolerate the increased energy and strength demands, impaired vision, poor balance, psychological or psychiatric problems, social situations, and other musculoskeletal conditions such as rheumatoid arthritis. Additionally, patients with amputations as the result of burns present unique challenges in the evaluation and design of prosthetic devices. Patients with large burns often have fragile healed or grafted skin on areas that would usually have pressure from the prosthetic socket or suspension system or from the control cables in an upper extremity prosthesis. In addition, burn patients may have contractures in joints proximal to the amputation, making the functional use of the prosthesis difficult. Likewise, hand burn contractures often make the donning and doffing of the prosthesis very difficult (Fig. 10–7). Patients with large burns or high-voltage electrical injuries may have multiple amputations that will complicate the prosthetic plan and limit functional gains.

The postoperative period is the time to promote wound healing, control incision and phantom pain, maintain joint ROM, explore the patient's and family's feelings about change in body image, and obtain adequate funding for the prosthesis and training. The preprosthetic program includes residual limb shrinkage and shaping, desensitization, preservation of ROM, increasing muscle strength, instruction in proper hygiene of the limb, maximizing functional independence, orientation to prosthetic options, and exploration of patient goals regarding the future.

Specialized teams with expertise in the management of amputation and prosthetics can provide consultation and invaluable assistance with the treatment of amputees. Their involvement can include recommendations regarding the type and

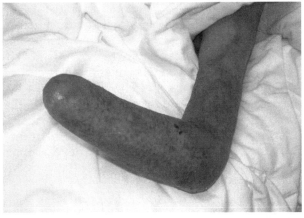 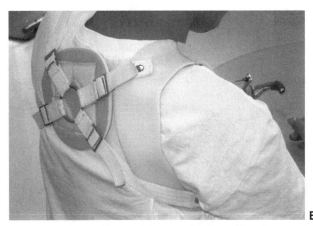

A   B

Figure 10–7. **A:** Management of amputations after burn injuries is complicated by problems with wound healing on the amputated extremity and contractures at proximal joints. **B:** The prosthetic design needs to accommodate the fragile skin proximal to the residual limb.

level of amputation, referral to a prosthetist, matching patients with peers for one-to-one support and counseling, or referral to amputee support groups. Psychological adaptation to amputation involves the loss of function, loss of sensation, and altered body image. Initial patient concerns center on pain, safety, and disfigurement and gradually shift to social reintegration and acceptance, sexual adjustment, and vocational concerns.

NEUROLOGIC INJURIES

Neurologic injuries to peripheral nerves are common after major burn injuries and are frequently not diagnosed. The exact incidence of peripheral nerve injuries is not known but has been reported to be up to about 30% of individuals followed prospectively (46–51). There is a greater incidence of neurologic injuries in individuals with burns of >20% TBSA (49). Predisposing risk factors include an injury caused by electricity, history of alcohol abuse, patient age, and greater number of days in the intensive care unit (ICU) (51).

Focal neuropathies can be caused by direct thermal or electrical injury to the nerves; pressure resulting from patient positioning, splinting or dressings; and stretching during ROM exercises or transfers. The peroneal nerve is at risk if the patient is maintained in a frog-leg position with hip and knee flexion and the foot internally rotated, causing a stretch of the nerve. The ulnar nerve can be compromised if the upper extremity is positioned in elbow flexion and forearm pronation, such as with the extremity positioned on pillows. Positioning of the shoulder to prevent contractures can result in a brachial plexus injury. Shoulder positioning in 90 or more degrees of abduction and in full external rotation will stretch the brachial plexus. If the shoulder

is also positioned in 30 degrees of horizontal adduction, the brachial plexus is not at risk of injury and the shoulder joint/axilla is still maintained on a position of stretch (49). Focal neuropathies are also caused by compartment syndrome after circumferential burns or electrical injury.

Peripheral polyneuropathies are another neurologic injury after a burn that is often not diagnosed. In a study of 88 burn patients with symptoms of weakness or sensory loss, a generalized peripheral neuropathy was diagnosed in 46 subjects (52%) by electrodiagnostic examination (49). Another study of 55 burn patients revealed a generalized distal axonal neuropathy in 9% (50). The peripheral neuropathy can occur early in the recovery from the injury. In a study of 17 subjects with >10% TBSA, 41% had evidence of peripheral neuropathy within 7 days of injury (52). The cause of the peripheral neuropathy is not known but may be due to inflammatory changes or metabolic or nutritional abnormalities.

Injury to multiple individual nerves, or mononeuritis multiplex, has also been described in patients after burn injuries (50,53). In one study, mononeuritis multiplex was diagnosed in 16% of patients with peripheral polyneuropathy (50), and in another study, it was diagnosed in 69% of such patients (48).

Once a peripheral neuropathy is recognized, splinting combined with an exercise regimen provides the keystone for effective rehabilitation. Splints are used for protection and to preserve or attain functional passive range of motion (PROM). A disruption of a localized peripheral nerve results in a relatively predictable loss, and it is helpful to not just design splints for the specific muscles involved, but to consider loss in terms of functional patterns (54). Splints must be used in tandem with exercise and sensory re-education.

A focal peripheral neuropathy may result from improper patient positioning and other treatments, and prevention is critical to avoid nerve injury. The patient should avoid prolonged elbow flexion and pronation (ulnar nerve), frog-leg positioning (peroneal nerve), and proning with arms overhead/shoulder retraction (brachial plexus). Also, care must be taken with the use of tourniquets, restraints, blood pressure cuffs, injection sites, skeletal traction, and tight, constricting dressings.

HETEROTOPIC OSSIFICATION

Heterotopic ossification (HO) is the development of mature bone in the soft tissue surrounding joints and often occurs after traumatic injuries, including severe burn injuries. Heterotopic ossification can be diagnosed by x-ray if there is calcification present, but early evidence of HO can be detected by bone scan. Since burn patients frequently develop decreased ROM due to contracture of the skin and underlying joint, the diagnosis of HO may not be considered until it results in a significant decrease in ROM and function. The incidence of functionally significant HO is reported to be 1% to 2% (55–59).

After other traumatic injuries such as spinal cord injury, HO primarily affects the larger joints, but HO after burn injuries frequently develops in the elbows (58,60) (Fig. 10–8). The etiology and contributing factors in the development of heterotopic ossification after burn injuries is unknown.

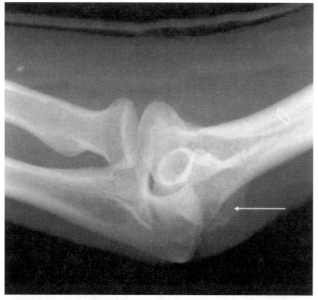

Figure 10–8. Heterotopic ossification often develops in the elbow after burn injuries. In this example, the heterotopic bone is seen posterior to the elbow joint.

Suggested contributing factors include size, depth, and location of burn, immobilization, microtraumas, metabolic disturbances, and prolonged open wounds. A case-control study by Logsetty et al. (61) demonstrated a strong correlation between open wounds at the elbow and HO formation, in which days to wound closure in the HO group far outnumbered that of the non-HO group. They propose that the prolonged inflammatory response of the open wound causes abnormal calcium deposition, and that more aggressive wound closure may decrease the incidence of HO.

The treatment of HO includes ROM exercises, medications, radiation, and surgical resection. The use of ROM, both passive and active, should be performed within a pain-free range and should be started as soon as possible following diagnosis of HO. Crawford (55) proposed that PROM beyond the pain-free ROM to joints with HO might enhance the ossification process by creating local hemorrhages, triggering an inflammatory response, which, in turn, leads to increased activity of osteoblasts. Treatment with medications such as nonsteroidal anti-inflammatory medications or etidronate has not been studied in burn patients but is recommended based on the response to treatment in other diagnostic groups (62,63).

Surgical resection of elbow HO can result in significant gains in ROM and function (59,64). Indications for surgical resection include significant functional limitation, a total arc of elbow ROM of <50 degrees (64), and entrapment of the ulnar nerve (56,65). Postoperative treatment includes active assisted ROM on the first or second postoperative day (59,64) and adequate pain management. Following resection of HO in the elbow, O'Neill and Baryza (66) recommend a clear postoperative protocol. Their standardized postoperative treatment plan consists of 3 days in a flexion cast, followed by 2 weeks of progressive CPM use (2 to 3 hours per day) and active range of motion (AROM) exercises twice daily. Treatment continues with the use of alternating elbow flexion and extension splints.

REHABILITATION OF DIFFICULT AREAS

Burn injuries to the face, neck, axilla, hands, knee, and foot/ankle present certain unique challenges to the treatment team. Burns to these areas require specialized treatment plans and close coordination of the treatment team.

Face

Burns to the face present the biggest challenge to the treatment team during the acute care, rehabilitation, and reconstruction phases. Deformities occur in the T-shaped area comprising the eyes, nose, lips, and mouth, where the complex contours make preserving ROM with exercise and fitting facial orthoses and garments difficult. A balance between pressure and exercise must be established to optimize both cosmetic and functional outcome.

Facial surgical reconstruction is usually planned after reconstruction of the extremities is completed, since the face reconstruction plan will not succeed if the patient cannot use his or her hands or feet (67). Fabric and/or rigid face masks are used for initial pressure and postreconstruction. Fabric face masks provide adequate compression over convex surfaces; however, they tend to tent over concave areas and require custom inserts for compression. Transparent facial orthoses (TFO) are fabricated over a positive plaster bust of the face from high temperature materials such as UVEX (cellulose acetate butyrate) and W-clear (Fig. 10–9). Fabrication of a compression face mask using silicone thermoplastic sheeting yields advantages of both fabric and rigid masks (68).

Burns of the head, face, and neck are especially problematic in pediatric patients because of the resultant deformities and the effect on normal growth and development (69). Fricke (70) reported that the direction of mandibular growth changed from a normal forward and downward orientation to a mainly downward direction when children wore face masks. Garment face masks appeared to affect facial growth more during the early stages of healing and reconstruction. It is recommended that infants and children be recasted and remeasured more frequently because of distortion of facial features and alteration of bony structures (69).

Eyelids

The common problem with eyelids is ectropion of the lower lid caused by contraction of the scar over the cheek area, pulling the lower eyelid down with eversion of the lid. Manual stretching exercises will help prevent or treat ectropion. Early surgical release is recommended because the ectropion can result in other complications such as eye irritation, corneal damage, and constant tearing due to change in shape of the lid near the tear ducts. Reconstruction can be done using FTSG taken from the postauricular area (71). Temporary tarsorrhaphy may be used to immobilize the lid and maintain a stretch to prevent contraction. Following grafting, custom-made silicone splints may be fit into a face mask or made to fit special eyewear to provide pressure to the medial canthal folds.

Ears

Because of their exposed position, the ears are at risk for severe burns with subsequent development of chondritis (72). If the burn exposes just the perichondrium, the wound will granulate and epithelialize. If the burn penetrates the perichondrium, it will not heal and will require debridement and late reconstruction.

Early positioning to eliminate pressure can prevent further damage to the delicate structure of the ears. Reconstruction does not start with early surgical intervention but with the preservation of tissue that is not already irreparably damaged (73). Pillows should be avoided. The use of a towel roll or an egg crate foam positioner is effective to position the head and prevent pressure to the ears, as well as to occiput. Thermoplastic molded ear protectors can also be used to protect the ears in patients with burns.

Rosenthal (73) uses a combination of procedures, including cutaneous flap, composite flap coverage, skin grafting, or excision of skin and/or cartilage with primary closure to preserve the individual components of the ear. Eriksson (72) suggests reconstruction of the external ear in three steps: (i) release of the scar contracture, (ii) construction of a scaffold of the ear, and (iii) coverage with skin graft. Reconstruction of the entire ear is problematic because of the lack of a technique to re-create the

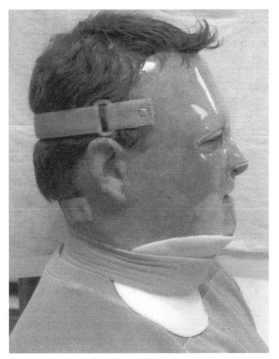

Figure 10–9. Transparent facial orthoses and neck conformers provide pressure to the face and neck area.

framework of the ear. Bone-anchored prosthetic ears can provide a solution to this problem. Surgery is done in two stages: first, implants are placed in the temporal bone, and then abutments are attached 3 months later for the slip on or magnetic attachments.

Nose

Deformity of the nose usually involves retraction of the alar margins as contracting forces shorten the nose and cause alar flaring (67,74). These areas can be reconstructed with a turn-down flap of scar tissue followed by an FTSG that covers the entire tip of the nose. If there is loss of tissue on the alar rim, the alar rim can be lowered and maintained by using a composite graft from the ear.

Nostril stenosis may be released with skin grafts. In the patient who requires reconstruction for obstructed nostrils, dilators work well and are worn for at least 6 months to maintain the correction. Proper fitting of a face mask around the patient's nasal structures can be challenging. Care must be taken not to cause further complications by adding pressure to the bridge of the nose.

Lips and Mouth

Deformities of the lip and mouth include microstomia, lower lip ectropion with eversion of the mucosa and flat chin, and thinning of the upper lip with loss of the cupid's-bow shape and flattened philtrum (67). Microstomia poses a major functional problem for proper oral hygiene, eating, speech, facial expression, dentistry, and intubation, and may warrant urgent reconstruction. Treatment of microstomia includes the use of stacked tongue blades, thermoplastic cones, microstomia prevention appliances (MPAs), and appliances custom made by an orthodontist to stretch the tissues surrounding the mouth. More than 20 appliances have been designed to prevent microstomia; however, these mouth appliances are effective only with cooperative patients (69). Some appliances allow for only either horizontal or vertical stretching of the perioral skin, but the Therabite Jaw Motion Rehabilitation System provides an ideal splint for static or dynamic stretching in all directions (75) (Fig. 10–10). It provides mouthpieces of varying sizes (pediatric and adult), a bite plate to distribute pressure, and an arc of motion simulating that of the normal jaw.

Reconstruction of the upper lip usually involves resurfacing of the lip with good quality FTSG and preservation of anatomic landmarks if they are recognizable (74). Surgery to reconstruct deformities of the lower lip and chin are completed after the

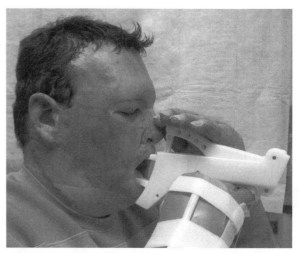

Figure 10–10. A Therabite is used to treat microstomia and can be used independently by patients.

scar is mature and may involve release of the everted lip, trimming of the obicularis muscle to create a better chin contour, and grafting by aesthetic unit (74).

Neck

Even with the best acute care, exercise, and splints, deformity of the chin angle and contractures of the neck can occur. During acute care, therapy options may be limited by tracheostomies, central lines, and ventilator tubing. Positioning of the neck in extension can be accomplished with the use of pillows under the scapulae, short mattresses, airbeds in which pressure can be manipulated, or specially shaped cushions.

Creative positioning techniques must be implemented for pediatric patients. Older children may lie prone while reading, playing games, or watching television to increase neck extension. Neck positioning in extension during the use of video games decreases the need for one-to-one interventions and increases leisure independence, self-confidence, and frustration tolerance (76). Younger children may benefit from caregivers' playing "peek-a-boo" and hanging mobiles at the head of the crib to encourage extension or at the side of the crib to facilitate rotation (69).

Neck conformers or splints extend from below the mandible and off the chin, with flaring of the splint edge away from the chin to allow normal lip closure and mandibular growth in children (69) (Fig. 10–9). This design also directs more pressure to the neck for better contouring. Bunchman et al. (77) showed a decrease from 37% to 9% in incidence and severity of neck contractures with the use of neck conformers. In those patients who demonstrate full neck ROM and require only pressure therapy to flatten scars,

Mepiform self-adhesive silicone (78) or Silipos neck wraps (79) are great options. Secondary problems associated with neck contractures include facial distortions, drooling, eating and swallowing difficulties, dental deterioration, difficulty with intubation for surgery, unsafe driving, and pull on pectoral and/or axillary regions (29,69).

Reconstructive procedures for neck contractures may include a combination of release and resurfacing with skin grafts, tissue expanders, or flaps (67, 74,80–82). After surgery the patient must be vigilant with exercises, positioning, splinting, and pressure devices.

Axilla

Contractures of the axilla can affect posture, self-care, work, and recreational tasks. Early treatment is the best defense in the prevention of contractures. Prevention is difficult, however, as most daily activities do not require full ROM of the shoulder. Early treatment for burns of the axilla includes positioning, splinting, and ROM exercises.

Ideal positioning of the shoulder is 90 degrees of shoulder abduction with external rotation and slight forward flexion. This positioning can be achieved by suspension from IV poles, slings, or positioning with troughs, pillows, traction, and bedside tables. Proper positioning with younger patients is achieved with prophylactic splints and the use of custom-made foam positioning devices. Careful attention to shoulder positioning is necessary to avoid stretch and injury of the brachial plexus.

The typical shoulder splint used is an axillary conformer, better known as an "airplane" splint. Postoperative and preventative positioning may need to be used for 6 to 12 months to prevent recurrence of contracture. A study by Huang et al. (83) reported 95% of patients developed axillary contracture without the use of splints, compared to 32% of patients when splints and pressure garments were used for longer than 12 months. Upper-extremity "spica" casts are effective positioners for pediatric patients and can be bivalved for continued use as a maintenance splint. Patients can be independent with donning their axillary splints with use of an abdominal binder to secure the splint around the trunk (31). An alternative splint is the abduction pillow, which can be positioned to hold the shoulder at either 45 or 90 degrees of abduction and has an extension to support the distal extremity (Fig. 10–11).

Contractures of the axilla may include, in order of increasing severity, just the anterior fold or posterior fold, both anterior and posterior axillary folds, or both folds and the axillary dome (13). Correction of axillary contractures may involve multiple Z-plasties,

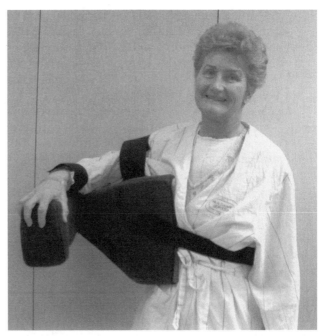

Figure 10–11. The axillary abduction splint is used to treat contractures of the axilla.

VY-plasties, and early local flaps. Severe contractures are best managed with regional flaps. If the contracture is released leaving a large tissue deficit, an STSG is used.

As with other reconstructive procedures, axillary releases require the patient to continue with an aggressive therapy program of splinting, positioning, pressure, and exercise.

Hands

The hand is at great risk for burn injury due to its position of exposure (84). The typical hand burn is to the dorsal surface as a result of exposure and thinner skin, but contact burns can occur on the palmer surface.

An established deformity of the hand is a surgical challenge, and prevention of contractures is much preferred. The best preventative measure lies in the initial treatment. The hand should be continuously elevated above heart level for edema management with frequent AROM (85). The dilemma of splinting for preserving or increasing motion at the expense of aggravating edema is a problem during initial treatment. Also, care must be taken not to further apply constricting forces to areas with borderline circulation and drainage status.

Joint tightness, tendon adhesions, and skin shortening are related to the length of time it takes for a wound to heal. Early wound coverage yields the best functional result due to shortened healing time. With early grafting the vicious cycle of pain, edema, and stiffness from immobilization recedes more rapidly and motion can be preserved before contractures become fixed. The ultimate goal of treatment of any hand injury is normal function with stability, maximum flexibility, and good sensibility.

The classic hand deformity is the intrinsic minus or "claw hand," which manifests as flattening of the transverse metacarpal arch and longitudinal arches, with metacarpophalangeal (MCP) extension/hyperextension, proximal interphalangeal (PIP) and distal interphalangeal (DIP) flexion, and thumb adduction. The claw hand develops as a result of the hindering of movement by pain and intrinsic muscle edema, leading to an imbalance of intrinsic and extrinsic muscles, with eventual contracture of the collateral ligaments (86).

Since the tendency for contracture is toward the claw deformity, a resting hand splint should place the hand in the "anti-claw" position. This type of splint positions the wrist in 30 degrees of extension, MCPs in 70 to 90 degrees flexion, and interphalangeals (IPs) in full extension. If the patient is awake and actively participating in a therapy program, the splint is worn at night and during rest periods. In those patients who are not yet able to adhere to the therapy program, it is worn at all times except during wound care and PROM. Hand splints can also include a dynamic or progressive stretching component to provide joint stretch (Fig. 10–12).

Acquired deformities of the fingers include the boutonniere, swan neck, and mallet finger. Boutonniere deformities can develop in deep burns of the PIP joint, which disrupt the extensor tendon insertion into the dorsal base of the middle phalanx (Fig. 10–13). The lateral bands slip volar to the

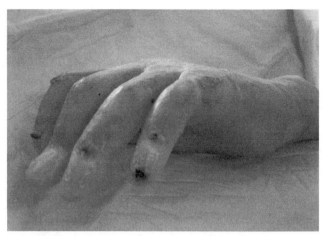

Figure 10–13. The boutonniere deformity is caused by injury to the extensor tendon of the finger.

axis of the PIP joint and become flexors of the PIP. The resultant boutonniere deformity is flexion of the PIP joint and hyperextension of the DIP joint. Finger gutter or wire-foam splints, plaster finger casts, or buddy taping may help correct the deformity. If surgery is indicated, PIP and DIP arthrodesis at approximately 60 degrees of flexion is a reliable and functional treatment option (87).

Swan neck deformities present as PIP hyperextension with DIP flexion. Mallet fingers present as a flexion posture of the DIP, in which there is complete passive but incomplete active extension of the DIP joint caused by damage to the extensor tendon. Finger gutter or wire-foam splints, finger casts, or buddy tape may help correct these deformities as well; however, if surgery is indicated, arthrodesis can be performed in both cases.

Other deformities of the hand can be classified into palmar contractures, web space deformities (web space contractures, thumb adduction contractures, and syndactyly), and amputation deformities (87). Palmar contractures usually occur in young children who grab or fall into hot objects such as curling irons, campfires, wood burning stoves, and oven doors. Early prophylactic splinting and scar management are keys to prevention of contractures. Patients are fit with extension splints that position the wrist in at least 30 degrees of extension and fingers in full extension. Silicone putty elastomer is a convenient way to ensure correct placement by forming an imprint of the child's hand, and it aids in scar management. For the patient who is not compliant with wearing the splints, use of cohesive bandages for fastening, clamshell splints, casts, and long-arm splints may be indicated. It must be remembered, however, that noninvolved joints should be allowed to continue to move.

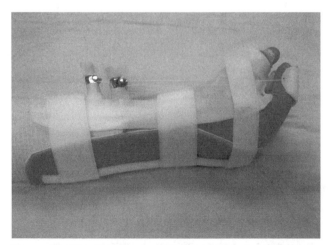

Figure 10–12. This hand splint places the wrist and fingers in a functional position and also allows for progressive stretching of the fingers into flexion.

If surgery is indicated for release of palmar contracture and possible grafting, the patient will need to continue to wear a pan extension splint including all of the fingers or individual finger gutter/foam-wire extension splints for maintenance and prevention of recurrence until the new graft has matured. Custom gloves are difficult to fit on small pediatric patients' hands and can make pressure therapy challenging. Cohesive wraps are a nice alternative to a custom glove, and parents can easily be taught to do the wrapping at home. Continuation of the pan extension splints with elastomer insert may be all the pressure therapy that is needed.

Web space deformities may involve a scar band on the dorsal aspect of the web space. Early treatment consists of use of peanut-shaped Velfoam, Webril, or silicone inserts (putty elastomer, Oto-form-K, Silipos web spacers). If surgery is indicated to deepen the web space, VY-plasty or Tanzer flaps are used (87). Pure web space contractures involve just the skin. Adduction contractures, however, usually include muscle fibrosis and commonly occur in the first web space. "L-shaped" first web space splints used with silicone inserts can be easily adjusted as range increases. The patient is also taught self-ROM exercises and scar massage for prevention. Burn syndactyly is a web space deformity in which two digits fuse together because of a loss of lateral skin. After release and reconstruction, measures must be taken to ensure separation of the fingers with pressure garments and inserts, splints, positioning, and exercise.

Extensive burns to the hand may require partial amputation of the thumb or digits. Reconstructive procedures in such cases may involve lengthening of the digits (phalangization) or thumb (pollicization) by deepening web spaces, or a toe-to-thumb transfer (87). In patients with unilateral injury and extensive tissue damage, amputation is an alternative that leads to most rapid rehabilitation. If bilateral hand injuries are involved, salvage may be justified to have a sensate helper hand versus two insensate prosthetic terminal devices.

Deep hand burns with exposed tendons and joints that cannot be grafted will require local and distal flaps, free tissue transfers, or a combination of techniques (88–90). Unfortunately, these burns are frequently associated with large surface area burns, resulting in limited availability of flaps and decreased patient tolerance for the extensive procedures required. Abdominal and groin flaps can be used; however, they are bulky and require later division of the digits. The use of the Millard "crane" flap, in which the hand is buried in abdominal tissue for several weeks to encourage granulation, then removed and grafted, has been shown to result in equivalent total active movement of the hand when compared to traditional abdominal flaps (89). Patients with crane flaps did not need to endure additional surgical procedures for debulking of flaps and separation of digits.

Patients with crane flaps and grafting are fit with regular pressure gloves and splints as indicated. Patients with bulky flaps are seen for instruction in cohesive bandage pressure wrapping to decrease edema and then possibly fit with a custom glove. A plaster mold of the affected hand sent to the glove manufacturer helps with improving fit of the custom glove. Following each surgical procedure, new custom pressure gloves and splints/inserts will need to be fabricated.

Elbow

Flexion contractures of the elbow commonly result from extensive injury with delayed healing, decreased patient cooperation, and scar bands across the antecubital fossa. To prevent contractures, early grafting and mobilization are often indicated, which may also help to decrease the incidence of heterotopic ossification (61). Even with the best of care and a cooperative patient, a linear scar band across the antecubital fossa can produce contractures despite a vigilant splint and exercise program. Also, patients with massive burns involving multiple joints will be at higher risk to develop elbow contractures because of the multiplicity of areas to manage. In addition, heterotopic ossification is frequently seen at the elbow and should be considered as a cause of contractures.

Improvement of elbow mobility is the most important indicator for correction of elbow contractures (13). The normal flexion-extension arc is 0 to 145 degrees, and an arc of 30 to 130 degrees is ample for independence in all ADL. Therefore, a patient demonstrating less than a 30-degree extension contracture is within functional limits and probably does not require correction. Release of an elbow contracture may improve shoulder and wrist mobility if a scar extends across these joints and may further increase functional independence.

Following scar release, the patient is fit with an elbow extension splint that is worn at all times until 5 to 7 days after surgery. The splint will then be used for maintenance at night. Dynamic splints may be indicated if the elbow joint capsule is tight and simple release of skin does not adequately increase extension. The joint active system (JAS) enables static progressive stretch of joint contractures as it applies stretch incrementally through a single 30-minute-per-day, patient-controlled therapy session, and it allows stress relaxation of contracted tissue (91).

Knee

The underlying theme to prevention of contracture and deformity of the lower extremity is early management such as escharotomies as indicated, aggressive wound care with early excision and grafting, leg elevation, and early ambulation (92). Additional interventions include the use of CPM devices, prevention of peripheral neuropathies with proper positioning to prevent peroneal neuropathy, use of splints and casts to prevent Achilles tendon shortening, and maintenance of skin integrity to prevent heel pressure sores.

Dependency of the lower extremities and possible destruction of the lymphatic system present unique problems to rehabilitation and reconstruction of the lower extremities (92). Vascular support is critical, initially in the form of TED hose or figure-eight–wrapped Ace bandages, and, later, tubular dressings or custom-made pressure stockings. When mobilizing and ambulating, patients are instructed to activate the lower-extremity muscle pump and never stand in one place. Dangling of the legs at the edge of the bed may be helpful initially for patients mobilizing for the first time; however, is not recommended for common practice. Widespread destruction of the lymphatic system compounds the problem because it results in the tendency for graft loss with ambulation, chronic edema formation, pain, and prolonged period of immature scar (92).

Surgical reconstruction of the knee is often not necessary for a good functional outcome. Leman (29) hypothesizes that early ambulation protocols, emphasis on cardiopulmonary endurance activities, effect of gravity on posture, effectiveness of contracture prevention techniques that allow function, and frequent standing and walking emphasizing normal lower extremity function all contribute to less need for later reconstruction. Occasionally, deformities of the lower extremity such as popliteal contractures and soft tissue defects after burns with exposed deep structures will require reconstruction. Popliteal contractures may be treated with local skin flaps, or scar release and grafts. Deep tissue defects require flaps, and unstable scars require resurfacing with grafts. Following surgery, prefabricated knee immobilizers or custom-made knee splints are indicated. Use of Unna boots allows early ambulation postoperatively and serves as a good initial pressure bandage until custom garments are fit (93–96).

Foot and Ankle

Deformities of the ankle include contracture of the Achilles tendon and soft tissue deficits. Achilles tendon shortening can be prevented with early splinting and positioning; however, preventing pressure necrosis of the heel or area under the metatarsals can be challenging. Continuous monitoring by all staff for proper positioning of the ankle and frequent skin checks are necessary to maintain skin integrity. Exposed Achilles tendons can be treated with local flaps. External fixation devices as used in orthopaedic surgery can be used for positioning of the ankle until wound closure is achieved.

Deformities of the foot include flexion or extension contractures of the toes and web space deformities. Both flexion and extension contractures of the toes are first treated with splints, exercises, and inserts in shoes. If surgery is warranted, the toes are released and k-wires are frequently used for immobilization until the grafts are secure. Fiberglass walking casts allow ambulation as well as immobilization and provision of vascular support and pressure to the grafts.

Postoperative splints, silicone inserts, and pressure socks may be used. Parry et al. (97) describe the use of dynamic toe flexion splints to progressively splint individual toes into metatarsal flexion, which results in normal gait and the ability to wear normal athletic shoes. It is recommended that shoes be worn for 24 hours with sufficient pressure to prevent recurrence of contractures. As with web space deformities of the hand, recommended treatment of toe webs include peanut-shaped foam inserts, silicone, and a foot "glove" to separate the toes.

ELECTRICAL INJURIES

Electrical injuries are injuries that have unique acute care and rehabilitation problems not seen with thermal injuries. The severity of injury is not characterized by the size of the skin lesion since a large degree of tissue damage can occur between the contact points. The severity can be partially determined by the voltage of the electricity with less than 1,000 volts comprising low voltage and greater than 1,000 volts, high voltage. Occupational injuries are a common cause of electrical injury. In data from 1992 to 1998, in the United States, an average of 381 individuals die per year and 5,467 individuals miss days of work because of electrical injuries (98). Acute complications can include cardiac arrest or arrhythmia, myoglobinuria, and compartment syndrome. Other complications include a risk of limb loss and neurologic injury.

The body's resistance to electrical current is lowest in neurologic tissue. As a result, exposure to electrical current poses the threat of direct injury to the brain, spinal cord, or peripheral nerves. Individuals with electrical injuries are at increased risk of peripheral nerve injuries that can occur even in low-voltage injuries with minimal cutaneous damage (51). In a study of cases of low-voltage electrical injuries, Smith documents persistent symptoms of peripheral nerve injury that improved with surgical decompression. Examination of the perineural tissue demonstrated tissue fibrosis (99).

Individuals that sustain an electrical injury are at risk for developing a central nervous system injury such as a brain injury or spinal cord injury. The symptoms of the injury are often present immediately after the injury, but the onset of symptoms may be delayed by several hours or days. In reviews of admissions with electrical injuries, spinal cord injury has been reported with a delayed onset up to 4 weeks after injury (100–104). MRI of the spinal cord may or may not demonstrate abnormalities. In one case, pathologic examination of the spinal cord several months after injury demonstrated localized degeneration of myelin sheaths consistent with a transverse myelitis (105).

A cardiac arrest can result in anoxic brain injury, but a brain injury can also occur as a result of the electrical injury. In some cases, there is evidence of brain injury on diagnostic imaging (106–108), but in other cases, brain imaging shows normal findings. Individuals sustaining electrical injuries often report an array of physical, cognitive, and emotional complaints. In a study of 63 patients after electrical injury, 49% complained of parasthesias and 48% headaches, and other frequent complaints included muscle spasms, weakness, balance problems, and pain. Almost half of the patients complained of concentration, word-finding, and emotional problems (109). A progressive decline in cognitive function over time has also been reported (110).

Lightning injuries are rare but can cause significant injury from the high current and heat generated. Cherington (111) classifies sequelae of lightning injuries into four groups. Group 1 are injuries that cause immediate but transient neurologic symptoms such as amnesia, confusion, paresthesia, and weakness. Individuals in Group 2 have immediate and prolonged or permanent symptoms that can be caused by multiple etiologies. Individuals who have a cardiac arrest are at risk of a hypoxic encephalopathy. Brain injuries include intracranial hemorrhages in the basal ganglia and brainstem, cerebral infarction, and cerebellar dysfunction (112–115). Spinal cord injuries (116) and peripheral nerve injuries are also seen after a lighting strike. In one case of a pathologic examination of the spinal cord 4 months postinjury, there was evidence of widespread myelin degeneration (117). Individuals in Group 3 include those with possible delayed neurologic syndromes,

and Group 4 includes injuries caused by associated trauma that did not result directly from the electrical current.

PAIN MANAGEMENT

Controlling pain presents a challenge from initial emergency room care through the rehabilitation phase of care. Burn pain is very likely the most difficult form of acute pain to treat from any type of etiology. Its treatment is problematic not only because the type of nociception inherent in a burn injury is likely to generate unusually high levels of pain, but also because the nature of standard burn care is likely to exacerbate whatever pain is present. Wound care and therapies can generate pain that is equivalent or exceeds that experienced by the patient at the time of the injury. Pain, in addition to being a source of outright suffering in patients, can interfere with wound care and therapies, as well as lengthen hospitalization. Moreover, the amount of pain experienced by hospitalized children and adults with burn injuries appears associated with long-term posttraumatic stress and general emotional distress (118,119). As such, there are practical as well as humanitarian reasons to control burn pain aggressively (120).

In terms of treatment, pain during hospitalization can be classified as background (that which is present while the patient is at rest and is of lower intensity and longer duration), procedural (more intense, short-lived pain generated by wound care or therapies), breakthrough (spiking of pain levels that exceed what current levels of drugs are about to control), and postoperative (121,122). Chronic pain is that which lasts >6 months; this type can be a challenge for outpatient therapy. Most burn pain results from direct tissue damage. However, it is important to be aware that neuropathic pain may be present, particularly in patients with amputations or peripheral nerve injuries. Neuropathic pain is often treated differently than conventional burn pain.

PHARMACOLOGIC APPROACHES

Early in patient care, particularly during intensive care, pharmacologic approaches are the standard of treatment. Moreover, opioid agonists (i.e., morphine-based drugs) form the cornerstone of pharmacologic treatment. Typical strategies involve treating background pain with continuous infusion morphine (during ICU stays when IV access is convenient) or slow release versions of oral morphine derivatives (e.g., methadone, time-release narcotics).

Procedural pain is treated with more potent, shorter-acting opioid agonists such as fentanyl or hydro-morphone (Dilaudid) (123). Again, the route of administration of such drugs depends on access routes and on the placement of the patient. Patient-controlled analgesia (PCA) often presents an attractive pain control option, particularly after surgery (124–126).

A number of nonopioid analgesics can play an important role in pain control. Oral nonsteroidal anti-inflammatory drugs and aspirin can play a useful role, but typically for less severe injuries or when burn injuries have largely healed (127,128). Anti-anxiety agents can be used to supplement opioids during procedural pain. Midazolam hydrochloride (Versed) may be administered during wound care for a patient with IV access, and patients can be dosed with oral benzodiazepines (e.g., lorazepam, diazepam) 30 minutes prior to wound care or troublesome therapies (129,130). Anesthetics, administered typically under the supervision of an anesthesiologist, can be useful and might include inhaled nitrous oxide, ketamine, or propofol (131). Such agents are typically reserved for the most severe types of procedures (e.g., staple removal). When pain is of neuropathic origin (i.e., from nerve damage), nonopioid therapies are often essential, such as carbamazepine (Tegretol) or gabepentin (Neurontin).

NONPHARMACOLOGIC APPROACHES

Perhaps the most powerful types of nonpharmacologic interventions are to avoid unnecessary elements of care that may cause pain. Adequately soaking dressings can ease the pain of their removal, and the use of caustic antiseptic agents can be minimized. Providing calm care and offering patients some control during painful procedures can facilitate comfort during therapies and wound care.

Psychological techniques for control of acute pain can include hypnosis, cognitive behavioral techniques, distraction, and operant (learning) approaches. Hypnosis has been found to reduce burn pain in over a dozen studies. With this modality, a clinician typically works with patients before wound care or therapies and provides posthypnotic suggestions for comfort. Cognitive-behavioral interventions work by restructuring patients' thoughts about pain. For example, patients may be taught that the sensations during therapy may *hurt* but will not *harm* them (132). Distraction techniques may be as simple as movies, computer games, or conversation during painful procedures, or as elaborate as immersive virtual reality. A recent series of studies indicates that placing patients in a virtual world can dramatically reduce pain during wound care and therapies (133). Hypnosis is another powerful technique that operates through psychological techniques and is particularly well suited for burn injuries (134,135).

Behavioral (learning) techniques have a particularly important role in burn rehabilitation. Patients who are overwhelmed and resistant to therapies may show amazing progress with the quota system (136,137). The quota system rewards activity with rest after patients have reached predetermined markers of therapeutic activity (quotas) that is well within their capacity. In establishing quotas, therapists exercise patients for three sessions to the point of fatigue and then record the duration or number of repetitions. The average of these three sessions is calculated and then 80% of that average serves as a starting point. For example, a patient may walk 150, 50, and 100 ft over 3 sessions. The average (100 ft) is calculated, and 80% of that (80 ft) serves as the starting point. The therapist then increases exercise by 5% each session. An important factor is that even when patients feel that they can keep exercising, increments are kept at 5%. This practice keeps exercise increments at steady rates and avoids overwhelming the patient.

Patients with chronic pain often respond well to techniques in which their pain behavior is ignored (their pain behavior, but not them) and they are distracted from pain. While acute pain necessitates immediate clinical attention, chronic pain often requires a reversal of strategies both in terms of medications and clinician response.

PSYCHOSOCIAL CONSEQUENCES OF BURN INJURIES

Although numerous studies have reported on rates of psychiatric sequelae in burn injuries, such statistics are rarely useful in treating patients (138). The nature of a burn injury cannot predict a patient's emotional response. Psychological reactions are more an interactive function of the patient's pre-injury personality, their social support, the complications of the burn injury, and their coping ability.

Anxiety and depression are the most common psychological problems resulting from burn injuries. Anxiety is often overlooked because clinicians prematurely diagnose depression. Early in care, clinicians should be favoring the use of anxiolytic agents such as benzodiazepines (e.g., diazepam, lorazepam, and midazolam) rather than antidepressants. Depression becomes more of an issue in the long-term rehabilitation of the patient and is far more likely in patients who have a history of depression. A tearful patient who has had a few "down" days is not automatically a candidate for antidepressants. However, when a patient shows a depressed mood for two weeks, shows guilt and self-deprecating cognitions (e.g., "I am worthless"), and shows vegetative signs (changes in appetite and sleep), then treatment for depression should be strongly considered (139). The current literature suggests that a combination of psychotherapy and pharmacology (antidepressants) represents the most efficacious approach to depression (140).

The stage of burn care (i.e., intensive care, acute, rehabilitation) largely dictates the nature of psychological problems demonstrated by burn patients. Early intensive care brings concerns of survival, intense pain, and primitive defenses (e.g., denial). Patients should be emotionally supported and encouraged to feel better about the "here and now" rather than to focus on the future. As they improve, patients become more cognitively capable of assessing the impact of their injuries. Enhanced education and brief psychotherapy is increasingly warranted. Long-term rehabilitation produces a minority of patients that may require more aggressive psychotherapy or pharmacotherapy.

Although no problems can be generalized to all burn survivors, disfigurement and cosmetic concerns typically represent the most serious psychological challenges for patients. The impact of burn scars may range from a minor irritation over the change of appearance to a devastating change in self-perception resulting in social isolation. Treatment for disfigurement is particularly challenging because we cannot tell who will have a negative reaction to their changed appearance, and at what phase of their recovery. Potential interventions include preparing the patient for societal responses during hospitalization, facilitating connections with peer-support groups, and psychotherapy for related poor self-esteem. A particularly promising approach has been social skills training developed by the Changing Faces organization in Great Britain (141).

Efforts towards community reintegration can be particularly important to a patient's emotional recovery. Community outings during hospitalization can help prepare patients for the physical and psychological challenges that occur after discharge. School re-entry programs can prevent teasing and negative reactions in children that occur out of fear and ignorance (142). Vocational counseling can be crucial to re-introducing patients to the work force at an acceptable pace, as well as educating them to the benefits that are possible.

SLEEP PROBLEMS

A huge proportion of burn outpatients suffer from sleep problems. Sleep is disrupted by pain, itching, excessive fatigue, medications, and changes in sleep cycles. Treatment ideally first focuses on sleep hygiene. Sleep hygiene techniques involve re-establishing sleep cycles (avoiding daytime naps, avoiding caffeine and alcohol late at night, and teaching patients to use the bed as a stimulus for sleep [e.g., no television]). Failing such educational/behavioral techniques, the relatively new short-acting benzodiazepines usually provide patients with the ability to fall asleep with minimal hangover effects. If this class of drugs fails, or the patient is depressed, sedating antidepressant medications may be of use, particularly in keeping the patient asleep (143).

COMPLIANCE AND DIFFICULT PATIENTS

Certain types of burn patients provide unique challenges to even the most capable of health care providers. It is important to point out that many patients who undergo burn hospitalization for longer than a week can show a period of poor sleep, irritability, and intense fatigue. Such reactions usually dissipate within the first few months postdischarge. Pacing the patients appropriately and not overwhelming them during this period becomes particularly important. The quota system discussed above is certainly one of the most powerful tools available to therapists to deal with an overwhelmed patient.

Often rehabilitation health professionals are challenged with the task of convincing patients to adhere to treatment recommendations. Motivational interviewing (MI) is a particularly effective strategy to encourage motivation in patients. MI was originally designed as an approach for addictive behaviors but has been found to be effective with a number of issues. Motivational interviewing assumes that patients will be ambivalent about changing their behavior and relies on techniques such as reflective listening to help patients clarify their thoughts and feelings (144). MI techniques can be summarized with the acronym FRAMES: Feedback, Responsibility, Advice, Menu of options, Empathy, and Self-efficacy.

Clinicians using MI techniques might provide *feedback* about the patient's medical condition and risks of not practicing things. ("You have a burned axilla. The chances are good that if you do not maintain active range of motion, the burn will scar and contract and you will require release surgery to use your arm.") *Responsibility* for behavior changed is put clearly on the patient. ("No one, including me, can make you do your exercises. It is totally your choice as to whether or not you will do them.") Non-judgmental *advice* can be given as long as the patient is not confronted or pushed. ("My advice is to find some way to set up your life so that you are able to attend therapy sessions and do your exercises.") Patients are presented with a *menu of options* for change or several opportunities for change. ("You might want to visit me twice a week, or perhaps you might want to try daily exercises with one visit a week.") *Empathy* involves reflective listening to clarify that you are aware of the patient's ambivalence (repeating what the patient has said and adding, "I don't blame you"). ("You find performing these actions very difficult, and I don't blame you.") *Self-efficacy* communicates that you believe that change is possible. ("I know it is hard, but I have seen patients with worse injuries avoid surgery; it really is possible.") The clinician can use any combination of these steps, in any order. Active listening and reflecting back to the patient remains the most critical component of this approach.

Personality disorders present an ongoing challenge to patient management. Personality disorders are enduring personality characteristics that prove to be dysfunctional to a person's life. Various types of personality disorders (e.g., paranoid, obsessive-compulsive, antisocial, narcissistic, and borderline) are defined as Axis II disorders in the *Diagnostic and Statistical Manual of Mental Disorders*, Fourth Edition, Text Revision (DSM-IV-TR) (139). The point to be made about personality disorders is that the burn staff cannot change such patients. The key to management is to recognize the personality disorder and interact with the patient in a manner that is effective with their ingrained characteristics. Although space limitations prevent discussing all the personality disorders, patients with borderline personalities can provide a useful example. Such patients often are repeatedly admitted to burn or other wards for para-suicide attempts. They can present emotionally labile, challenging behavior to the staff. As surprising as it sounds, setting very rigid limits (e.g., "We will not admit you if you do this again") and providing excessive mental health support for such patients is actually counteractive. Excessive limits can result in escalating patient behavior, and too much mental health attention can encourage re-admissions. Rather, the burn unit staff should (i) treat on an outpatient basis when possible, (ii) play down the role of the personality disorder, and (iii) treat the injury in a calm, matter-of-fact manner (145).

OUTCOME MEASUREMENT AFTER BURN INJURIES

Measuring functional outcome for patients with burn injury is at an early stage. First of all, there is not firm agreement on conceptualizing the severity of a burn injury. Such variables as total burn surface area, length of hospitalization, and the number of surgeries have been proposed in the literature. However, they have been found to be poor predictors of outcome. The American Medical Association (AMA) impairment ratings have been proposed but are labor intensive, and no study has related them to outcome (146). With respect to outcome, a variety of domains have been considered. The Functional Independence Measure (FIM) has been used in burn injury and a number of disabilities but has been found to lack sensitivity to long-term change in burn patients (147). Health-related quality of life has been measured with the Sickness Impact Profile (SIP) and the SF-36 Health Survey (148,149). Although the SIP is likely more appropriate to burn injuries than the SF-36, neither has been found to be sensitive to the full spectrum of outcome issues specific to burn injuries. The Burn Specific Health Scale (150) is much more sensitive to burn injuries but, because it is specific to burn injuries, does not allow for comparison with other medical populations. Time off work has been measured in a few studies. One study reported the use of the Community Integration Scale as a measure of this dimension of outcome (151). Finally, several studies have presented on emotional recovery, and thus far, the Brief Symptom Inventory (152) seems to be the most useful measure of generic emotional outcome in adults with burn injuries.

The ultimate measure of the effectiveness of burn therapy is the burn survivor's functional outcome—that is, returning a burn survivor to society in such a condition that he or she can function in daily work, school, recreational, and social activities. These activities must be *meaningful* or valuable to the patient and family, *practical* or applicable to the patient, and *sustainable* over time in which the functional ability achieved during the course of therapy is maintained outside the clinical environment (153).

Function refers to more than just independence in activities of daily living and mobility. Function must be viewed from beyond performance in the physical domain and include the burn survivor's psychological and social performances as well. Esselman et al. (151) found that burn survivors have significant difficulties with community integration due to burn and non-burn-related factors, as measured by the Community Integration Questionnaire (CIQ), which scores home integration, social integration, and productivity.

Despite major progress in survival rates in burn care, there is still little information on vocational outcomes for burn survivors (154,155). In a study by Brych et al. (154) examining time off work and return to work rates, it was concluded that people with large burns or burns of the upper extremities would benefit most from vocation-related interventions. Saffle et al. (155) examined return to work and the influence of burn size, health care coverage, and other factors affecting return to work and failure to return to work. They suggest that returning to work is not a natural consequence of successful burn treatment, and that future success in burn rehabilitation must include returning patients to productive lifestyles.

A vocational rehabilitation counselor is yet another important player on the treatment team. Interventions include patient interviews and completion of vocational history, liaison with employers and agencies, assistance with job change or job adaptation, and vocational retraining arrangements. A working knowledge of labor laws and long-term follow-up on vocational and productivity issues are important.

REFERENCES

1. Brigham PA, McLoughlin E. Burn incidence and medial care use in the United States: Estimates, trends and data sources. *J Burn Care Rehabil.* 1996;17:95–107.
2. National Center for Health Statistics. *Health, United States 1996-97 and injury chartbook.* Hyattsville, MD: DHHS Publication; 1997.
3. Saffle JR, Davis B, Williams P. Recent outcomes in the treatment of burn injury in the United States: A report from the American Burn Association patient registry. *J Burn Care Rehabil.* 1995;16:219–232.
4. Pruitt BA Jr, Goodwin CW, Mason AD. Epidemiological, demographic, and outcome characteristics of burn injury. In: Herndon DN, ed. *Total burn care.* 2nd ed. New York, NY: WB Saunders; 2002:16–30.
5. Han H, Mustoe TA. Structure and function of skin. In: Achauer BM, Eriksson E, eds. *Plastic surgery indications, operations and outcomes.* St. Louis, MO: Mosby; 2000:23–35.
6. Lund CC, Browder NC. Estimation of areas of burns. *Surg Gynecol Obstet.* 1944;79:352–358.
7. Williams WG. Pathophysiology of the burn wound. In: Herndon DN, ed. *Total burn care.* 2nd ed. New York, NY: WB Saunders; 2002:514–522.
8. Committee on Trauma. Guidelines for the operation of burn units. In: *Resources for the optimal care of the injured patient.* Chicago, IL: American College of Surgeons; 1999:55–62.
9. Miller SF, Staley MJ, Richard RL. Surgical management of the burn patient. In: Richard RL, Staley MJ, eds. *Burn care and rehabilitation: Principles and practice.* Philadelphia, PA: FA Davis Co; 1994: 177–197.
10. Heimbach DM, Warden GD, Luterman A, et al. Multicenter postapproval clinical trial of integra dermal regeneration template for burn treatment. *J Burn Care Rehabil.* 2003;24:42–48.
11. Ryan CM, Schoenfeld DA, Malloy M, et al. Use of Integra artificial skin is associated with decreased length of stay for severely injured adult burn survivors. *J Burn Care Rehabil.* 2002;23:311–317.
12. Robson MC. Overview of burn reconstruction. In: Herndon DN, ed. *Total burn care.* 2nd ed. New York, NY: WB Saunders; 2002:620–627.
13. Kurtzman LC, Stern PJ. Upper extremity burn contractures. *Hand Clin.* 1990;6(2):261–279.
14. Bombaro KM, Engrav LH, Carrougher GJ, et al. What is the prevalence of hypertrophic scarring following burns? *Burns.* 2003;29:299–302.
15. Deitch EA, Wheelahan TM, Rose MP, et al. Hypertrophic burn scars: Analysis of variables. *J Trauma.* 1983;23:895–898.
16. Miles WK, Grigsby L. Remodeling of scar tissue in the burned hand. In: Hunter JM, Schneider LH, Mackin EJ, et al., eds. *Rehabilitation of the Hand: Surgery and Therapy.* 3rd ed. St. Louis, MO: CV Mosby Company; 1990.
17. Mann R, Yeong EK, Moore ML, et al. Do custom-fitted pressure garments provide adequate pressure? *J Burn Care Rehabil.* 1997;18(3):247–249.
18. Groce A, Meyers-Paal R, Herndon DN, et al. Are your thoughts of facial pressure transparent? *J Burn Care Rehabil.* 1999;20:478–481.
19. Moore ML, Engrav LH, Calderon J, et al. Effectiveness of custom pressure garments in wound management: A prospective trial within wound and with verified pressure. *J Burn Care Rehabil.* 2000;21:S177.
20. Malick MH, Carr JP. Flexible elastomer molds in burn scar control. *Am J Occup Ther.* 1980;34(9):603–608.
21. Mann R, Yeong EK, Moore ML, et al. A new tool to measure pressure under burn garments. *J Burn Care Rehabil.* 1997;18(2):160–163.
22. Stewart R, Bhagwanjee AM, Mbakaza Y, et al. Pressure garment adherence in adult patient with burn injuries: An analysis of patient and clinician perceptions. *Am J Occup Ther.* 2000;54(6):598–606.
23. Rosser P. Adherence to pressure garment therapy of post traumatic burn injury. *J Burn Care Rehabil.* 2000;21:S178.
24. Richard RL, Staley MJ. *Burn care and rehabilitation principles and practice.* Philadelphia, PA: FA David Company; 1994.
25. Von Prince K, Curreri W, Pruitt B. Application of fingernail hooks in splinting burned hands. *Am J Occup Ther.* 1970;24(8):556–559.
26. Larson DL, Abston S, Dobrkovsky M, et al. *The prevention and correction of burn scar contracture and hypertrophy.* Galveston, TX: Shriners Burn Institute & University of Texas Medical Branch; 1973.

27. Fishwick GM, Tobin DG. Splinting the burned hand with primary excision and early grafting. *Am J Occup Ther.* 1978;32(3):182–183.

28. Rivers EA, Strate RG, Solem LD. The transparent face mask. *Am J Occup Ther.* 1979;33(2):108–113.

29. Leman CJ. Splints and accessories following burn reconstruction. *Clin Plast Surg.* 1992;19(3):721–731.

30. Costa BA, Nakamura DY, Engrav LH. Self "riveting" silicone to make palm burn splints. *J Burn Care Rehabil.* 1999;20:S250.

31. Costa BA, Nelson BJ, Nakamura DY, et al. An axillary conformer enabling independent application. *J Burn Care Rehabil.* 1999;20:S251.

32. Gripp CL, Salvaggio J, Fratianne RB. Use of burn intensive care unit gymnasium as an adjunct to therapy. *J Burn Care Rehabil.* 1995;16:160–161.

33. Silverberg R, Johnson J, Moffat M. The effects of soft tissue mobilization on the immature burn scar: Results of a pilot study. *J Burn Care Rehabil.* 1996;17(3):252–259.

34. Patino O, Novick C, Merlo A, et al. Massage in hypertrophic scars. *J Burn Care Rehabil.* 1998;20:268–271.

35. Field T, Peck M, Krugman S, et al. Burn injuries benefit from massage therapy. *J Burn Care Rehabil.* 1998;19(3):241–244.

36. Melchert-McKearnan K, Deitz J, Engel JM, et al. Children with burn injuries: Purposeful activity versus rote exercises. *Am J Occup Ther.* 2000;54(4):381–390.

37. Zablotny C, Forte-Andric M, Gowland C. Serial casting: Clinical applications for the adult head-injured patient. *J Head Trauma Rehabil.* 1987;2(2):46–52.

38. Richard R, Miller S, Staley M, et al. Multimodal versus progressive treatment techniques to correct burn scar contractures. *J Burn Care Rehabil.* 2000;21:S194.

39. Marmer L. The versatile art of plaster casting. *Advance for occupational therapists.* 1993;9(23):11.

40. Johnson J, Silverberg R. Serial casting of the lower extremity to correct contractures during the acute phase of burn care. *Phys Ther.* 1995;75(4):262–266.

41. Costa BA, Robinson CA, Moore ML, et al. Use of footplate in lower extremity serial casting. *J Burn Care Rehabil.* 2001;22:S142.

42. Costa BA, Moore ML, Engrav LH. Shovel cast: A new technique to correct MCP extension contracture in children. *J Burn Care Rehabil.* 2000;21:S239.

43. Costa BA, Foster K, Mann R, et al. Bubble cast. *J Burn Care Rehabil.* 1997;18:S176.

44. Hunt JL, Purdue GF. Epidemiology of major amputations in a burn unit: A high morbidity and high mortality injury. *J Burn Care Rehabil.* 2001;22:S113.

45. Kucan JO, Bash D. Reconstruction of the burned foot. *Clin Plast Surg.* 1992;19(3):705–719.

46. Henderson B, Koepke GH, Feller I. Peripheral polyneuropathy among patients with burns. *Arch Phys Med Rehabil.* 1971;52:149–151.

47. Helm PA, Johnson ER, Carlton AM. Peripheral neurological problems in acute burn patient. *Burns.* 1977;3:123–125.

48. Marquez S, Turley JE, Peters WJ. Neuropathy in burn patients. *Brain.* 1993;116:471–483.

49. Helm PA, Pandian G, Heck E. Neuromuscular problems in the burn patient: Cause and prevention. *Arch Phys Med Rehabil.* 1985;66:451–453.

50. Khedr EM, Khedr T, el-Oteify MA, et al. Peripheral neuropathy in burn patients. *Burns.* 1997;23:579–583.

51. Kowalske K, Holavanahalli R, Helm P. Neuropathy after burn injury. *J Burn Care Rehabil.* 2001;22:353–357.

52. Margherita AJ, Robinson LR, Heimbach DM, et al. Burn-associated peripheral polyneuropathy: A search for causative factors. *Am J Phys Med Rehabil.* 1995;74(1):28–32.

53. Dagum AB, Peters WJ, Neligan PC, et al. Severe multiple mononeuropathy in patients with major thermal burns. *J Burn Care Rehabil.* 1993;14:440–445.

54. Fess EE. Rehabilitation of the patient with peripheral nerve injury. *Hand Clin.* 1986;2(1):207–215.

55. Crawford CM, Varghese G, Mani MM, et al. Heterotopic ossification: Are range of motion exercises contraindicated? *J Burn Care Rehabil.* 1986;7:323–327.

56. Vorenkamp SE, Nelson TL. Ulnar nerve entrapment due to heterotopic bone formation after a severe burn. *J Hand Surg.* 1987;12:378–380.

57. Elledge ES, Smith AA, McManus WF, et al. Heterotopic bone formation in burned patients. *J Trauma.* 1988;28(5):684–687.

58. Peterson SL, Mani MM, Crawford CM, et al. Postburn heterotopic ossification: Insights for management decision making. *J Trauma.* 1989;29(3):365–369.

59. Djurickovic S, Meek RN, Snelling CF, et al. Range of motion and complications after postburn heterotopic bone excision about the elbow. *J Trauma.* 1996;41(5):825–830.

60. Holguin PH, Rico AA, Garcia JP, et al. Elbow anchylosis due to postburn heterotopic ossification. *J Burn Care Rehabil.* 1996;17:150–154.

61. Logsetty S, Costa BA, Moore ML, et al. Heterotopic ossification: A function of the time to burn wound closure [abstract]. *Proceedings of American College of Surgeons.* Washington, DC; 1999.

62. Banovac K. The effect of etidronate on late development of heterotopic ossification after spinal cord injury. *J Spinal Cord Med.* 2000;23(1):40–44.

63. Barthel T, Baumann B, Noth U, et al. Prophylaxis of heterotopic ossification after total hip arthroplasty. *Acta Orthop Scand.* 2002;73:611–614.

64. Gaur A, Sinclair M, Caruso I, et al. Heterotopic ossification around the elbow following burns in children: Results after excision. *J Bone Joint Surg.* 2003;85:1538–1543.

65. Brooke MM, Heard DL, deLateur BJ, et al. Heterotopic ossification and peripheral nerve entrapment: Early diagnosis and excision. *Arch Phys Med Rehabil.* 1991;72:425–429.

66. O'Neill K, Baryza MJ. Post-operative treatment of elbow heterotopic ossification. *J Burn Care Rehabil.* 1999;20:S254.

67. Engrav LH, Donelan MB. Face burns: Acute care and reconstruction. *Op Tech Plastic Reconstr Surg.* 1997;4(2):53–85.

68. Bradford BA, Breault LG, Schneid T, et al. Silicone thermoplastic sheeting for treatment of facial scars: An improved technique. *J Prosthodont.* 1999;8(2):138–141.

69. Staley M, Richard R, Billmire D, et al. Head/face/neck burns: Therapist considerations for the pediatric patient. *J Burn Care Rehabil.* 1997;18(2):164–171.

70. Fricke NB, Omnell ML, Dutcher KA, et al. Skeletal and dental disturbances in children after facial burns and pressure garments use: A 4-year follow up. *J Burn Care Rehabil.* 1999;20(3):239–249.

71. Achauer BM, Adair SR. Acute and reconstructive management of the burned eyelid. *Clin Plast Surg.* 2000;27(1):87–96.

72. Eriksson E, Vogt PM. Ear reconstruction. *Clin Plast Surg.* 1992;19(3):637–643.

73. Rosenthal JS. The thermally injured ear: A systematic approach to reconstruction. *Clin Plast Surg.* 1992; 19(3):645–661.

74. Achauer BM. Reconstructing the burned face. *Clin Plast Surg.* 1992;19:623–636.

75. Costa BA, Nakamura DY, Mann R, et al. The Therabite jaw motion rehabilitation system. *J Burn Care Rehabil.* 1995;27:203.

76. Foley K, Kaulkin C, Greenhalgh DG, et al. Video games: A method to maintain extension after neck contracture release. *J Burn Care Rehabil.* 2000;21: S242.

77. Bunchman HH, Huang TT, Larson DL, et al. Prevention and management of contractures in patients with burns of the neck. *Am J Surg.* 1975;130:700–703.

78. Cain VJ, McMahon LR, O'Donnell FJ, et al. Effectiveness of a silicone adherent dressing on post-burns and other traumatic scars. *J Burn Care Rehabil.* 2001; 22:S45.

79. Nakamura DY, Costa BS, Mann R, et al. Silipos™ neck wraps. *J Burn Care Rehabil.* 1998;19(2):181–182.

80. Jacobson D, Achauer B, Celikiz B, et al. Tissue expansion for the correction of burn contracture of the neck. *J Burn Care Rehabil.* 1998;19:S211.

81. Maclennan SE, Corcoran JF, Neale HW. Tissue expansion in head and neck burn reconstruction. *Clin Plast Surg.* 2000;27:121–132.

82. McCauley RL, Owiesy F, Dhanaraj P. Management of grade IV burn scar contractures of the neck in children. *J Burn Care Rehabil.* 2001;22:S90.

83. Huang TT, Blackwell SJ, Lewis SR. Ten years' experience in managing patients with burn contractures of axilla, elbow, wrist and knee joints. *Plast Reconstr Surg.* 1978;61(1):70–76.

84. Celikoz B, Achauer BM, VanderKam VM. Hot-press hand burn treatment. *J Burn Care Rehabil.* 1998; 19(2):128–130.

85. Salisbury RE. Soft tissue injuries of the hand. *Hand Clin.* 1986;2(1):25–32.

86. American Society of Surgery of the Hand. *The hand: Examination and diagnosis.* 3rd ed. New York, NY: Churchill Livingstone; 1990.

87. Achauer BM, ed. *Burn reconstruction.* New York, NY: Thieme Medical Publishers; 1991.

88. Nuchtern JG, Engrav LH, Nakamura DY, et al. Treatment of fourth-degree hand burns. *J Burn Care Rehabil.* 1995;16(1):36–42.

89. Matsumura H, Engrav LH, Nakamura DY, et al. The use of the Millard "crane" flap for deep hand burns with exposed tendons and joints. *J Burn Care Rehabil.* 1999;20(4):316–319.

90. Tredgett EE. Management of the acutely burned upper extremity. *Hand Clin.* 2000;16(2):187–203.

91. Gamage T, Haynes L, Hartford CE. The use of static progressive stretch on the burn joint contractures. *J Burn Care Rehabil.* 1999;20:S180.

92. Witt PD, Achauer BM. Lower extremity. In: Achauer BM, ed. *Burn reconstruction.* New York, NY: Thieme Medical Publishers, 1991:134–147.

93. Harnar T, Engrav LH, Marvin JA, et al. Dr. Paul Unna's boot and early ambulation after skin grafting the leg: A survey of burn centers and a report of 20 cases. *Plast Reconstr Surg.* 1982;69:359–360.

94. Grube BJ, Heimbach DM, Engrav LH. Molten metal burns to the lower extremity. *J Burn Care Rehabil.* 1987;8(5):403–405.

95. Ainsworth P, Blanche C, Dyess DL, et al. The evaluation of the Unna boot in lower leg autografts. *Wounds, A Compend Clin Res Pract.* 1991;3(5):195–197.

96. Cox GW, Griswold JA. Outpatient skin grafting of extremity burn wound with the use of Unna boot compression dressings. *J Burn Care Rehabil.* 1993; 14(4):455–457.

97. Parry I, Doyle W, Foley K, et al. Post-operative splint for dorsal toe contracture release. *J Burn Care Rehabil.* 2000;21:S260.

98. Cawley JC, Homce GT. Occupational electrical injuries in the United States, 1992-1998, and recommendations for safety research. *J Safety Res.* 2003; 34(3):241–248.

99. Smith MA, Muehlberger T, Dellon AL. Peripheral nerve compression associated with low-voltage electrical injury without associated significant cutaneous burn. *Plast Reconstr Surg.* 2002;109:137–144.

100. Varghese G, Mani MM, Redford JB. Spinal cord injuries following electrical accidents. *Paraplegia.* 1986;24:159–166.

101. Ratnayake B, Emmanuel ER, Walker CC. Neurological sequelae following a high voltage electrical burn. *Burns.* 1996;22:574–577.

102. Arevalo JM, Lorente JA, Balseiro-Gomex J. Spinal cord injury after electrical trauma treated in a burn unit. *Burns.* 1999;25(5):449–452.

103. Breugem CC, Van Hertum W, Groenevelt F. High voltage electrical injury leading to a delayed onset tetraplegia, with recovery. *Ann N Y Acad Sci.* 1999; 888:131–136.

104. Kalita J, Jose M, Misra UK. Myelopathy and amnesia following accidental electrical injury. *Spinal Cord.* 2002;40:253–255.

105. Levine NS, Atkins A, McKeel DW Jr. Spinal cord injury following electrical accidents: Case reports. *J Trauma.* 1975;15:459–463.

106. Gans M, Glaser JS. Homonymous hemianopia following electrical injury. *J Clin Neuroophthalmol.* 1986;6:218–221.

107. Iob I, Salar G, Ori C, et al. Accidental high voltage electrocution: A rare neurosurgical problem. *Acta Neurochir (Wein).* 1986;83:151–153.

108. Sure U, Kleihues P. Intracerebral venous thrombosis and hematoma secondary to high-voltage brain injury. *J Trauma.* 1997;42(6):1161–1164.

109. Pliskin NH, Capelli-Schellpfeffer M, Law RT, et al. Neuropsychological symptom presentation after electrical injury. *J Trauma.* 1998;44(4):709–715.

110. Martin TA, Salvatore NF, Johnstone B. Cognitive decline over time following electrical injury. *Brain Inj.* 2003;17(9):817–823.

111. Cherington M. Neurologic manifestations of lightning strikes. *Neurology.* 2003;60:182–185.

112. Stanley LD, Suss RA. Intracerebral hematoma secondary to lightning stroke: Case report and review of the literature. *Neurosurgery.* 1985;16:686–688.

113. Cherington M, Yarnell P, Hallmark D. MRI in lightning encephalopathy. *Neurology.* 1993;43:1437–1438.

114. Janus TJ, Barrash J. Neurologic and neurobehavioral effects of electric and lightning injuries. *J Burn Care Rehabil.* 1996;17:409–415.

115. Van Zomeren AH, ten Duis HJ, Minderhoud JM, et al. Lightning stroke and neuropsychological impairment: Cases and questions. *J Neurol Neurosurg Psychiatry.* 1998;64:763–769.

116. Cherington M, Yarnell P, Lammereste D. Lighting strikes: Nature of neurological damage in patients evaluated in hospital emergency departments. *Ann Emerg Med.* 1992;21(5):575–578.

117. Davidson GS, Deck JH. Delayed myelopathy following lightning strike: A demyelinating process. *Acta Neuropathol.* 1988;77(1):104–108.

118. Ptacek JT, Patterson DR, Montgomery BK, et al. Pain, coping, and adjustment in patients with severe burns: Preliminary findings from a prospective study. *J Pain Symptom Manage.* 1995;10:446–455.

119. Saxe G, Stoddard F, Courtney D, et al. Relationship between acute morphine and the course of PTSD in children with burns. *J Am Acad Child Adolesc Psychiatry.* 2001;40(8):915–921.

120. Melzack R. The tragedy of needless pain. *Sci Am.* 1990;262(2):27–33.

121. Choiniere M, Melzack R, Rondeau J, et al. The pain of burns: Characteristics and correlates. *J Trauma.* 1989;29(11):1531–1539.

122. Patterson D, Sharar S. Burn pain. In: Loeser J, ed. *Bonica's management of pain.* 3rd ed. Philadelphia, PA: Lippincott Williams & Wilkins; 2001:780–787.

123. Sharar SR, Bratton SL, Carrougher GJ, et al. A comparison of oral transmucosal fentanyl citrate and oral hydromorphone for inpatient pediatric burn wound care analgesia. *J Burn Care Rehabil.* 1998;19(6):516–521.

124. Baskett PJ, Hyland J, Deane M, et al. Analgesia for burns dressing in children. A dose-finding study for phenoperidine and droperidol with and without 50 percent nitrous oxide and oxygen. *Br J Anaesth.* 1969;41:684–688.

125. Choiniere M, Grenier R, Paquette C. Patient-controlled analgesia: A double-blind study in burn patients. *Anaesthesia.* 1992;47(6):467–472.

126. Filkins SA, Cosgrav P, Marvin JA. Self-administered anesthesia: A method of pain control. *J Burn Care Rehabil.* 1981;2:33–34.

127. Lee JJ, Marvin JA, Heimbach DM. Effectiveness of nalbuphine for relief of burn debridement pain. *J Burn Care Rehabil.* 1989;10(3):241–246.

128. Moiniche S, Pedersen JL, Kehlet H. Topical ketorolac has no antinociceptive or anti-inflammatory effect in thermal injury. *Burns.* 1994;20:483–496.

129. Egan KJ, Ready LB, Nessly M, et al. Self-administration of midazolam for postoperative anxiety: A double blinded study. *Pain.* 1992;49(1):3–8.

130. Patterson DR, Ptacek JT, Carrougher GJ, et al. Lorazepam as an adjunct to opioid analgesics in the treatment of burn pain. *Pain.* 1997;72:367–374.

131. Dimick P, Helvig E, Heimbach D, et al. Anesthesia-assisted procedures in a burn intensive care unit procedure room: Benefits and complications. *J Burn Care Rehabil.* 1993;14(4):446–449.

132. Patterson DR. Non-opioid-based approaches to burn pain. *J Burn Care Rehabil.* 1995;16(3):372–376.

133. Hoffman HG, Doctor JN, Patterson DR, et al. Use of virtual reality as an adjunctive treatment of adolescent burn pain during wound care: A case report. *Pain.* 2000;85(1–2):305–309.

134. Patterson DR, Jensen M. Hypnosis and clinical pain. *Psychol Bull.* 2003;129(4):495–521.

135. Patterson DR, Ptacek JT. Baseline pain as a moderator of hypnotic analgesia for burn injury treatment. *J Consult Clin Psychol.* 1997;65(1):60–67.

136. Ehde DM, Patterson DR, Fordyce WE. The quota system in burn rehabilitation. *J Burn Care Rehabil.* 1998;19(5):436–440.

137. Fordyce WE. *Behavioral methods for chronic pain and illness.* St. Louis, MO: Mosby–Year Book; 1976.

138. Patterson DR, Everett JJ, Bombardier CH, et al. Psychological effects of severe burn injuries. *Psychol Bull.* 1993;113(2):362–378.

139. American Psychiatric Association. *Diagnostic and statistical manual of mental disorders.* 4th ed. Washington, DC: American Psychiatric Association; 1994.

140. Patterson DR, Ford GR. Burn injuries. In: Frank RG, Elliott TR, eds. *Handbook of rehabilitation psychology.* Washington, DC: American Psychological Association; 2000:145–162.

141. Partridge J. *When burns affect the way you look.* London, UK: Changing Faces, 1997.

142. Meyer WJ III, Marvin JA, Patterson DR, et al. Management of pain and other discomforts in burned patients. In: Herndon DN, ed. *Total burn care.* 2nd ed. New York, NY: WB Saunders; 2002; London, UK: Harcourt Publishers Limited; 2002:747–765.

143. Jaffe S, Patterson DR. Treating sleep problems in patients with burn injuries. *J Burn Care Rehabil.* 2004;25(3):294–305.

144. Miller WR, Rollnick S. *Motivational interviewing: Preparing people to change addictive behavior.* New York, NY: The Guilford Press; 1991.

145. Wiechman SA, Ehde DM, Wilson BL, et al. The management of self-inflicted burn injuries and disruptive behavior for patients with borderline personality disorder. *J Burn Care Rehabil.* 2000;21(4):310–317.

146. Costa BA, Engrav LH, Holavanahalli R, et al. Impairment after burns: A two-center, prospective report. *Burns.* 2003;29(7):671–675.

147. Kowalske K, Holavanahalli R, Esselman P, et al. Functional improvement post burn including its relationship to burn characteristics. *J Burn Care Rehabil.* 1998;19:S150.

148. Doctor JN, Patterson DR, Mann R. Health outcome for burn survivors. *J Burn Care Rehabil.* 1997;18(6):490–495.

149. Williams RM, Doctor J, Patterson DR, et al. Health outcomes for burn survivors: A two-year follow-up. *Rehabil Psychol.* 2003;48(3):189–194.

150. Kildal M, Andersson G, Fugl-Meyer AR, et al. Development of a brief version of the burn specific health scale (BSHS-B). *J Trauma.* 2001;51:740–746.

151. Esselman P, Ptacek J, Kowalske K, et al. Community integration after burn injuries. *J Burn Care Rehabil.* 2001;22:221–227.

152. Derogatis LR, Melisaratos N. The brief symptom inventory: An introductory report. *Psychol Med.* 1983;13:595–605.

153. Staley M, Richard R, Warden GD, et al. Functional outcomes for the patient with burn injuries. *J Burn Care Rehabil.* 1996;17(4):362–368.

154. Brych SB, Engrav LH, Rivara FP, et al. Time off work and return to work rates after burns: Systematic review of the literature and a large two-center series. *J Burn Care Rehabil.* 2001;22:401–405.

155. Saffle JR, Tuohig GM, Sullivan JJ, et al. Return to work as a measure of outcome in adults hospitalized for acute burn treatment. *J Burn Care Rehabil.* 1996;17(4):353–361.

11

Chronic Pain Management in Patients with a History of Trauma

James P. Robinson and Mark P. Jensen

This chapter focuses on the management of chronic pain among individuals who have sustained significant trauma—especially trauma to the musculoskeletal system or the nervous system. It does not address strategies for managing such patients in the period immediately following injury, or during the postoperative period following procedures. The modal patient for purposes of this chapter is one who has sustained a traumatic spinal cord injury (SCI) at the T8 level 6 months ago, has undergone initial spine stabilization surgery and initial rehabilitation, and reports persistent, diffuse pain below the level of the lesion.

The evaluation and management of chronic pain in patients with a history of trauma is important for two primary reasons. First, chronic pain is a serious problem for many patients who have sustained significant trauma. For example, cross-sectional surveys indicate that 60% to 80% of persons with spinal cord injury report chronic pain (1–6), and this pain is rated as severe in 20% to 40% of cases (2,4,6). Similar surveys indicate that about 50% to 80% of persons with acquired amputation experience pain (7–10), and that about 25% of such persons experience ongoing, severe pain (11). Second, there is good evidence of significant morbidity associated with chronic pain in trauma patients. For example, survey studies indicate that the presence or severity of pain in persons with SCI is associated with increased depression and psychological distress (2,3,12), unemployment (2), and sleep difficulty (13). Amputation-related pain has similarly been shown

to be negatively associated with functioning, including measures of daily and work activities (14,15).

Managing chronic pain in trauma patients does not create any new problems over and above the management of chronic pain in other settings. However, this is no cause for comfort, because chronic pain management is difficult in any setting. One factor that contributes to the difficulty of treating chronic pain is the fact that pain is a personal experience that cannot be fully confirmed by a physician or any other third party. Thus, clinicians treating patients with chronic pain are faced with uncertainty about how to interpret patients' pain complaints. This ambiguity becomes especially challenging when patients demand high doses of opiates to control pain or report a level of incapacitation that appears to be excessive relative to the severity of the injury. Moreover, even if the ambiguities regarding pain assessment could be resolved, clinicians are still confronted by endless ambiguity regarding appropriate therapies.

Several factors contribute to the ambiguity associated with pain treatment. Most therapies for chronic pain have not been subjected to rigorous research on effectiveness or have failed to show efficacy in appropriately designed research. In addition, even therapies that have been validated in the treatment of chronic pain tend to produce only partial and inconsistent therapeutic effects. As a result, chronic pain tends to persist despite what appears to be appropriate therapy (16); both clinicians and patients are often left with the difficult task of identifying small improvements in a problem that tends to persist, and that varies significantly across time even without treatment. In addition, multiple factors moderate patients' responses to treatments. As a result, it is difficult to define therapeutic interventions that are robust over patients who differ in medical diagnosis, pathophysiologic processes underlying their pain (17), age, gender, and psychosocial variables. Finally, the patients with chronic pain who become challenging are precisely those who have not profited from standard therapies. Clinicians can anticipate that whenever they treat a patient who has failed to benefit from first-line and second-line therapies for a chronic pain problem, they will have to make therapeutic decisions that have not (yet) been validated by scientific evidence.

Our goals for this chapter are to describe some of the difficulties physicians are likely to encounter when they treat chronic pain in trauma patients and to outline treatment strategies that will maximize the probability of successful outcomes. We note at the outset that we make no attempt to describe therapies for chronic pain exhaustively (see 18,19). Rather, we will describe general strategies for pain management and will use case examples to illustrate the complexities that occur in the treatment of chronic pain in trauma patients.

TREATING SYMPTOMS VERSUS TREATING "UPSTREAM" PATHOLOGY

Pain is a cardinal symptom of many illnesses and injuries. Medical training and the traditional medical model emphasize that physicians should look beyond symptoms to the underlying biological abnormality thought to be causing the symptoms and provide treatment that reverses this abnormality. In the best case, the patient's symptoms should resolve without any additional treatments once the underlying biological disturbance has been reversed. Common examples include appendectomy for a patient who presents with right lower quadrant pain secondary to appendicitis, and angioplasty for a patient who presents with chest pain secondary to cardiac ischemia.

The logic of looking past pain and treating underlying biological abnormalities is so ingrained that many physicians have trouble thinking about pain in any other way. In the real world, however, there are multiple settings in which treatment must be directed toward pain rather than toward a hypothesized biological abnormality that is thought to drive pain. For example, the goal of surgical anesthesia is to prevent patients from experiencing agonizing pain during surgical procedures.

Chronic pain represents another condition for which it is often most appropriate to treat pain directly rather than to look for "upstream" pathology. A major reason for taking this approach is that both neurobiologic research (20,21) and clinical research (22,23) indicate that pain often becomes autonomous over time, so that its association with a definable disease or injury becomes less clear. A key process leading to this dissociation between pain experience and definable injury or disease is *sensitization* of the peripheral or central nervous system (24). Turk et al. (25) describe the implications of sensitization as follows: "A major implication of recent research on sensitization is that the failure of medical and surgical investigation to account for a given pain may result not from looking in the wrong place, but from looking at the wrong time. That is, the investigations may be directed toward the organ or body part that was historically responsible for the individual's pain, but they may be unrevealing because the pain, having been initiated by an injury or illness in the past, is now relatively independent."

A practical implication of research on sensitization is that attempts to find the underlying "pain generator" in a patient with chronic pain are often unproductive. In fact, such efforts can often be counterproductive, because, like the pot of gold at the end of the rainbow, a single specific cause for chronic pain is rarely found. And as physicians search for specific biological causes of patients' pain, both they and the patients may devalue management strategies that may effectively treat pain as a symptom.

PROCESSES UNDERLYING CHRONIC PAIN

Various systems have been developed to classify chronic pain on the basis of its presumed underlying pathophysiology (17). There is no single system that is universally accepted. We favor the following categories:

NOCICEPTIVE PAIN

This is the "normal" pain that is usually seen in acute injuries. In nociceptive pain, a patient's pain experience is driven by activity in nociceptors, the sensory afferents that typically signal impending tissue injury (26). An example is persistent pain associated with degenerative joint disease of the knee following a fracture of the joint.

PAIN SECONDARY TO ALTERED FUNCTIONING OF PERIPHERAL NERVES

Peripheral Neuropathic Pain

This type of pain occurs when peripheral nerves have been damaged. The patient will typically experience pain and paresthesias in the part of his body that is normally innervated by the damaged nerve. In cases of this type, the patient's pain experience is based on an injury, but the physiologic abnormality underlying the pain is in a nerve rather than in the part of the body identified as painful. An example is pain experienced in the distal aspect of the leg following an injury to the L5 or S1 nerve root (27).

Pain Based on Sensitization of Peripheral Nerves

In this type of pain, a peripheral nerve becomes hyperactive following injury, even though there is no evidence that the nerve has been injured (28).

PAIN SECONDARY TO ALTERED CENTRAL NERVOUS SYTEM FUNCTIONING

Pain Secondary to Central Nervous System Injury

This type of pain is based on damage to the central nervous system (CNS). Examples include the "thalamic syndrome" that occurs following stroke or brain injury and the persistent pain that SCI patients often report below the level of their lesion (29).

Pain Based on Central Nervous System Sensitization

Animal research during the past 20 years has convincingly demonstrated that a nociceptive barrage can lead to sensitization of an organism's CNS (26,30). Most of this research has examined changes in the dorsal horn of the spinal cord, but it is likely that changes occur throughout the CNS in response to nociceptive barrage. The net effect of these changes is that following injury the organism responds excessively to new stimulation of the previously injured area, even when the new stimulation is nonnoxious.

PAIN SECONDARY TO, OR INFLUENCED BY, PSYCHOLOGICAL FACTORS

In this type of pain, psychological factors such as anticipation of further injury or desire to influence the behavior of others affect a patient's experience of pain and/or communication about pain (31).

A few comments about the previously mentioned categories are in order. First, it is typical for chronic pain to be based on some mixture of the processes described in the previous paragraphs, rather than being entirely explainable in terms of just one. Second, hypotheses about which of these processes play a dominant role in a patient's pain have implications for the diagnostic work-up. For example, if a clinician believes that the patient's pain is based on ongoing nociception, it would be appropriate to perform a thorough diagnostic evaluation in the hope that a treatable abnormality can be found. In contrast, if the clinician concludes that the patient's pain is driven by CNS sensitization, it makes little sense to perform an exhaustive diagnostic evaluation. Third, judgments about the pathophysiology underlying a patient's pain also have implications for the type of therapy that is likely to help. For example, nonsteroidal anti-inflammatory drugs (NSAIDs) are most likely to help in nociceptive pain, whereas tricyclic antidepressants and antiseizure medications can be helpful in neuropathic pain.

Fourth, it is difficult to classify some types of pain that are commonly encountered clinically in terms of the previously mentioned categories. A striking example is myofascial pain. This might be construed as nociceptive pain, based on the "energy crisis" model of Simons (32). Alternatively, it might be construed as a form of hyperalgesia that reflects CNS sensitization (22).

Fifth, it is important to note that chronic pain is often dissociated from the definable tissue dysfunction that physicians typically search for when a patient presents with pain. In fact, only nociceptive pain has a straightforward relation to tissue injury at the site where the pain is experienced. In all of the other categories described above, tissue injury is separated from the site where pain is experienced either in space (e.g., radicular pain) or in time (e.g., pain based on peripheral or central nervous system sensitization).

Finally, even for pain problems that have a clear physiological basis, once pain becomes chronic, psychological factors often play a significant role in the impact that pain has on patient functioning (33). Thus, it is often the case that factors such as pain-coping strategies used, thoughts and fears about pain, and the patient's social environment should be thoroughly considered, and addressed as appropriate, in order to maximize patient functioning in the face of chronic pain.

PERSPECTIVES ON PAIN: FIRST PERSON VERSUS THIRD PERSON

Scarry made a profound observation about pain when she stated, "To have pain is to have certainty.

To hear about another person's pain is to have doubt" (34). For the person experiencing pain, pain has immediacy and is accepted at face value as an indicator of bodily dysfunction. In fact, most patients would be puzzled or insulted if someone asked them whether the pain was "real," or whether it really reflected some abnormality in the functioning of their bodies. In our culture, patients typically seek medical help to get rid of pain and expect physicians to manage their pain by first identifying its biological cause, and then treating that cause to eliminate the pain.

The situation is strikingly different for the physician evaluating a patient's pain. Physicians who are experienced in chronic pain recognize that pain behaviors (i.e., the verbal and nonverbal behaviors that communicate pain to others) are a complex function of multiple factors. The problem of interpreting pain behavior can be likened to solving an equation with multiple unknowns; in other words. solving the following equation:

$$PB = f(X_1, X_2, X_3.....................X_n)$$

Where PB = a patient's observable pain behaviors, and $X_1....X_n$ represent the multiple factors that contribute to these pain behaviors.

Because of uncertainty about the many causes of pain behavior in any one patient, clinicians are often left with a disquieting set of questions when evaluating a patient who complains of pain. Should the patient undergo a work-up to determine if the pain is based on some injury or dysfunction of an organ or body part? Might the underlying biological problem be an acute one that warrants an urgent work-up? Is the patient exaggerating pain? If so, is the exaggeration based on excessive fear, a desire to get drugs or otherwise manipulate the physician, the patient's prior experience of getting attention when he or she communicates pain (i.e., learning history), or some unknown additional "X" factor? How disabling is the pain? Does the severity of the patient's reported pain or the degree of disability that the patient reports make sense on the basis of medical assessment?

Uncertainty regarding how to construe a patient's pain problem is likely to be greatly augmented by the interactions that clinicians and their patients have with practitioners of alternative medicine. A substantial proportion of patients with chronic pain seek input from practitioners of alternative or complementary medicine, including chiropractors, massage therapists, acupuncturists, and naturopaths (35,36). These practitioners generally have strong views regarding the pathophysiology underlying

pain and the appropriateness of various therapies that may be different from those based on standard western medical practice. For example, physicians might be puzzled by the chiropractic concept of a subluxation or the acupuncture concepts of yin and yang. A clinician's confidence in their own explanatory models may well be shaken when patients state that they have gotten significant relief from treatment by practitioners of alternative/complementary medicine.

A GENERAL STRATEGY FOR ADDRESSING PATIENTS' REPORTS OF PAIN

Clinicians should give careful thought to their philosophic approach to patients with chronic pain and their strategies for managing his or her condition. Forethought is required mainly because they will be challenged as they manage chronic pain in patients who have sustained major trauma. The challenge is likely to be particularly uncomfortable for clinicians who have not done any "mental homework" about the management of chronic pain.

There are several reasons why the treatment of chronic pain patients is challenging. First, as noted above, clinicians will frequently be confused about the factors underlying their patient's pain behaviors. Even clinicians who think they understand these factors qualitatively will often be puzzled about the apparently devastating effects they have on a patient's ability to function. Second, clinicians often feel pushed by patients with chronic pain. For example, patients may insist that only high dose opiates control their pain or ask their attending physician to certify that they are entitled to various kinds of disability benefits because of their pain (37). Third, clinicians will likely find the treatment of chronic pain humbling. Diagnostic skills may seem irrelevant, because patients will often present with pain that bears no simple relation to definable derangement of organs or tissues. Another humbling discovery is that the responses of patients to pain treatments are highly variable, so that physicians cannot be confident that their prescriptions will really help any one patient.

Many physicians respond to these uncertainties by adopting one of two extreme positions. Some take the reports of patients at face value, without any critical analysis. These physicians are at risk to perform multiple unnecessary diagnostic work-ups, and to advocate disability benefits for patients when they are not really needed. At the opposite extreme, some physicians develop a cynical, withholding perspective toward patients with chronic pain. They (implicitly) take the position that the patients are exaggerating their distress and do not really deserve aggressive treatment for their pain complaints.

We suggest a more subtle approach to patients with chronic pain. It is based on several premises.

As described previously, pain behaviors are typically the product of a variety of factors, and the mix differs from patient to patient. Thus, clinicians should avoid simple conceptual models that embody the assumption that all pain behaviors are driven by the same (few) dynamics in all patients.

Clinicians should remember that chronic pain can have enormously detrimental effects on patient functioning (16,38).

While patients with chronic pain sometimes overstate their incapacitation and underestimate their ability to cope (see the following paragraph), most experts in chronic pain believe that frank malingering is rare. In fact, the tragedy of chronic pain is that everyone involved in it loses—including the insurance and disability carriers who pay benefits, the physicians who treat the pain, and (especially) the patients themselves.

The fact that many patients with chronic pain perceive themselves as having no options provides a therapeutic opportunity for physicians. Both patients and physicians often construe the complaints of pain patients in one of two ways—either patients are telling the truth and deserve enormous deference from the physician (and others, such as disability agencies), or they are lying (i.e., malingering). Rarely do patients or physicians think of a third option—namely, that in a fundamental sense patients are often *incorrect* in their appraisals regarding their pain. This third approach might seem odd at first. Because pain is a subjective experience, how could a patient be incorrect in his or her appraisals regarding pain? The answer is that patients' appraisals regarding pain involve multiple assumptions about what will or might occur under certain circumstances. Patients often incorrectly assume the worst. For example, they might assume that if they carry out activities that produce pain, they will inevitably retard their recovery; or they might assume that they are unable to perform activities that they actually are capable of performing (39). Once physicians recognize that patients with pain are often incorrect in their appraisals, they are in a position to (gently) challenge patients' assertions about pain without impugning their character. In fact, most experts in chronic pain believe that a major role of physicians is to educate patients regarding the complexities of pain and to help patients see ways that they can

overcome hurdles that they have perceived as overwhelming (40,41).

One of the most important errors in patients' perceptions is their tendency to be exquisitely sensitive to aggravations of their pain or deterioration in their functioning, while remaining relatively unaware of modest improvements. One practical consequence of this perceptual bias is that patients often dismiss as ineffective treatments that do in fact produce benefit, but not complete resolution of pain.

Pain leads many patients to be desperate. They may grasp onto treatments that produce short-term relief, even when the long-term effects of the treatments are equivocal or even harmful. The most obvious setting where this dynamic plays out is the arena of opiate prescriptions. However, patients with chronic pain are heavy consumers of not only opiates but also of a variety of palliative therapies, including physical therapy, chiropractic treatment, bed (or recliner) rest, and massage.

Physicians who operate on the basis of the previously described premises will gently challenge patients' statements about their pain without implying that the patients are liars or malingerers. They will emphasize the devastating impact that chronic pain can have on patients' quality of life but also help them understand that they can improve their situations greatly by learning how to better manage their pain, by reversing the secondary effects of chronic injuries or illnesses, and by becoming resourceful in finding ways to limit the impact that pain has on their ability to function.

TREATMENT OF CHRONIC PAIN: GENERAL PRINCIPLES

Usually, an overall strategy for treatment will be multifaceted—that is, physicians will approach the patient's pain problem from a variety of perspectives simultaneously. Physicians will probably do a better job if they consider a wide range of strategies and issues that might be relevant.

The first question is whether the patient's pain is a symptom that will resolve with treatment of an upstream biological abnormality or a problem that needs direct treatment.

Within direct treatment approaches, physicians should be aware of different perspectives and approaches. The major ones are as follows:

1. **Palliation.** In this approach, pain reduction is essentially the only goal of treatment. The patient is not expected or required to change

behavior in any way. Examples of this approach include immediate postoperative treatment and sometimes treatment of terminally ill patients.

2. **Rehabilitation.** In the rehabilitation approach, the patient is expected to take an active role to improve his or her level of functioning, and to optimize a variety of factors that may contribute to pain relief. The rationale for this approach is twofold. First, it embodies the assumption that improvements in functional status are worthwhile even if the patient does not experience (or report) any changes in pain. Second, it assumes that if patients work to improve their functional status, they will often eventually experience pain reduction or at least be able to do more despite their pain. An example of this approach is the multidisciplinary rehabilitative care that is often provided to injured workers with chronic low back pain (42,43).

3. **Environmental Modification.** The physician may conclude that changes need to be made in the environment of the patient in order for the patient to achieve an optimal balance between functional capabilities and pain control. The physician may then support a wide range of supportive devices and services, such as crutches or other assistive devices for ambulation, a disability parking sticker, or services of a chore worker.

As noted previously, ambiguity regarding the assessment and treatment of chronic pain abounds.

Chronic pain tends to be chronic. That is, treatments for chronic pain rarely lead to a complete resolution of symptoms or permit a patient to completely return to his or her pre-injury level of function (16). An implication of this somber statement is that the physician and the patient must be prepared to accept modest goals that are short of total cure and must be willing and able to note small improvements as they occur. Physicians will often need to educate the patient to give up an "absolutist" view of pain and embrace and use interventions that produce limited decreases in pain.

The context in which treatment is provided is extremely important. This point can best be grasped by contrast. A patient who is septic from a staphylococcal infection will typically respond dramatically to appropriate antibiotic therapy. This response will occur regardless of the patient's opinions about antibiotics or the quality of his or her relationship with the physician who prescribes the antibiotics. In contrast, the effectiveness of most treatments for chronic pain depends to a large degree on the context within which they are provided. Thus, a patient's response to a treatment will depend heavily on the patient's attitudes toward the treating physician, his or her expectations about what the treatment is intended to change, what changes represent early indicators of a positive response, and what responsibilities he or she has while undergoing the treatment. These patient attitudes and expectations are, in turn, influenced by the content and style of physician communications.

There are at least two reasons for this dependence on context. First, as noted above, virtually no chronic pain treatment is so potent that it predictably produces large reductions in pain in all patients. Second, because so many factors affect pain, patients must be careful not to counterbalance the positive effects of a treatment with negative effects of other changes in their life. For example, if a patient starts a new medication that reduces pain and responds to this pain relief by dramatically increasing activity level without any preparation, that patient is likely to experience a flare-up of pain and might well conclude that the drug was ineffective. An entirely different outcome might occur if the physician who prescribed the medication also provided information about how the patient should approach the challenge of increasing his or her activity level after experiencing some pain relief.

One important aspect of the context surrounding treatment is the patient's conceptual model regarding his or her chronic pain. Many people implicitly assume that they should reduce their use of a painful body part and should rely on physicians to pinpoint the cause of the pain and treat it effectively. These assumptions are usually valid for acute pain but are counterproductive for chronic pain. As demonstrated in multidisciplinary pain rehabilitation programs, people with chronic pain manage their problems better if they have a more accurate conceptual model that incorporates the limits of medical/surgical therapies for chronic pain and emphasizes the importance of self-management, including regular moderate use of the affected body part.

A related point is that patients with chronic pain must be active participants in treatment if they are to maximize their chance of improvement. Patients who passively expect the physician to solve their pain problem are likely to be disappointed.

Effective treatment of chronic pain often needs to be multidisciplinary. A major reason for this is that both the factors influencing pain and the effects of pain span multiple domains. For example, it is not at all uncommon for a patient with chronic pain to have problems with depression, work disability, substance abuse, and marital discord. It is virtually impossible for a physician to keep track of all these domains, much less to intervene effectively in all of them. Multidisciplinary pain centers began about 35 years ago in large part because of the multiplicity of the problems associated with chronic pain (42). Physicians will not have the opportunity to send all of their patients with chronic pain to multidisciplinary pain centers, but they need to consider how to incorporate some concepts from multidisciplinary treatment into their office practice. For example, physicians should try to forge links with physical therapists (PTs), vocational rehabilitation counselors, and psychologists who are experienced in treating chronic pain and associated disability.

AN ALGORITHM FOR TREATING CHRONIC PAIN

Figure 11–1 shows a general algorithm that is often appropriate for the treatment of chronic pain in patients who have experienced trauma. Obviously, physicians need to be flexible and individualize treatment based on the needs of specific patients,

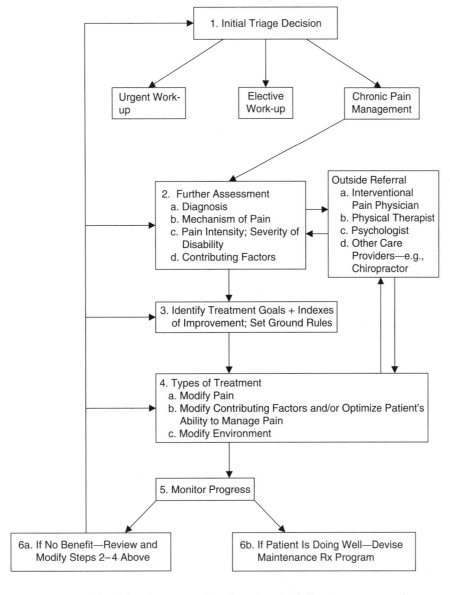

Figure 11–1. Algorithm for managing chronic pain following trauma.

but the broad approach shown in the algorithm can be a useful guide.

INITIAL TRIAGE DECISION

First, the treating physician needs to decide whether or not to go "upstream" from the patient's pain and look for and then treat a modifiable pathophysiologic process that might underlie the pain. This implies a diagnostic work-up as the first step. In some instances, a work-up is urgently needed. Examples include a traumatic brain injury (TBI) patient with suspected deep vein thrombosis or an SCI patient with suspected pyelonephritis and impending sepsis. Alternatively, the physician may determine that the patient needs a diagnostic work-up, but that there is no medical emergency. This is usually the situation encountered in patients who complain of pain that appears to reflect dysfunction in the musculoskeletal system (e.g., shoulder pain in a paraplegic) or the peripheral nervous system (e.g., suspected carpal tunnel syndrome). In these situations, the physician has the luxury of observing a patient for at least several days and making a decision to do a diagnostic work-up only if symptoms persist.

FURTHER ASSESSMENT FOR PURPOSES OF PAIN MANAGEMENT

If the physician decides that a pain management approach is the most appropriate general strategy for treating the patient's pain, the work of assessing the pain is by no means finished.

The physician still needs to consider (or make) a diagnosis based on the *International Classification of Diseases, Ninth Revision (ICD-9)*. However, it is important to remember that diagnostic labels are often misleading in patients with chronic pain. One reason for this is that the processes underlying pain become blurred when the pain becomes chronic. For example, while basic scientists have given us a rather detailed picture of the pathophysiology underlying symptoms in acute lumbar radiculopathies, our understanding of the mechanisms underlying pain in chronic lumbar radiculopathies is much more limited (27). Physicians can mislead both themselves and their patients if they take the position that they understand the pain problem in detail because they have attached a diagnostic label to it. A related point is that in chronic pain, diagnoses rarely provide much insight into the degree of disability that a patient shows. For example, some individuals with a diagnosis of chronic lumbar radiculopathy are productive in all major arenas of their lives, while others are virtually bed-bound.

The physician should also attempt to ascertain mechanisms underlying the patient's pain. As already discussed, this is not an easy task, and it is often the case that multiple processes underlie the patient's pain. However, if a primary pain mechanism can be identified, this will have substantial implications for treatment. For example, if the patient is determined to have neuropathic pain, it would be rational to be vigorous in prescribing pharmacologic agents such as tricyclic antidepressants and antiseizure medications, since these have demonstrable efficacy in the treatment of neuropathic pain (44,45). Alternatively, if it is concluded that a patient's activity restrictions are driven primarily by an irrational fear of reinjury, intervention by a psychologist should be prominent in the treatment plan.

It is crucial to go beyond the medical evaluation implied in making a diagnosis and to consider the ways in which the patient is affected by pain. We believe that this more detailed analysis should cover four domains: (i) pain severity; (ii) the emotional impact of pain; (iii) limitations in the patient's ability to engage in daily activities because of pain; and (iv) limitations in participation in important social roles such as employment. There are two key things physicians should keep in mind as they go through this more detailed analysis. First, the treatment plan needs to be anchored in an understanding of how the patient is affected by his or her pain. For example, if the patient is disabled from work because of pain, the pain treatment plan for that patient is unlikely to be successful unless it addresses the issue of return to work. Second, a traditional medical evaluation of chronic pain does not assess how severely a patient is impacted by the pain.

Finally, physicians need to consider a variety of factors other than the traumatic injury and its direct sequelae that may be contributing factors to the patient's pain and consequent disability/dysfunction. In essence, the physician needs a "laundry list" of factors that combine with a traumatic injury to overwhelm a patient (46). In particular, it is important to assess other factors that are potentially modifiable in a pain treatment program that emphasizes rehabilitation. For example, most patients become severely deconditioned during the time when they receive initial treatment for their trauma. In general, patients feel better and function better when the effects of deconditioning have been reversed. As another example, a patient who has gone through severe trauma may have posttraumatic stress disorder, or an excessive sense of vulnerability to reinjury. Such a patient will frequently function better and report less pain if these psychological issues are effectively addressed.

As shown in Figure 11–1, input may be needed from other physicians or various allied health professionals while performing a more thorough evaluation of a patient in preparation for a pain management treatment program. Similarly, input from various health care professionals may be needed as the treatment program is implemented (see step 2 and step 4 of the algorithm).

IDENTIFY TREATMENT GOALS AND INDEXES OF IMPROVEMENT; SET GROUND RULES

Several issues are important regarding the goals of pain treatment. First, it is important to remember that treatment will rarely produce complete symptom resolution in a patient with chronic pain, especially when the patient also has residuals from the trauma that limit activity tolerances in ways that have nothing to do with pain. For example, a patient with a traumatic amputation of the right-upper extremity will certainly have activity limitations because of the amputation and may have additional limitations because of phantom limb pain. Second, knowing that patients can ignore improvements that fall short of a cure (complete pain relief), it is important to establish measurable markers, so that the patient can be aware of small changes as they occur. Third, although self-reported pain reduction is an important indicator of improvement, other outcome indicators that are objective (such as return to work), or that rely on the perceptions of people other than the patient (e.g., input from the patient's significant other), are also important to keep track of when possible. These alternative types of information are needed to avoid getting bogged down in the (sometimes) biased perceptions of patients with pain—that is, their tendency to focus on pain rather than on functional capabilities, and their tendency to focus on aggravations of pain while ignoring improvements.

It is also important to set ground rules for treatment. These should spell out the obligations/responsibilities of the patient. This is particularly important if the treatment plan involves opiates. We strongly recommend that any patient being treated with long-term opiate therapy sign a contract that outlines ground rules and consequences if the ground rules are violated (47,48).

TYPES OF TREATMENT
Reduce Pain

As noted above, a focus on pain reduction is most consistent with a palliative model of pain treatment.

The most obvious type of intervention that a physician might order to produce pain reduction is the prescription of medications. It is beyond the scope of this chapter to review the multiple categories of medications that might produce amelioration of chronic pain. But physicians treating patients with chronic pain should be aware of the role of tricyclic antidepressants and antiseizure medications in the management of neuropathic pain, and of the role of NSAIDs and corticosteroids in treating pain associated with inflammation. These medications are by no means simple to use in the management of chronic pain, but in terms of complexity, they pale by comparison to the opiates.

Until the 1990s, disciplinary boards generally took the position that it was inappropriate for physicians to provide long-term opiate therapy for patients with chronic nonmalignant pain. The regulatory climate has changed dramatically during the past 15 years, and, although physicians should know the policies and regulations in the area where they practice, the odds are good that physicians will not face sanctions if they provide long-term opiate therapy to patients with chronic pain (49). The removal of regulatory pressure has given physicians a new tool in treating chronic pain but has also created new ambiguities. It is beyond the scope of this chapter to summarize the lengthy and sometimes acrimonious debate that has gone on during the past 15 years about the appropriate role of opiates in chronic nonmalignant pain. We will thus limit ourselves to a few general statements. These should be taken as our best understanding of pros and cons of opiate therapy, based on our review of relevant literature and our clinical experience. It is by no means the final word on the subject, because there is no universally accepted final word.

First, opiates are effective analgesics in that they do reduce pain, although they rarely eliminate pain completely. They can be viewed as akin to broad spectrum antibiotics, in the sense that they have some beneficial effect on virtually any kind of pain. Some research suggests that they are less effective in neuropathic pain than other kinds of pain (50), but on balance the scientific literature supports the conclusion that they can be effective analgesics even for this type of pain (51). At least in the short run, opiates are the most reliable pain relievers we have. Second, although well-designed trials to assess the efficacy of long-term opiate use are virtually nonexistent, results from case series (52,53) and relatively short randomized controlled trials (RCTs) on chronic pain patients (54–58) support the conclusion that prolonged opiate therapy can benefit some patients with chronic pain. However, a countervailing concern is that when opiates are used over long periods, there is a significant danger that patients will develop opioid tolerance. Tolerance can reliably be induced in laboratory animals (59,60), and there is persuasive evidence that it occurs in at least some humans with chronic pain (51,61). If a physician tries to overcome this tolerance by progressively increasing a patient's opiate dose, an uncomfortable situation can develop in which the patient ends up on an enormous dosage of an opiate but still complains of severe, disabling pain. Third, a subset of patients will engage in grossly inappropriate behaviors regarding their opiates. As a practical matter, if you make long-term opiate therapy a part of your practice, you will inevitably be "burned" by patients who forge prescriptions, sell their drugs on the street, get opiate prescriptions from multiple practitioners simultaneously, alter their drugs to get a "high" (e.g., grind up oxycodone [OxyContin] tablets), or engage in other inappropriate drug-related behaviors (47,62). Each individual physician needs to decide whether the benefit that responsible patients derive from opiate use is substantial enough to make up for the stress the physician is bound to experience as he or she interacts with opiate abusers. Finally, even responsible patients often seem to overvalue opiates, in the sense that they report benefit from the medications but do not demonstrate obvious functional improvement that convinces you that they are actually benefiting from opiate use.

There are several nonpharmacologic treatments that are best viewed as palliative, pain-relieving therapies. These treatments include passive physical therapy, massage, hypnosis and relaxation training, transcutaneous electric nerve stimulation (TENS) units, acupuncture, and trigger point injections. While it is beyond the scope of this chapter to discuss these treatments in any detail, some patients respond well to one or more of these treatments, and so they are worth considering for any patient for whom pain reduction is a goal.

It is difficult to define the appropriate use of palliative treatments in chronic pain. Patients with chronic pain will usually emphasize pain relief as the most important treatment goal. However, physicians with experience in treating chronic pain will probably have different priorities. For example, while pain relief is undoubtedly *one* important goal of treatment, physicians should also be concerned about the patient's ability to function physically, emotionally, and interpersonally.

Some negotiation is often needed to prioritize the possible goals of treatment. Even physicians who tend to focus on functional improvement should acknowledge the patient's concerns about pain relief in order to maintain rapport. Sometimes it is appropriate to provide pain control therapies that are linked with a physical therapy program that focuses on functional restoration. For example, it might be reasonable to link sympathetic blocks with active physical therapy in a patient with complex regional pain syndrome, or to provide opiates to a low back pain patient as he or she goes through a functionally oriented physical therapy program.

Modify Contributing Factors and/or Optimize Patient's Ability to Manage Pain

Rehabilitative therapies often focus on optimizing a patient's ability to function despite limitations imposed by an illness or injury. For example, functionally oriented physical therapy can help a trauma patient reverse secondary effects of an injury, such as joint contractures and disuse atrophy of muscles. At a more subtle level, functionally oriented physical therapy can help patients regain confidence that they can trust their bodies, and that their bodies can recover from the injury the patients sustained.

A variety of psychological therapies are consistent with a rehabilitative model of pain treatment. They include cognitive therapies that help patients understand the complexities of interactions between emotional stress and pain; those that counter the tendency of some patients to view their pain problem as a simple mechanical problem that needs to be fixed before the patient can be expected to increase his or her activity level; those that counter the tendency of some patients to experience disabling anxiety ("catastrophizing") about their pain; and those that focus on pacing and practical problem solving about ways in which patients can accomplish necessary tasks without paying an enormous price in the form of increased pain (33).

Modify the Environment

Even if a trauma patient with chronic pain participates fully in a treatment program designed to reduce pain and improve function, it may well be that he or she will have significant residual limitations. In that situation, the ability of the patient to meet real-world challenges will often depend on environmental modifications that permit functioning despite physical limitations and pain.

Physiatrists are already familiar with many kinds of environmental modifications and assistive devices that improve the function of people with disabilities. Many of these are relevant to patients with chronic pain; for example, some of these patients may need canes, orthoses, or modifications to their homes. Patients with chronic pain may also need more subtle environmental accommodations, such as work stations that are ergonomically designed, or the approval of work supervisors to take short breaks at strategic intervals during work shifts.

MONITOR PROGRESS

Even physicians who have taken the time to identify treatment goals as recommended previously will often find it difficult to monitor the progress of a patient with chronic pain. One major reason for this difficulty is that there is no way to directly assess a major target of treatment—the intensity of the patient's pain. Patients' reports about pain are often ephemeral and enigmatic. Some patients will say they are feeling better but will remain extremely inactive and demonstrate no measurable functional improvement. Others will continue to complain of pain, but will show remarkable progress as they go through a functionally oriented treatment program.

Another complication is the difficulty of monitoring several different parameters at once in order to determine whether, on balance, the patient is improving. It is difficult for any single clinician to monitor a patient with respect to pain intensity, illness beliefs, possible side effects of medications, functional improvement in physical therapy and/or daily activities, progress in vocational rehabilitation, and amelioration of depression. Yet all of these parameters may be relevant to the broad question of whether the patient is improving, and to decisions about future treatment. Because of the multiple domains that are relevant to chronic pain, it is often best to have the patient's progress assessed in multidisciplinary team meetings.

Regardless of the resources that are available for assessing a patient, or the parameters that the physician believes are most important to monitor, it is crucial to monitor patients on an ongoing basis. As noted above, pain may distort patients' perceptions in ways that lead them to underestimate their abilities and to overvalue treatments that produce short-term symptom amelioration but no long-term benefit. Independent information about a patient's progress is needed in order to know when to discontinue these treatments. More generally, physicians who have carefully monitored a patient's progress will be in a better position to determine when the patient has achieved maximal medical benefit from various therapies and what level of activity can be expected of him or her after the condition stabilizes.

Review and Modify the Treatment Plan if the Patient Has Not Benefited

One reason for carefully monitoring patients is that despite efforts to treat pain and functioning with a carefully reasoned treatment plan, some patients will fail to improve. Given the uncertainties that have been described regarding the treatment of chronic pain, this should not be surprising.

If the patient is not getting benefit from the treatment program, the decisions you made in steps 1 through 4 in the algorithm will need to be reconsidered. For example, if a patient with low back pain reports worsening lower extremity pain during a functional restoration program, the patient's lumbar spine may need to be re-imaged, the patient may need to be referred to an interventional pain specialist, the medication regimen may need to be changed, or the patient may need to be referred to a psychologist for assessment and recommendations concerning psychological factors that may be contributing to the pain problem. The general point is that because of the uncertainty about whether any individual patient will respond positively to a treatment plan, some degree of flexibility is needed, and physicians need to be willing to carefully reconsider their decision making in patients who are doing poorly.

Devise Maintenance Treatment If Patient Is Doing Well

If serial monitoring reveals that the patient has reached a plateau in response to a treatment program and has attained a satisfactory level of function and pain control, the physician is in a position to discontinue high-intensity therapies. However, in doing so, it is important to remember that chronic pain tends to be *chronic* (63). The patient may no longer need intensive treatment, but he or she will probably continue to need at least low-level monitoring and perhaps medication management. Often this kind of maintenance care can best be carried out by a primary care physician, but both the patient and the primary care provider may need some intermittent consultation with a specialist in rehabilitation medicine.

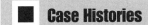

■ Case Histories

General Comments

The following four case histories illustrate some of the issues that arise in the management of pain in individuals with a history of trauma. One point that should be noted is the diversity of approaches that may be used. The frustrating reality is that there is essentially no conclusive research that tells us which therapies or combinations of therapies to prescribe for patients with various chronic pain problems. The best that we can do is make intelligent choices among a long list of possibilities and establish a method of monitoring the patient to see if a therapy is working.

Because of space limitations, only certain features of patients' problems are presented, and only a limited set of interventions are discussed. In actual clinical practice, however, physicians are likely to face more complicated situations than the ones described here. A key issue is that patients with chronic pain after trauma are likely to have psychosocial problems and disability problems that interact with their pain. Thus, a variety of skills in rehabilitation will be needed. For example, it is important to be aware of vocational problems and be vigilant for evidence of emotional distress and/or significant interpersonal problems. The clinical situation may well be complicated further by pre-injury problems; for example, the history of substance abuse in case number 1.

As a general rule, treatment of chronic pain is most likely to be successful if it addresses several domains at once (e.g., medical, psychological, disability), and if the patient makes a commitment to functional goals beyond simply achieving pain control. As a practical matter, regardless of the medications that are prescribed, patients should have (or have had) the benefit of a functionally oriented physical therapy program and be compliant with a self-directed follow-up exercise program. Another practical issue is that treatment of pain is unlikely to be successful unless the patient resolves work disability problems brought on by the injury. Although these multiple dimensions of trauma-induced chronic pain are not systematically discussed in the cases that follow, they should be considered when treating such patients.

Another oversimplification in the examples that follow is that they imply that medication trials are easy to supervise and lead to unequivocal answers. In fact, just the opposite is often the case. Despite efforts to identify indices of improvement, involve people who know the patient well, and spend a great deal of time explaining the rationale for various medications, it is not always possible to determine whether or not a trial has produced any benefit.

Case Number 1

Background

A 23-year-old woman was the driver of a vehicle that was involved in an accident 1 year ago. She sustained an acute flexion injury to her spine, with burst fracture of the T8 vertebral body and incomplete T8 paraplegia. During her initial management, she underwent an instrumented fusion from T6 through T10. This fusion appears to be stable, and the patient has no significant midback pain. She does, however, complain of diffuse burning pain in both lower extremities. At the time of the initial evaluation (1 year postaccident), she is taking nabumetone 1,000 mg per day and sustained-release oxycodone (oxycontin) 160 mg three times per day (t.i.d.) for pain control. She reports that she has been on opiates ever since her motor vehicle accident, and review of records confirms this.

Past history is noteworthy in that the patient abused both alcohol and street drugs prior to her motor vehicle crash (MVC). In fact, her blood alcohol level at the time of her MVC was 250 mg per dL. She indicates that she has been through a drug rehabilitation program during the past year and is now clean and sober.

Treatment

You start by meeting with the patient and her sister, with whom she lives. The patient reports that despite her pain medication regimen, she is having severe lower-extremity pain, and that she spends several hours per day lying down because of pain. The three of you agree to use time out of bed as an indicator of improved pain control. You have the patient sign an opiate treatment contract. You first ask her to stop her nabumetone and have her and her sister observe the effect on her functioning. Two weeks later, they report that there was no apparent change in her pain after discontinuation of nabumetone, so you do not prescribe nabumetone or any other NSAID for long-term use (although you suggest that the patient take ibuprofen 600 mg four times per day [q.i.d.] for acute pain flare-ups). You then gradually change her from oxycodone 480 mg per day to methadone 200 mg per day over a 4-week period.

You give the methadone in the form of a pain cocktail, so that the patient is blind to the dose. Over the next 6 months, and as agreed with the patient, you gradually reduce the dose of the methadone in the cocktail, so that the patient stabilizes at 80 mg of methadone per day. She tolerates this drug taper well. Because the patient reports significant symptoms of depression, you start her on citalopram 20 mg per day. The patient and her sister report that this medication leads to a reduction in her irritability and sense of hopelessness, although it does not affect her pain. You start her on amitriptyline for presumed neuropathic pain. However, even at low dosages (20 to 30 mg per day) the patient reports severe sedation and no pain relief. You stop the amitriptyline and prescribe gabapentin, building up to a dosage of 600 mg q.i.d. The patient tolerates this well, and she and her sister report that after starting gabapentin she is spending more time out of bed.

Eight months after you start treating the patient, she is on a stable medication regimen of methadone 80 mg per day, gabapentin 600 mg q.i.d., and citalopram 20 mg per day, and she consistently reports at least moderate pain relief relative to the pain she initially experienced. She then calls your office one day after hours, reporting a marked increase in her lower-extremity pain. She also says that for the past 2 days her urine has been foul-smelling, and her lower-extremity spasticity has been worse. She does not have a thermometer at her home but believes she is running fevers. You advise her to go to a local emergency room. You later talk on the phone with the emergency room physician, who suspects pyelonephritis, and learn that the patient is febrile to 103°. The plan is to admit her to the hospital for IV antibiotic therapy. The patient is admitted, started on antibiotic therapy, and given a patient-controlled analgesia (PCA) system for IV morphine. She defervesces over the next 24 hours. As her pyelonephritis resolves, her pain returns to baseline. After she is discharged from the hospital, you have her return to the medication regimen she was following before her admission.

Discussion

This patient probably had a central neuropathic type of pain. In such a patient, it is appropriate to prescribe tricyclic antidepressants and antiseizure medications, since both of these groups have demonstrated efficacy in controlling neuropathic pain (44,45). You should be aware that both types of medications can cause significant side effects. This patient showed very poor tolerance for amitriptyline, but tolerated gabapentin better, and she did report some pain relief from it.

Several key issues in this case involve opiates. Regardless of the pros and cons of chronic opiate therapy for nonmalignant pain in the abstract (see the previous discussion), this patient has specific issues that deserve comment. One is a history of drug and alcohol abuse. Most experts in pain management believe that such a history does not preclude the prescription of long-term opiate therapy, but clearly caution and careful observation are required if you do decide to prescribe them. This patient comes to you on sustained-release oxycodone (oxycontin). Because oxycontin can be ground up or otherwise altered to produce a drug "high," it is a poor choice in a patient with a history of substance abuse. If opiates are to be prescribed for such a patient, methadone is, in our opinion, the best choice. The main reason for choosing methadone is that it is an inherently long-acting drug. Thus, a patient cannot alter it in a way that changes its pharmacokinetics.

A second issue is that the patient comes to you on a very high dosage of oxycodone. It is not unusual for trauma patients to be treated aggressively with opiates right after injury and to be continued on them if they report ongoing pain. This prescribing pattern causes significant problems for a new physician who assumes care later on. It is virtually impossible to know how a patient might respond to a lower dose of an opiate, or

to complete discontinuation of the opiate, when you have seen her only when she is on a high dosage. Recognizing that there is no clear-cut research evidence about the efficacy of high-dosage opiate therapy, we recommend that this type of treatment be avoided (64). Although it is certainly possible that a patient might fail to get reasonable pain relief from moderate dosages of opiates but respond very well to high dosages, we think it is far more likely that patients slide into high opiate dosages because of a number of other issues, including unrecognized tolerance, desperate grasping for any intervention that offers a glimmer of pain relief, or reliance on the sedative effects of an opiate rather than its analgesic effect. In any case, we believe a physician should make a determined effort to reduce the opiate dosage in a patient who enters treatment on a high dosage regimen. In this example, the physician starts by converting the patient from oxycodone to a roughly equi-analgesic dose of methadone and then slowly tapers the methadone. The methadone is delivered by way of a pain cocktail in order to reduce the symbolic value that patients may place on opiates, and to minimize the chance that they experience increased pain during opiate tapers because they have conditioned responses to cues associated with opiate consumption (65,66).

This patient's high dosage of opiates also complicates the issue of switching to another opiate medication. Although there are published tables showing equivalent dosages among different opiates (67), it is important to be aware that the equivalences are very imprecise, and that there is very likely to be significant patient-to-patient variation in the response to changing from one opiate to another. Thus, when switching a patient from a high dosage of oxycodone to a high dosage of methadone, there is a significant risk of underdosing or overdosing. One way to minimize this risk is to make the conversion from one opiate to another (e.g., from oxycodone to methadone) in small steps. A simple strategy is to start by reducing the patient's oxycodone by 25% and giving her 25% of what is judged to be an equivalent dosage of methadone. The published data suggest that methadone is two to three times more potent than oxycodone. For the present patient, this means you would initially reduce her oxycodone from 480 mg per day to 360 mg per day and start her on methadone 40 mg per day. If she becomes agitated and demonstrates subtle signs of opiate withdrawal on this regimen, you will know that she is less responsive to methadone than standard tables would lead you to believe. In contrast, if she becomes sedated, you will know that she is extremely sensitive to methadone and that you should err on the low side when converting from oxycodone to methadone. With this information in hand, you can gradually reduce her oxycodone in 120-mg-per-day steps until her entire dose of oxycodone has been replaced by methadone.

Another issue relates to the appropriateness of opiates in the treatment of neuropathic pain. Some investigators have argued that opiates are effective for some kinds of pain, but not for neuropathic pain (50). However, more recent research indicates that although opiates are most likely to be helpful in acute nociceptive pain, they are effective enough against pain of any pathophysiologic origin to warrant consideration (51). This broad effectiveness is in contrast to other types of medications, which have narrower spectrums of action; for example, against neuropathic pain (tricyclic antidepressants and antiseizure medications) or pain secondary to inflammation (NSAIDs). The practical bottom line is that it is appropriate to consider opiates in any patient with refractory pain.

This case history also sheds light on the appropriate use of nonsteroidal anti-inflammatories in the management of chronic pain. Some patients are put on NSAIDs more or less permanently, without any obvious rationale.

Finally, the case highlights the point that you always must be alert to acute medical problems that may be contributing to a patient's pain. The general rule is that when increased pain is associated with other evidence of pathology (e.g., fever), you should consider the possibility of a medical work-up.

Case Number 2

Background

A 19-year-old man was involved in an accident while driving a motorcycle. He was not wearing a helmet. He hit his head against a telephone pole during the accident and sustained a skull fracture with intracerebral bleed. He was comatose for 10 days afterward. He did not sustain any other significant injuries in the accident. After his coma resolved, he demonstrated significant cognitive difficulties, along with right-sided paresis and spasticity. He reports diffuse pain in his right lower extremity. There is no obvious orthopaedic reason for this.

Treatment

You first evaluate the patient 4 weeks after his accident, when he is transferred to your rehabilitation facility. At that time he is taking oxycodone/acetaminophen (Tylox) (5/500) up to 12 tablets per day for pain control. He is on no other medications.

The patient is started in a vigorous gait training and general functional restoration program in physical therapy. You use feedback about his physical therapy performance and feedback from nursing staff and his speech therapist to monitor his pain control and overall progress.

Baseline cognitive assessment reveals that the patient is capable of understanding your standard opiate contract and appears to have sufficient impulse control to follow through on commitments that he makes. You have the patient sign an opiate treatment contract and change him from oxycodone/acetaminophen to extended-release

morphine sulfate (MS Contin) 30 mg twice per day (b.i.d.). Once this regimen is stabilized, you add piroxicam 20 mg per day. The patient and nursing staff report improved pain control, so you keep him on this regimen. You give him a trial on gabapentin, but nursing staff reports significant deterioration in his mental status, so the gabapentin is discontinued. You then prescribe carbamazepine and gradually increase the dose to 200 mg t.i.d. Because the patient does not demonstrate or report any mental status problems on carbamazepine, he reports significant pain relief, and the PTs report improved performance in his therapies, you continue him on this medication.

You address the patient's spasticity with stretching and proprioceptive neuromuscular facilitation exercises in physical therapy. Also, you start him on baclofen. At high dosages, he demonstrates cognitive deterioration, but you find that these effects do not occur if his dosage is limited to 10 mg t.i.d. and he demonstrates adequate reduction in spasticity with this dosage. He reports a significant reduction in his right lower extremity pain when his spasticity is controlled.

Your patient lives with his parents after he is discharged from your facility. You continue to treat him. You learn that he is getting ahead on his morphine sulfate, so that he finishes your monthly prescriptions in about 25 days rather than 30. You have a conference with the patient and his parents. The patient acknowledges that he has trouble resisting the temptation to take extra morphine sulfate when his pain level is high. Also, he reports that he sometimes forgets whether he has taken morphine sulfate or his other medications. He and his parents are comfortable with a plan in which they keep possession of all his medications and set out doses for him. This plan goes well in the sense that there are no more requests for early refills of medications.

Discussion

The patient in this case was thought to have neuropathic pain, because of the pain's widespread nature and the absence of any obvious orthopaedic condition to explain it. Medications appropriate for neuropathic pain were prescribed, and carbamazepine produced significant benefit. But as is the case with many patients, this individual's pain was probably multifactorial, as demonstrated by his positive response to piroxicam. One implication here is that if there is any reasonable chance that inflammation is contributing to a patient's pain—even when the pain is chronic—an NSAID is worth considering.

This case also raises complexities related to prescribing opiates. When you first see the patient, he is on high dosages of oxycodone/acetaminophen. This is a common situation and is problematic for two reasons. First, most pain experts believe that a patient who may receive long-term opiate therapy is better served by a long-acting opiate than by a short-acting one. Second, combination drugs like oxycodone/acetaminophen expose patients to the risk of liver toxicity from excessive doses of acetaminophen.

Another dilemma regarding opiates comes later, when the patient starts running ahead on his morphine sulfate prescriptions. One possibility would be to terminate opiate therapy on the grounds that the patient was non-compliant with your boundaries. However, the issue of how much responsibility this patient should assume is complicated by his organic brain syndrome and cognitive limitations. In the example, one possible solution was outlined—having a family member take physical control of a patient's medications. This option can produce serious strains between a patient and his significant others, but sometimes it is a reasonable way to resolve a difficult issue.

The case also highlights the problems that can occur when patients with CNS dysfunction are treated with centrally acting drugs. This patient shows a significant deterioration in cognitive functioning to gabapentin and baclofen. You should expect these kinds of problems in TBI patients. It is interesting to note that opiates appear to be less likely than other kinds of centrally acting drugs to produce cognitive dysfunction (68).

Finally, the case demonstrates the potential role of spasticity in aggravating pain in patients with CNS disorders. Treating spasticity is an example of treating an "upstream" problem that can contribute to pain.

Case Number 3

Background

A 34-year-old male roofer fell off a roof and sustained an L1 vertebral body fracture. There is no neurologic compromise. The patient was treated conservatively with bracing for several weeks. Radiography reveals his condition has stabilized, with no identifiable abnormality other than a 30% loss of height of the L1 vertebral body.

Treatment

You initially evaluate the patient 9 months after his injury. He reports severe pain at the thoracolumbar junction. He has no symptoms in his lower extremities. He is taking sustained-release oxycodone (oxycontin) 40 mg t.i.d. and diclofenac 75 mg b.i.d. for pain control. He is also on paroxetine 20 mg per day for "nerves." He has not returned to work since his accident and indicates that he spends most of his day lying in a reclining chair and watching TV. He has been through extensive physical therapy with no apparent benefit. He has undergone evaluation by an interventional pain physician. Diagnostic injections including medial branch blocks and discography at the thoracolumbar junction did not delineate any specific pain generator that might be a target for interventional therapy.

Treatment

You refer the patient to a multidisciplinary pain center. The patient subsequently goes through a 4-week pain management program in which he receives treatment 8 hours per day, 5 days per week. During this time, his opiates are tapered and then discontinued. The discharge summary from the pain management program indicates that the patient's physical capacities increased dramatically, and that his pain level decreased despite the fact that his oxycodone was discontinued completely. Also, he established the vocational goal of becoming a building inspector and was accepted by his workers' compensation carrier into a training program for this kind of work. The patient was continued on paroxetine during his pain center program. His diclofenac was briefly stopped twice but was restarted after the patient reported a sharp increase in pain.

When you re-evaluate the patient after he completes the pain management program, he does not demonstrate the guarding that you saw before he participated. He is obviously more confident and expresses optimism that he will be able to return to work. He indicates that he feels clearer mentally now that he is off oxycodone and believes that his pain control is good enough that he can function without opiates, as long as he is scrupulous about following through with the daily exercises he learned in the pain management program. You agree to monitor him as he goes through his vocational training and to resume management of his paroxetine and diclofenac, with the proviso that he will take diclofenac only intermittently.

Discussion

Case number 3 highlights the fact that multidisciplinary rehabilitative treatment can make an enormous difference for a patient with chronic pain. Research on multidisciplinary rehabilitative treatment has demonstrated its efficacy (43), particularly in the setting of low back pain. This patient demonstrated substantial functional gains with multidisciplinary treatment, was tapered completely off his opiates, and developed a vocational plan.

Multidisciplinary pain centers are particularly effective in getting patients off opiates. This is an important matter. Now that physicians are (for the most part) free from disciplinary action for prescribing opiates, it is common to see patients with chronic pain who are on opiates indefinitely. It is difficult for a treating physician to taper such a patient off opiates without gravely damaging rapport with the patient. In contrast, at a pain center patients usually can be tapered off opiates uneventfully. It may be appropriate for their treating physicians to restart opiate therapy after patients complete pain center treatment, but at least the patients get a clean slate with respect to opiates as they go through pain center treatment, get an opportunity to see how they feel and how they function when drug-free, and reverse their tolerance, so that they are likely to respond to lower doses if opiate therapy is reintroduced later.

This case also raises questions about the appropriate role of NSAIDs in a patient with chronic musculoskeletal pain. Many of these patients report pain relief with NSAIDs over long periods of time. Unfortunately, prolonged, continuous use of NSAIDs puts them at risk for gastrointestinal, renal, and hepatic toxicity. One option in this difficult situation is to urge patients to take NSAIDs intermittently. If you do put a patient on continuous long-term NSAID therapy, you should consult guidelines established by the American College of Rheumatology regarding monitoring for potential problems (69).

Case Number 4

Background

A 46-year-old woman slipped on ice and fractured her right tibia. She underwent open reduction and internal fixation of the fracture. She appears to have made a satisfactory recovery from an orthopaedic standpoint, but within a few days of her accident she reported severe, diffuse pain in the distal right lower extremity. Along with this, she developed diffuse swelling of the right foot. The right foot was also cool, cyanotic, and diaphoretic. A diagnostic work-up did not reveal any orthopaedic abnormality in the right ankle/foot or any vascular abnormality to account for her symptoms. She was given a diagnosis of reflex sympathetic dystrophy (complex regional pain syndrome).

You first evaluate the patient 6 months after her injury. At that time, she reports that she wears a rigid boot over her right foot and ankle essentially all day long and uses axillary crutches to ambulate. She is on 30 mg q.i.d. of morphine sulfate for pain control; she does not take any other medications. She readily acknowledges significant depression because of her ongoing pain and activity restrictions.

On physical examination, the patient demonstrates findings of complex regional pain syndrome (CRPS) as described above. Also noteworthy is the fact that she is extremely guarded in the use of her right lower extremity, and hypersensitive to stimulation of it. For example, she winces and withdraws to gentle stroking of her foot and distal leg and shows severe, pain-inhibited weakness during manual muscle testing in the right lower extremity. She is unwilling to put her right foot on the floor when asked to walk without her boot.

Treatment

You discuss the significance of CRPS with her and emphasize that her best chance of getting substantial functional improvement will be to undergo therapies to produce at least partial pain relief and use the respite to start mobilizing her right lower extremity with a progressive exercise program. You refer her to a physical therapist who is familiar with CRPS. You instruct the physical therapist to perform a careful functional assessment initially

and to monitor the patient's functional improvement as she goes through therapeutic trials to control her pain better. Also, you ask the therapist to start a desensitization program on the patient in order to deal with her cutaneous hypersensitivity. The desensitization program consists of stimulating the hypersensitive areas with progressively rougher materials.

Over the next 4 months, you supervise trials on several different medications, including NSAIDS, opiates, tricyclic antidepressants, antiseizure medications, mexilitine, prednisone, phenoxybenzamine, and transdermal clonidine. These produce modest and inconsistent improvement, as indicated both by the patient and by the physical therapist who is monitoring her performance. The one medication that does make a substantial difference is fluoxetine, which helps the patient's emotional distress.

Also, you refer the patient to an interventional pain physician for a series of lumbar sympathetic blocks. These are scheduled in a way that is coordinated with the patient's physical therapy sessions. Specifically, she gets a lumbar sympathetic block in the morning and a physical therapy session the same day in the afternoon. The goal is to establish a pattern that will permit the patient to convert pain control into functional improvement. She does in fact demonstrate improved function in the physical therapy sessions that follow sympathetic blocks, but her performance returns to baseline within a few days after a block, and she does not show progressive improvement over a series of four such blocks.

At the end of 7 months, the patient is no longer using crutches and does not wear her boot all day long, but she is still severely limited in ambulation and reports only slightly less pain than when she started treatment with you. You then refer her back to the interventional pain specialist for a trial on spinal cord stimulation. The patient undergoes placement of temporary leads and reports virtually complete relief from her pain during the trial. She then undergoes placement of a permanent spinal cord stimulator. Four months later, she is able to ambulate without her boot, and her walking tolerance has increased to approximately two blocks. Also, she has been able to resume work as an office manager. But she still reports significant right lower extremity pain and continues to take a combination of morphine sulfate 30 mg b.i.d. plus nortriptyline 75 mg every night at bedtime (q.h.s.), along with fluoxetine 40 mg per day.

Discussion

The pathophysiology underlying CRPS is not well understood. Many observers believe that CNS sensitization is crucial to its development (70), but the exact pathophysiology remains a mystery. The mystery is especially deep when CRPS develops after a relatively modest orthopaedic problem and persists long after the orthopaedic problem has resolved.

In the face of the above uncertainty, pharmacologic treatment of CRPS is often empirical, with a wide range of options used. In this example, the patient was stabilized on an opiate, a tricyclic antidepressant (for presumed neuropathic pain), and a selective serotonin re-uptake inhibitor (SSRI) antidepressant (to treat her depression rather than her pain).

There is almost unanimous agreement among physicians who treat CRPS that patients must overcome their activity aversion and start progressively mobilizing their affected limb if they are to have much of a chance of a good recovery. Thus, interventional therapies such as medications and nerve blocks are often linked closely with active physical therapy.

An interventional pain specialist played a major role in the treatment of this patient. While the use of interventional therapies in CRPS or any other chronic pain syndrome remains controversial, some patients do report impressive responses to interventions such as spinal cord stimulation. Because of the potential for interventional therapies to benefit patients with chronic pain syndromes, you need to be familiar enough with them to provide appropriate guidance to your patients and to interface appropriately with interventional pain specialists. Note, though, that the patient in this example was by no means pain-free after placement of a spinal cord stimulator and continued to need pharmacologic support. This is typical of a patient with CRPS.

CONCLUSIONS

We have attempted in this chapter to provide a realistic picture of the complexities and ambiguities involved in treating chronic pain in people who have sustained significant trauma. In order to treat these patients effectively, it is important to remain flexible in assessments (that is, to avoid putting every patient in the same conceptual pigeonhole), be resourceful in the use of therapies, be able to achieve some balance between catering to all the demands that patients will make and hostilely rejecting them, and be willing to tolerate the inevitable treatment failures that will occur.

Many physicians are tempted to run the other way when they think about managing chronic pain in patients who have experienced trauma. We believe that there are several important reasons to avoid this impulse and make an effort to develop skill in pain management. First, chronic pain is an extremely common problem in trauma patients. Second, chronic pain has enormous consequences for the quality of life of these patients. Conversely, effective treatment of chronic pain can have an enormously positive influence on patients' attempts

to return to reasonably normal functioning following serious traumas. Finally, many of the concepts we have elaborated in this chapter for treating chronic pain are entirely consistent with general concepts of rehabilitation medicine. Thus, your training as a physiatrist gives you tools that are generally not available to other medical specialists, and that can, with moderate effort, be adapted to the treatment of chronic pain.

REFERENCES

1. Finnerup NB, Johannesen IL, Sindrup SH, et al. Pain and dysesthesia in patients with spinal cord injury: A postal survey. *Spinal Cord.* 2001;39:256–262.
2. Ravenscroft A, Ahmed YS, Burnside IG. Chronic pain after SCI: A patient survey. *Spinal Cord.* 2000;38:611–614.
3. Rintala DH, Loubser PG, Castro J, et al. Chronic pain in a community-based sample of men with spinal cord injury: Prevalence, severity, and relationship with impairment, disability, handicap, and subjective well-being. *Arch Phys Med Rehabil.* 1998;79:604–614.
4. Siddall PJ, Taylor DA, McClelland JM, et al. Pain report and the relationship of pain to physical factors in the first 6 months following spinal cord injury. *Pain.* 1999;81:187–197.
5. Turner JA, Cardenas DD. Chronic pain problems in individuals with spinal cord injuries. *Semin Clin Neuropsychiatry.* 1999;4:186–194.
6. Turner JA, Cardenas DD, Warms CA, et al. Chronic pain associated with spinal cord injuries: A community survey. *Arch Phys Med Rehabil.* 2001;82:501–508.
7. Ehde DM, Czerniecki JM, Smith DG, et al. Chronic phantom sensations, phantom pain, residual limb pain, and other regional pain after lower limb amputation. *Arch Phys Med Rehabil.* 2000;81:1039–1044.
8. Jensen TS, Krebs B, Nielson J, et al. Immediate and long-term phantom limb pain in amputees: Incidence, clinical characteristics and relationship to pre-amputation limb pain. *Pain.* 1985;21:267–278.
9. Kooijman CM, Dijkstra PU, Geertzen JHB, et al. Phantom pain and phantom sensations in upper limb amputees: An epidemiological study. *Pain.* 2000;87:33–41.
10. Wilkins KL, McGrath PJ, Finley GA, et al. Phantom limb sensations and phantom limb pain in child and adolescent amputees. *Pain.* 1998;78:7–12.
11. Pezzin LE, Dillingham TR, MacKenzie EJ. Rehabilitation and the long-term outcomes of persons with trauma-related amputations. *Arch Phys Med Rehabil.* 2000;81:292–300.
12. Barrett H, McClelland JM, Rutkowski SB, et al. Pain characteristics in patients admitted to hospital with complications after spinal cord injury. *Arch Phys Med Rehabil.* 2003;84:789–795.
13. Widerström-Noga EG, Felipe-Cuervo E, Yezierski R. Chronic pain after spinal injury: Interference with sleep and daily activities. *Arch Phys Med Rehabil.* 2001;82:1571–1577.
14. Ehde DM, Smith DG, Czerniecki JM, et al. Back pain as a secondary disability in persons with lower limb amputations. *Arch Phys Med Rehabil.* 2001;82:731–734.

15. Jensen MP, Smith DG, Ehde DM, et al. Pain site and the effects of amputation pain: Further clarification of the meaning of mild, moderate, and severe pain. *Pain*. 2001;91:317–322.

16. Robinson JP, Fulton-Kehoe D, Franklin GM. Functional limitations among injured workers 4.5 years after undergoing pain center treatment. *Arch Phys Med Rehabil*. 2002;83(11):1669.

17. Woolf CJ, Max MB. Mechanism-based pain diagnosis. *Anesthesiology*. 2001;95:241–249.

18. Loeser JD, ed. *Bonica's management of pain*. 3rd ed. Philadelphia, PA: Lippincott Williams & Wilkins; 2001.

19. Wall PD, Melzack R, eds. *Textbook of pain*. 4th ed. New York, NY: Churchill Livingstone; 1999.

20. Terman GW, Bonica JJ. Spinal mechanisms and their modulation. In: Loeser JD, ed. *Bonica's management of pain*. 3rd ed. Philadelphia, PA: Lippincott Williams & Wilkins; 2001.

21. Dubner R. Neuronal plasticity in the spinal and medullary dorsal horns: A possible role in central pain mechanisms. In: Casey KL, ed. *Pain and central nervous system disease*. New York, NY: Raven Press; 1991.

22. Curatolo M, Petersen-Felix S, Arendt-Nielsen L, et al. Central hypersensitivity in chronic pain after whiplash injury. *Clin J Pain*. 2001;17(4):306–315.

23. Sorensen J, Graven-Nielsen T, Henriksson KG, et al. Hyperexcitability in fibromyalgia. *J Rheumatol*. 1998; 25(1):152–155.

24. Melzack R, Coderre TJ, Katz J, et al. Central neuroplasticity and pathological pain. *Ann N Y Acad Sci*. 2001;933:157–174.

25. Turk DC, Robinson JP, Loeser JD. Pain. In: Cocchiarella L, Andersson GBJ, eds. *Guides to the evaluation of permanent impairment*. 5th ed. Chicago, IL: AMA Press; 2001.

26. Doubell TP, Mannion RJ, Woolf CJ. The dorsal horn: State-dependent sensory processing, plasticity and the generation of pain. In: Wall PD, Melzack R, eds. *Textbook of pain*. 4th ed. New York, NY: Churchill Livingstone; 1999.

27. Robinson JP, Brown PB, Fisk JD. Pathophysiology of lumbar radiculopathies and the pharmacology of epidural corticosteroids and local anesthetics. *Phys Med Rehabil Clin N Am*. 1995;6(4):671–690.

28. Byers MR, Bonica JJ. Peripheral pain mechanisms and nociceptor plasticity. In: Loeser JD, ed. *Bonica's management of pain*. 3rd ed. Philadelphia, PA: Lippincott Williams & Wilkins; 2001.

29. Boivie J. Central pain. In: Wall PD, Melzack R, eds. *Textbook of pain*. 4th ed. New York, NY: Churchill Livingstone; 1999.

30. Hoheisel U, Mense S. Long-term changes in discharge behaviour of cat dorsal horn neurones following noxious stimulation of deep tissues. *Pain*. 1989; 36:239–247.

31. Turk DC, Flor H. Chronic pain: A biobehavioral perspective. In: Gatchel RJ, Turk DC, eds. *Psychosocial factors in pain: Critical perspectives*. New York, NY: Guilford Press; 1999:18–34.

32. Mense S, Simons DG. *Muscle pain*. Philadelphia, PA: Lippincott Williams & Wilkins; 2001.

33. Gatchel RJ, Turk DC. *Psychosocial factors in pain: Critical perspectives*. New York, NY: Guilford Press; 1999.

34. Scarry E. *The body in pain*. New York, NY: Oxford University Press; 1985.

35. Haetzman M, Elliott AM, Smith BH, et al. Chronic pain and the use of conventional and alternative therapy. *Fam Pract*. 2003;20(2):147–154.

36. Wolsko PM, Eisenberg DM, Davis RB, et al. Patterns and perceptions of care for treatment of back and neck pain: Results of a national survey. *Spine*. 2003; 28(3):292–297; discussion 298.

37. Robinson JP. Disability evaluation in painful conditions. In: Turk DC, Melzack R, eds. *Handbook of pain assessment*, 2nd ed. New York, NY: The Guilford Press; 2001.

38. Osterweis M, Kleinman A, Mechanic D, eds. *Pain and disability*. Washington, DC: National Academy Press; 1987.

39. Hidding A, van Santen M, De Klerk E, et al. Comparison between self-report measures and clinical observations of functional disability in ankylosing spondylitis, rheumatoid arthritis and fibromyalgia. *J Rheumatol*. 1994;21(5):818–823.

40. Deyo RA, Phillips WR. Low back pain: A primary care challenge. *Spine*. 1996;21:2826–2832.

41. Borkan J, Van Tulder M, Reis S, et al. Advances in the field of low back pain in primary care. *Spine*. 2002; 27:E128–E132.

42. Loeser JD. Multidisciplinary pain programs. In: Loeser JD, ed. *Bonica's management of pain*. 3rd ed. Philadelphia, PA: Lippincott Williams & Wilkins; 2001.

43. Guzman J, Esmail R, Karjalainen K, et al. Multidisciplinary rehabilitation for chronic low back pain: Systematic review. *BMJ*. 2001;322:1511–1516.

44. Max MB. Antidepressants as analgesics. In: Fields HL, Liebeskind JC, eds. *Pharmacological approaches to the treatment of chronic pain: New concepts and critical issues*. Seattle, WA: IASP Press; 1994.

45. Rowbotham MC, Petersen KL, Davies PS. Recent developments in the treatment of neuropathic pain. In: Devor M, Rowbotham MC, Wiesenfeld-Hallin Z, eds. *Proceedings of the 9th world congress on pain*. Seattle, WA: IASP Press; 2000.

46. Robinson JP. Disability management in primary care. In: McCarberg B, Passik SD, eds. *Expert guide to pain management*. American College of Physicians; 2005.

47. Portenoy RK. Opioid therapy for chronic nonmalignant pain: A review of the critical issues. *J Pain Symptom Manage*. 1996;11:203–217.

48. Schug SA, Merry AF, Acland RH. Treatment principles for the use of opioids in pain of nonmalignant origin. *Drugs*. 1991;42:228–239.

49. Hoffman DE, Tarzian AJ. Achieving the right balance in oversight of physician opioid prescribing for pain: The role of state medical boards. *J Law Med Ethics*. 2003;31:21–23.

50. Arner S, Meyerson BA. Lack of analgesic effect of opioids on neuropathic and idiopathic forms of pain. *Pain*. 1988;33:11–23.

51. Kalso E. Opioids for chronic noncancer pain. In: Dostrovsky JO, Carr DB, Koltzenburg M, eds. *Proceedings of the 10th World Congress on Pain*. Seattle, WA: IASP Press; 2003:751–765.

52. Tennant FS, Uelman GF. Narcotic maintenance for chronic pain: Medical and legal guidelines. *Postgrad Med*. 1983;73:81–94.

53. Portenoy RK, Foley KM. Chronic use of opioid analgesics in non-malignant pain: Report of 58 cases. *Pain*. 1986;25:171–186.

54. Arkinstall W, Sandler A, Goughnour B, et al. Efficacy of controlled-release codeine in chronic non-malignant pain: A randomized, placebo-controlled clinical trial. *Pain*. 1995;62:169–178.

55. Jamison RN, Raymond SA, Slawsby EA, et al. Opioid therapy for chronic noncancer back pain. *Spine*. 1998; 23:2591–2600.

56. Moulin EM, Iezzi A, Amireh R, et al. Randomized trial of oral morphine for chronic non-cancer pain. *Lancet.* 1996;347:143–147.

57. Peloso PM, Bellamy N, Bensen W, et al. Double blind randomized placebo control trial of controlled release codeine in the treatment of osteoarthritis of the hip or knee. *J Rheumatol.* 2000;27:764–771.

58. Roth SH, Fleischmann RM, Burch FX, et al. Around-the-clock, controlled-release oxycodone therapy for osteoarthritis-related pain. *Arch Intern Med.* 2000;160:853–860.

59. Sharif RN, Osborne M, Coderre TJ, et al. Attenuation of morphine tolerance after antisense oligonucleotide knock-down of spinal mGluR1. *Br J Pharmacol.* 2002;136(6):865–872.

60. von Zastrow M, Svingos A, Haberstock-Debic H, et al. Regulated endocytosis of opioid receptors: Cellular mechanisms and proposed roles in physiological adaptation to opiate drugs. *Curr Opin Neurobiol.* 2003;13(3):348–353.

61. Rapp SE, Ready LB, Nessly ML. Acute pain management in patients with prior opioid consumption: A case-controlled retrospective review. *Pain.* 1995;61(2):195–201.

62. Chabal C, Erjavec MK, Jacobson L, et al. Prescription opiate abuse in chronic pain patients: Clinical criteria, incidence, and predictors. *Clin J Pain.* 1997;13(2):150–155.

63. Turk DC. Are pain syndromes acute or chronic diseases? *Clin J Pain.* 2000;16(4):279–280.

64. Ballantyne JC, Mao J. Opioid therapy for chronic pain. *N Engl J Med.* 2003;349:1943–1953.

65. Ader R. Conditioned responses in pharmacotherapy research. *Psychol Med.* 1993;23(2):297–299.

66. Fordyce WE. *Behavioral methods for chronic pain and illness.* St. Louis, MO: Mosby; 1976.

67. Miyoshi HR, Leckgand SG. Systemic opioid analgesics. In: Loeser JD, ed. *Bonica's management of pain.* 3rd ed. Philadelphia, PA: Lippincott Williams & Wilkins; 2001.

68. Zacny JP. A review of the effects of opioids on psychomotor and cognitive functioning in humans. *Exp Clin Psychopharmacol.* 1995;3:432–466.

69. American College of Rheumatology. Guidelines for monitoring drug therapy in rheumatoid arthritis. Available at: http://www.rheumatology.org/publications/guidelines/ra-drug/ra-drug.asp?aud=mem. Accessed January 22, 2004.

70. Baron R, Binder A, Schattschneider J. Pathophysiology and treatment of complex regional pain syndromes. In: Dostrovsky JO, Carr DB, Koltzenburg M, eds. *Proceedings of the 10th world congress on pain.* Seattle, WA: IASP Press; 2003.

12

Management of Substance Abuse after Trauma

Charles H. Bombardier

OVERVIEW

Substance abuse, especially alcohol intoxication, is the underlying cause of nearly half of traumatic injuries in the United States (1). It is tempting to assume that alcohol-related injuries are largely due to isolated episodes of intoxication among otherwise normal drinkers. However, large-scale survey data among trauma patients indicate that 75% of intoxicated patients have a prior history of clinically significant alcohol-related life problems and 26% of non intoxicated patients will also admit to significant pre-injury alcohol problems (2). Given the pattern revealed by this data, it is not surprising that alcoholism is also reported to be the most prevalent chronic disease among trauma survivors (3). Furthermore, prospective controlled studies reveal that injured problem drinkers are subsequently more likely to be reinjured, rehospitalized, and die compared to normal controls (4–6). Despite the prevalence and importance of substance abuse among trauma survivors, effective screening and interventions for substance use disorders are conspicuously absent from many trauma rehabilitation programs (1).

This chapter will examine what is known about substance abuse disorders among people with traumatic brain injury (TBI) and spinal cord injury (SCI). Rates of alcohol problems are particularly high among persons with traumatic injuries, including TBI (7) and SCI (8). Therefore, TBI and SCI will be used as examples of disabling conditions in which alcohol-related problems play a significant role. Studies from the general trauma literature will be used to

supplement the review when data on people with SCI and TBI are limited. While the focus of this chapter will be on substance abuse, the quantity and quality of data on alcohol-related problems exceed the data on other drug use problems. Consequently, in this chapter, data on alcohol will dominate and other drug use will be discussed when possible.

Links between alcohol problems and these two forms of acquired disability will be described in terms of the prevalence and effects on outcome. The chapter will describe the major ways alcohol problems and models of treatment are conceptualized, including how persistent stereotypes and myths about substance abuse may interfere with implementation of effective screening and intervention programs. Practical strategies for screening, assessing, and intervening in alcohol-related problems within the context of rehabilitation will be discussed with an emphasis on seeing rehabilitation as a window of opportunity for intervening in these problems. Rehabilitation physicians, nurses, psychologists, and others without extensive training in addictions can play useful roles in preventing return to substance abuse following rehabilitation.

THE PREVALENCE AND IMPACT OF ALCOHOL AND DRUG ABUSE IN PEOPLE WITH TRAUMATIC BRAIN INJURY AND SPINAL CORD INJURY

There are two major reasons why alcohol problems merit special attention among people with TBI and SCI. The first reason is the sheer prevalence of alcohol-related problems in these populations. The second is the potential that alcohol may contribute to poor recovery or secondary complications. In the following section, prevalence will be described in terms of pre-injury alcohol problems, intoxication at the time of injury, and postinjury alcohol problems.

Pre-injury Alcohol and Drug Abuse

Corrigan (7) reviewed the literature on alcohol and TBI and found that the occurrence of pre-injury alcohol abuse or dependence ranged from 16% to 66%. The most rigorous studies and those conducted in rehabilitation settings produced the highest occurrence rates, between 44% and 66%. Most recently researchers found 59% of consecutive inpatients with TBI were considered "at-risk" drinkers (9). In terms of pre-injury drug use this study reported that 31.4% used illicit drugs within the 3-month period before their injury (9). Only 27% of this sample abstained from alcohol or drugs or used alcohol normally. The data on drinking before SCI are more limited. Persons with SCI report greater than average pre-injury alcohol consumption, and 35% to 49% report a history of significant alcohol problems (8,10).

Much larger studies of pre-injury alcohol problems have been conducted on general trauma patients. Rivara and colleagues (2) found that 44% of consecutive trauma admissions scored in the "alcoholic" range on a brief screening measure. A similar study (11) found that 24% of all admissions met diagnostic criteria for current alcohol dependence (28% for males and 15% for females) while 17.7% met criteria for drug dependence.

Substance Use at the Time of Injury

Another indication of alcohol- or drug-related problems among people with TBI or SCI can be derived from toxicology data at the time of injury. Among patients with TBI, Corrigan (7) found that rates of alcohol intoxication (blood alcohol level >100 mg per dL) ranged from 36% to 51% among the seven studies reviewed. Bombardier et al. (9) reported that toxicology data on 114 of 137 consecutive patients with TBI revealed 23.7% tested positive for marijuana, 13.2% for cocaine, and 8.8% for amphetamine. A total of 37.7% tested positive for one or more illicit drugs. Alcohol intoxication rates reported in the SCI literature are 40% (12) and 36% (13). Among general trauma patients Rivara et al. (2) found that 47% had a positive blood alcohol test while 36% were intoxicated. Toxicology assays from a large sample of general trauma patients revealed 16% tested positive for opiates, 14% for cocaine, 11% for marijuana, 1% for phencyclidine, and 0.1% for amphetamine (11). Data on toxicology assays for opiates should be interpreted cautiously, since opiates are commonly used in emergency medical management of trauma.

Postinjury Substance Abuse and Problems

Longitudinal surveys of alcohol use and alcohol problems among persons with TBI and SCI show that drinking declines during the months immediately following injury (14,15) followed by increased drinking during the first and second years after injury, at least for people with TBI (14,16). At 1 year after injury, about one quarter of people with TBI report heavy drinking, significant alcohol-related problems, or both (16,17). This represents 1-year remission rates of 31% to 56%. Pre-injury alcohol use and problems are highly predictive of use and problems in the year following injury (17). Some people begin problem drinking for the first time following their injury (18,19), though this pattern appears to occur in only about 7% of normal drinkers (17). Alcohol consumption after TBI may be somewhat higher than in the general population (20,21), whereas abuse, but not use of alcohol, seems more frequent in people with SCI than in the general population (20). Drinking rates may be particularly high among selected groups such as vocational rehabilitation clients (22), those in postacute care rehabilitation programs (23), and among veterans with SCI (24).

Taken together, rates of lifetime alcohol abuse or dependence approach 50% in people with TBI or SCI, while current dependence is nearly 25%. The prevalence of pre-injury alcohol dependence is roughly three to six times higher than in the general population (25,26). For many persons, there is a natural remission in problem drinking after trauma. This period of remission appears stable for many and probably is not dependent on formal treatment (14). This "natural recovery" is known to occur on a widespread basis without formal help in community samples of people with alcohol problems, often in response to changes in health (27). As will be discussed later, natural recovery may represent spontaneous healing processes that can be exploited in the context of rehabilitation. On the other hand, a significant fraction of people with alcohol dependency resume problem drinking, probably as the person achieves greater independence and has increased access to alcohol. Little is known about what triggers relapse into problem drinking or drug use after injury. People in postacute and vocational rehabilitation settings may have especially high rates of alcohol abuse, possibly because alcohol problems interfere with achievement of community integration goals and necessitate additional psychosocial services. These settings may represent important opportunities for interventions.

THE EFFECT OF SUBSTANCE ABUSE ON OUTCOMES

Alcohol Intoxication

Studies of the effects of alcohol intoxication on neurologic outcomes provide mixed results. Some studies have shown that alcohol intoxication at the time of TBI is associated with poorer short-term outcomes such as longer length of coma, longer period of agitation (28), and greater cognitive impairment postinjury (29,30). Other studies of persons with TBI have found no relationship between blood alcohol level and neurologic outcome (31,32). Alcohol may have both neuroprotective and neurotoxic effects in the context of acute TBI (33). In the case of SCI, both animal (34) and human studies (13) suggest that alcohol intoxication may be associated with more severe injury.

Pre-injury Alcohol Problems

A pre-jury pattern of chronic alcohol abuse or dependence is predictive of numerous negative outcomes after TBI and SCI. Pre-injury alcohol abuse is associated with increased risk of mortality and more severe brain lesions (7). A history of alcohol abuse is thought to increase the risk of recurrent TBI (35,36) and is associated with development of posttraumatic seizures (37) and cerebral atrophy (38). Several studies report poorer cognitive recovery among those with a history of significant alcohol-related problems (39–42). In the best controlled study, patients with a history of alcohol abuse demonstrated poorer neuropsychological test performance 1 month and 1 year postinjury (42). Similarly, pre-injury alcohol problems predict poorer community integration (43) and deterioration of emotional and behavioral functioning during the postacute recovery phase (44). It should be noted that since many of these studies were not able to completely control for potential confounding factors, the precise role pre-injury alcohol abuse plays in poorer outcomes remains ambiguous (42).

SCI patients with a history of pre-injury problem drinking may be at greater risk for postinjury medical complications, and this may be due to differences in rehabilitation participation or rate of functional gain. Those with premorbid alcohol problems have been found to spend less time in productive activities such as rehabilitation therapies (45). A history of problem drinking is associated with 36% less average functional independence measure (FIM) improvement per day compared to normal drinkers (46). Heinemann and Hawkins (47) reported that individuals with a history of significant alcohol problems who abstained after injury had higher rates of urinary tract infections and pressure ulcers, as well as greater depression and lower acceptance of disability compared to all other subjects combined. Elliott et al. (48) found that at 1 to 3 years post-SCI, the odds of pressure ulcer occurrence for those with a history of significant alcohol problems was >2.5 times greater than for those without such a history. People with SCI and a history of alcohol problems have significantly higher rates of suicide (49).

The general trauma literature also demonstrates that a history of significant alcohol-related problems confers an increased risk of reinjury, rehospitalization, and death following the index injury. One longitudinal study of substance-abusing patients found that within 5 years of an initial injury requiring hospitalization, 44% had been reinjured and 20% had died due to recurrent trauma, mostly substance abuse–related (4). In another study, patients with indications of significant alcohol-related problems were more than twice as likely to be readmitted for traumatic injuries compared to case controls without comorbid alcohol-related problems (6). There is little reason to think these findings would not generalize to people who sustain TBI or SCI.

Postinjury Alcohol Use or Abuse

It is widely suspected that even moderate alcohol consumption after TBI may dampen neurological recovery and magnify cognitive impairments (23). Yet there is surprisingly little empirical research in this area. Clearly, alcoholism can cause cognitive impairment, including permanent brain damage (50). Cognitive impairment also can develop in heavy "social drinkers," and the effects are roughly dose-dependent (51). The only study of brain function influenced by drinking after TBI found that event-related potentials are more impaired among persons with TBI who also abused alcohol than among persons who only had a TBI or only abused alcohol (52). Support for the idea that TBI magnifies the acute neurocognitive effects of alcohol comes from self-reports of increased sensitivity to alcohol (53) and the finding that alcohol intoxication and TBI produce similar neuropsychological impairments (54).

Regarding persons with SCI living in the community, alcohol abuse is associated with poorer subjective health, higher levels of depressive symptoms, and more life stress (20). Marijuana use is also associated with greater occurrence of depressive symptoms and life stress (20). Krause (55) speculates that return to drinking may interfere with health maintenance behaviors secondary to impaired judgment, coordination, and memory. Curiously, people with pre-injury alcohol problems who *abstained* from alcohol after injury have been found to be at increased risk for developing pressure sores (47).

Taken together, the relevant literature could be interpreted to suggest that alcohol intoxication at the time of injury is most likely to affect early indicators of cognitive function, but that with time and physical recovery, the influence of intoxication on cognitive functioning diminishes. The effect of pre-injury alcohol abuse and problems on postinjury outcomes is the most well-established finding. However, even this relationship remains controversial because of the potential confounding effects of numerous variables including education level and pre-injury socioeconomic status, as well as postinjury drinking. Extremely little is known about the additional risks attributable to alcohol use or abuse that occurs after TBI or SCI. Studies are needed that examine the differential impact on outcomes of pre-injury alcohol abuse, intoxication at the time of injury, and postinjury alcohol use. The effects of alcohol on cognition, behavior, complications (e.g., seizures), and functional recovery after TBI merit further research. Studies are needed on the effects of alcohol on immune functioning, sexual functioning, depression, rehabilitation participation, and self-care after SCI. The effects of drug abuse in people with TBI or SCI are largely unknown.

MODELS OF ADDICTION AND INTERVENTIONS

HISTORICAL PERSPECTIVE: COMPETING MODELS OF ALCOHOLISM

Alcoholism can be conceptualized in categorical terms as a disease or as a continuum of alcohol-related problems. The prevailing disease model is represented by the *Diagnostic and Statistical Manual of Mental Disorders*, Fourth Edition (DSM-IV) (56), definition of alcohol dependence. The disease model views alcoholics as qualitatively different from nonalcoholic persons. That is, persons with alcoholism are thought to have a medical or psychological defect resulting in behaviors such as excessive consumption. Traditionally alcoholism is believed to be progressive and can only be put in remission through abstinence. Nonalcoholics are assumed to have no such defect and to experience no adverse consequences from alcohol.

The emphasis on alcoholism as a disease follows a historical pattern similar to that of other medical conditions:

As a 1990 report from the Institute of Medicine (IOM) explains, "The historical record also suggests that treatment for any problem tends to originate as a result of attention being drawn to severe cases. Initially, treatment consists of applying to these cases the existing remedies that are available when the problem is first recognized. *As time passes, however, it becomes increasingly clear that (a) cases other than severe cases exist and (b) other methods can be used to deal with them...Thus, it is not surprising to find the same progression in the treatment of persons with alcohol problems*" [italics added] (57).

Much contemporary theory and research on alcoholism has moved away from the categorical disease model and toward a continuum model that holds that alcohol-related problems occur along a spectrum of severity (58). Although it is predicated upon the disease model, the *DSM-IV* recognizes gradations of alcoholism other than dependence through the diagnosis of alcohol abuse (56). The IOM report (57) is notable for moving even farther from the disease model by explicitly adopting a terminology of "alcohol problems" that are expressed along numerous dimensions.

In the IOM report, a triangle diagram was developed to represent this continuum of alcohol problems (Fig. 12–1). The area of the triangle depicts the entire United States population with regard to alcohol consumption and alcohol-related problems. The figure illustrates a number of important conceptual shifts that are relevant to the issue of alcohol and disability.

First, prototypical alcoholics represent a minority of Americans with alcohol problems. A larger proportion of Americans consumes hazardous amounts of alcohol and incurs significant harm from alcohol use without meeting criteria for alcoholism or seeking help. Second, the IOM model emphasizes that there are no clear boundaries between normal use and abuse of alcohol or between alcohol abuse and dependence. Third, individuals seem to shift back and forth along the continuum. Among persons with alcoholism, consumption and the degree of alcohol-related problems vary significantly over the course of the person's lifetime (59). Moreover, the majority of the shifting that occurs is probably not attributable to treatment (27). Finally, the continuum model provides a more appropriate framework through which to view the modal person with alcoholism, and someone with mild to moderate problems with alcohol, whom rehabilitation staff will encounter.

COMMON MYTHS ABOUT SUBSTANCE ABUSE

A number of widely held assumptions appear to conflict with the contemporary literature on addictive behaviors and could interfere with potential

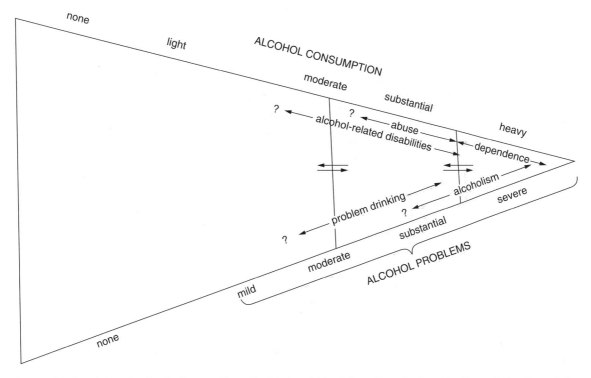

Figure 12–1. A terminological map. (From Institute of Medicine. *Broadening the Base of Treatment for Alcohol Problems*. Washington, DC: National Academy Press; 1990, with permission.)

innovations in clinical care. First, there is the belief that patients must acknowledge they have an alcohol problem before they can change their drinking. Yet, accepting that one is an "alcoholic" is not only unrelated to treatment outcomes but generates unnecessary resistance as the person naturally rejects a stigmatizing label (60). A nonjudgmental attitude on the part of the therapist and avoiding labels is thought to facilitate greater motivation to change and more valid self-reporting (60).

Next, there is a belief that alcoholism is a "disease of denial" and that denial is a personality trait of people with alcoholism. Numerous studies conducted over many years have failed to find systematic differences between alcoholics and nonalcoholics on measures of denial (60). Instead, carefully controlled studies have shown that patient denial varies as a function of *therapist* behaviors (61). Therapists whose style is to confront their patients with evidence of their drinking problem elicit more denial and resistive behavior from their clients. Therapists who are more empathic, listen reflectively, and communicate acceptance of their client's problems elicit less resistance and denial (61). The traditional confrontation-of-denial approach is correlated with poorer outcomes, including higher levels of drinking 1 year after this type of counseling (61). Recent survey data from people undergoing rehabilitation

for TBI indicated that 45% of at-risk drinkers endorsed wanting to change their problem drinking, 32% reported they were contemplating change, and only 23% reported they were not thinking about change (9). Contrary to the disease-of-denial concept, greater readiness to change was correlated with more severe alcohol-related problems, greater signs of alcohol dependence, and higher levels of alcohol consumption.

Not wanting to engage in formal treatment or attend self-help groups such as Alcoholics Anonymous (AA) is often interpreted as evidence of denial. Yet, most people with psychological problems, including those with addictions, do not seek professional help (62). In fact, the plethora of self-help guides confirms that not wanting help is a characteristic endemic in American culture. Interpreting not wanting help as an indication of denial only pathologizes and blames the patient for a condition most of us seem to have: preferring to change on our own.

Not wanting professional help does not necessarily mean not wanting to change. In people with recent TBI and comorbid alcohol-related problems, <20% wanted to try attending Alcoholics Anonymous or treatment, whereas nearly 70% wanted to change their alcohol use on their own (9). Pressure to enter treatment or attend AA hinges on the assumption that formal help is necessary for recovery. However, the research literature shows that there are many routes to recovery and that most people literally recover on their own. Controlled research has shown that people with alcohol problems can benefit as much from a self-help guide as from formal treatment (63). Even more surprising is a finding from two independent population surveys of problem drinkers who recovered from their alcohol problem for at least 1 year. These surveys found that 77% of those who recovered from their problem drinking did so without treatment, any other professional help, or even AA (27).

The research on recovery without treatment, on the efficacy of self-help materials, and on the efficacy of brief alcohol interventions indicates that those seeking to facilitate recovery from substance abuse problems in the context of rehabilitation have many more potentially effective tools to achieve this goal. With regard to brief interventions, a review of 44 controlled studies showed that brief interventions of one to three sessions produce significant change and are often as effective as more intensive treatment (64). In fact, there is more evidence for the efficacy of brief interventions than for the effectiveness of any other treatment modality (65). More than a decade ago, the IOM convened a conference that recognized specialized substance abuse treatment programs were not capable of addressing the problems of substance abuse in this country (57). They suggested that screening and brief interventions conducted in a variety of community settings by nonspecialists had considerably more potential to be effective from a public health perspective.

Finally, there is a belief that lifetime abstinence is the only acceptable goal for people with alcohol problems. There is little question that lifetime abstinence is the best option for many persons with alcohol problems. However, there are also good reasons to support moderate drinking when this is the person's treatment goal. Requiring a commitment to abstinence at the outset of an intervention may unnecessarily exclude individuals who could make other meaningful changes in their drinking (66). Giving the client choices in the process of setting treatment goals is considered more therapeutic and enhances adherence to treatment (66). Many patients who initially refuse abstinence will reconsider it after a trial of moderate drinking fails (67). Some people with a history of problem drinking achieve good long-term outcomes through moderate use of alcohol (68).

In summary, these common assumptions have little support when one considers the empirical literature on the broader population of persons with alcohol problems. What emerges is hopefully a sense that alcohol-related problems are more treatable than typically assumed, that a variety of treatments may be effective, and that there may be opportunities for nonspecialists to provide valuable interventions within the context of comprehensive rehabilitation.

SCREENING AND ASSESSMENT

GENERAL CONSIDERATIONS

There are several reasons to advocate for universal screening for substance abuse problems in the context of rehabilitation. As noted above, substance abuse is prevalent and influences important outcomes relevant to rehabilitation, yet health care providers are notoriously poor at detecting substance abuse problems without the systematic use of valid screening measures. Clinical detection has not been well studied in rehabilitation settings; however, a survey of rehabilitation staff indicated they believe that on average 22% of rehabilitation patients have substance abuse problems (69), whereas screening studies suggest the actual rate is two to three times higher (7,8). Research in acute trauma care showed that 23% of acutely intoxicated patients were not detected by their physicians, and staff identified chronic alcohol problems in less than half of the patients with such problems (70). In the same study, staff also incorrectly labeled 26% of patients as alcoholic. Clinical judgment in primary care settings also tends to have poor sensitivity for alcohol abuse or dependence (18% to 44%) but good specificity (96% to 99%) (71). Clinical judgment regarding the presence or absence of substance abuse is subject to systematic biases based on sex, appearance, insurance status, and socioeconomic status (70).

As described earlier, accurate identification of people with pre-injury problem drinking is an excellent way of predicting those at risk for problem drinking 1 year after injury (9). Identification of problem drinkers also may identify people at risk for slower rate of functional improvement within inpatient rehabilitation (46). Blood alcohol and other toxicology screening can help identify those with substance abuse (1); however, simple self-report measures tend to be more sensitive and specific (71). A number of studies show that it is feasible to administer self-report screening measures even within acute care medical, surgical, and rehabilitation settings (9,11, 72). Perhaps the most important reason to implement universal screening, however, is to identify people in need of interventions aimed at preventing return to substance abuse.

Some clinicians may be reluctant to institute alcohol screening and assessment procedures because of concerns about federal confidentiality laws and insurance coverage. Before undertaking alcohol screening,

Table 12-1	Commonly Used Screening Measures				
Measure	Items	Cut Score	Time	Comments	
CAGE (79)	4	>1	1–2 min	Easy to administer; more specific for alcohol dependence; no consumption items	
AUDIT (84)	10	>7	2–5 min	Measures consumption, consequences, and dependence; more sensitive to alcohol abuse	
SMAST (81,82)	13	>2	5–7 min	Measures consequences in more detail	
RAPS (80)	5	>0	1–2 min	More valid screen for alcohol dependence among women and minority persons; no consumption items	

staff should become familiar with federal law (73) that describes rules regarding protection of health information related to alcohol and drug abuse. Laws regarding potential exclusion of coverage for alcohol- or drug-related injuries vary by state. A thorough discussion of these laws is beyond the scope of this chapter; however Rivara et al. (74) provide an excellent review, as well as practical advice for managing substance abuse–related confidentiality and insurance coverage issues.

Another potential barrier to systematic screening is clinician doubt about the validity of self-reported alcohol screening or assessment data. Considerable attention has been paid to this issue in the substance abuse literature, and extensive reviews have concluded that persons with alcohol problems generally provide reliable and valid reports if proper measures and procedures are used (75). With regard to people with TBI, where the validity of alcohol screening measures may be even more controversial, Sander, Witol, and Kreutzer (76) have demonstrated very good agreement (>90%) between self-reported and independent observer ratings of alcohol use.

Numerous procedures for maximizing the validity of self-reports have been described (77,78). Generally, interviews should be conducted in clinical settings when the subject is alcohol-free and given reassurances of confidentiality. Alcohol screening measures should be embedded within the context of a larger battery of health-related assessments, and emphasis should be placed on alcohol use as one of several behavioral risk factors that might affect health or well-being. Adjunctive biomedical data such as blood alcohol levels or liver function tests can enhance validity. Any alcohol-related assessments should be conducted in a nonjudgmental fashion, avoiding terms such as "alcoholism" or similar labels. Screening batteries that include a measure of recent alcohol use have the advantage of being able to distinguish patients with current versus lifetime alcohol-related problems.

PRACTICAL SCREENING MEASURES

There are a number of brief screening measures that have been found to be reliable and valid indicators of significant alcohol-related problems (see Tables 12-1 and 12-2). One valid tool for identifying people with alcohol dependence is the CAGE questionnaire (79). The CAGE acronym stands for four questions: Have you ever felt you should *cut* down on your drinking? Have you ever felt *annoyed* by someone criticizing your drinking? Have you ever felt bad or *guilty* about your drinking? Have you

Table 12-2	Clinical Utility of Screening Measures			
	Criterion Category			
	Current At-Risk Drinking		Current Alcohol Dependence	
Measure	Sensitivity	Specificity	Sensitivity	Specificity
AUDIT	74%	88%	74%	89%
CAGE	54%	91%	84%	90%
RAPS	55%	79%	93%	87%
SMAST	68%[a]	92%[a]	100%[a]	85%[a]

[a]Based on one study.
From Fiellin DA, Reid MC, O'Connor PG. Screening for alcohol problems in primary care: A systematic review. *Arch Intern Med*. 2000;160(13):1977–1989; Cherpitel CJ. A brief screening instrument for problem drinking in the emergency room: The RAPS4. Rapid Alcohol Problems Screen. *J Stud Alcohol*. 2000;61(3): 447–449, with permission.

ever had a drink first thing in the morning (*eye opener*) to steady your nerves or to get rid of a hangover? Each affirmative response is scored 1 point, and a total score of 2 or greater is considered clinically significant. The CAGE has been used extensively in medical settings and requires only about 1 minute to administer. The CAGE has documented internal consistency and criteria-related validity mostly related to identification of people with alcohol dependence (75).

The RAPS4 is a newer measure designed to perform equally well among women and different ethnic groups and to be brief enough to use in hospital emergency departments (80). RAPS is an acronym for four questions: During the past year have you had a feeling of guilt or remorse after drinking (*remorse*)? During the last year has a friend or family member ever told you about things you said or did while drinking that you could not remember (*amnesia*)? During the past year have you failed to do what was normally expected of you because of drinking (*perform*)? Do you sometimes take a drink in the morning when you first get up (*starter*)? The sensitivity of the RAPS4 as an indicator of alcohol dependence was found to be equivalent for males and females and across ethnic groups (80). However, performance was not equivalent across groups when the measure was used to detect harmful drinking or abuse.

The Michigan Alcoholism Screening Test (MAST) (81) is a 25-item list of common signs and symptoms of generic alcoholism. While this measure has enjoyed wide use, it may be too long for many trauma rehabilitation settings. However, the 13-item Short MAST (SMAST) (82) has been found to be nearly as sensitive as the complete MAST among patients with TBI (83). A drawback of the SMAST, as well as the CAGE and RAPS, is that none include information on recent alcohol consumption. It cannot be determined from these measures alone whether the person's alcohol abuse or dependence is current or in remission. Therefore, it is advisable to include questions on alcohol consumption after these measures, especially as a follow-up to a positive screen.

The Alcohol Use Disorders Identification Test (AUDIT) is a 10-item measure developed by the World Health Organization to promote early identification of problem drinking in primary care medical settings (84). An advantage of the AUDIT is that it measures all three primary domains of alcoholism—alcohol consumption, alcohol-related life problems, and alcohol dependence symptoms—culminating in a single risk score. A cut-off of 8 is recommended (84). The AUDIT requires 2 minutes to administer and approximately 1 minute to score. The AUDIT is most appropriate in settings where it is desirable to identify people with alcohol abuse or risky

use, rather than alcohol dependence (71). Patients can even complete the AUDIT online at www.alcoholscreening.org and receive feedback and advice tailored to their particular drinking profile.

Screening for drug abuse is less advanced. The Drug Abuse Screening Test-10 is a relatively brief self-report measure of drug use–related problems. It has been used in a number of settings and has demonstrated good reliability, temporal stability, and validity (85). Another option is a very brief screening test for alcohol and other drug problems referred to as the Two-Item Conjoint Screening (TICS) (86). The two questions are "In the last year have you ever drunk or used drugs more than you meant to?" and "Have you felt you wanted or needed to cut down on your drinking or drug use in the last year?" At least one positive response had a sensitivity and specificity of 81% for an independently diagnosed substance abuse disorder in a primary care medical population. Respondents with zero positive responses had a 7.4% chance of having a substance abuse disorder, while among those with one positive response 45.0% had a substance abuse disorder, and 75.0% of those with two affirmative responses had a substance abuse diagnosis (86).

In summary, universal screening for alcohol-related problems is highly recommended, can be conducted with very little investment in clinical time, and can be used to predict a variety of clinical outcomes among people with recent TBI and SCI. Whenever possible, both drinking problems and recent alcohol consumption should be measured in order to determine whether alcohol-related problems are current or in remission. When recommended procedures are used, screening measures produce valid results and can be conducted with nearly every person.

ASSESSING SUBSTANCE USE PATTERNS

More detailed assessment of substance related factors may be useful for persons who screen positive for a substance use disorder. Further assessment can be used to make appropriate diagnoses and understand the person's problems more thoroughly. A detailed assessment also can help motivate people with substance abuse problems to change, because it provides an opportunity to review the effects of alcohol or drugs in their life within a supportive and confidential atmosphere. Assessment can be used to match treatment plans to the specific needs of the individual. For example, Turner et al. (87) showed that TBI and SCI patients on rehabilitation fall into four general groups with regard to alcohol use and problems (Table 12-3). One group representing 18% of the sample appeared alcohol-dependent and might require more intensive treatment and follow-up in

| Table 12-3 | Summary of Interventions Matched to Patient Drinking Subtype |

	Recommended Intervention Strategies			
Drinker Subtype	Education	Motivational Interviewing	Comprehensive Treatment	Relapse Prevention
I Alcohol dependence	X	X	X	X
II Alcohol abuse	X	X		
III Alcohol dependence in full or partial remission	X			X
IV Normal drinkers/ abstainers	X			

From Turner AT, Bombardier CH, Rimmele CT. A typology of alcohol use patterns among persons with recent TBI or SCI: Implications for treatment matching. *Arch Phys Med Rehabil.* 2003;84:362, with permission.

order to achieve abstinence. A second group (21%) was characterized by high levels of consumption but lower levels of alcohol-related problems and symptoms of dependence. For this group, brief interventions may be sufficient as a means of initiating a reduction in drinking or abstinence. A third group (15%) appeared to consist of alcohol-dependent persons who were in remission, partial remission, or relapse from their substance use disorder. For these persons relapse prevention types of interventions may be most useful. The fourth group (46%) contained normal drinkers and nondrinkers.

Assessment should include at least three core dimensions: drinking patterns, symptoms of dependence, and alcohol-related life problems (57). Assessment also frequently covers diagnostic criteria, drug use, motivation to change, and other factors related to tailoring treatment. Selected measures for assessing each of the aforementioned areas will be reviewed in the text that follows. Measures were chosen primarily on the basis of good psychometric properties as well as brevity and ease of use.

Drinking Patterns

There are four general procedures for eliciting information on alcohol use: the Quantity Frequency Variability Index (QFVI), the grid method, timeline follow-back, and drinking diaries (88). The QFVI measures the number of drinking occasions that occur over a fixed time interval and the number of drinks consumed on a typical drinking occasion. Separate questions may be used to cover beer, wine, and distilled spirits, as well as the frequency of binge-drinking episodes. In the grid method, a typical drinking week is reconstructed by assessing alcohol consumption during the morning, afternoon,

and evening of each day. The time line follow-back method samples drinking during a specific time period by using a calendar and specific memory anchor points to prompt recall of daily drinking. Finally, alcohol use can be measured with a daily drinking diary. An advantage of this method is that it minimizes reliance on memory and the subjective averaging needed to respond to "typical day" drinking questions (88).

Alcohol Dependence

The Alcohol Dependence Scale (ADS) (89) consists of 25 questions that can be self-administered in less than 10 minutes. The ADS focuses on symptoms of dependence over the past year. It is the most psychometrically sound measure of dependence, with established reliability, validity, and normative data (88). The Severity of Alcohol Dependence Questionnaire (SADQ) (90) is a 20-item measure that takes about 5 minutes to complete. It measures the frequency of dependence symptoms associated with a 30-day period of heavy drinking. The briefest recommended measure is the Short Alcohol Dependence Data (SADD) (91) questionnaire that includes only 15 items. This measure has established validity and is sensitive to early signs of dependence (92).

Alcohol-related Life Problems

The Drinker's Inventory of Consequences (DrInC) (93) is a 50-item scale designed to assess negative life events that are specifically attributable to alcohol. This measure has good psychometric properties and detailed norms on people seeking help for alcohol-related problems. The DrInC has five subscales: physical, interpersonal, intrapersonal, impulse control, and social responsibility. The measure includes a control scale to check on unreliable reporting, a feature that may be especially desirable among patients with cognitive impairment.

Alcohol Diagnosis

One of the most widely used diagnostic measures is the alcohol section from the *Structured Clinical Interview for DSM, Patient Edition* (SCID-P) (94). The interview requires training, takes 15 to 20 minutes, and permits a diagnosis of alcohol abuse as well as mild, moderate, or severe dependence (88). An alternative diagnostic measure is the alcohol section of the *National Institute of Mental Health Diagnostic Interview Schedule* (95). It contains 30 questions written to be asked exactly as written, requires about 15 to 20 minutes to administer, and captures a range of severity from mild to moderate symptoms (88).

Drug Use

Drug use can be assessed using the previously mentioned Drug Abuse Screening Test (DAST-10) (85) or with the 28-item original version (96). The original DAST has demonstrated an overall accuracy of 85% when compared to a *DSM-III* diagnosis of drug abuse or dependence. A cutoff score of 6 or more results in the best diagnostic accuracy (96).

Readiness to Change

Several measures of readiness to change are available based on the transtheoretical stages of change model (62). These measures are designed to predict acceptance of treatment as well as to help tailor the initial treatment approach. The transtheoretical model characterizes motivation to change as a spiral continuum from precontemplation (not considering change) through contemplation (ambivalent about change), determination (getting ready for change), action (making behavioral changes), maintenance (continuing change), and relapse (reverting to prechange behaviors). The University of Rhode Island Change Assessment Scale (URICA) (97) consists of 32 items that measure readiness to change "your problem." The measure has been used in a number of studies and has a stable factor structure (88). The Stages of Change and Treatment Eagerness Scale (98) is available in longer (40-item) and shorter (20-item) forms with good internal consistency, factor structure, and test-retest reliability (88). Finally, the shortest measure is the 12-item Readiness to Change Questionnaire (RTC) (99) that was designed for use in medical settings as part of a brief opportunistic intervention for problem drinkers. This measure has been used successfully among people with TBI and SCI (10,100). In subsequent analyses it was also shortened to ten items and rescaled to produce a more coherent linear measure of readiness to change that correlated meaningfully with independent measures of alcohol abuse severity among rehabilitation patients (101).

Comprehensive Measures

Some measures are designed to cover all the critical domains in a single multidimensional inventory. The strongest, most researched comprehensive measure is the Alcohol Use Inventory (AUI) (102). The AUI is made up of 228 items yielding 17 primary scales on such dimensions as motivation for and styles of drinking, physical dependence, loss of behavioral control, and readiness for change (88). The AUI can be completed in about 1 hour and scored by hand or computer. Another well-regarded omnibus measure is the Addiction Severity Index (ASI) (103). The ASI is a structured interview comprised of 8 subscales that takes about 40 minutes to complete. Subscales include life problems, medical, legal, employment/support, alcohol, other drugs, family/social, and psychiatric status.

To summarize, a wide range of measures exist to assess alcohol problems. Choice of measures will depend on clinical needs, time constraints, and who can perform the assessments and their level of training. Attention should be paid to the time frame referred to in the measure (typically lifetime or recent). In persons with TBI, memory impairment may complicate recall depending on the time frame (104). More thorough assessment may help trigger change, can provide data for diagnostic purposes, and may aid the process of tailoring treatment to match patient needs.

MODELS OF SERVICE DELIVERY

A number of factors can influence the means by which substance abuse–related problems are addressed within rehabilitation. These include the clinical resources present at a given institution, base rates of patients with substance abuse problems, and the severity or complexity of substance abuse problems in the patient population, as well as the availability and accessibility of specialized substance abuse treatment resources outside the rehabilitation program. Given the prevalence and impact of substance abuse in this population, as well as recent recommendations such as that offered by the National Institutes of Health (NIH) conference on TBI rehabilitation, which stated "substance abuse evaluation and treatment should be a component of rehabilitation treatment programs" (105), no institution claiming to provide comprehensive rehabilitation services should fail to have some process for managing this comorbid condition.

There are at least four broad approaches to providing substance abuse treatment in rehabilitation settings. Approaches differ in the extent to which they focus on treating substance abuse problems within rehabilitation versus referring these individuals elsewhere for treatment. While additional staff and training may be required in order to treat substance abuse problems within rehabilitation, referring them elsewhere is also problematic. Follow-through with substance abuse treatment referrals is often poor (75), and there may be major barriers to specialized treatment, such as physical, cognitive, and financial inaccessibility.

One approach is to have appropriate rehabilitation staff become skilled in a single effective treatment modality and treat all affected patients with that model. Having physiatrists provide advice and a medical rationale not to drink or having rehabilitation psychologists implement brief motivational interventions would fit into this category.

Another approach is to use initial screening or assessment data to match patients to different levels or types of treatment depending on the severity of the patient's alcohol problem or their treatment preferences. Table 12-3 depicts the four types of drinkers found among rehabilitation inpatients described earlier and the intervention strategies recommended for each type (87). Some interventions such as relapse prevention skills training and brief interventions can be conducted within rehabilitation, while for more dependent or complex patients, referral to outside agencies may be made for comprehensive treatment.

A third approach is to screen patients for substance use disorders and attempt to refer all those meeting criteria for substance abuse or dependence to outside treatment programs. Gentilello et al. (106) describe the use of this model to successfully induce a series of 17 general trauma patients to accept outpatient alcoholism treatment.

A fourth approach is to use a "stepped care" model. Stepped care involves providing a small dose of therapy (e.g., brief intervention during an inpatient stay) to all at-risk patients, followed by reassessment and more intensive treatment only if the person fails to meet a predetermined clinical goal, such as abstinence (107). Implementation of a stepped-care model would require planned outpatient follow-up visits for substance abuse as part of the person's overall rehabilitation program.

Whatever treatment model is adopted, the program will need to address the special challenges of providing opportunistic interventions. Traditionally medical treatment involves a patient having obvious or self-identified problems and seeking professional help. With opportunistic interventions, the health care provider identifies a different problem, one not necessarily related to the primary medical problem and one about which the patient may not be concerned nor want treatment for. Therefore, opportunistic interventions involve greater challenges in establishing a rationale for further assessment or treatment and eliciting the patient's cooperation (Table 12-4).

It is in this context that the transtheoretical stages of change model introduced earlier can be useful. For example, if a person who abuses alcohol presents in "precontemplation," not aware of a problem nor interested in changing, the clinician's initial goal should not be to encourage the person to change his

Table 12-4	The Context and Process of Substance Abuse Screening
How To Do It	**How Not To Do It**
Screen everyone and reassure patients that screening is standard care for all patients.	Screen selectively and make patients feel they are being singled out for special scrutiny.
Embed screening questions within existing assessments of other relevant health risk behaviors, such as smoking and medication use, that are normally conducted by core rehabilitation team members.	Separate alcohol-related questions into special assessments that are conducted outside the normal initial assessments, out of the blue, without reference to a larger concern about health and recovery.
Present alcohol screening as having to do with the health and recovery of people with TBI.	Frame alcohol screening as a unique moral or personality issue unrelated to their primary medical problems
Ask screening questions in a neutral tone of nonjudgmental concern or curiosity, the way you might ask about someone's history of prior TBI.	Remain skeptical, adopt an interrogatory style, and assume patients will always deny or minimize alcohol-related problems except under detailed scrutiny.
Ask these questions in private; clarify confidentiality and how the information will be used before the assessment.	Assume that patients need no reassurances or explanations in order to trust you with potentially stigmatizing information.
Delay screening until the patient is out of posttraumatic amnesia and not intoxicated.	Screen patients regardless of mental status or intoxication.
Use valid measures with specific cutoff scores to judge what is a significant alcohol problem.	Rely on your own personal screening questions and "clinical judgment."

or her drinking, but to raise the person's awareness of the problem so as to establish a basis for considering behavior change. Similarly, if the person abusing alcohol presents in "contemplation," that is, ambivalent about changing his or her drinking, the clinician's initial goal should be to explore that person's ambivalence, possibly by examining the costs and benefits of changing. Assuming that either of these hypothetical persons wants to make behavior changes and will simply follow advice to change ignores their stage of change and may lead to poorer outcomes. Studies on client resistance suggest that if clinicians press for change in people who are not in the action phase, resistance to change or ambivalence may be exacerbated (60).

EDUCATION AND POLICIES

Before discussing specific interventions the role of policies and educational approaches will be described. Policies have become more commonplace and are often developed to manage the most egregious substance abuse problems. By itself, educating patients about substance abuse is unlikely to be an effective intervention (65), but it can set the stage for other interventions and can fit well within or alongside existing rehabilitation-related educational programs.

Substance abuse policies can be useful when dealing with drinking or illicit drug use that may occur during the rehabilitation program (69). Policies also may be useful in cases with unusual pain problems, suspected medication-seeking behaviors, and escalating dosages of psychoactive medications, especially narcotics. A typical policy may be structured as a behavioral contract between the patient and attending physician. Patients may be asked to agree not to use drugs other than those ordered for them, to participate in all therapies, to permit toxicology screens as needed, to notify staff when leaving and returning to the unit, not to tamper with IV access, to accept methadone if ordered, and to accept narcotics or other psychoactive medications on a scheduled rather than an as-needed (prn) basis. In return, the physician agrees to address problems with pain, withdrawal, and addiction with appropriate medications and therapies, and to provide access to ongoing rehabilitation.

The policy can then specify potential consequences or actions that will occur if alcohol or illicit drug use is suspected. The first step is typically toxicology screening and withholding medications when there is thought to be potential for overdose or adverse drug-drug interactions. Outside pass privileges may be restricted or withdrawn. Visitors may also be restricted or some may visit only when supervised

by staff. Though it rarely may be enforced, early discharge can be threatened if the infractions are serious enough to abrogate the patient-physician relationship.

Educating rehabilitation patients about alcohol and drug use after SCI or TBI is a logical extension of the traditional rehabilitation model. Education is also an important ingredient in more comprehensive effective interventions. Education should be used to help patients understand the role of substance use (if any) in the onset of their injuries, to explain how substance use may affect them differently given their current impairments or disabilities, and to highlight the potential benefits of moderation or abstinence as part of their overall recovery process. Information that is personally relevant to the concerns of people with SCI or TBI can help tip the balance toward change among patients who are contemplating stopping alcohol or drug use. To that end, Tables 12-5 and 12-6 are patient education pamphlets summarizing the research literature that explains the risks of alcohol use and the benefits of abstinence after SCI and TBI.

TREATMENT: BACKGROUND ISSUES

In the United States, treatment for substance abuse has developed largely independent of scientific scrutiny. As a result, the most commonly used therapies are the ones with the *least* empirical support, and effectiveness is *inversely* related to cost (65). Fortunately, empirical reviews and meta-analyses are available as a rational guide to clinical care (65). In the following sections, several effective alcohol interventions will be described with an emphasis on how they may be utilized in rehabilitation settings. Therapies with the highest cumulative evidence for their efficacy are (in rank order) brief interventions, social skills training, motivational enhancement, and the community reinforcement approach (65). It is worth noting that a number of therapies have documented *in*effectiveness (65). These include educational lectures/films, general psychotherapy, general alcohol counseling, relaxation therapy, and anti-anxiety medications.

In the context of discussing substance abuse treatment, Alcoholics Anonymous (AA) merits special mention. AA has not been studied in a way that permits firm conclusions about its efficacy as a stand-alone treatment (65). While the popular press is replete with testimonials to the efficacy of AA, the absence of controlled studies leaves major questions unresolved such as selection biases, dropout rates, and the magnitude of spontaneous recovery in those who do not attend. Nevertheless, a large multisite study has been conducted that compared a therapy designed to facilitate participation in AA (as well as

Table 12-5	Alcohol and Your Health after Spinal Cord Injury

Alcohol and Immune Functioning
- Alcohol lowers the body's ability to fight off infection.
- One drink temporarily lowers immune function, and regular drinking lowers immune function even more.
- It takes 2 months of not drinking for the immune system to return to normal.
- Drinking alcohol may increase the risk of urinary tract and skin infections.

Alcohol and Bladder Function
- Alcohol causes the body to lose water, filling the bladder and causing dehydration.
- Drinking alcohol may cause overfilling and stretching of the bladder.
- Stretching the bladder can damage the kidneys, the organs that filter waste from the blood.
- Overfilling the bladder can also cause autonomic dysreflexia, a dangerous increase in blood pressure.
- Dehydration increases the risk of developing pressure sores.

Alcohol and Sex
- Alcohol reduces testosterone (the male sex hormone) production in males.
- Alcohol reduces sexual desire and sexual satisfaction.
- Alcohol reduces sexual performance in men (erection and ejaculation).
- Abstinence from alcohol improves sexual ability and sexual activity.

Alcohol and Injury Severity
- Alcohol in the blood at the time of injury seems to make SCI worse and reduces potential for recovery.
- SCI survivors are at higher risk of being injured again; drinking puts them at even higher risk of reinjury.

Alcohol and Other Medications
- Alcohol may cause bad reactions when used with medications for pain, spasticity, and infections.
- Alcohol can either magnify or interfere with the effects of prescribed medications by affecting your liver.

Alcohol and Mental Health
- Alcohol use is associated with depression, self-neglect, and suicide in persons with SCI.
- Drinking may be a warning sign that other help is needed.

AA attendance) to cognitive-behavioral therapy or motivation enhancement therapy (108). The results of this study indicated that those randomized to AA facilitation had slightly higher abstinence rates 3 years after the intervention. These findings are promising; however, the effectiveness of AA participation without the therapy facilitation component remains unknown.

Table 12-6	Alcohol and Your Health after Traumatic Brain Injury

Alcohol and Brain Injury Recovery
- Recovery from brain injury continues for at least 1 to 2 y after injury.
- Alcohol may slow or stop brain injury recovery, possibly by interfering with dendritic sprouting (neurons making new connections with each other).
- Not drinking is one way to give the brain the best chance to heal.

Alcohol, Brain Injury, and Seizures
- Traumatic brain injury puts survivors at risk for developing seizures (epilepsy).
- Alcohol lowers the seizure threshold and may trigger seizures.
- Not drinking can reduce the risk of developing posttraumatic seizures.

Alcohol and the Risk of Having Another Brain Injury
- After one brain injury, survivors are at higher risk (3 to 8 times higher) of having another brain injury.
- Drinking alcohol puts survivors at even higher risk for having a second brain injury.
- Not drinking can reduce the risk of having another brain injury.

Alcohol and Mental Functioning
- Alcohol and brain injury have similar effects on memory, mental speed, balance, and thinking.
- Alcohol seems to magnify the negative effects of brain injury.
- Alcohol may affect brain injury survivors more than it did before their injury.
- The negative mental effects of alcohol can last from days to weeks after drinking stops.
- Not drinking is one way to maximize your mental abilities.

Alcohol and Sex
- Alcohol reduces testosterone production in males.
- Alcohol reduces sexual desire in men and women.
- Alcohol reduces sexual performance in men (erection and ejaculation).
- Alcohol reduces sexual satisfaction in men and women.
- Abstinence from alcohol improves sexual ability and sexual activity in men and women.

During the initial surge of interest in TBI and alcoholism, many brain injury professionals believed that AA was not effective for persons with TBI (23), in part because of the somewhat abstract nature of the concepts used. Nevertheless, the brain injury association supported the development of materials to assist people with TBI who wanted to participate in AA (109). AA deserves consideration also because it can be difficult to find treatment programs in the community that offer viable alternatives to the 12-step model (110). Therefore, when the patient is interested in attending AA or other 12-step programs, it seems prudent to support this plan and, whenever possible, educate sponsors and provide psychological services or cognitive remediation aimed at maximizing the patient's ability to participate in and benefit from 12-step programs.

TREATMENT: OUTCOME STUDIES AMONG PATIENTS WITH TRAUMATIC BRAIN INJURY OR SPINAL CORD INJURY

There have been no randomized controlled studies of substance abuse interventions on rehabilitation patients published to date. Yet much can be learned from the existing studies from within rehabilitation in conjunction with the much stronger empirical literature in the substance abuse field more generally.

Blackerby and Baumgarten (111) were among the first to envision a model treatment program for people with dual diagnoses of TBI and substance abuse. Within a residential treatment facility they began with lectures on alcohol and drug use followed by a combined program of AA and cognitive behavior therapy provided individually as well as in small groups. Preliminary outcome data on seven clients who were in the program for an average of 3.4 months indicated that 90 to 180 days after discharge, three of seven patients were sober, three were not, and the outcome for one was unknown.

Jones (112) reported outcomes from the Vineland National Center, a combined TBI rehabilitation and substance abuse program offering residential and outpatient services, support groups, early intervention, and prevention services. The program design included an initial evaluation, a focus on wellness, positive reinforcement and low confrontation, interdisciplinary service provision, coping skills training, and transitional services to promote transfer of skills back into the person's own community. The author reports preliminary outcomes from 100 clients 6 months after discharge. About 66% of clients were reportedly abstinent from all alcohol or other drug use; 59.4% were living independently (versus 34.4% prior to admission); and the percentage of persons with paid employment improved from 9.4% to 37.5%.

Corrigan, Lamb-Hart, and Rust (19) describe the TBI Network, a community-based program for people with TBI that involves coordination of resources and services, not only to address substance abuse problems but also unemployment and other rehabilitation needs. The TBI Network includes several core services: comprehensive assessment, integrated service planning, and service coordination and monitoring. Supplemental services include screening, outreach, education, assistance accessing resources, and emotional support. The authors report an in-depth analysis of the first 37 referrals that were screened. From assessment to 6 months, alcohol use declined by 77%; quantity consumed per occasion declined by 33% among those still using alcohol; frequency of other drug use dropped by 89%; and the number of those abstaining from drugs and alcohol increased almost threefold. Large increases were also observed on numerous indicators of employment status. In a follow-up study of 72 clients followed for at least 1 year, increased abstinence rates and improved vocational outcomes were reported (113). Better outcomes were associated with involvement of a community team and being referred to the program within 3 months after injury.

Delmonico et al. (114) described a group treatment model for people undergoing acute or post-acute care rehabilitation for TBI. However, no systematic outcome data were reported.

Bombardier and Rimmele (10) developed a two-session version of motivational interviewing for use in people with TBI during inpatient rehabilitation. Fifteen patients screened positive for current alcohol abuse and were approached; 12 (80%) consented and were treated. One-year outcome data were obtained on nine participants. Results showed that 89% of treated subjects reported consuming no alcohol during a typical week. However, the proportional reduction in drinking observed in the treatment group was not significantly different from a historical comparison group in which 50% reported no current drinking at follow-up.

Most recently, the effects of systematic motivational counseling (SMC) were tested among outpatients with TBI (115). Forty participants received 12 SMC sessions and were compared to 54 participants from another institution that received no motivational or substance abuse treatment. SMC focused on the subject's personal goals and concerns in various areas of their lives and helped them formulate and carry out plans to address these concerns. After the intervention, the SMC group showed improvement in motivational structure, reduced negative affect, and reduced substance abuse, whereas the comparison group did not demonstrate these changes.

There are fewer published treatment studies among people with SCI. Early work in this area was conducted by Sweeney and Foote (116). They reported on the development of an inpatient multimodal therapeutic community model of treatment at the Long Beach Veterans Administration Medical Center (VAMC). Outcome data from their center indicated that 56% of former patients were not using drugs. A similar program at the Bronx VAMC was developed (117). Krause (55) described a program for inpatients with SCI that included biweekly group therapy, individual psychotherapy, recreational outings, in-house AA, and family therapy. No outcome data were presented; however, practical problems with institutional acceptance, staff enabling, and patient noncompliance were discussed.

TREATMENT: SELECTED EMPIRICALLY SUPPORTED INTERVENTIONS

Advice

Giving at-risk patients brief advice on abstaining or reducing drinking is possible for any physician who works with these patient populations. Numerous controlled studies in medical settings have shown that brief physician advice results in significant, lasting decreases in drinking (75). For example, a recent randomized controlled study showed that two 10- to 15-minute interactions with a primary care physician resulted in a 40% reduction in alcohol consumption among problem drinkers measured 1 year later (118). Advice may be more effective when it is combined with self-help materials or personalized feedback and information about the adverse health effects of alcohol (75). Several self-help guides have been published (119,120), including one written specifically for persons with TBI (121). A guide to physicians who want to provide their patients with advice regarding alcohol problems is available on the Web at http://www.niaaa.nih.gov/publications/physicn/htm. This model uses a simple four-step approach: (i) *Ask* about alcohol use. (ii) *Assess* for alcohol-related problems. (iii) *Advise* appropriate action based on risk. (iv) *Monitor* patient progress.

Brief Interventions

Brief interventions have been used in a variety of settings, both as a stand-alone treatment and a means of enhancing the effects of subsequent treatments (92). The effective elements of brief interventions have been summarized by the acronym FRAMES (64). These key elements are *feedback, responsibility, advice, a menu of options, empathy,* and *self-efficacy.* Following the FRAMES model, the patient typically

undergoes some systematic assessment, and based on results, the patient is provided with personally relevant feedback that includes the impairment or risks associated with past and future drinking. The therapist emphasizes the patient's personal responsibility for change, provides clear advice to make a change in drinking, and gives a menu of alternative strategies for changing problem drinking. This information is provided with empathy and understanding, not confrontation, in such a way as to reinforce the patient's hope, self-efficacy, or optimism.

The most widely researched model of brief interventions is motivational interviewing (60,122). Reviews and meta-analyses of interventions based on motivational interviewing support the efficacy and applicability of this intervention (123,124). Numerous authors have recommended motivational interviewing as a potentially effective intervention among rehabilitation patients (100,112,125), and two studies have described adaptations of this method in people with TBI (100,115). In another relevant study, Gentilello and colleagues (72) randomized 366 general trauma patients to a 30-minute motivational interview, while 396 controls received usual care during their acute care medical/surgical hospital stay. At 12 months postinjury, the intervention group not only reduced their alcohol consumption significantly more than the control group (21.8 drinks per week versus 6.7 drinks) but there was also a significantly greater reduction in reinjury and rehospitalization in the intervention group versus the control group.

In summary, brief interventions have considerable potential as a means of preventing return to substance abuse following TBI and SCI. Existing data suggest these interventions are able to be conducted within rehabilitation settings, are acceptable to patients, and fit with the needs and expectations of a large segment of patients with substance abuse problems within rehabilitation (9,87). Detailed training manuals and workshops are available for clinicians to learn motivational interviewing (60,122). Although many rehabilitation psychologists do not have extensive training in substance abuse, by virtue of their general psychological training they are in a good position to learn the additional skills needed to address substance abuse using brief interventions.

Coping and Social Skills Training

This approach to alcohol treatment has evolved out of a social learning perspective on alcoholism (126). The underlying assumption is that persons with alcohol problems lack adequate skills to regulate positive and negative moods and to cope with social and interpersonal situations such as work, marriage, and parenting. Core interpersonal treatment modules include drink refusal skills, giving positive feedback, giving criticism, receiving criticism about substance use, listening skills, conversation skills, developing sober supports, and conflict resolution. Core mood regulation topics include managing negative thinking and coping with drinking-related beliefs, triggers, and cravings. Coping and social skills training has been adapted for persons with TBI and is highly recommended for those with significant alcohol dependence (110).

Relapse Prevention

Relapse prevention is an influential cognitive-behavioral self-management program originally designed to complement traditional treatments by anticipating and planning to cope with relapse (66). The relapse prevention model includes three major components: behavioral skills training, cognitive interventions, and lifestyle change. Alcoholism is reconceptualized as an over learned maladaptive habit, and relapse becomes a natural phase of behavior change that can be anticipated. As noted above, relapse prevention is relevant for a significant fraction of rehabilitation patients with a history of substance abuse; however, this model involves the use of abstract and metaphorical content that may need to be adapted for persons with cognitive impairment.

Community Reinforcement Approach

The Community Reinforcement Approach (CRA) is a behaviorally based intervention that emphasizes the use of natural reinforcers in the patient's environment (e.g., family, spouse, friends, work, leisure activities) to facilitate change in drinking behavior (127). The CRA begins with a traditional behavioral analysis of drinking and nondrinking behaviors (127). Rather than requiring clients to make a commitment to lifelong abstinence, CRA therapists negotiate a period of "time out" from drinking that may include the use of disulfiram (Antabuse). The CRA includes special procedures to address marital/relationship issues, vocational training, lack of social support, and the absence of nondrinking recreational alternatives (127). This approach has been shown to be effective in four out of four outcome studies (65).

A promising application of CRA is when it is used with the concerned friends or family members of people with alcoholism who refuse to seek treatment (128). Concerned others can be trained to use behavior management skills, communication skills, and assertiveness to help the person with alcoholism seek treatment. A randomized controlled trial of this method showed a dramatic increase in treatment participation compared to two other types

of interventions and significantly decreased drinking even before the subject entered treatment (128). The intervention also reduced distress among the concerned others who participated.

To summarize, recent innovations in theory and treatment should make it possible for every rehabilitation program to provide on-site interventions. The types and intensity of interventions as well as the staff who provide treatment will vary depending on the individual site or program. Legitimate, potentially efficacious interventions range from brief advice provided by a rehabilitation physician or psychologist to intensive interdisciplinary coping skills treatment specifically tailored for persons with neurologic impairments. Alcohol interventions will likely be more effective to the extent they are woven into the daily fabric of a given rehabilitation program and to the extent that the substance abuse intervention focuses on enhancing rehabilitation outcomes, general health, and well-being, rather than solely on reducing alcohol or drug use.

CONCLUSIONS

Substance abuse is the major cause underlying traumatically induced disability, and rehabilitation represents a window of opportunity to intervene in substance abuse problems for people with TBI and SCI. While rehabilitation programs report improved attention to substance abuse issues, more can be done (69). Currently, only 67% of surveyed programs support universal screening, 53% provide substance abuse education to their patients, and 69% provide easy access to substance abuse counselors (69).

A key to providing better alcohol-related services for persons with traumatic disabilities is improving access to effective treatment. Rehabilitation programs can do a great deal to promote access to treatment through systematic screening and by bringing empirically valid treatment approaches into the acute and postacute care rehabilitation settings in which people with traumatic disabilities are usually seen. When it is not feasible to bring substance abuse interventions into rehabilitation programs, staff can forge effective relationships with outside treatment facilities to which they can refer more severely affected patients who are willing to consider formal treatment.

Physiatrists and other rehabilitation professionals can facilitate implementation of effective programs in several ways. We can become more familiar with current thinking in the area of addictive behavior. In doing so we can help dispel counterproductive myths and shed new light on these problems. Clinicians, especially physiatrists, rehabilitation psychologists, social workers, and nurses can expand their clinical expertise to include alcohol- and drug-related problems. There is a tendency to think that substance abuse problems are qualitatively different than other behavior problems and that treating addictions requires unique skills and experiences. However, current theory and research emphasize that alcohol and drug problems are behaviors that respond to the same psychological principles as other disorders such as anxiety and depression (58). Using empirically validated treatments, rehabilitation professionals can design treatment programs that fit within rehabilitation and meet the needs of traumatically injured and disabled persons where they are, physically, cognitively, and motivationally. Finally, we can conduct research to determine if the treatment approaches we have tailored and the programs to which we refer are effective.

ACKNOWLEDGMENTS

Background work for this chapter was supported by the National Center for Injury Prevention and Control and the Disabilities Prevention Program, the National Center for Environmental Health (R49/CCR011714; Charles H. Bombardier, P.I.) and the National Institute on Disability and Rehabilitation Research, Department of Education (Northwest Regional Spinal Cord Injury System, Grant Number H133N50025, Diana Cardenas, P.I.). The contents of this chapter are solely the responsibility of the author and do not necessarily represent the official views of the NCIPC, NCEH or NIDRR. Gratitude is expressed to Johanna Brown for editorial help.

REFERENCES

1. Gentilello L, Donovan D, Dunn C, et al. Alcohol interventions in trauma centers: Current practice and future directions. *J Am Med Assoc.* 1995;274: 1043–1048.
2. Rivara FP, Jurkovich GJ, Gurney JG, et al. The magnitude of acute and chronic alcohol abuse in trauma patients. *Arch Surg.* 1993;128(8):907–912.
3. Morris JAJ, MacKenzie EJ, Edelstein SL. The effect of preexisting conditions on mortality in trauma patients. *J Am Med Assoc.* 1990;263:1942–1946.
4. Sims DW, Bivins BA, Obeid FN, et al. Urban trauma: A chronic recurrent disease. *J Trauma.* 1989;29(7): 940–946; discussion 946–947.
5. National Institute on Alcoholism and Alcohol Abuse. *Screening for alcoholism in primary care settings.* Rockville, MD: Alcohol, Drug Abuse, and Mental Health Administration; 1987.
6. Rivara FP, Koepsell TD, Jurkovich GJ, et al. The effects of alcohol abuse on readmission for trauma. *J Am Med Assoc.* 1993;270:1962–1964.
7. Corrigan J. Substance abuse as a mediating factor in outcome from traumatic brain injury. *Arch Phys Med Rehabil.* 1995;76:302–309.
8. Heinemann A, Keen M, Donohue R, et al. Alcohol use in persons with recent spinal cord injuries. *Arch Phys Med Rehabil.* 1988;69:619–624.
9. Bombardier CH, Rimmele CT, Zintel H. The magnitude and correlates of alcohol and drug use before traumatic brain injury. *Arch Phys Med Rehabil.* 2002; 83(12):1765–1773.
10. Bombardier CH, Rimmele C. Alcohol use and readiness to change after spinal cord injury. *Arch Phys Med Rehabil.* 1998;79:1110–1115.
11. Soderstrom CA, Smith GS, Dischinger PC, et al. Psychoactive substance use disorders among seriously injured trauma center patients. *J Am Med Assoc.* 1997;277(22):1769–1774.
12. Heinemann A, Schnoll S, Brandt M, et al. Toxicology screening in acute spinal cord injury. *Alcohol Clin Exp Res.* 1988;12:815–819.
13. Kiwerski J, Krauski M. Influence of alcohol intake on the course and consequences of spinal cord injury. *Int J Rehabil Res.* 1992;15:240–245.
14. Dikmen S, Machmer J, Donovan D, et al. Alcohol use before and after traumatic head injury. *Ann Emerg Med.* 1995;26:167–176.
15. Heinemann AW, Doll MD, Armstrong KJ, et al. Substance use and receipt of treatment by persons with long-term spinal cord injuries. *Arch Phys Med Rehabil.* 1991;72:482–487.
16. Kreutzer JS, Witol AD, Sander AM, et al. A prospective longitudinal multicenter analysis of alcohol use patterns among persons with traumatic brain injury. *J Head Trauma Rehabil.* 1996;11(5):58–69.
17. Bombardier CH, Dikmen S, Temkin N, et al. The natural history of drinking and alcohol-related problems after traumatic brain injury. *Arch Phys Med Rehabil.* 2003;84:185–191.
18. Heinemann A, Doll M, Schnoll S. Treatment of alcohol abuse in persons with recent spinal cord injuries. *Alcohol Health Res World.* 1989;13:1110–1117.
19. Corrigan JD, Lamb-Hart GL, Rust E. A programme of intervention for substance abuse following traumatic brain injury. *Brain Inj.* 1995;9(3):221–236.
20. Kreutzer JS, Witol AD, Marwitz JH. Alcohol and drug use among young persons with traumatic brain injury. *J Learn Disabil.* 1996;29(6):643–651.
21. Young M, Rintala D, Rossi C, et al. Alcohol and marijuana use in a community-based sample with spinal cord injury. *Arch Phys Med Rehabil.* 1995;76:525–532.
22. Kreutzer J, Wehman P, Harris J, et al. Substance abuse and crime patterns among persons with traumatic brain injury referred for supported employment. *Brain Inj.* 1991;5:177–187.
23. National Head Injury Foundation. *Substance abuse task force white paper.* Southborough, MA: The Foundation; 1988.
24. Kirubakaran V, Kumar V, Powell B, et al. Survey of alcohol and drug misuse in spinal cord injured veterans. *J Stud Alcohol.* 1986;47:223–227.
25. Kessler RC, McGonagle KA, Zhao S, et al. Lifetime and 12-month prevalence of DSM-III-R psychiatric disorders in the United States. Results from the National Comorbidity Survey. *Arch Gen Psychiatry.* 1994;51(1):8–19.

26. Grant BF, Harford TC, Dawnson DA, et al. Prevalence of DSM-IV alcohol abuse and dependence. *Alcohol Health Res World.* 1994;18:243–248.

27. Sobell L, Cunninghavm J, Sobell M. Recovery from alcohol problems with and without treatment: Prevalence in two population surveys. *Am J Public Health.* 1996;86:966–972.

28. Sparadeo F, Gil D. Effects of prior alcohol use on head injury recovery. *J Head Trauma Rehabil.* 1989;4:75–82.

29. Bombardier CH, Thurber C. Blood alcohol level and early cognitive status after traumatic brain injury. *Brain Inj.* 1998;12:725–734.

30. Tate PS, Freed DM, Bombardier CH, et al. Traumatic brain injury: Influence of blood alcohol level on post-acute cognitive function. *Brain Inj.* 1999; 13(10):767–784.

31. Kaplan C, Corrigan J. Effect of blood alcohol level on recovery from severe closed head injury. *Brain Inj.* 1992;6:337–349.

32. Ruff R, Marshall L, Klauber M, et al. Alcohol abuse and neurological outcome of the severely head injured. *J Head Trauma Rehabil.* 1990;5:21–31.

33. Kelly D. Alcohol and head injury: An issue revisited. *J Neurotrauma.* 1995;12:883–890.

34. Halt P, Swanson R, Faden A. Alcohol exacerbates behavioral and neurochemical effects of rat spinal cord trauma. *Arch Neurol.* 1992;49:1178–1184.

35. Annegers J, Grabow J, Kurland L, et al. The incidence, causes and secular trends of head trauma in Olmstead County, Minnesota. *Neurology.* 1980;30:912–919.

36. Salcido R, Costich J. Recurrent traumatic brain injury. *Brain Inj.* 1992;6:293–298.

37. Freedland E, McMicken D, D'Onofrio G. Alcohol and trauma. *Emerg Med Clin North Am.* 1993;11:225–239.

38. Ronty H, Ahonen A, Tolonen U, et al. Cerebral trauma and alcohol abuse. *Eur J Clin Invest.* 1993;23:182–187.

39. Brooks N, Symington C, Beattie A, et al. Alcohol and other predictors of cognitive recovery after severe head injury. *Brain Inj.* 1989;3(3):235–246.

40. Sparadeo F, Strauss D, Barth J. The incidence, impact and treatment of substance abuse in head trauma rehabilitation. *J Head Trauma Rehabil.* 1990;5:1–8.

41. Solomon D, Malloy P. Alcohol, head injury and neuropsychological function. *Neuropsychol Rev.* 1992; 3:249–280.

42. Dikmen S, Donovan D, Loberg T, et al. Alcohol use and its effects on neuropsychological outcome in head injury. *Neuropsychology.* 1993;7:296–305.

43. Burke W, Weselowski M, Guth W. Comprehensive head injury rehabilitation: An outcome study. *Brain Inj.* 1988;2:313–322.

44. Dunlop T, Udvarhelyi G, Stedem A, et al. Comparison of patients with and without emotional/behavioral deterioration during the first year after traumatic brain injury. *J Neuropsychiatry Clin Neurosci.* 1991;3:150–156.

45. Heinemann A, Goranson N, Ginsberg K, et al. Alcohol use and activity patterns following spinal cord injury. *Rehabil Psychol.* 1989;34:191–206.

46. Bombardier CH, Stroud M, Esselman P, et al. Do pre-injury alcohol problems predict poorer rehabilitation progress in persons with spinal cord injury? *Arch Phys Med Rehabil.* 2004;85:1488–1492.

47. Heinemann A, Hawkins D. Substance abuse and medical complications following spinal cord injury. *Rehabil Psychol.* 1995;40:125–141.

48. Elliott TR, Kurylo M, Chen Y, et al. Alcohol abuse history and adjustment following spinal cord injury. *Rehabil Psychol.* 2002;47(3):278–290.

49. Charlifue S, Gerhart K. Behavioral and demographic predictors of suicide after spinal cord injury. *Arch Phys Med Rehabil.* 1991;72:488–492.

50. Rourke S, Loberg T. The neurobehavioral correlates of alcoholism. In: Grant I, Adams K, eds. *Neuropsychological assessment of neuropsychiatric disorders.* New York, NY: Oxford University Press; 1996:423–485.

51. Parsons O, Nixon S. Cognitive functioning in sober social drinkers: A review of the research since 1986. *J Stud Alcohol.* 1998;59:180–190.

52. Baguley I, Felmingham K, Lahz S, et al. Alcohol abuse and traumatic brain injury: Effect on event-related potentials. *Arch Phys Med Rehabil.* 1997;78: 1248–1253.

53. Oddy M, Coughlin T, Tyerman A. Social adjustment after closed head injury. *J Neurol Neurosurg Psychiatry.* 1985;48:564–568.

54. Peterson J, Rothfleisch J, Zelazo P, et al. Acute alcohol intoxication and cognitive functioning. *J Stud Alcohol.* 1990;51:114–122.

55. Krause J. Delivery of substance abuse services during spinal cord injury rehabilitation. *NeuroRehabilitation.* 1992;2:45–51.

56. American Psychiatric Association. *Diagnostic and statistical manual of mental disorders.* 4th ed. Washington, DC: Author; 1994.

57. Institute of Medicine. *Broadening the base of treatment for alcohol problems.* Washington, DC: National Academy Press; 1990.

58. Miller W, Brown S. Why psychologists should treat alcohol and drug problems. *Am Psychol.* 1997;52: 1269–1279.

59. Valliant G. *The natural history of alcoholism: Causes, patterns and paths to recovery.* Cambridge, MA: Harvard University Press; 1983.

60. Miller WR, Rollnick S. *Motivational interviewing: Preparing people to change addictive behavior.* New York, NY: Guilford; 1991.

61. Miller WR, Benefield G, Tonigan J. Enhancing motivation for change in problem drinking: A controlled comparison of two therapist styles. *J Consult Clin Psychol.* 1993;61:455–461.

62. Prochaska J, DiClemente C, Norcross J. In search of how people change. *Am Psychol.* 1992;47:1102–1114.

63. Miller W, Gribskov C, Mortell R. Effectiveness of a self-control manual for problem drinkers with and without therapist contact. *Int J Addict.* 1981;16: 1247–1254.

64. Bien T, Miller W, Tonigan J. Brief interventions for alcohol problems: A review. *Addiction.* 1993;88: 315–335.

65. Miller W, Brown J, Simpson T, et al. What works? A methodological analysis of the alcohol treatment outcome literature. In: Hester R, Miller W, eds. *Handbook of alcoholism treatment approaches: Effective alternatives.* Boston, MA: Allyn & Bacon; 1995:12–44.

66. Dimeff L, Marlatt A. Relapse prevention. In: Hester R, Miller W, eds. *Handbook of alcoholism treatment approaches: Effective alternatives.* Boston, MA: Allyn & Bacon; 1995:148–159.

67. Miller WR, Page A. Warm turkey: Other routes to abstinence. *J Subst Abuse.* 1991;8:227–232.

68. Sanchez-Craig M, Wilkinson DA, Davila R. Empirically based guidelines for moderate drinking: One-year results from three studies with problem drinkers. *Am J Public Health.* 1995;85(6):823–828.

69. Basford JR, Rohe DE, Barnes CP, et al. Substance abuse attitudes and policies in US rehabilitation training programs: A comparison of 1985 and 2000. *Arch Phys Med Rehabil.* 2002;83(4):517–522.

70. Gentilello LM, Villaveces A, Ries RR, et al. Detection of acute alcohol intoxication and chronic alcohol dependence by trauma center staff. *J Trauma.* 1999; 47:1131–1139.

71. Fiellin DA, Reid MC, O'Connor PG. Screening for alcohol problems in primary care: A systematic review. *Arch Intern Med.* 2000;160(13):1977–1989.

72. Gentilello L, Rivara F, Donovan D, et al. Alcohol interventions in a trauma center as a means of reducing the risk of injury recurrence. *Ann Surg.* 1999;230: 473–483.

73. United States Public Health Service. *Code of federal regulations, Part II: Confidentiality of alcohol and drug abuse patient records.* Washington, DC: Author; 1989.

74. Rivara FP, Tollefson S, Tesh E, et al. Screening trauma patients for alcohol problems: Are insurance companies barriers? *J Trauma.* 2000;48(1):115–118.

75. Cooney NL, Zweben A, Fleming MF. Screening for alcohol problems and at-risk drinking in health-care settings. In: Hester RK, Miller WR, eds. *Handbook of alcoholism treatment approaches: Effective alternatives.* Boston, MA: Allyn & Bacon; 1995:45–60.

76. Sander A, Witol A, Kreutzer J. Concordance of patients' and caregivers' reports of alcohol use after traumatic brain injury. *Arch Phys Med Rehabil.* 1997; 78:138–142.

77. Babor TF, Brown J, Del Boca FK. Validity of self-reports in applied research on addictive behaviors: Fact or fiction? *Addict Behav.* 1990;12:5–32.

78. Sobell LC, Sobell MB. Self report issues in alcohol abuse: State of the art and future directions. *Behav Assess.* 1990;12:77–90.

79. Ewing J. Detecting alcoholism: The CAGE questionnaire. *J Am Med Assoc.* 1984;252:1905–1907.

80. Cherpitel CJ. A brief screening instrument for problem drinking in the emergency room: The RAPS4. Rapid Alcohol Problems Screen. *J Stud Alcohol.* 2000;61(3):447–449.

81. Selzer JL. The Michigan Alcoholism Screening Test: The quest for a new diagnostic instrument. *Am J Psychiatry.* 1971;127:89–94.

82. Selzer M, Vinokur A, van Rooijen L. A self-administered Short Michigan Alcoholism Screening Test (SMAST). *J Stud Alcohol.* 1975;36:127–132.

83. Bombardier CH, Kilmer J, Ehde D. Screening for alcoholism among persons with recent traumatic brain injury. *Rehabil Psychol.* 1997;42:259–271.

84. Allen J, Litten R, Fertig J, et al. A review of research on the Alcohol Use Disorders Identification Test (AUDIT). *Alcohol Clin Exp Res.* 1997;21:613–619.

85. French MT, Roebuck MC, McGeary KA, et al. Using the Drug Abuse Screening Test (DAST-10) to analyze health services utilization and cost for substance users in a community-based setting. *Subst Use Misuse.* 2001;36(6&7):927–946.

86. Brown RL, Leonard T, Saunders LA, et al. A two-item conjoint screen for alcohol and other drug problems. *J Am Board Fam Pract.* 2001;14:95–106.

87. Turner A, Bombardier CH, Rimmele CT. A typology of alcohol use patterns among persons with recent TBI or SCI: Implications for treatment matching. *Arch Phys Med Rehabil.* 2003;84:358–364.

88. Miller WR, Westerberg VS, Waldron HB. Evaluating alcohol problems in adults and adolescents. In: Hester R, Miller W, eds. *Handbook of alcoholism treatment approaches: Effective alternatives.* Boston, MA: Allyn & Bacon; 1995:61–88.

89. Skinner HA, Horn JL. *Alcohol Dependence Scale (ADS) user's guide.* Toronto, Canada: Addiction Research Foundation; 1984.

90. Stockwell T, Hodgson R, Edwards G, et al. The development of a questionnaire to measure severity of alcohol dependence. *Br J Addict Alcohol Other Drugs.* 1979;74(1):79–87.

91. Davidson R, Raistrick D. The validity of the Short Alcohol Dependence Data (SADD) questionnaire. *Br J Addict.* 1986;81:217–222.

92. Heather N. Brief intervention strategies. In: Hester R, Miller W, eds. *Handbook of alcoholism treatment approaches: Effective alternatives.* Boston, MA: Allyn & Bacon; 1995:105–122.

93. Miller WR, Tonigan JS, Longabaugh R. The drinker's inventory of consequences: An instrument for assessing the adverse consequences of alcohol abuse. *Test manual,* Project MATCH Monograph Series. Rockville, MD: Project National Institute on Alcohol Abuse and Alcoholism; 1994.

94. Spitzer RL, Williams JB, Gibbon M, et al. *Structured clinical interview for DSM-IV-patient edition.* Washington, DC: American Psychiatric Press; 1996.

95. Robbins L, Helzer J, Cottler L. *NIMH diagnostic interview schedule: Version III—revised (DIS–III–R).* St. Louis, MO: Washington University Press; 1989.

96. Gavin DR, Ross HE, Skinner HA. Diagnostic validity of the drug abuse screening test in the assessment of DSM-III drug disorders. *Br J Addict.* 1989;84:301–307.

97. McConnaughy EA, Prochaska JO, Velicer WF. Stages of change in psychotherapy: Measurement and sample profiles. *Psychother Theo Res Prac.* 1983;20: 368–375.

98. Miller W. The Stages of Change Readiness and Treatment Eagerness Scale (SOCRATES, Version 6.0). Unpublished instrument. Center on Alcoholism, Substance Abuse, and Addictions (CASAA). Albuquerque, NM: University of New Mexico Press; 1993.

99. Rollnick S, Heather N, Gold R, et al. Development of a short "readiness to change" questionnaire for use in brief, opportunistic interventions among excessive drinkers. *Br J Addict.* 1992;87:743–754.

100. Bombardier CH, Ehde D, Kilmer J. Readiness to change alcohol drinking habits after traumatic brain injury. *Arch Phys Med Rehabil.* 1997;78(6):592–596.

101. Bombardier CH, Heinemann AW. The construct validity of the readiness to change questionnaire for persons with TBI. *J Head Trauma Rehabil.* 2000; 15(1):696–709.

102. Horn JL, Wanberg KW, Foster FM. *Guide to the alcohol use inventory.* Minneapolis, MN: National Computer Systems; 1987.

103. McLellan AT, Luborsky L, O'Brien CP, et al. An improved evaluation instrument for substance abuse patients: The addiction severity index. *J Nerv Ment Dis.* 1980;168:26–33.

104. Corrigan J, Rust E, Lamb-Hart G. The nature and extent of substance abuse problems in persons with

traumatic brain injury. *J Head Trauma Rehabil.* 1995; 10:29–46.

105. NIH Consensus Development Panel. Consensus conference. Rehabilitation of persons with traumatic brain injury. NIH Consensus Development Panel on Rehabilitation of Persons with Traumatic Brain Injury. *J Am Med Assoc.* 1999;282(10):974–983.

106. Gentilello L, Duggan P, Drummnd D, et al. Major injury as a unique opportunity to initiate treatment in the alcoholic. *J Surg.* 1988;156:558–561.

107. Marlatt A, Taupert S. Harm reduction: Reducing the risk of addictive behaviors. In: Baer J, Marlatt A, eds. *Addictive behaviors across the life span: Prevention, treatment, and policy issues.* Newbury Park, CA: Sage Publications; 1993:243–273.

108. Project MATCH Research Group. Matching alcoholism treatments to client heterogeneity: Project MATCH three year drinking outcomes. *Alcohol Clin Exp Res.* 1998;22:1300–1311.

109. Peterman W. *Substance abuse counseling strategies for head injury survivors.* Southborough, MA: National Head Injury Foundation Substance Abuse Task Force; 1987.

110. Langley M, Kiley D. Prevention of substance abuse in persons with neurological disabilities. *NeuroRehabilitation.* 1992;2:52–64.

111. Blackerby WF, Baumgarten A. A model treatment program for the head-injured substance abuser: Preliminary findings. *J Head Trauma Rehabil.* 1990;5:47–59.

112. Jones G. Substance abuse treatment for persons with brain injuries. *NeuroRehabilitation.* 1992;2:27–34.

113. Bogner JA, Corrigan JD, Spafford DE, et al. Integrating substance abuse treatment and vocational rehabilitation after traumatic brain injury. *J Head Trauma Rehabil.* 1997;12(5):57–71.

114. Delmonico RL, Hanley-Peterson P, Englander J. Group psychotherapy for persons with traumatic brain injury: Management of frustration and substance abuse. *J Head Trauma Rehabil.* 1998;13(6): 10–22.

115. Cox W, Heinimann A, Miranti S, et al. Outcomes of systematic motivational counseling for substance use following traumatic brain injury. *J Addict Dis.* 2003;22:93–110.

116. Sweeney TT, Foote JE. Treatment of drug and alcohol abuse in spinal cord injury veterans. *Int J Addict.* 1982;17(5):897–904.

117. Radnitz CL, Tirch D. Substance misuse in individuals with spinal cord injury. *Int J Addict.* 1995;30(9): 1117–1140.

118. Fleming M, Barry K, Manwell L, et al. Brief physician advice for problem alcohol drinkers. *J Am Med Assoc.* 1997;277:1039–1045.

119. Miller W, Munoz R. *How to control your drinking.* Revised ed. Albuquerque, NM: University of New Mexico Press; 1982.

120. Kishline A. *Moderate drinking: The moderation management guide for people who want to reduce their drinking.* New York, NY: Crown Trade Paperbacks; 1994.

121. Karol R, Sparadeo F. Alcohol, drugs and brain injury: A survivor's workbook. Alberta, Canada: Alberta Alcohol and Drug Abuse Commission; 1991.

122. Miller WR, Rollnick S. *Motivational interviewing: Preparing people for change.* 2nd ed. New York, NY: The Guilford Press; 2002.

123. Dunn C, Deroo L, Rivara FP. The use of brief interventions adapted from motivational interviewing across behavioral domains: A systematic review. *Addiction.* 2001;96(12):1725–1742.

124. Noonan WC, Moyers TB. Motivational interviewing: A review. *J Subst Misuse.* 1997;2:8–16.

125. Langley MJ, Lindsay WP, Lam CS, et al. A comprehensive alcohol abuse treatment programme for persons with traumatic brain injury. *Brain Inj.* 1990; 4(1):77–86.

126. Monti PM, Rohsenow DJ, Colby SM, et al. Coping and social skills training. In: Hester R, Miller W, eds. *Handbook of alcoholism treatment approaches: Effective alternatives.* Boston, MA: Allyn & Bacon; 1995: 221–241.

127. Smith J, Meyers R. The community reinforcement approach. In: Hester R, Miller W, eds. *Handbook of alcoholism treatment approaches: Effective alternatives.* Boston, MA: Allyn & Bacon; 1995:251–266.

128. Miller WR, Meyers RJ, Tonigan JS. Engaging the unmotivated in treatment for alcohol problems: A comparison of three strategies for intervention through family members. *J Consult Clin Psychol.* 1999;67(5):688–697.

13

Adjustment to Trauma

Dawn M. Ehde and Rhonda M. Williams

The consequences of traumatic injuries are enormously varied and are detectable at different levels. At the most visible level, these experiences may result in physical disability or impairment in function, or perhaps the loss of or damage to a person's loved ones, property, or livelihood. At a slightly less visible level, traumatic experiences can result in psychological effects, ranging from anger and frustration to symptoms such as intrusive thoughts, emotional numbing, depression, and anxiety. The most hidden and elusive consequences of trauma may include an alteration in the way the traumatized person organizes and utilizes existing and novel information and a forced and substantial reorganization of existing cherished belief structures and ways of thinking (1).

For the majority of people, however, trauma presents a transient disruption. They experience the temporary upheaval of the trauma, injury, or loss, ultimately maintaining their health and ability to function in work and social relationships. In the psychological literature, this phenomenon of human capacity to thrive after aversive events is often referred to as resilience. As articulated by Bonanno (2), "the term *recovery* connotes a trajectory in which normal human functioning temporarily gives way to threshold or subthreshold psychopathology and then gradually returns to pre-event levels. By contrast, *resilience* reflects the ability to maintain a stable equilibrium" in the face of loss or highly disruptive events.

Our goals in this chapter are to describe not only disruptions in psychological functioning but also resilient responses that may occur in adults following a traumatic injury. We will review some of the misconceptions that are commonly held about the psychological effects of trauma. We will also point out some of the shortcomings of the literature that we believe constrain our understanding of the full breadth of psychological experiences that may occur after a traumatic injury. We will highlight aspects of traumatic events, characteristics of survivors, and the environments that influence the risk of disruption caused by trauma. We will discuss ways to assess trauma and facilitate both resilience and recovery. Finally, we hope to impress upon the reader that while caring for persons who have experienced trauma requires sensitivity and a willingness to be exposed to the most tragic and devastating human experiences, it more often provides an opportunity to marvel at that which is the best of human nature—resilience, strength, courage, forgiveness, and growth. For this reason, we encourage the use of the term trauma *survivors* instead of *patients* or *victims*.

DEFINITIONS OF TRAUMA AND TRAUMATIC EVENTS

In its simplest terms, psychological trauma is defined as "a psychic or behavioral state resulting from mental or emotional stress or physical injury." In the *Diagnostic and Statistical Manual of Mental Disorders*, Fourth Edition (DSM-IV) (3), a traumatic event (required for the diagnosis of acute stress disorder or post-traumatic stress disorder) involves either the experiencing or witnessing of "an event that involved actual or threatened death or serious injury, or a threat to the physical integrity of self or others." Such events are generally so extreme, severe, powerful, harmful, or threatening that they demand extraordinary coping efforts. They usually subject people to extreme terror, horror, fright, threat to life, and feelings of helplessness, vulnerability, loss of control, and uncertainty.

By these definitions, essentially all patients seen in an acute hospitalization setting for medical treatment of traumatic injuries, possibly some of their family members or friends, and some of the staff have experienced psychological trauma. These populations would include (i) individuals who have been injured in or exposed to a recent sudden, unpredictable event, such as a motor vehicle crash (MVC), accident, shooting, or natural disaster; (ii) individuals who have been injured by or exposed to a prolonged, repeated stressor, such as domestic violence; (iii) individuals who have experienced prolonged duress associated with chronic medical illness, causing cumulative impact and a feeling of being traumatized but without the specific traumatic event; and (iv) individuals exposed to "vicarious trauma," such as the health care providers who treat trauma patients, or persons who witness traumatic events but are not endangered or physically injured by them. Exposure to a "near miss" can also inflict a disruption in well-being. Many times these various types of survivors overlap; they are not mutually exclusive (4).

TERMINOLOGY RELEVANT TO UNDERSTANDING PSYCHOLOGICAL RESPONSES TO TRAUMA

A variety of psychological and psychiatric terms are commonly used when discussing psychological reactions to trauma. Too often, these terms are used inaccurately. Thus, a brief discussion as well as some definitions of relevant terminology are warranted.

Clinicians and researchers often use the term *depression* imprecisely to describe any of a number of psychological experiences after trauma, including formal diagnosable disorders, subclinical symptoms, and distressed or tearful mood, and they use it interchangeably with a variety of words, including agitated, sad, and upset. Indeed, according to the *Diagnostic and Statistical Manual of Mental Disorders*, Fourth Edition (3), there are several formal disorders or diagnoses that are more likely to occur after a major trauma, including mood disorders (e.g., major depressive disorder [MDD]), adjustment disorders, and post-traumatic stress disorder (PTSD). Accurate diagnosis is important to differentiate these disorders from one another and from subclinical levels of symptomatology.

To illustrate the importance of precise terminology, we offer the criteria for major depressive episode

(MDE), so that these might be contrasted against the more imprecise label of *depression*. MDE involves much more than depressed mood, anhedonia, or distress. Symptoms of MDE include (i) depressed mood; (ii) significantly diminished pleasure or interest in activities (sometimes referred to as anhedonia); (iii) decreased or increased appetite and/or significant weight loss or weight gain; (iv) insomnia or hypersomnia; (v) psychomotor agitation or retardation; (vi) decreased concentration or indecisiveness; (vii) decreased energy or fatigue; (viii) feelings of excessive guilt or worthlessness; and (ix) recurrent suicidal ideation with or without a plan and/or recurrent preoccupation with death. To be diagnosed with an MDE, an individual must have a minimum of five of the nine symptoms, one of which must be depressed mood or anhedonia. In addition, the symptoms must be experienced most of the time for a minimum of 2 weeks. These symptoms must also cause impairment in functioning and not be attributable to a medical condition or medications. If a person experiences at least one MDE, they meet diagnostic criteria for major depressive disorder.

As pointed out by others (5), too often in research self-report measures of depressive symptoms (e.g., Beck Depression Inventory [6], Center for Epidemiological Studies-Depression [CES-D] [7]) are thought to provide a measure of a diagnosable MDD. Many of these self-report measures do not include adequate time referents or measures of the functional impairment that are key to diagnosing an MDD, however. Although such self-report measures are quite valuable for describing the presence, severity, and characteristics of psychological distress and depressive symptoms, they do not constitute a diagnosis of MDD. As noted by Elliott and Frank (5), these self-report measures of depressive symptoms may be better viewed as measures of depressive symptoms or psychological distress. A diagnosis of major depressive disorder is best obtained through a clinical interview that includes an assessment of the specific MDD criteria, including the impairment in functioning that is required by the *DSM-IV*. In psychiatric research, the norm is to use standardized diagnostic interviews, which are typically administered by a mental health professional or someone else trained in the administration of the tool.

Although beyond the scope of this chapter, a number of authors (5,8,9) have pointed out the importance of distinguishing depressed mood, depressive symptoms, and MDD from one another and the semantic, conceptual, theoretical, and clinical problems that can occur when such distinctions are not made. Thus, in this chapter we will use the term *depressed mood* to specifically mean a mood state characterized by feeling depressed, blue, sad, or empty. We will use *major depressive disorder* or *MDD* to represent a *DSM-IV*–based diagnosis of this mood disorder. For all other subthreshold levels of depressive symptoms, we will use the term *depressive symptoms*.

The term *post-traumatic stress disorder* is another term that is frequently used imprecisely in the literature and by clinicians. In our opinion, the term *posttraumatic stress disorder* or *PTSD* should be reserved for the actual anxiety disorder described in the *DSM-IV* (3). The diagnostic criteria for PTSD can be found in Table 13-1. As seen in the table, a diagnosis of PTSD involves not only exposure to a traumatic event (criterion A) but also a number and pattern of symptoms involving re-experiencing the trauma (criterion B), avoidance of things associated with the trauma (criterion C), numbing of overall responsiveness (criterion C), and symptoms of increased arousal (criterion D). It is important to note that according to *DSM-IV* criteria, an individual cannot be diagnosed with PTSD within the first month after a traumatic event, as the symptoms must be present for >1 month. In this chapter we will use the term PTSD only when referring to an actual *DSM-IV* diagnosis of the anxiety disorder PTSD.

A number of self-report measures of post-traumatic stress *symptoms* also exist. We recommend that clinicians and researchers avoid labeling the results of such measures as PTSD unless the measures truly allow diagnosis of the disorder. This recommendation does not negate the use of such symptom measures, as they can provide worthwhile information regarding the post-traumatic anxiety

---

Table 13-1 *DSM-IV* Diagnostic Criteria for Post-traumatic Stress Disorder

A. The person has been exposed to a traumatic event in which both of the following were present:
  1. The person experienced, witnessed, or was confronted with an event or events that involved actual or threatened death or serious injury, or a threat to the physical integrity of self or others.
  2. The person's response involved intense fear, helplessness, or horror.[a]
B. The traumatic event is persistently re-experienced in one (or more) of the following ways:
  1. Recurrent and intrusive distressing recollections of the event, including images, thoughts, or perceptions [b]
  2. Recurrent distressing dreams of the event[c]
  3. Acting or feeling as if the traumatic event were recurring (includes a sense of reliving the experience, illusions, hallucinations, and dissociative flashback episodes, including those that occur on awakening or when intoxicated) [d]
  4. Intense psychological distress at exposure to internal or external cues that symbolize or resemble an aspect of the traumatic event
  5. Physiologic reactivity on exposure to internal or external cues that symbolize or resemble an aspect of the traumatic event
C. Persistent avoidance of stimuli associated with the trauma and numbing of general responsiveness (not present before the trauma), as indicated by three (or more) of the following:
  1. Efforts to avoid thoughts, feelings, or conversations associated with the trauma
  2. Efforts to avoid activities, places, or people that arouse recollections of the trauma
  3. Inability to recall an important aspect of the trauma
  4. Markedly diminished interest or participation in significant activities
  5. Feeling of detachment or estrangement from others
  6. Restricted range of affect (e.g., unable to have loving feelings)
  7. Sense of a foreshortened future (e.g., does not expect to have a career, marriage, children, or a normal life span)
D. Persistent symptoms of increased arousal (not present before the trauma), as indicated by two (or more) of the following:
  1. Difficulty in falling or staying asleep
  2. Irritability or outbursts of anger
  3. Difficulty in concentrating
  4. Hypervigilance
  5. Exaggerated startle response
E. The duration of the disturbance (symptoms in criteria B, C, and D) is >1 mo.
F. The disturbance causes clinically significant distress or impairment in social, occupational, or other important areas of functioning.

Specify if
Acute: if duration of symptoms is <3 mo
Chronic: if duration of symptoms is ≥3 mo

Specify if
With Delayed Onset: if onset of symptoms is at least 6 mo after the stressor

---

[a] In children, this may be expressed instead by disorganized or agitated behavior.
[b] In young children, repetitive play may occur in which themes or aspects of the trauma are expressed.
[c] In children, there may be frightening dreams without recognizable content.
[d] In young children, trauma-specific re-enactment may occur.
From American Psychiatric Association. *Diagnostic and statistical manual of mental disorders.* 4th ed. Washington, DC: American Psychiatric Association; 1994, with permission.

experience, including symptom description and severity. Indeed, as will be discussed later in this chapter, many individuals who have experienced a traumatic injury do not meet criteria for a *DSM-IV* diagnosis of PTSD and yet experience a number of the symptoms included in this syndrome. We will refer to such subthreshold symptoms as *post-traumatic stress (PTS) symptoms*.

Another anxiety disorder of relevance to this chapter is acute stress disorder (ASD). ASD is a diagnosis new to the *DSM-IV*; the diagnostic criteria for ASD are listed in Table 13-2. In its current formulation, ASD describes an anxiety disorder characteristic of acute psychological reactions to trauma that involve not only the intrusive, avoidant, and arousal symptoms characteristic of PTSD but also dissociative symptoms (criterion B). Dissociative symptoms involve alterations in perceptions of the self and external world such that one may feel detached from one's thoughts or body (*depersonalization*) or feel that external events are unreal (*derealization*). Emotional numbing, being in a daze, and difficulties recalling aspects of the trauma are also considered signs of dissociation. ASD thus shares some of the symptoms of PTSD but emphasizes the dissociative symptoms that may occur following trauma. The disorder is also limited to an onset within and maximum duration of 4 weeks after the traumatic

event (criterion G). We will use *ASD* to refer to a *DSM-IV* diagnosis of acute stress disorder.

Since being added to the *DSM-IV*, a number of concerns have been raised regarding the value of the ASD diagnosis in accurately describing early pathologic post-traumatic stress phenomenon (10–12). ASD's emphasis on dissociative responses has been criticized (12), as such emphasis implies that dissociative symptoms are integral to the immediate psychological response to trauma, a conclusion that has been questioned. Despite its limitations, given its inclusion in the *DSM-IV*, we include a review of ASD as it pertains to traumatic injury later in this chapter.

In addition to terms describing psychopathologic states, we will use several terms from the positive psychology literature. By *positive emotion* we mean a positive feeling or affective state, which may include subjective feelings, physiologic changes, and observable expressions. In contrast, *mood* pertains to a pervasive and persistent emotion. Moods tend to be more long-lasting and all-encompassing than positive emotions.

Recently research has shown that many individuals not only persevere but thrive in spite of adversity, trauma, tragedy, or loss. This process of adapting well to or bouncing back from significant challenges is known as *resilience*. It involves the ability to maintain healthy levels of psychological well-being and

---

Table 13-2	*DSM-IV* Diagnostic Criteria for Acute Stress Disorder

A. The person has been exposed to a traumatic event in which both of the following were present:
  1. The person experienced, witnessed, or was confronted with an event or events that involved actual or threatened death or serious injury, or a threat to the physical integrity of self or others.
  2. The person's response involved intense fear, helplessness, or horror.

B. Either while experiencing or after experiencing the distressing event, the individual has three (or more) of the following dissociative symptoms:
  1. A subjective sense of numbing, detachment, or absence of emotional responsiveness
  2. A reduction in awareness of his or her surroundings (e.g., "being in a daze")
  3. Derealization
  4. Depersonalization
  5. Dissociative amnesia (e.g., inability to recall an important aspect of the trauma)

C. The traumatic event is persistently re-experienced in at least one of the following ways: recurrent images, thoughts, dreams, illusions, flashback episodes, a sense of reliving the experience, or distress on exposure to reminders of the traumatic event.

D. Marked avoidance of stimuli that arouse recollections of the trauma (e.g., thoughts, feelings, conversations, activities, places, and people) is present.

E. Marked symptoms of anxiety or increased arousal (e.g., difficulty sleeping, irritability, poor concentration, hypervigilance, exaggerated startle response, motor restlessness) are present.

F. The disturbance causes clinically significant distress or impairment in social, occupational, or other important areas of functioning or impairs the individual's ability to pursue some necessary task, such as obtaining necessary assistance or mobilizing personal resources by telling family members about the traumatic experience.

G. The disturbance lasts for a minimum of 2 d and a maximum of 4 wk and occurs within 4 wk of the traumatic event.

H. The disturbance is not due to the direct physiologic effects of a substance (e.g., a drug of abuse, a medication) or a general medical condition, is not better accounted for by brief psychotic disorder, and is not merely an exacerbation of a pre-existing Axis I or Axis II disorder.

From American Psychiatric Association. *Diagnostic and statistical manual of mental disorders*. 4th ed. Washington, DC: American Psychiatric Association; 1994, with permission.

functioning in the face of trauma or loss. Another construct that has been examined in the psychology literature is *post-traumatic growth*, defined as positive psychological changes resulting from or in response to a challenging circumstance such as a traumatic event (13). Post-traumatic growth can be manifested in a variety of ways, including but not limited to having an increased appreciation for life, feeling increased personal strength, experiencing improved interpersonal relationships, changing life priorities, gaining positive spiritual changes, or finding new meaning and purpose in life. Other terms for such positive changes exist in the literature and include *stress-related growth* (14), *positive adjustment, positive adaptation, thriving,* and *adversarial growth* (15). All of these terms suggest that positive changes can come from a challenging or adverse life experience, an idea that is important but under-recognized in the trauma rehabilitation literature.

PSYCHOLOGY OF TRAUMA: THEORETICAL APPROACHES

As society has become more sensitive to the impact of trauma and more skilled in treating problems that arise from it, trauma has become the subject of much research and intervention. While this is a positive step, in many cultures and in recent decades, health professionals have focused on psychological disorders that arise from trauma and on their treatment while losing sight of the more prevalent phenomenon of resilience. In fact, some have adopted the perspective that if someone is not outwardly demonstrating difficulties following a loss or trauma, this is a pathologic absence, often labeled with terms such as *avoidance, denial,* or *delayed grief response* (2,16). Many theories have been developed in an attempt to understand and explain psychopathologic reactions to trauma. We present three main theories—behavioral, psychodynamic, and cognitive—as useful tools that can help us understand the way that some people experience trauma.

BEHAVIORAL THEORIES

In their simplest terms, behavioral conditioning theories (17,18) suggest that trauma responses are learned through experience or observation of others and then reinforced. Positive reinforcement might occur if one is rewarded with sympathy, attention, or care in response to a certain reaction to trauma. Negative reinforcement might occur if an aversive outcome is avoided or removed by demonstrating certain responses to trauma. Although this may sound simple, such responses can become deeply ingrained and are rarely deliberate. For example, it is understandable that a woman who was raped might experience terror in circumstances that reminded her of those in which she was raped. To cope with this, she might avoid such circumstances, thus negatively reinforcing her fear and response to the trauma. Partial empirical support for this theory is obtained from the treatment literature, as one of the most effective treatments for severe fears and avoidance behaviors following trauma is a behavioral intervention that involves graded, increasing exposure to the feared stimulus while simultaneously managing fear and anxiety (19). Thus, over time, the trauma survivor is increasingly able to tolerate the feared stimulus.

PSYCHODYNAMIC THEORIES

Other theories of trauma are more psychodynamic in nature (20,21). A psychodynamic approach notes the presence of an unconscious mind and suggests that things which are too difficult, unpleasant, or threatening are kept from the conscious mind through a variety of adaptive defenses. An example of a specific psychodynamic theory of trauma comes from Horowitz (20), who suggests that traumas are eventually processed by alternating exposure to or immersion in the conscious experience of the trauma with avoidance, denial, or numbing (i.e., the trauma goes back into the unconscious or subconscious). Horowitz's theory proposes that when a person experiences an overwhelmingly stressful or traumatic experience, he or she subconsciously "titrates" their exposure to the experience by alternating between intrusive thoughts and numbing or avoidant thoughts. In this manner, the person is able to manage their emotions associated with the experience and process them effectively. As a person successfully processes, or copes with an experience, intrusive thoughts and avoidant or numbing behaviors should diminish. By cycling through these two different states (immersion or intrusion into the conscious re-experiencing and avoiding or denying), the experience eventually becomes less distressing and can be tolerated.

COGNITIVE THEORIES

Cognitive theories are based on the observation and assumption that human beings have a basic inclination to make sense of the world and to assign meaning and organization to life experiences. Some cognitive theories describe a "normal" or pretrauma cognitive state in which humans function effectively through the use of core beliefs about the nature of the world, justice, themselves, and other people (22).

Exposure to trauma may shatter or violate one's core beliefs such as the belief in one's own invulnerability or worth, the belief in the safety of the world, the belief that events are orderly, predictable, controllable, and fair, or the belief that life is meaningful. Thus, making sense of traumatic experiences can be particularly challenging, requiring a unique type of cognitive processing at an emotional and cognitive level (4,23). One goal of such cognitive processing may be to find acceptable meaning in the trauma, on both an emotional and cognitive level (24–26), and to focus on different types of mental evidence to support these more positive meanings (27,28). Traumatized individuals may also seek to understand and adapt to an experience that violates their core beliefs by reframing the experience in a way that fits with their pre-existing beliefs more closely, or by challenging, reconsidering, and possibly altering core beliefs.

Several types of thought patterns have been observed and described among those who fail to cope with trauma, and these thought patterns may exist for many years following the traumatic experience. For example, some continue to search for meaning but fail to find satisfactory resolution (23); some experience a persistent need for information after factual information had been provided (29); some continue to have intrusive ideation (30); some make unfavorable comparisons between life as it is and what it might have been had the traumatic event not occurred (4); some engage in continual comparisons between aspects of life after the stressful event versus how it was before the traumatic event (31); some see themselves as blameworthy (32); and some view themselves as victims and at risk with little expectation or hope that things will improve or change, thus remaining hypervigilant (33).

One of the more recent cognitive approaches to understanding trauma is called the constructive narrative perspective (4,28) and is based on the survivor's narrative account of the experience and the subjective meaning ascribed to the experience. In this approach, survivors' storylike narratives of events include descriptions of behavioral and emotional reactions, explanations, and predictions. These accounts are created in an effort to infuse these experiences with some coherence and meaning and to help survivors make sense of the world and their place in it. As individuals "process" the trauma, their narrative about the event changes. Thus far research has not determined whether changing the narrative account causally contributes to improved adjustment, whether changes in adjustment lead to changes in the narrative, or whether some third factor mediates both of these changes. It is likely that the narratives are dynamically interactive and interdependently connected with adjustment.

SUMMARY

Each of the theoretical approaches described above provides a useful framework for clinicians and scientists to conceptualize adjustment to trauma. However, we caution against the universal application of these or any other theories that prescribe a certain sequence of experience in response to a trauma. Universal application of a particular theoretical approach may increase the likelihood of viewing survivor responses in a pathologic fashion (if they do not conform to the theory of choice), underestimate the importance and prevalence of resilience, and lead the clinician to overly influence the adjustment process.

COMMON PSYCHOLOGICAL RESPONSES TO TRAUMA

What is a "normal" reaction to having just sustained a traumatic, potentially life-threatening, life-altering injury? What is a "normal" response to undergoing intensive medical and rehabilitation interventions following injury? What is a "normal" reaction to the onset of a disability acquired due to a sudden traumatic injury? As will be described in this chapter, there is no universal psychological response to experiencing a traumatic event. However, the literature has suggested that there are a number of common psychological reactions that may occur following a trauma. What follows is a description of common acute and long-term psychological responses to a traumatic event. For the purposes of this discussion, we will define "acute" reactions as those occurring within the first few days and weeks after a trauma. For most survivors of physical trauma, this time period involves a period of hospitalization and medical rehabilitation. "Long-term" reactions will include those psychological states that are present after the acute rehabilitation period and, for many, during the time when the survivor is likely reintegrating back into the community.

METHODOLOGICAL ISSUES

Before describing acute and long-term psychological responses to trauma, several methodological and theoretical constraints of the relevant trauma literature must be noted, as they strongly shape the current knowledge of such responses. First, with a few exceptions (some of which will be described later in this chapter), most of the research that has been conducted on psychological responses to traumatic injuries has been done from a disease model of human functioning that focuses primarily on the prevalence or absence of psychopathologic reactions to injury. Seldom have other possible psychological responses such as positive emotions, resilience, or post-traumatic growth been empirically examined following injury. This tendency to focus on "negative" emotional reactions has previously been described by several authors (34–36) in the broader disability literature, which has also focused primarily on negative emotional states. Although there is growing interest in nonpathologic reactions to trauma and disability (34), our current empirical understanding of psychological responses to traumatic injury, particularly nonpathologic responses, is nonetheless constrained by such viewpoints.

A second constraint stemming from the focus on psychopathologic models for research on psychological responses to trauma is a tendency for research to focus primarily on individual characteristics of the person who was injured. For example, when using such a model to study depression following spinal cord injury, a researcher might examine demographic, personality, behavioral, or injury severity factors as predictors of depression. Although such research has value, it neglects to include important environmental factors (36,37). Thus, most of the literature examining factors that influence one's psychological responses to trauma is on individual or injury characteristics and does not examine the impact of environmental factors (e.g., the health care system, financial resources, societal attitudes, physical barriers) that may significantly influence such responses.

In describing psychological responses to traumatic injury, this chapter draws primarily from the body of research that has been done on psychological reactions to a few specific injuries, including spinal cord injury, traumatic brain injury, amputations, and burns. Although research on psychological responses to these injuries is growing, many unanswered questions remain about the psychology of traumatic injuries. As such, our conceptualizations of psychological responses and adaptation to traumatic injury were also informed by the large body of knowledge that exists about psychological responses to other traumatic events (not necessarily involving personal injury), such as violent crimes, war zone experiences, and natural disasters. These literatures not only focus on the psychopathologic conditions but also on other psychological responses, including resilience, that occur following a trauma such as a rape or natural disaster.

ACUTE RESPONSES

Individuals who have suffered a trauma may experience any of a range of psychological reactions in response to injury. For many, these symptoms are a normal response to having experienced an unusual or abnormal life event. What follows in this section is a description of potential physical, emotional, cognitive, and behavioral responses after injury, focusing on the acute phase of medical care and rehabilitation. The prevalence of psychopathologic disorders will also be reviewed, followed by a discussion on the potential for other psychological responses during the acute phase.

Physical Responses

In the initial hours and days following a trauma, individuals may experience physical symptoms such as fatigue, sleep disturbances, nightmares, changes in appetite, muscle tension, exaggerated startle response, hyperarousal, and somatic complaints (e.g., nausea, diarrhea, or pain) as part of a reaction to the traumatic event. For example, several studies have suggested that 50% to 75% of patients hospitalized with an acute burn injury have difficulties falling or maintaining sleep (38–40) and approximately 25% to 33% have nightmares (39,40) during hospitalization. It is difficult, if not impossible, to differentiate when a physical response, such as insomnia, is caused by the psychological effects of the trauma versus the injury (e.g., pain, limited mobility), medical treatment (side effects of medication), or environmental factors (frequent awakenings by hospital staff for medical procedures).

Emotional Responses

Although the majority of persons do not experience significant long-term emotional distress, even after a significant injury such as a burn injury (41), the acute "normal" emotional response to trauma is thought to be one of immediate and considerable distress (42). In a rare study (43) of the immediate emotional experiences of hospitalized physical injury survivors, 45% of a randomly selected sample of trauma patients ($n = 269$) demonstrated high levels of emotional distress while on the surgical ward. As described in the broader trauma literature, any of a range of emotions may accompany the sudden onset of a traumatic injury, such as anxiety, fear, helplessness, depression, sadness, grief, irritability, anger, guilt, despair, or anguish. The research on acute emotional reactions following traumatic injury has primarily focused on depressive and post-traumatic stress symptoms, and thus little is known about the nature or incidence of other potential emotional responses.

In addition to increased feelings of emotional distress, survivors of a recent trauma may also report what has been categorized in the *DSM-IV* as dissociative symptoms (3). Dissociative symptoms involve feelings of emotional detachment, emotional numbing, or an absence of emotional responsiveness. Feelings of derealization or depersonaliziation may be present; individuals may describe feeling as if they are living in a dream, a daze, or a stupor. In some cases, an individual may experience dissociative amnesia, which involves amnesia for all or part of the traumatic event. It is important not to misidentify the various injury, treatment, and environmental factors associated with having a traumatic injury as symptoms of dissociation. For example, a loss of consciousness at the time of a brain injury and subsequent post-traumatic amnesia should not be confused with dissociative amnesia. Medications may cause an individual to feel detached, numb, or dazed. In one study (39) of patients hospitalized for an acute burn injury, 26% met the *DSM-IV* dissociative criterion of acute stress disorder, meaning that they endorsed three or more of the five dissociative symptoms included in this symptom cluster.

In addition to the negative emotional states most commonly described in the literature, positive emotions can and do occur in the aftermath immediately following traumatic injury. Many health care professionals have witnessed positive emotions such as joy, hope, and humor in the newly injured trauma survivors with whom they have worked. Unfortunately, empirical descriptions of such responses after traumatic injury are absent in the literature.

Cognitive Responses

The general literature on trauma has documented a number of cognitive changes that can occur in the immediate aftermath of a traumatic event. These include difficulties concentrating, disorientation, confusion, distractibility, and subjective memory difficulties (4). In addition, intrusive thoughts of or recollections about the trauma itself are also common. For example, persons who have experienced a burn injury in a house fire may find images and thoughts about the circumstances surrounding the fire "intruding" into their mind, even when actively trying to focus on something else (such as a visitor). Some may experience sudden recollections of the trauma in which they feel as if they are re-experiencing the event; frequently these recollections are distressing. For example, in one study (40), 52% of 172 adults assessed on the first day of hospitalization for an acute burn injury reported distressing recollections of the trauma. It is also possible that an individual may be preoccupied with the traumatic event, frequently thinking about or ruminating on the event. This preoccupation and rumination may or may not be distressing to the individual experiencing it. An increased perception of vulnerability,

a preoccupation with self-blame, and thoughts of the world being an unsafe place are also found in some persons who are newly injured. Congruent with the cognitive and psychodynamic theories described above, these thoughts may represent both symptoms of distress or difficulty as well as coping efforts and progress.

Behavioral Responses

A number of potential behavioral responses have been described in the general literature as common following a trauma and are not necessarily associated with poor adjustment or outcome. Individuals may respond to a trauma with social withdrawal or isolation. It can be difficult to physically withdraw from or avoid others when in a hospital environment, so social withdrawal, when present, may take on other forms, such as a reduction in interacting with others or limiting of the environment. For example, patients who respond with withdrawal behavior may isolate themselves in their room or not go on therapeutic recreation outings. Avoidance behavior can occur, and what is avoided can take various forms, including avoidance of feelings, avoidance of reminders of the trauma, or avoidance of discussion about the event. For example, a person who suffered an injury in a motor vehicle collision may avoid looking at pictures of the damaged car, avoid thinking about the collision, or avoid talking about the events surrounding the trauma. Less commonly, some patients may avoid aspects of medical care, not because of the aversiveness or unpleasantness of the care itself (such as a painful procedure) but because the medical care reminds them of their trauma. Conversely, others may respond by talking frequently about the trauma, including the events leading up to, during, and after, in considerable detail. Such individuals appear to have a need to tell and retell their story to themselves and/or others. At times this can be quite uncomfortable for those around the patient, particularly if they have heard the story before and find it distressing or unpleasant.

Similar to the emotional aspects of traumatic responses, individuals can also exhibit behaviors in the acute period that are positive, although this area, too, has received far less empirical attention than the "negative" behaviors. Rather than withdrawing from others, for example, persons may respond to trauma by seeking support from and affiliation with others (44). It is not uncommon to see individuals who are injured re-establishing contact or relationships with family members with whom they were estranged. Individuals who were recently traumatized may also report intentions to change or demonstrate actual changes in unhealthy behaviors such as substance abuse (see Chapter 12 for a discussion on substance use and abuse following trauma). Other positive behaviors are likely, although rarely described in the literature.

Prevalence of Psychopathology during the Acute Phase

Given the literature's focus on psychopathology after traumatic injury, most studies of acute psychological responses to traumatic injury have examined the prevalence of depressive symptoms, MDD, and anxiety (primarily ASD or PTS symptoms). Table 13-3 summarizes recent studies describing the prevalence of depressive symptoms and MDD in adults who had experienced a traumatic injury, specifically spinal cord injury (SCI), traumatic brain injury (TBI), or burn injury. It also includes a few studies of mixed etiology trauma cases hospitalized on trauma surgical services following intentional and unintentional injury. Table 13-3 is not an exhaustive list of all studies done in this area, as such a review is beyond the scope of this chapter. We included studies that met several criteria: (i) sample size larger than 50 participants; (ii) use of standardized and/or well-described, replicable measures; (iii) clearly specified time points at which the data were collected; (iv) inclusion of prevalence data in the results; (v) published after 1994, the year in which the *DSM-IV* was published and ASD was included in it. Studies of post-traumatic psychopathology following motor vehicle collisions that included persons without personal injury were not included. We also excluded samples that consisted exclusively of veterans, as they may not be representative of the broader injury population.

As shown in Table 13-3, across injury categories, depressive symptoms were reported by a sizable subset of persons who had recently experienced a traumatic injury. For example, in a longitudinal study of 283 adults admitted consecutively to a level I trauma center for moderate to severe traumatic brain injury, Dikmen et al. (45) found that nearly half (46%) of the sample endorsed a clinically significant level of depressive symptoms at 1 month post–brain injury, and of these,15% scored in the severe depressive symptom range. It is difficult to compare the specific rates of depressive symptoms across the various studies in Table 13-3 because of the variability in the measures used and in the time postinjury the assessments were conducted. In spite of these restrictions, clinically significant levels of depressive symptoms appeared prevalent in the other injury samples, including a study that excluded persons with a *Diagnostic and Statistical Manual of Mental Disorders*, Third Edition, Revised (DSM-III-R) diagnosis of MDD at the time of the trauma (46). In general, these rates are much higher

Table 13-3	Rates of Depressive Symptoms and Major Depressive Disorder in Adult Injury Samples			
Study	**Sample**	**Assessment (in Time Post Injury)**	**Used Diagnostic Interview**	**Results**
Wiechman et al., 2001 (67)	151 adults with burn injury	1 mo 1 y 2 y	No	54% had moderate to severe depressive symptoms at 1 mo 43% had moderate to severe depressive symptoms at 2 y
Zatzick et al., 2002 (68)	101 randomly selected trauma patients on a surgery service	While inpatient 1 y	No	41% had severe depressive symptoms in hospital
Zatzick et al., 2002 (69)	269 randomly selected trauma patients on acute surgery service	While hospitalized 1, 4, 12 mo	No	41% had significant depressive symptomatology (CES-D >27) while hospitalized and did not report rates of depressive symptoms for other time points
Ptacek et al., 2002 (46)	209 prospective sample with new burn injury Excluded those with preburn psychiatric diagnoses	Within 24 h of admission to burn center, 5 d, 10 d later, 1 mo post-discharge	No	d 1: 35% moderate, 17% severe depressive symptoms d 5: 23% moderate, 10% severe d 10: 8% moderate, 7% severe 1 mo postdc: 22% moderate, 13% severe (note significant attrition at 1 mo: $n = 30$)
Blanchard et al., 2004 (53)	132 survivors of MVCs Naturalist follow-up	14 mo	Yes	16% had MDD at 14 mo
Dikmen et al., 2004 (45)	283 consecutively admitted patients with moderate to severe TBI	1 mo, 6 mo, 12 mo, & 3–5 y	No	1 mo: 31% had moderate and 15% had severe depressive symptoms 6 mo: 22% moderate, 12% severe 1 y: 19% moderate, 12% severe 3–5 y: 17% moderate, 10% severe

dc, discharge; CES-D, Center for Epidemiological Studies-Depression; MDD, major depressive disorder; MVC, motor vehicle crash; TBI, traumatic brain injury.

than rates of depressive symptoms found in the general population (47) or primary care populations (48).

A concern often raised when assessing depressive symptoms in persons with a recent injury is that somatic and cognitive symptoms secondary to the injury inflate scores. Two main approaches have been developed to address this concern, the "inclusive" diagnostic approach, which counts depressive symptoms regardless of etiology, and the etiologic approach, which counts symptoms only if they are not clearly and fully accounted for by a medical condition (49). Using the more conservative etiologic approach, Dikmen et al. (45) found that the elevated depressive scale scores in their TBI sample did not reflect merely the somatic and cognitive symptoms of brain injury, as depressed affect, a lack of positive affect, and interpersonal problems were also present and contributed to the elevated scores. More work examining this diagnostic issue is needed in trauma populations.

Table 13-4 summarizes recent studies describing the prevalence of ASD and post-traumatic stress symptoms in samples of adults with traumatic injuries. The same criteria used in selecting studies to include in Table 13-3 were used for selecting the studies in Table 13-4. Only a few studies exist on ASD in survivors of traumatic injuries. Given this, as well as the potential limitations inherent in the construct of ASD noted in the literature, we must be cautious in drawing too many conclusions about ASD in trauma populations. It appears that ASD as it is currently defined likely occurs in 20% or less of survivors of traumatic injury. A recent review of post-traumatic disorders following traumatic injury (50) suggested a similar rate for survivors of traumatic injuries.

Aside from ASD, a few of the studies reviewed suggest that a number of post-traumatic stress symptoms are present in a sizable proportion of traumatic injury survivors during the immediate aftermath following injury. For example, in one study, persons with a new burn injury ($n = 172$) were asked to complete a post-traumatic stress symptom checklist within 24 hours of admission to a burn center (40). Of these, more than half (55%) reported sleep disturbance and nearly half (48%) reported difficulties concentrating. Nearly a third of the sample reported flashbacks (32%), exaggerated startle response (31%), and nightmares (30%) within the first 24 hours after the burn. Only 10% reported no symptoms of post-traumatic stress in this sample. In another sample of burn survivors (39) who were assessed within 2 weeks of their injuries, a considerable portion of the patients experienced distress at reminders of the injury (40%), intrusive recollections of the trauma (39%), and nightmares (29%). Many also reported avoidance of stimuli reminiscent of the burn injury, including avoidance of feelings (51%), thoughts (50%), and talking about the trauma (27%). Insomnia (76%), irritability (44%), hypervigilance (37%), and exaggerated startle response (33%) were also common. Taken together, these results suggest that post-traumatic stress symptoms, including re-experiencing the trauma, increased arousal, and avoidance, can occur but are not universally experienced after a traumatic injury.

Other Psychological Responses during the Acute Phase

A paucity of research exists in the empirical literature about the phenomenology of other types of acute psychological responses to traumatic injury besides depressive symptoms, ASD, and post-traumatic stress symptoms. Little is known empirically about other types of acute anxiety such as anxiety related to medical procedures. Given that subthreshold levels of depressive and post-traumatic stress symptoms can occur in a number of acutely injured adults, psychological distress and suffering can occur even in the absence of a diagnosable *DSM-IV* disorder.

In most studies of acute emotional responses to traumatic injury, half or more of the survivors did *not* have clinically significant levels of depressive and post-traumatic stress symptoms. Regrettably, we know very little about this majority, that is, those survivors who do not report significant emotional distress following an acute traumatic injury. It is quite likely that many individuals who have suffered a traumatic injury respond with a variety of non-pathologic responses, such as positive emotions and resilience, in the immediate aftermath of trauma.

Summary

In the immediate aftermath of a traumatic injury, depressive symptoms, post-traumatic stress symptoms, and, to a lesser degree, ASD are common but not universal. Very little is known about the more than half of the survivors of traumatic injuries who do not have significant distress in the acute phase following their injuries. In addition, our understanding of other acute psychological experiences besides depressive symptoms and post-traumatic stress is limited by the focus on psychopathology and lack of research on more positive experiences. We suspect that most of the acute psychological responses to trauma are "normal" reactions to highly abnormal events, but this hypothesis remains to be tested empirically in traumatically injured samples.

Table 13-4	Rates of Acute Stress Disorder, Post-traumatic Stress Symptoms, and Post-traumatic Stress Disorder in Adult Injury Samples

Study	Sample	Assessment (in Time Post Injury)	Used Diagnostic Interview	Results
Bryant & Harvey, 1995 (70)	56 patients hospitalized following MVC[a]	12 mo	No	46% had significant PTS symptoms
Ehlers et al., 1998 (71)	967 consecutive patients presenting to emergency clinic after MVC	immediate 3 mo 1 y	No but able to compute PTSD	23% had PTSD at 3 mo 17% at 1 y
Bryant & Harvey, 1998 (72)	79 consecutive adults with mild TBI	1 & 6 mo post injury	Yes	14% had ASD within 1 mo of injury 24% satisfied criteria for PTSD at 1 mo 24% had PTSD 82% of those with ASD had PTSD at 6 mo as compared to 11%
Ehde et al., 1999 (40)	172 adults with burn injury Excluded persons with Axis I mental disorders at time of injury	Within 24 h of admission to burn center	No	10% reported no PTS symptoms 24% met criteria for all three PTSD symptom clusters
Ehde et al., 2000 (73)	172 prospective sample of adults with burn injury Excluded persons with Axis I mental disorders at time of injury	While inpatient 1 mo 1 y	No	21% met criteria for all three PTSD symptom clusters at 1 mo 19% met criteria for all three PTSD symptom clusters at 1 y
Kennedy & Evans, 2001 (74)	85 inpatients at SCI center	6–24 wk post injury	No	14% had high levels of PTS symptoms No difference in PTS symptoms between those with & those without post-traumatic amnesia; those with high levels of PTS also scored high on state anxiety and depressive symptoms
Difede, et al., 2002 (39)	83 consecutive cases of hospitalized adults with burn injury	Within 2 wk 6 mo postburn	Yes	19% met *DSM-IV* criteria for ASD at 2 wk 21% met acute PTSD criteria (except time criteria) at 2 wk 36% had PTSD at 6 mo 89% of those with ASD while hosp had PTSD at 6 mo; only 1 person who had ASD did not develop PTSD at 6 mo 24% had prior psychiatric history
Zatzick et al., 2002 (69)	269 randomly selected trauma patients on acute surgery service	While hospitalized 1, 4, 12 mo	No	31% had significant PTS symptomatology (45 >27) while hospitalized 41% at 1 mo, 40% at 4 mo, 30% at 12 mo had significant PTS symptoms
Zatzick et al., 2002 (68)	101 randomly selected trauma patients on a surgery service	While inpatient 1 y	No	30% met symptomatic criteria for PTSD at 1 y
Nielson, 2003 (75)	69 consecutively admitted cases of SCI	Acute care rehabilitation	No	20% had significant PTS symptoms
Blanchard et al., 2004 (53)	132 survivors of MVCs Naturalist follow-up	1 to 4 mo 14 mo	Yes	14% had PTSD at 14 mo 53% of those with PTSD at 14 mo also had MDD
Zatzick et al., 2004 (43)	269 randomly selected trauma patients on surgery service	Acute care hospitalization	No	20% met symptomatic criteria for ASD

ASD, acute stress disorder; PTS, post-traumatic stress; PTSD, post-traumatic stress disorder; MDD, major depressive disorder; MVC, motor vehicle crash; SCI, spinal cord injury; TBI, traumatic brain injury; hosp, hospitalized.
[a]Only MVC studies in which personal injury were sustained were included. Studies in which persons may not have been injured were excluded.

LONG-TERM PSYCHOLOGICAL RESPONSES TO TRAUMA

The long-term psychological outcomes most frequently studied after a traumatic injury have overwhelmingly been depressive symptoms, depressive disorders, and post-traumatic stress disorder. Few studies have examined other psychological disorders, and even fewer have investigated positive outcomes. What follows is a brief overview of this research, along with a summary of what remains to be investigated with respect to long-term psychological responses to traumatic injury.

Prevalence of Psychopathology after the Acute Injury Period

A number of empirical studies, as shown in Table 13-3, as well as several reviews have examined long-term rates of depressive symptomatology and MDD after injury, including amputation (51), burn injury (8), traumatic brain injury (52), and spinal cord injury (5). Comparing rates across injury groups or at specific time points after the onset of injuries is difficult given the methodological variability in the depressive symptom measures, the cut-offs used by researchers to ascertain levels of clinically significant symptoms, and the varied assessment time points. Nonetheless, it is apparent from reviewing these studies that the rates of depressive symptomatology and MDD are higher than rates in the general population (47) and other medical populations, including primary care populations (48). In general, the rate of moderate or severe depressive symptoms appears to range roughly between 20% and 45% for persons who are 1 year or more past the onset of their injury. We found only one study (53) that used *DSM-IV* criteria for diagnosing an actual MDD. Interestingly, the rate of MDD in this study of survivors of MVC was lower—14%—than rates of reported "significant" depressive symptoms in the other studies.

Post-traumatic stress disorder is the most frequently studied anxiety disorder in survivors of traumatic injuries. As shown in Table 13-4, there is considerable variability in the rates of PTSD symptoms and PTSD itself following injury. As noted in a recent review (50), a number of methodologic issues may contribute to the disparate findings in the injury literature. First, few studies attempt to differentiate whether the post-traumatic stress symptoms (e.g., difficulty concentrating) are directly attributable to the psychological trauma (e.g., post-traumatic anxiety), the effects of the injury (e.g., cognitive sequelae of head injury), or the treatment (e.g., medications). Second, few studies measured

the occurrence of distress and disability (criterion F of *DSM-IV* PTSD), and few indicated whether samples were representative of the larger population from which they were drawn. Finally, we suggest that the variability of measures used for and timing of assessing PTSD also potentially contribute to the inconsistent PTSD rates in the trauma injury literature.

Depressive and post-traumatic stress disorders are not the only psychiatric conditions that may arise from a traumatic event. Increased rates of other psychiatric disorders, including generalized anxiety disorder, substance abuse disorders, and phobias, were reported in a meta-analysis of psychopathology following civilian trauma (54). The available literature on other psychiatric conditions following traumatic injuries is sparse, and, when available, methodological limitations make drawing conclusions difficult (for a review, see O'Donnell et al. [50]). In the broader trauma literature, it is well established that other psychiatric disorders are frequently found in survivors with PTSD (55). A recent study (53) of survivors of personal injury motor vehicle collisions found high rates of comorbid psychiatric conditions in survivors with PTSD between 1 and 2 years after the collision. For example, of persons with PTSD, 53% had a concurrent major depressive disorder, 26% had a concurrent generalized anxiety disorder, and 42% had any concurrent anxiety disorder (in addition to PTSD). Surprisingly, Blanchard et al. found strikingly similar high rates of comorbid conditions not only in individuals seeking treatment for PTSD but also in their naturalistic follow-up sample. Thus, when PTSD is present, assessment of other potential disorders is indicated.

Some persons develop specific fears in response to circumstances of the traumatic event that caused the injury. For example, a person who sustained an injury in a fall from a ladder may develop a fear of heights, ladders, ledges, or all three. At their most severe levels, these specific fears may meet *DSM-IV* diagnostic criteria for an anxiety disorder known as specific phobia. A specific phobia may be present if (i) the fear triggered by the feared situation (e.g., driving) or anticipation of the situation is persistent, excessive, and/or unreasonable and the person recognizes that the fear is excessive or unreasonable; (ii) exposure to the feared stimulus triggers a significant anxiety response, including possibly a panic attack; (iii) the feared situation is avoided or tolerated but with extreme anxiety; (iv) the anxiety, avoidance, or distress caused by the fear interferes considerably with the person's functioning (3).

Survivors of motor vehicle collisions may develop specific fears about driving, being a passenger in a vehicle, or crossing streets, for example. In a rare study (56) that included a question about such fears,

38% of motor vehicle collision survivors ($n = 149$) reported a fear of driving 1 year after discharge from a trauma center. This type of fear is sometimes referred to as travel anxiety, travel phobia, accident phobia, or driving phobia (57). Our understanding of this phenomenon is limited by a lack of empirical studies in the area. One study (58) of injured and non-injured adults presenting to an emergency department following MVCs reported rates of "phobic travel anxiety" (measured by a self-report questionnaire) of 22% and 16% at 3 and 12 months, respectively, postinjury. In our clinical experience, this fear and its effects on the individual experiencing it can range considerably. Our impression is that some degree of travel-related fear is commonly but not universally experienced by survivors of a travel-related traumatic injury. For many, it appears to gradually dissipate with time and exposure to the feared situation (e.g., riding in a car, crossing a street). However, we have noticed that, for some, the fears may persist and develop into a specific phobia. Research on the assorted fears and phobias found after injury is needed.

Other Long-term Psychological Responses

In addition to the formal psychological disorders that may occur following trauma, a few studies have examined other psychological responses to trauma. One unique study combining quantitative and qualitative research methods (59) asked injury survivors ($n = 97$) what concerned them the most since being injured. They were interviewed and asked to respond to this question in the hospital and at 1, 4, and 12 months after the trauma as well as to complete measures of post-traumatic stress symptoms and functional limitations. Their findings revealed that 99% of their sample identified at least one post-traumatic concern in the first year. Over the course of the year, the frequency of concerns decreased, as did post-traumatic stress symptoms and functional limitations. Physical health concerns (e.g., worried about future and current health, self-care, physical limitations) were of primary concern, followed by psychological concerns (e.g., distress, struggles with substance abuse, body image concerns, fear regarding safety), and employment/financial concerns (worried about finances, employment, ability to provide for self or family).

One recent study (60) examined "positive by-products" of spinal cord injury using the Perceived Benefits Scale (PBS) (61). The PBS requires respondents to rate 30 positive items that are delineated into eight subscales: increased self-efficacy, increased faith in people, increased compassion, increased spirituality, increased community closeness, increased family closeness, positive lifestyle changes, and material gain. Respondents (42 persons between 18 and 36 months post spinal cord injury) were also asked whether they had experienced other benefits as a result of the spinal cord injury. A majority (79%) of participants reported at least one positive by-product; the average number of positive benefits in the sample was 2.28 (SD = 1.83). The most frequently reported positive by-products from the SCI were increased family closeness and increased compassion. The least frequently reported were material gain and community closeness. Additional by-products were reported and grouped into several categories that included gaining new attitudes/perspectives, improved views of self, improved views of persons with disabilities, increased gratitude, and increased helping of others. Although the authors noted several limitations in this study, including uncertainty about the representativeness of the sample and its size, it remains an important study for its focus on nonpathologic outcomes to spinal cord injury. Other less rigorous studies have described positive outcomes in other areas, such as brain injury (44); however, more studies in other injury populations are needed.

Natural History of Psychological Responses

The theories of trauma described earlier describe a variety of possible mechanisms by which individuals may cope with a trauma over time. For example, coping strategies may be learned and reinforced (behavioral approach), psychic distress gradually reduced to a tolerable level (psychodynamic approach), or core beliefs altered and meaning found (cognitive approach). It is probable that the normative response following a traumatic injury is to experience a range of psychological symptoms, including post-traumatic stress symptoms, in the initial aftermath followed by a remittance of most or all symptoms in the following months (62). We hypothesize that similar to noninjured trauma survivors, many individuals will not only show a lack of psychological distress but also show evidence of positive responses such as resilience, positive emotions, and post-traumatic growth during and after the trauma. Given that rates of psychopathology are higher in trauma samples, it is also likely that an important subset of individuals after trauma will suffer considerable psychological distress that interferes with their functioning. Research testing these and other hypotheses about the natural history of traumatic responses to injury are needed.

Summary

Much of the literature on long-term emotional experiences after traumatic injury is limited in its focus on psychopathologic states. In particular, we know little about the nature, range, frequency, profile, or natural history of positive emotions, resilience, and post-traumatic growth after injury. In most studies of emotional responses to traumatic injury, more than half of the samples do *not* report clinically notable levels of psychopathology. Yet, we know very little about this majority, that is, those who did not report significant emotional distress. For example, we do not know if these nondistressed individuals experience a lack of distress, a lack of positive emotions, the presence of positive emotions, or some combination of these states. In the broader psychological and trauma literatures, it has been repeatedly documented that positive psychological emotions and outcomes are experienced by persons facing tremendous changes, stressors, and loss (2,63). Much empirical work remains to be done if our understanding of the full range of responses to traumatic injury is to grow.

DEBUNKING MYTHS ABOUT PSYCHOLOGICAL RESPONSES TO TRAUMA

The general public as well as many health care professionals holds strong assumptions about how individuals should respond to a traumatic event such as an injury or loss. These assumptions are most likely influenced by a number of factors, including popular theories about loss, clinical lore, and culture. Research has shown, repeatedly, however, that many of these assumptions are simply not true but are instead misconceptions or myths; for further reading on these myths and relevant research, see (9,36,64). Thus, when discussing psychological responses to injury, it is important to be wary of several of these myths.

Perhaps the biggest myth about adaptation to trauma is that adjustment occurs by means of a predictable "stage model" process that is common among most persons. Of these, the most widely known "stage model" of coping was proposed by Kubler-Ross (65), who suggested that people respond to trauma or major loss in five sequential stages: denial, anger, bargaining, depression, and acceptance. In their excellent review, Wortman and Silver (64) note that not all individuals experience all of the stages, nor do they necessarily progress through the stages in the same order, instead bouncing back and forth between reactions. Moreover, they observed that individuals often demonstrate concurrent emotional reactions that do not occur in a linear fashion, may skip entire emotional experiences or stages, and may also have positive emotional experiences that are not usually represented in these stage theories.

Finally, a sizable minority of survivors do not achieve the "acceptance" or "recovery" stage. Although certainly stage theories of loss have been useful in describing many of the reactions that can occur following loss, the adjustment process does not follow such rules. In fact, Elizabeth Kubler-Ross herself later noted that she did not anticipate that people would ascribe to her theory so rigidly; she meant it to be a useful framework for conceptualizing loss.

In a similar vein, another common myth commonly seen in health care and rehabilitation settings is that intense psychological distress is inevitable and must be "worked through" in order to adapt to the injury and consequent disability. In the disability literature this assumption has been referred to as the "requirement of mourning" (9,36,37). Inherent in this myth is the notion that an injury or disability represents a "loss" and that a process of mourning the loss is necessary for resolution (9,36,37). A related myth, identified by Wortman and Silver (64) is the inaccurate assumption that severe distress is necessary, and it is abnormal not to experience severe distress. This myth assumes that it is somehow "therapeutic" to be depressed following a trauma or loss and that confronting the realities of the situation is necessary for healthy adaptation. It further assumes that one is "denying" the situation if the person is not depressed following the loss and that severe distress will "surface" later if not experienced early on. However, research has shown that this is simply not true (2,64,66). In contrast, psychological distress is not an inevitable consequence of trauma, as shown in Tables 13-3 and 13-4. Indeed, the majority of injury survivors do *not* experience significant psychological distress after injury.

A more recent review (76) tested three additional assumptions about coping with sudden, traumatic loss: (i) that people confronting such losses inevitably search for meaning; (ii) that over time most are able to find meaning and put the issue aside; and (iii) that finding meaning is critical for adjustment or healing. These authors found evidence that refuted each of these assumptions. First, they found that there is a significant subset of individuals who do not search for meaning and yet appear relatively well adjusted to their losses. In fact, endless search for meaning may be a hallmark of poor coping. Second, fewer than half of the respondents in each of the samples studied reported finding any meaning in their loss, even more than a year after the event. Finally, while those who found meaning were better adjusted than those who searched but were unable to find meaning, many were unable to put the issue of meaning aside and move on. Rather, they continued to pursue the issue of meaning as fervently as those who searched but did not find meaning. While other studies have shown that benefit finding and meaning making are common and important after loss or trauma (77–80), these findings suggest that there may be an optimal level of such activities, beyond which little additional benefit is gained.

Finally, it is commonly assumed that everyone who has experienced a trauma or loss "recovers" from or resolves the emotional effects of the loss. Further, this recovery is thought to occur within a prescribed period of time, most commonly, one year. However, the research has shown that adapting to a loss is not as neat and orderly as this myth assumes. In fact, as observed by Wortman and Silver (64), a sizable minority of individuals continue to exhibit considerable distress long after loss. This has been replicated repeatedly in the injury literature, which has shown that depressive symptoms, MDD, and PTSD are prevalent in a considerable subset of persons long after they have suffered their injuries. Thus, it is not clear that everyone "accepts" his or her injury or disability, nor is it evident that such "acceptance" is necessary for psychological health.

In addition to these myths, it is also worth noting that health care providers may be poor judges of their patients' distress levels. In a study (81) of 50 patients hospitalized for burns and 75 members of the burn staff, staff tended to overestimate depression and underestimate optimism in their patients. Moreover, the more experienced nurses and occupational and physical therapists were less accurate in estimating depression and optimism than their less experienced counterparts. Similar findings have been noted among persons with new spinal cord injuries and their care providers (82).

FACTORS INFLUENCING PSYCHOLOGICAL RESPONSES TO AND RECOVERY FROM TRAUMA

A large body of research exists on biopsychosocial factors associated with the development of post-traumatic psychopathology, particularly PTSD. As summarized in Table 13-5, one's response to a traumatic event depends on multiple factors, including (i) objective aspects of the traumatic event; (ii) biologic, psychological, and cognitive peritraumatic responses; (iii) individual factors, including the resources and difficulties the individual brings to the situation as well as the subjective experience and meaning that the trauma holds for the individual; and (iv) characteristics of the post-traumatic environment, including the social and cultural environment. A recent meta-analysis of predictors of PTSD in adults found that prior trauma history, prior psychological disorders, family history of psychopathology,

perceived life threat during the trauma, poor post-trauma social support, peritraumatic emotional responses, and peritraumatic dissociation were all associated with increased risk of PTSD. However, of these factors, peritraumatic dissociation was the strongest predictor of PTSD development, while family history and prior trauma were the weakest predictors of PTSD, although still significant (83). A brief synopsis of predictors described in the general trauma literature is provided in Table 13-5.

Aspects of the Trauma

In general, traumatic events that are severe, sudden, unexpected, prolonged, repetitive, or the result of intentional human actions are highly predictive of the development of PTSD (4). Proximity to and responsibility for the trauma have also been associated with greater risk of PTSD. Specifically, increasing risk is generally associated with each of the following roles in a trauma—witness, participant, target, and agent (4). That said, this is not always the case, highlighting the importance of subjective meaning. For example, in one study (84) comparing survivors of MVCs who were responsible for their accidents with survivors of MVCs who were not, survivors who were not responsible were more likely to report long-term distress and to have PTSD at 1 year than those who were responsible, even when controlling for injury severity. Drivers who were not responsible reported more concerns that they would experience a similar collision again in the future. The authors hypothesized that drivers not responsible may have suffered a loss of confidence in their ability to control future driving experiences. In contrast, some studies in the general trauma literature have found that the perception of personal responsibility for a trauma is associated with increased risk of PTSD (4).

Injury factors have also been examined for their potential role in psychopathology following trauma. It is frequently assumed in our culture that the more severe the injury and subsequent disability, the more likely an individual will be to suffer from psychopathology after trauma. However, the preponderance of available research suggests that the severity of injury is a poor predictor of who will and will not develop post-traumatic psychopathology across a variety of injury types (50,69,84,85). Considerable debate in the literature exists regarding whether individuals who have sustained TBI can develop PTSD, given survivors of TBI typically have a loss of consciousness, post-traumatic amnesia, or both during the time the trauma occurs. A proportion of survivors of TBI report intrusive and avoidance symptoms despite being amnestic of their trauma (86). In his review of the evidence for and against PTSD

Table 13-5	Factors Associated with Increased Vulnerability to PTSD after Trauma

CHARACTERISTICS OF THE TRAUMA
- Increased proximity to trauma
- Longer duration of exposure to stressor or trauma
- Trauma was the result of an intentional or deliberate act
- Witnessing physical violence or massive injuries
- Witnessing violent or sudden death of others, especially loved ones
- Witnessing significant property damage
- Learning of one's exposure to further potential threats, continued risk
- Irreversibility of resource losses
- Escape blocked or experienced impossible choices
- Constant reminders, chronic exposure to reminders of the event, absence of a "safety" signal
- Uncertainty about further future injury (e.g., exposed to noxious agents, long-term consequences unknown)
- Immediate loss of access to social support (i.e., separated from loved ones during trauma, significant disruption in social network)

FACTORS RELATED TO THE SURVIVOR
- Trauma perceived as unexpected, unpredictable, sudden
- Trauma perceived as intensely threatening to life or bodily integrity of self or family
- Perceived lack of control
- Perception of personal responsibility or self-blame
- Lack of social support
- Prior history of mental illness, presence of comorbidity
- Prior history of adjustment problems to stressors of traumatic events
- Prior exposure to traumatic events, particularly those that may be "re-activated" by current trauma
- Premorbid marital or familial distress, financial distress, or other major life stressor

CHARACTERISTICS OF THE PERITRAUMATIC RESPONSE AND ENVIRONMENT
- Intense initial emotional reactions, such as panic or dissociation
- Feelings of helplessness during and after the trauma
- Lack of safety or inadequate removal of threat
- Immediate negative social consequences (i.e., separation from loved ones)
- Inability to resume normal routines or exposure to continued adversity
- Perceived lack of assistance
- Provision of assistance that made things worse
- Lack of information
- Provision of information that is inconsistent, confusing, or contradictory
- Mitigating factors, such as unwanted media presence, litigation, logistical problems

SOCIAL/CONTEXTUAL FACTORS
- Unsupportive views from community (e.g., stigmatizing)
- "Secondary victimization" whereby survivor experiences repeated trauma in the course of coping with initial trauma
- "Marginalized" social status (e.g., geographically isolated, homeless, lacking financial or social resources)
- Stress reactions of significant others
- Lack of community solidarity or group cohesion

after brain injury, Bryant (87) describes several potential mechanisms, including neurobiologic contributors, which may explain why PTSD has been reported in persons with TBI. Thus, we caution against uniformly viewing a loss of consciousness or post-traumatic amnesia as protective factors for PTSD after brain injury.

Peritraumatic Responses

Evidence is increasingly mounting for neurobiologic factors, including neural sensitization and ongoing sympathetic nervous system activation, as potentially important mediators of PTSD (62). Experiencing marked psychological distress, such as panic attacks or dissociation, may lead to subsequent anxiety, including panic attacks and PTSD.

Numerous studies in the trauma literature, including the injury literature, have looked at the relationship between initial symptoms of ASD and/or post-traumatic stress symptoms and the subsequent development of PTSD. Findings are contrary, however; one recent review (62) concluded that the literature lacks consensus on the value of such symptoms in predicting PTSD, while a recent meta-analysis (83) indicated that peritraumatic dissociation is the strongest predictor of PTSD.

Individual's cognitive responses to the traumatic event have also been implicated as potential mediators between the trauma and post-traumatic psychological functioning. Excessively negative appraisals of the trauma and/or subsequent consequences have been shown to be associated with PTSD. For example, in one study, negative or catastrophic thinking in the first 3 months after a trauma predicted PTSD at one year as well as chronic PTSD (71). Coping with the trauma by using wishful thinking (e.g., wishing the trauma had not occurred) has also been associated with poorer outcomes after a traumatic injury (88). Other types of coping strategies, such as coping through avoidance behavior, have also been associated with higher rates of post-traumatic stress after injury (70,89).

Individual Factors

Characteristics of the survivor's premorbid history, functioning, and environment may also play a role in an individual's vulnerability to PTSD. A prior history of psychiatric disorder, prior exposure to trauma, and premorbid stressors have been associated with post-traumatic psychological difficulties. For example, limited evidence suggests that previous trauma experience is associated with increased difficulty in adjusting to subsequent trauma (4). This cumulative toll has been particularly well demonstrated among soldiers, where each additional battle experience makes him or her more susceptible to subsequent psychiatric distress (90). Survivors of trauma, including traumatic injuries, often have a premorbid history of trauma (39,69). Thus, in clinical settings, persons who may require special consideration are those with a military combat history, those who have a history of rape, domestic violence, or sexual or other abuse, those with a history of prior traumatic injuries or motor vehicle collisions, and those who are refugees from other countries who have been exposed to prolonged or widespread trauma.

Some gender differences have been observed in response to trauma, including traumatic injury. After a trauma, women report higher incidence of psychological symptoms, especially anxiety and depression, while men evidence an increased number of physician visits, physical symptoms, hospital referrals, belligerence, and alcohol use (4). In two samples of survivors of mixed-injury etiology, female gender was associated with higher post-traumatic stress symptoms (43,69). Women also evidence greater sensitivity to the stress of others, referred to as "network stress" (91), and are more often called upon to provide emotional support (4). Women report more comfort in self-disclosing and more benefit from talking with others than men (27).

Environmental and Contextual Factors

Social and cultural factors, such as lack of social support, perceived stigma or marginalization from society, and ongoing barriers that interfere with resumption of normal routines are also associated with increased risk for post-traumatic psychopathology. Those who experienced a lack of assistance in the face of trauma, who were faced with unhelpful behavior from witnesses, who have been faced with negative reactions from others or significant stress reactions from loved ones, or who have been deprived of accurate information and relief from immediate threat are at increased risk for post-traumatic psychological difficulties. The reader is referred to Meichenbaum's comprehensive PTSD treatment manual (4) for a more in-depth review of factors associated with increased difficulty recovering from trauma.

WHAT ABOUT RESILIENCE?

Psychological resilience after injury has been woefully neglected in the empirical literature. Authors have alluded to its presence in injury populations when describing those who do not suffer from psychopathology after injury as resilient. However, theoretically driven investigations of resilience are lacking. Given resilience is likely the norm, rather than the exception, after trauma, a few points from the noninjury resilience literature merit discussion. First, resilience is increasingly being recognized as common after adversity, loss, and trauma (2). For example, recent prospective studies have shown repeatedly that 50% or more of bereaved individuals experience low levels of distress after loss (66). This proportion is strikingly similar to the proportion of adults not experiencing significant distress in Tables 13-3 and 13-4 of this chapter. Resilience also appears to be the norm, rather than the exception, in survivors of violent and life-threatening events such as assault (92), terrorism (93,94), and natural disasters (80). Second, being resilient does not mean that a person never experiences difficulty, discouragement, intrusive thoughts about the trauma, or emotional distress. Such experiences are common following loss or trauma and may in fact be part of the resilience process (2). However, in resilient individuals, such experiences are typically transient, co-occur with positive emotions, and do not significantly interfere with functioning (95). Third, although certain personality traits such as hardiness may predispose some individuals to resilience (96,97), resilience is most likely not merely a personality characteristic that individuals either have or do not have. Rather, resilience appears to consist of thoughts and actions, many of which may be learned, nurtured, and practiced by anyone who seeks resilience. A number of factors likely contribute to resilience and include the following: (i) supportive relationships; (ii) the ability to problem solve difficulties with realistic plans; (iii) good interpersonal communication skills; (iv) the ability to cope with strong negative emotions; and (v) self-efficacy (98). Finally, as observed by Bonanno in his review (2), there is no one path or strategy to resilience. Thus far, the evidence suggests that resilience may be maintained or achieved through a variety of mechanisms, including some that are often considered "unhealthy" such as using repression of emotions to cope with distressing events.

PROMOTING RESILIENCE AND PSYCHOLOGICAL HEALTH AFTER TRAUMA: ASSESSMENT, ISSUES, AND INTERVENTIONS

Considerable methodologically rigorous research exists in the general trauma literature on effective interventions for treating psychopathologic conditions, primarily PTSD, following trauma. This literature, as well as the few intervention studies conducted for injury-related concerns, will form the basis of our recommendations regarding treatment. First, we will discuss issues relevant to the assessment of traumatic reactions in the rehabilitation setting. We will then review two of the most common ways people naturally deal with trauma: by seeking support from others and by talking about the trauma (*disclosure*). We will also briefly review the literature on one type of trauma intervention, *debriefing*, that, although frequently applied, does not have empirical support in the literature. After describing what not to do, we will provide an overview of empirically supported interventions for post-traumatic stress conditions. We will conclude with a list of specific strategies for facilitating resilience and decreasing normal distress that rehabilitation staff and other health care professionals may consider when working with survivors of physical trauma.

Because a number of reviews (52,99) regarding the pharmacologic and psychological treatment of mood disorders, primarily depressive disorders, are available in the rehabilitation literature, they will not be reviewed here.

ASSESSMENT OF IMPACT OF TRAUMA

It is a complicated matter to thoroughly assess the psychological impact of a trauma, requiring sensitivity, skill, and training. Inquiring about the trauma may be distressing and further traumatizing to the survivor, particularly if multiple providers are asking similar questions, if the "interviewer" is perceived as insensitive or voyeuristic, if the material is highly personal, distressing, or sensitive, or if the rationale for the assessment is unclear. The trauma can impact a range of different life domains and can vary markedly depending on the assessment time point. Thorough assessment should include the survivor, as well as immediate family members or others who might have been involved in the trauma. Treatment may need to be integrated with assessment immediately. Assessment in the acute stage may overestimate the presence of psychological distress associated with trauma and result in unnecessary or even iatrogenic treatment or recommendations. Finally, in an acute medical setting, immediate assessment may be complicated by medical factors, such as traumatic brain injury, delirium, pain, medications, or other mental status changes that interfere with memory for the event. These are some of a myriad of reasons why we recommend against routine psychological assessment for psychological adjustment to trauma in acute settings, and we particularly caution providers who are not mental health professionals against assessing for impact of trauma beyond the physical realm.

That said, it is clearly important to monitor survivors' psychological well-being and provide services in a timely and effective manner if indicated. When should adjustment to trauma be formally assessed? How should it be assessed, and by whom? We propose that in acute medical settings, symptoms such as sleep disturbance, occasional emotional expressions of distress, fear, or anger, periods of transient withdrawal or refusal to engage, or attempts to control one's surroundings and increase safety be accommodated with sensitivity if possible and monitored but not necessarily viewed as signs of adjustment difficulties. Survivors who confide their experiences or concerns to care providers can be provided with empathy and support, and, if indicated, a referral to a mental health provider. Indications for consulting a psychologist, social worker, psychiatrist, or chaplain with specific training in trauma for assessment or treatment would include the following:

1. The patient or his or her family member requests input or help from a mental health professional;
2. The patient (or his or her family member) reports persistent symptoms of dissociation, intrusive thoughts/ruminations, nightmares, marked anxiety, fear, or sadness related to the trauma;
3. The patient reports suicidal or homicidal ideation;
4. The mental health provider has learned enough of the circumstances surrounding the trauma to identify it as high risk, and further evaluation is indicated. Aspects of a trauma that increase risk of adjustment problems are discussed elsewhere in this chapter.

There are many ways to assess psychological reactions to trauma, including formalized screening tools as well as clinically oriented discussions or interviews. A thorough review of available assessment tools and necessary interview questions is beyond the scope of this chapter, and the reader is referred to two comprehensive texts that describe such assessments, the *Clinical Handbook/Practical Therapist Manual for Assessing and Treating Adults with Post-Traumatic Stress Disorder* (4) and *After the Crash: Psychological Assessment and Treatment of Survivors of Motor Vehicle Accidents* (57).

THE ROLE OF SOCIAL SUPPORT IN ADAPTING TO TRAUMA

Social support is a complex phenomenon, comprised of a person's social networks, perceived availability and quality of support, support provided and supportive behaviors, and aversive (unhelpful) support. A comprehensive review of the role of social support in adaptation to trauma is beyond the scope of this chapter. Nevertheless, it is important to mention that a trauma can result in both increases and decreases in social networks and support. It may also disrupt the lives of close friends and families, and for some, contribute to any of a variety of interpersonal challenges such as increased conflict in relationships. For example, in the TBI literature there are numerous studies documenting the disrupted social relationships that can occur after a brain injury. Changes described include losses of old friends, difficulties forming new social contacts, and fewer leisure and social activities (52). Therefore, social support should be evaluated as part of a trauma assessment and viewed as an area of potential difficulty as well as an immense potential resource.

Disruption in social support following trauma is associated with increased likelihood of adjustment difficulties, while good social support in the aftermath of trauma may buffer the individual against the negative consequences of stress, depression, and pain (100,101). Research has repeatedly shown that having a network of caring and supportive relationships both within and outside the family plays a key role in being resilient (98). The most helpful support is likely to be that which matches the stressor or the person's needs in a given situation. For example, social support may be tangible (e.g., financial help, transportation, child care), emotional, companionship, information, or affection, depending on the specific needs of the affected individual.

It is important to treat trauma in a social context and involve family in treatment after trauma. For example, Malt (102) notes that in a 3-year follow-up study of adults injured in traffic accidents, 25% of close relatives reported impaired psychological health in themselves as a consequence of injury to their loved one. Members of the survivor's social support network may experience their own unique stressors as a result of the trauma, such as having to independently manage the home, finances, and children during an extended hospitalization, having to make medical decisions for an incapacitated loved one, or experiencing anxiety over medical procedures or injuries (i.e., threatened loss of family member). Providing support and care to the affected family members may benefit both the family and the survivor.

DO YOU HAVE TO TALK ABOUT A TRAUMA IN ORDER TO RECOVER?

Empirical evidence suggests that when confronted with major life difficulties or trauma, most people are naturally inclined to talk about their thoughts (103) and share their emotions (104,105). However, certain circumstances may dissuade individuals from disclosing to others. For example, people may not discuss their feelings if they perceive their experience or situation as socially unacceptable, desire to protect their audience, find such discussion painful or difficult, or perceive that the consequences of disclosure are severe or stigmatizing.

Many schools and methods of clinical psychotherapy incorporate disclosure or discussion of traumatic experiences as part of the therapeutic process. Indeed, dialog is the foundation of most clinical psychology practice. Such discussion can be desensitizing, cathartic, and can guide psychotherapists in the provision of support and insight. This is particularly relevant for persons whose presenting problems or diagnoses center around trauma.

The literature generally suggests that talking about a trauma can be of benefit to survivors, and that inhibition of such discussion (either based on intrinsic or extrinsic constraints) can be associated with detrimental outcomes. Pennebaker's Action-Inhibition Theory (106,107) suggests that to deliberately refrain from sharing and experiencing thoughts and emotions surrounding highly stressful or traumatic experiences (i.e., to inhibit) requires cognitive, behavioral, and physiologic work. Pennebaker proposes that the physiologic work associated with such inhibition may ultimately increase the risk of stress-related illness and may also prevent effective coping and adjustment. Information that is inhibited cannot be assimilated or forgotten and may emerge in intrusive thoughts or lead to avoidant behavior (108). Ironically, deliberately suppressing thoughts also may lead to increased frequency of the unwanted thoughts and to increased ruminations and worry (109).

Disclosing thoughts and emotions surrounding a traumatic experience either verbally or in writing has been conceptualized as the "antidote" to inhibition. Studies of such disclosure in an experimental context have provided compelling evidence supporting Pennebaker's theory (see Littrell [110] for a review). Essentially, existing studies suggest that disclosure of thoughts and feelings surrounding a traumatic experience results in improvement across some indicators of health (111–114), and in some studies, reduced disease outcome (115,116). In a meta-analysis of 13 randomized, controlled disclosure studies, Smyth (116) reported a mean weighted effect size of (Cohen's) $d = 0.47$ (r = 0.23, p <0.0001), which suggests that there is a causal relationship between written emotional expression and positive long-term health outcomes.

In sum, there are also multiple reasons why people ultimately choose to share personal information and why it appears to be associated with improved adjustment to trauma. Disclosing to an audience, even a symbolic audience, may facilitate the development of a coherent, complete story, generate multiple perspectives, foster insight, and generate emotional reactions. Such disclosure forces the speaker to consider the perspective, input, and reactions of the listener (27). Disclosure may help to (i) clarify ambiguous emotional sensations; (ii) articulate an emotional experience in language; (iii) redefine self-concept; (iv) preserve a sense of cultural integration and connectedness; (v) generate alternative perspectives; (vi) find meaning in the trauma; and (vii) receive problem-focused, emotion-focused, or perception-focused coping assistance (27,105). Talking to an audience may also help the individual control emotional reactions and defensiveness so that effective problem solving can take place (27,117).

Despite the potential benefits, there are several reasons why people frequently do not share personal information: (i) revealing struggles may elicit more rejection from others than acting as if you are coping well (118); (ii) disclosing may upset the listener (119); and (iii) people justifiably expect that the listener will make an unhelpful comment (120) or interrupt the individual's disclosures and switch to a more comfortable topic (118). For these reasons, many patients find disclosure in the context of a professional relationship particularly helpful. Professional therapists are less likely than family or friends to become upset by the survivor's disclosure; thus the survivor may be relieved of the sense of needing to be responsible for the therapist reaction. Second, therapists may educate clients and help them interpret, paraphrase, and identify things that are not clear or may require further processing (27). Therapy may increase participants' positive moods over the course of the intervention (121). Murray et al. (122) found that individuals participating in two 30-minute psychotherapy sessions reported greater cognitive change, positive emotions, self-esteem increases, and problem solving and adaptive behavior than individuals who participated in a written trauma group.

WHAT NOT TO DO: A CRITICAL REVIEW OF DEBRIEFING

While disclosure or discussion of a trauma may ultimately facilitate recovery, it is critical that this disclosure be at the time and pace selected by the survivor. Unfortunately, this is often not the case, with well-meaning family, friends, and providers often encouraging discussion and emotional expression immediately after the trauma. When conducted systematically by professionals or volunteers, this immediate discussion is often termed *crisis* or *psychological debriefing*. Debriefing is a popular early intervention for trauma that typically involves a single session with the aim of promoting emotional and cognitive processing of the trauma so that "resolution" may occur. Debriefing often entails education about common trauma reactions, a comprehensive review of the traumatic event, promotion of expressing emotions and thoughts about the trauma, and normalization of post-traumatic symptoms. Recent reviews (123,124) of the literature, however, suggest that crisis debriefing does not prevent PTSD and may actually increase the likelihood of psychiatric problems following trauma.

Debriefing interventions are sometimes used with survivors of physical trauma, despite the lack of empirical support for them. A recent study (125) examining their efficacy found that among a sample of those who experienced medical traumas, those who had a psychological debriefing intervention immediately after the trauma reported significantly worse outcome 3 years later (in terms of general psychiatric symptoms, travel anxiety, pain, physical problems, overall level of functioning, and financial problems). Patients who had initially reported high levels of intrusion and avoidance symptoms remained symptomatic if they had received the intervention but recovered if they did not receive the intervention. The intervention lasted approximately 1 hour and included a detailed review of the accident, the encouragement of appropriate emotional expression, and initial cognitive appraisal of the experience; that is, an appraisal of the subject's perceptions of the accident. The aim of the intervention was to promote the emotional and cognitive processes that, it was believed, would lead to resolution of the trauma. The intervention ended with the researcher giving information about common reactions to traumatic experience, stressing the value of talking about the experience rather than suppressing feelings and thoughts, and also stressing the importance of an early and graded return to normal travel. We suggest that this is an example of a misguided early intervention that is prematurely timed in terms of processing the trauma and gives survivors a message that something particular must be done to cope or that the person is at risk for poor outcome.

OVERVIEW OF EMPIRICALLY SUPPORTED INTERVENTIONS FOR POST-TRAUMATIC STRESS DISORDER AND TRAUMA

So what interventions are recommended when a person is determined to have PTSD or other significant trauma-related distress?

Although we recommend against crisis debriefing interventions, at least one other type of early intervention, cognitive behavioral therapy, shows promise for reducing immediate distress as well as preventing the development of chronic PTSD. As reviewed by Ehlers & Clark (123), several studies (126–128) support the early use of cognitive behavioral therapy (CBT) with trauma survivors identified as being at risk for having persistent PTSD. To qualify as "at risk" in these studies, patients had to have a diagnosis of ASD and/or have severe post-traumatic stress symptoms. Across studies, the CBT involved education about psychological effects of trauma, imaginary exposure to or reliving of the event, changing maladaptive thought patterns, and reversal of avoidance behaviors. Some of the interventions also included additional training in anxiety management skills such as relaxation training and positive self-talk. The interventions were brief, generally four to six 1- to 2-hour sessions. In these randomized clinical trials, the CBT interventions were superior to supportive counseling on measures of post-traumatic symptoms, anxiety, and depressive symptoms at posttreatment and at follow-up. Although these trials had some methodological limitations (123), their consistent finding that early CBT was helpful for survivors of various types of trauma is noteworthy. Given that a few of these studies were done with survivors of motor vehicle collisions (127,128) and mild head trauma (129), these interventions hold promise for the early treatment of survivors of physical trauma who may be at risk for post-traumatic psychopathology.

If PTSD is identified in a person who has experienced a traumatic injury, effective pharmacologic and psychotherapeutic interventions from the broader trauma literature are available for consideration. For a review of pharmacologic treatments for PTSD, the reader is referred to a 2000 Cochrane review on this topic (130). This review concluded that pharmacotherapy can be effective in treating PTSD and should be considered as part of the overall treatment plan. Although the largest trials showing efficacy were conducted with the selective serotonin reuptake inhibitors, sufficient evidence for recommending one particular class of medication over another does not exist.

Several recent meta-analyses (131,132) and reviews (19,133) have concluded that psychotherapeutic interventions, particularly cognitive-behavioral treatments, are effective in reducing PTSD and general psychiatric symptoms in persons with PTSD. CBT for PTSD typically involves elements of exposure, cognitive restructuring, and anxiety management skills. Exposure entails having the individual "expose" him- or herself to fear-producing stimuli such as memories of the traumatic event or situations that serve as reminders of the trauma. The exposure may occur by imagining the feared stimuli (e.g., imagining the accident, imagining driving a car) or by confronting the actual feared event (e.g., actually driving a car). Typically exposure is done gradually and systematically so that the individual first exposes him- or herself to a mildly anxiety-provoking stimuli, gradually working up to whatever is feared the most. A goal of exposure is to reduce anxiety associated with intrusive symptoms and reduce avoidance behavior. Cognitive restructuring involves helping the patient to identify negative and/or maladaptive thoughts and beliefs that contribute to the anxiety and replace such thoughts with more adaptive, realistic, or reassuring thoughts and beliefs. Anxiety management strategies can entail a variety of skills for decreasing anxiety, including but not limited to relaxation training, trauma education, problem solving, communication skills training, and stress reduction.

A popular but controversial treatment for PTSD is eye movement desensitization and reprocessing therapy (EMDR) (134). During EMDR, patients perform rhythmic, multisaccadic eye movements while recalling trauma related images and memories. With the exception of the eye movements, EMDR has in common with CBT several other therapeutic strategies, including desensitization and generating alternative cognitions and appraisals. EMDR has been criticized for its lack of theoretical foundation (19), particularly with respect to the justification for the eye movement component. Studies (19,135,136) comparing EMDR with and without the eye movements found that the effects were essentially equivalent, bringing into question the value of the eye movements. Some authors have concluded that there is limited support for EMDR in the literature (19), although a recent meta-analysis suggested otherwise

(136). Until further evidence is generated for EMDR, we recommend empirically supported CBT interventions over EMDR for survivors of physical trauma.

Cognitive behavioral interventions should be considered for the treatment of travel anxiety or phobia. Examples, primarily case studies, of CBT for travel phobia have been described in the literature, including the use of systematic desensitization (137), exposure (138), and virtual reality exposure therapy (139).

A variety of group interventions are occasionally offered to survivors of trauma. These interventions can take on many forms such as peer-led support groups, peer consultation, professionally led support groups, recreational groups, psychoeducational groups, or psychotherapeutic groups. The groups are sometimes organized by psychopathology diagnosis, such as PTSD, or by type of injury or disability, such as brain injury. While we hypothesize that such groups may be very helpful for some survivors of traumatic injuries, we cannot unconditionally recommend that all trauma survivors participate in group interventions for at least two reasons. First, the treatment literature lacks trials of the efficacy and effectiveness of such groups. While evidence exists supporting the efficacy of a few specific group interventions after trauma or disability such as a CBT intervention for depression after SCI (140), there is insufficient evidence to conclude that all group interventions are effective in promoting resilience and reducing distress in injury survivors. Second, in the cancer field, where support groups are commonplace, research has shown that support group interventions have as much potential to adversely affect attendees as they do to positively help them (141). Thus, in the absence of empirical evidence to guide the construction of group interventions after injury, we recommend that careful consideration be given to the type, nature, components, and targeted participants when forming group interventions. We hope to see more research on the efficacy and effectiveness of group interventions, as we believe they have the potential to be a cost-effective, beneficial form of service for addressing psychopathology and building resilience in survivors of trauma.

Although not typically conceptualized as an intervention for facilitating resilience, physical rehabilitation hypothetically has the potential to increase or maintain resilience in at least several ways. Rehabilitation often emphasizes problem solving to address challenges and barriers secondary to the injury, disability, and environment. Through realistic goal setting and attainment, self-efficacy may be increased, and with it, resilience bolstered. Opportunities for supportive social relationships, with rehabilitation professionals as well as other individuals with disabilities, may also exist. Therapeutic recreational activities may provide chances for positive emotions, leisure skill acquisition, and development of appropriate support and social contacts. To our knowledge, the effects of comprehensive rehabilitation on resilience or post-traumatic distress have not been examined.

SPECIFIC STRATEGIES FOR FACILITATION RESILIENCE AND PSYCHOLOGICAL HEALTH FOLLOWING INJURY

Although we recommend that persons with severe distress such as MDD or PTSD be evaluated and treated by a qualified mental health professional, there are many things rehabilitation staff can do to facilitate resilience in their trauma patients (and patients' families and loved ones) and to support those who are highly distressed. Some of these strategies are more relevant to the acute surgical and rehabilitation settings, some are more relevant to outpatient settings, and many will be helpful at all points of the rehabilitation continuum.

1. Provide regular, accurate medical information, as research has shown that survivors often perceive this as very helpful. Anxiety is often heightened more by what is not known but feared rather than by what is known. Provide regular opportunities for the patient and family to ask questions to ensure understanding of their medical condition and treatment.
2. Remember that although there are certainly commonalities and shared experiences amongst persons with trauma, individuals have a variety of styles in coping and a range of emotional reactions. No one reaction is "wrong" or "right" for all persons. Be aware and respectful of such individual differences as well as cultural differences that may influence responses.
3. Avoid the myths about responses to trauma described earlier in this chapter. Providers, family, and friends have the potential to hinder recovery after trauma by adhering to or conveying expectations about reactions based upon such misconceptions. The data and survivor experiences are invariably more complicated than stage theories suggest.
4. Avoid overinterpretation or pathologizing of psychological symptoms or distress. Keep in mind that most psychological reactions are transient, normal responses to highly abnormal situations. If in doubt about a patient's psychological responses or behavior, consult a mental health provider.

5. Do not attempt to provide psychotherapy, help the patient "process" the trauma, encourage the patient to have any particular reaction (e.g., get angry, cry, or grieve), or talk with patients about stages of recovery.

6. Maintain an empathic, nonjudgmental attitude towards the patient. Remember, one of the ways staff may cope with extremely disturbing things is by blaming or judging the patient—this can increase your own feeling of control or predictability in the world. However, such attitudes can get in the way of providing necessary care and support.

7. Reduce or minimize repeated traumatic, painful, or anxiety-provoking experiences in the hospital as much as feasible. Suggestions for doing this include the following:

   a. Provide the patient with as much control in procedures and care as he or she desires. Some may wish to participate in their medical care, for example, assisting with burn dressing changes, whereas others may prefer not to participate. Consider allowing the patient choice in when such procedures are done, if feasible.

   b. Keep the patient's room a "safe" place by conducting painful or anxiety-provoking procedures in a place other than their hospital room.

   c. Maximize acute pain control, particularly for procedures.

   d. Offer coping strategies such as hypnosis, relaxation training, imagery, or distraction as adjuncts to medical care, particularly for use during difficult procedures or for pain control.

8. Allow the patient to determine how much exposure or avoidance he or she wants with respect to reminders of the trauma, particularly in the acute period. Some may wish to talk about or face reminders of the trauma while others may not. Respect that in most cases, the patient will do what is best for him or her at that time. Do not inadvertently encourage avoidance behavior, as avoidance may lead to increased symptoms and distress over the long term. For example, a well-meaning provider may discourage a patient from talking about the accident, viewing pictures of the damaged motor vehicle, or looking at their injured body, even when the patient requests to do these things. At the same time, do not push the patient to talk about or "face" the trauma if he or she does not appear interested.

9. Help patients identify and meet rehabilitation goals that are realistic and provide opportunities for tangible successes. Successful goal attainment, even of small goals, can increase a sense of mastery and control and decrease feelings of helplessness.

10. Encourage opportunities for positive emotions during all phases of care. Opportunities for the survivor to enjoy humor, pleasant activities, or other positive experiences provide a number of benefits, including respite from the trauma and associated consequences.

11. Encourage and provide opportunities for social connections during rehabilitation. Social connections can take many forms such as recreational therapy outings, informal shared meals, peer support, scheduled activities, or activities with family or friends. Some survivors will find formal support groups beneficial. However, remember that not every group is helpful and not every survivor will be interested in or appropriate for a group.

12. Encourage family members to provide support in a variety of ways, keeping in mind that family members will respond differently to the traumatic injury of a loved one, too, and likely require support of their own. Some family members or friends may feel uncomfortable or helpless in the face of a traumatic event, and as a result, avoid the person who was injured. Others might feel pressure to help the injured one "process" the trauma or find meaning. In such cases, you may reassure them that the best emotional support they can provide is a nonjudgmental presence that allows the survivor to talk or not, depending on his or her needs. Whatever the family members' reactions, encourage listening, providing opportunities for positive emotions, and practical support.

13. If you witness other staff, family members, or friends responding in ways that are well intended but potentially unhelpful, consider talking with them about this. In doing so, it may help to acknowledge their concern and good intentions, followed by a suggestion of what they can do that may be helpful. In such circumstances you may also wish to discuss with the patient that others are going to have expectations about how he or she "should" react to the trauma, and that such expectations are not necessarily true. Reassure the patient it is normal to have a variety of reactions.

14. Ensure that your patients know how to seek help for post-traumatic emotional concerns, should they occur in the future. Consider having such information available in your health

care setting. The American Psychological Association's Help Center (www.helping.apa.org) has good information on finding resources.

CARING FOR THE CARE PROVIDERS WHO WORK WITH TRAUMA SURVIVORS

Providers who work with trauma survivors are often exposed vicariously to traumatic events, requiring personal and emotional strength in addition to professional and technical skills. Trauma may destroy (at least temporarily) some survivors' sense of mastery, and their immediate posttrauma needs may overwhelm those around them, implanting in the observers feelings of powerlessness, incompetence, helplessness, or resentment. Care providers confronted with gruesome injuries and the characteristics of the causal event may feel overwhelmed by feelings of hopelessness, empathy, anger, anxiety, or grief. Over time, care providers may come to feel cumulatively burdened with chronic stress associated with being in close proximity to trauma and its aftermath, a phenomenon described as "burnout," "vicarious trauma," or "secondary trauma." Signs of "burnout" may include the following: (i) avoiding or withdrawing from emotional connection with their patients; (ii) overly identifying with patients and becoming enmeshed in their lives, at times to the point of having difficulty separating one's personal from one's professional roles; (iii) experiencing distress, despair, cynicism, alienation, and physiological and psychological symptoms (e.g., fatigue, sleep disturbances); and (iv) a heightened sense of vulnerability.

Several strategies are recommended to help care providers cope with their professional responsibilities over time. First, providers are encouraged to cultivate self-awareness, which is critical for recognizing clients or situations that may pose particular challenges and require deliberate intervention. For example, nurses or therapists may find themselves particularly distressed when caring for a traumatically injured child the same age as their own, because they can empathize so greatly with the child's parent. Alternatively, a provider who is experiencing their own stressors (e.g., divorce, illness) may find themselves having difficulty caring for others who have been traumatized, because their psychological resources are already depleted. In challenging situations, it is important for providers to engage in personal self-management activities, as well as seek organizational support. Personal self-management activities might include increasing self-care (which may include professional support at times, such as psychotherapy), limiting the amount of trauma-related work, seeking social support, seeking healing or life-affirming activities and experiences, and deliberately recognizing professional limitations and responsibility. At a professional or organizational level, strategies might include maintaining collegial on-the-job support to reduce isolation, re-arranging patient loads or schedules to avoid over burdening staff members, and pursuing ongoing educational opportunities that focus on managing traumatized patients.

SUMMARY

After sustaining a traumatic injury, many individuals experience a variety of transient psychological symptoms that are likely normal reactions to highly abnormal life events. Research on psychopathology following trauma dominates the literature, even though the majority of persons who experience trauma do not suffer from psychopathology. When psychopathology is present after trauma, several evidence-based interventions, including cognitive behavioral psychotherapy, are available for implementation. Given the potentially negative impact of psychopathological states on health and well-being, research on MDD, ASD, PTSD, travel phobias, and other forms of psychological distress after injury should continue.

The study of positive psychological responses to trauma, including positive emotions, resilience, and post-traumatic growth, is long overdue. Research on these phenomena has the potential to not only close gaps in our knowledge about the full range of psychological responses to traumatic injury but also to inform the broader trauma, loss, growth, and resilience literatures. Theoretically driven, longitudinal studies of the broad range of responses, as well as potential risk and protective factors, will aid in developing strategies for identifying those at risk for maladaptive responses after injury. In addition, such information could lead to interventions for promoting resilience, preventing suffering due to psychopathology, and treating distress when it exists.

REFERENCES

1. MacLeod MD. Why did it happen to me? Social cognition processes in adjustment and recovery from criminal victimisation and illness. *Curr Psychol Res Rev.* 1999;18(1):18–31.
2. Bonanno GA. Loss, trauma, and human resilience: Have we underestimated the human capacity to thrive

after extremely aversive events? *Am Psychol*. 2004; 59(1):20–28.

3. American Psychiatric Association. *Diagnostic and statistical manual of mental disorders*. 4th ed. Washington, DC: American Psychiatric Association; 1994.

4. Meichenbaum D. *A clinical handbook/practical therapist manual for assessing and treating adults with post-traumatic stress disorder*. Waterloo, Ontario: Institute Press; 1994.

5. Elliott TR, Frank RG. Depression following spinal cord injury. *Arch Phys Med Rehabil*. 1996;77(8): 816–823.

6. Beck AT, Steer RA, Ball R, et al. Use of the beck anxiety and depression inventories for primary care with medical outpatients. *Assessment*. 1997;4(3):211–219.

7. Radloff LS. The CES-D scale: A self-report depression scale for research in the general population. *Appl Psychol Meas*. 1977;1(3):385–401.

8. Patterson DR, Everett JJ, Bombardier CH, et al. Psychological effects of severe burn injuries. *Psychol Bull*. 1993;113(2):362–378.

9. Trieschmann RB. *Spinal cord injuries: Psychological, social and vocational rehabilitation*. New York, New York: Demos; 1988.

10. Bryant RA, Harvey AG. Acute stress disorder: A critical review of diagnostic issues. *Clin Psychol Rev*. 1997;17(7):757–773.

11. Harvey AG, Bryant RA. Acute stress disorder: A synthesis and critique. *Psychol Bull*. 2002;128(6):886–902.

12. Marshall RD, Spitzer R, Liebowitz MR. Review and critique of the new *DSM-IV* diagnosis of acute stress disorder. *Am J Psychiatry*. 1999;156(11):1677–1685.

13. Tedeschi RG, Calhoun LG. Posttraumatic growth: Conceptual foundations and empirical evidence. *Psychol Inq*. 2004;15(1):1–18.

14. Park CL, Cohen LH, Murch RL. Assessment and prediction of stress-related growth. *J Pers*. 1996;64:71–105.

15. Linley PA, Joseph S. Positive change following trauma and adversity: A review. *J Trauma Stress*. 2004;17(1): 11–21.

16. Wortman CB, Silver RC. The myths of coping with loss. *J Consult Clin Psychol*. 1989;57(3):349–357.

17. Keane TM, Zimering RT, Caddell JM. A behavioral formulation of post-traumatic stress disorder in Vietnam veterans. *Behav Ther*. 1985;8:9–12.

18. Keane TM. Post-traumatic stress disorder: Current states and future directions. *Behav Ther*. 1989;20: 149–153.

19. Keane TM. Psychological and behavioral treatments of post-traumatic stress disorder. In: Nathan PE, Gorman JM, eds. *A guide to treatments that work*. New York, NY: Oxford University Press; 1998:398–407.

20. Horowitz MJ. Stress-response syndromes: A review of posttraumatic and adjustment disorders. *Hosp Community Psychiatry*. 1986;37(3):241–249.

21. Marmar CR. Brief dynamic psychotherapy of post-traumatic stress disorder. *Psychiatr Ann*. 1991;21: 405–414.

22. Janoff-Bulman R. *Shattered assumptions: Towards a new psychology of trauma*. New York, NY: Free Press; 1992.

23. Silver RL, Boon C, Stones MH. Searching for meaning in misfortune: Making sense of incest. *J Soc Issues*. 1983;39:81–102.

24. Dollinger SJ. The need for meaning following disaster: Attributions and emotional upset. *Pers Soc Psychol Bull*. 1986;12(3):300–310.

25. Janoff-Bulman R. Assumptive worlds and the stress of traumatic events: Applications of the schema construct. *Soc Cognit*. 1989;7(2):113–136.

26. Lehman DR, Wortman CB, Williams AF. Long-term effects of losing a spouse or child in a motor vehicle crash. *J Pers Soc Psychol*. 1987;52:218–231.

27. Clark LF. Stress and the cognitive-conversational benefits of social interaction. *J Soc Clin Psychol*. 1993; 12(1):25–55.

28. Meichenbaum D, Fong G. How individuals control their own minds: A constructive narrative perspective. In: Wegner DM, Pennebaker JW, eds. *Handbook of mental control*. Englewood Cliffs, NJ: Prentice Hall; 1993.

29. Winje D. Cognitive coping: The psychological significance of knowing what happened in the traumatic event. *J Trauma Stress*. 1998;11(4):627–643.

30. Baum A, Cohen L, Hall M. Control and intrusive memories as possible determinants of chronic stress. *Psychosom Med*. 1993;55:274–286.

31. Wortman CB, Silver RC. Coping with irrevocable loss. In: Van den Bos GR, Bryant BK, eds. *Cataclysma, crises, and catastrophes*. Washington, DC: American Psychological Association; 1987.

32. Janoff-Bulman R, Lang-Gunn L. Coping with disease, crime, and accidents: The role of self-blame attributions. In: Abramson LY, ed. *Social cognition and clinical psychology: A synthesis*. New York, NY: Guilford; 1988.

33. Foa E, Meadows EA. Psychosocial treatments for posttraumatic stress disorder: A critical review. *Annu Rev Psychol*. 1997;48:449–480.

34. Elliott TR, Kurylo M, Rivera P. Positive growth following acquired disability. In: Snyder CR, Lopez SJ, eds. *Handbook of positive psychology*. New York, NY: Oxford University Press; 2002:687–699.

35. Livneh H, Antonak R. *Psychosocial adaptation to chronic illness and disability*. Gaithersburg, MD: Aspen; 1997.

36. Olkin R. *What psychotherapists should know about disability*. New York, NY: Guilford Press; 1999.

37. Wright BA. *Physical disability: A psychosocial approach*. 2nd ed. New York, NY: Harper & Row; 1983.

38. Lawrence JW, Fauerbach J, Eudell E, et al. The 1998 clinical research award. Sleep disturbance after burn injury: A frequent yet understudied complication. *J Burn Care Rehabil*. 1998;19(6):480–486.

39. Difede J, Ptacek JT, Roberts J, et al. Acute stress disorder after burn injury: A predictor of posttraumatic stress disorder? *Psychosom Med*. 2002;64(5):826–834.

40. Ehde DM, Patterson DR, Wiechman SA, et al. Posttraumatic stress symptoms and distress following acute burn injury. *Burns*. 1999;25(7):587–592.

41. Williams RM, Doctor J, Patterson DR, et al. Health outcomes for burn survivors: A two-year follow-up. *Rehabil Psychol*. 2003;48(4):189–194.

42. Friedman MJ, Foa EB, Charney DS. Toward evidence-based early interventions for acutely traumatized adults and children. *Biol Psychiatry*. 2003;53(9): 765–768.

43. Zatzick D, Jurkovich G, Russo J, et al. Posttraumatic distress, alcohol disorders, and recurrent trauma across level 1 trauma centers. *J Trauma*. 2004;57(2): 360–366.

44. Adams N. Positive outcomes in families following traumatic brain injury. *ANZJFT*. 1996;17(2):75–84.

45. Dikmen SS, Bombardier CH, Machamer JE, et al. Natural history of depression in traumatic brain injury. *Arch Phys Med Rehabil*. 2004;85(9):1457–1464.

46. Ptacek JT, Patterson DR, Heimbach DM. Inpatient depression in persons with burns. *J Burn Care Rehabil.* 2002;23(1):1–9.

47. Eaton WW, Kessler LG. Rates of symptoms of depression in a national sample. *Am J Epidemiol.* 1981;114(4):528–538.

48. Coyne JC, Fechner-Bates S, Schwenk TL. Prevalence, nature, and comorbidity of depressive disorders in primary care. *Gen Hosp Psychiatry.* 1994; 16(4):267–276.

49. Williams JW, Noel PH, Cordes JA, et al. Is this patient clinically depressed? *JAMA.* 2002;287(9):1160–1170.

50. O'Donnell ML, Creamer M, Bryant RA, et al. Posttraumatic disorders following injury: An empirical and methodological review. *Clin Psychol Rev.* 2003; 23:587–603.

51. Horgan O, MacLachlan M. Psychosocial adjustment to lower limb amputation: A review. *Disabil Rehabil.* 2004;26(14/15):837–850.

52. Rosenthal M, Christensen BK, Ross TP. Depression following traumatic brain injury. *Arch Phys Med Rehabil.* 1998;79(1):90–103.

53. Blanchard EB, Hickling EJ, Freidenberg BM, et al. Two studies of psychiatric morbidity among motor vehicle accident survivors one year after the crash. *Behav Res Ther.* 2004;42:569–583.

54. Brown ES, Fulton MK, Wilkeson A, et al. The psychiatric sequelae of civilian trauma. *Compr Psychiatry.* 2000;41(1):19–23.

55. Brady KT, Killeen TK, Brewerton T, et al. Comorbidity of psychiatric disorders and posttraumatic stress disorder. *J Clin Psychiatry.* 2000;61(Suppl. 7):22–32.

56. Vingilis E, Larkin E, Stoduto G, et al. Psychosocial sequelae of motor vehicle collisions: A follow-up study. *Accid Anal Prev.* 1996;28(5):637–645.

57. Blanchard EB, Hickling EJ. *After the crash: Psychological assessment and treatment of survivors of motor vehicle accidents.* 2nd ed. Washington, DC: American Psychological Association; 2003.

58. Mayou R, Bryant B, Ehlers A. Prediction of psychological outcomes one year after a motor vehicle accident. *Am J Psychiatry.* 2001;158(8):1231–1238.

59. Zatzick DF, Kang SM, Hinton WL, et al. Posttraumatic concerns: A patient-centered approach to outcome assessment after traumatic physical injury. *Med Care.* 2001;39(4):327–339.

60. McMillen JC, Cook CL. The positive by-products of spinal cord injury and their correlates. *Rehabil Psychol.* 2003;48(2):77–85.

61. McMillen JC, Howard MO, Nower L, et al. The perceived benefits scales: Measuring perceived positive life changes following negative life events. *Soc Work Res.* 2001;22:173–187.

62. Bryant RA. Early predictors of posttraumatic stress disorder. *Biol Psychiatry.* 2003;53:789–795.

63. Foa E, Rothbaum BO, Kozak, MJ. Behavioral treatments of anxiety and depression. In: Kendall P, Watson D, eds. *Anxiety and depression: Distinctive and overlapping features.* San Diego, CA: Academic Press; 1989:413–454.

64. Wortman CB, Silver RC. The myths of coping with loss. *J Consult Clin Psychol.* 1989;57(3):349–357.

65. Kubler-Ross E. *On death and dying.* New York, NY: Macmillan; 1969.

66. Bonanno GA, Kaltman S. The varieties of grief experience. *Clin Psychol Rev.* 2001;21(5):705–734.

67. Wiechman SA, Ptacek JT, Patterson DR, et al. Rates, trends, and severity of depression after burn injuries. *J Burn Care Rehabil.* 2001;22(6):417–424.

68. Zatzick DF, Jurkovich GJ, Gentilello L, et al. Posttraumatic stress, problem drinking, and functional outcomes after injury. *Arch Surg.* 2002;137(2):200–205.

69. Zatzick DF, Kang SM, Muller HG, et al. Predicting posttraumatic distress in hospitalized trauma survivors with acute injuries. *Am J Psychiatry.* 2002; 159(6):941–946.

70. Bryant RA, Harvey AG. Avoidant coping style and post-traumatic stress following motor vehicle accidents. *Behav Res Ther.* 1995;33(6):631–635.

71. Ehlers A, Mayou RA, Bryant B. Psychological predictors of chronic posttraumatic stress disorder after motor vehicle accidents. *J Abnorm Psychol.* 1998; 107(3):508–519.

72. Bryant RA, Harvey AG. Relationship between acute stress disorder and posttraumatic stress disorder following mild traumatic brain injury. *Am J Psychiatry.* 1998;155(5):625–629.

73. Ehde DM, Patterson DR, Wiechman SA, et al. Posttraumatic stress symptoms and distress 1 year after burn injury. *J Burn Care Rehabil.* 2000;21(2):105–111.

74. Kennedy P, Evans, MJ. Evaluation of post traumatic distress in the first six months following SCI. *Spinal Cord.* 2001;39:381–386.

75. Nielsen MS. Post-traumatic stress disorder and emotional distress in persons with spinal cord lesion. *Spinal Cord.* 2003;41:296–302.

76. Davis CG, Wortman CB, Lehman DR, et al. Searching for meaning in loss: Are clinical assumptions correct? *Death Stud.* 2000;24(6):497–540.

77. Folkman S, Moskowitz JT. Positive affect and the other side of coping. *Am Psychol.* 2000;55(6):647–654.

78. Bower JE, Kemeny ME, Taylor SE, et al. Cognitive processing, discovery of meaning, CD4 decline, and AIDS-related mortality among bereaved HIV-seropositive men. *J Consult Clin Psychol.* 1998; 66(6):979–986.

79. Frazier P, Conlon A, Glaser T. Positive and negative life changes following sexual assault. *J Consult Clin Psychol.* 2001;69(6):1048–1055.

80. McMillen JC, Smith EM, Fisher R. Perceived benefit and mental health after three types of disaster. *J Consult Clin Psychol.* 1997;65:733–739.

81. Adcock RJ, Goldberg ML, Patterson DR, et al. Staff perceptions of emotional distress in patients with burn trauma. *Rehabil Psychol.* 2000;45(2):179–182.

82. Cushman LA, Dijkers M. Depressed mood in spinal cord injured patients: Staff perceptions and patient realities. *Arch Phys Med Rehabil.* 1990;71:191–196.

83. Ozer E, Best SR, Lipsey TL, et al. Predictors of posttraumatic stress disorder and symptoms in adults: A meta-analysis. *Psychol Bull.* 2003;129(1):52–73.

84. Delahanty DL, Herberman HB, Craig KJ, et al. Acute and chronic distress and posttraumatic stress disorder as a function of responsibility for serious motor vehicle accidents. *J Consult Clin Psychol.* 1997;65(4): 560–567.

85. Patterson DR, Goldberg ML, Ehde DM. Hypnosis in the treatment of patients with severe burns. *Am J Clin Hypn.* 1996;38(3):200–212; discussion 213.

86. Bryant RA, Harvey AG. Acute stress response: A comparison of head injured and non-head injured patients. *Psychol Med.* 1995;25(4):869–873.

87. Bryant RA. Posttraumatic stress disorder and traumatic brain injury: Can they co-exist? *Clin Psychol Rev.* 2001;21(6):931–948.

88. Tsay S, Halstead MT, McCrone S. Predictors of coping efficacy, negative moods and posttraumatic stress syndrome following major trauma. *Int J Nurs Pract.* 2001;7:74–83.

89. Fauerbach JA, Richter L, Lawrence JW. Regulating acute posttraumatic distress. *J Burn Care Rehabil.* 2002;23:249–257.

90. Solomon Z. *Combat stress reactions: The enduring toll of war.* New York, NY: Plenum Press; 1993.

91. Vrana S, Lauterbach O. Prevalence of traumatic events and post-traumatic psychological symptoms in a nonclinical sample of college students. *J Trauma Stress.* 1994;7:289–302.

92. Resnick HS, Kilpatrick DG, Dansky BS, et al. Prevalence of civilian trauma and posttraumatic stress disorder in a representative national sample of women. *J Consult Clin Psychol.* 1993;61:984–991.

93. Galer BS, Jensen MP. Development and preliminary validation of a pain measure specific to neuropathic pain: The neuropathic pain scale. *Neurology.* 1997;48(2):332–338.

94. Galea S, Vlahov D, Resnick H, et al. Trends of probably post-traumatic stress disorder in New York City after the September 11th terrorist attacks. *Am J Epidemiol.* 2003;158:514–524.

95. Bonanno GA, Wortman CB, Nesse RM. Prospective patterns of resilience and maladjustment during widowhood. *Psychol Aging.* 2004;19(2):260–271.

96. Kobasa SC, Maddi SR, Kahn S. Hardiness and health: A prospective study. *J Pers Soc Psychol.* 1982;42:168–177.

97. Florian V, Mikulincer M, Taubman O. Does hardiness contribute to mental health during a stressful real-life situation? The roles of appraisal and coping. *J Pers Soc Psychol.* 1995;68:687–695.

98. American Psychological Association. The road to resilience. Available at: http://www.apahelpcenter.org/featuredtopics/feature.php?id=6. Accessed 2004.

99. Elliott TR, Kennedy P. Treatment of depression following spinal cord injury: An evidence based review. *Rehabil Psychol.* 2004;49(2):134–139.

100. Cohen S, Gottlieb BH, Underwood LG. Social relationships and health. In: Cohen S, Gottlieb BH, Underwood LG, eds. *Social support measurement and intervention: A guide for health and social scientists.* New York, NY: Oxford University Press; 2000:3–25.

101. Williams RM, Ehde DM, Smith DG, et al. A two-year longitudinal study of social support following amputation. *Disabil Rehabil.* 2004;26(14/15):862–874.

102. Malt UF. Traumatic effects of accidents. In: Ursano RJ, McCaughey BG, Fullerton CS, eds. *Individual and community responses to trauma and disaster.* New York, NY: Cambridge University Press; 1994.

103. Stiles WB. Is it therapeutic to disclose? In: Pennebaker JW, ed. *Emotion, disclosure, and health.* Washington, DC: American Psychological Association; 1996.

104. Lepore SJ, Silver RC, Wortman CB, et al. Social constraints, intrusive thoughts, and depressive symptoms among bereaved mothers. *J Pers Soc Psychol.* 1996;70(2):271–282.

105. Rime B, Mesquita B, Philippot P, et al. Beyond the emotional event: Six studies on the social sharing of subjects. *Bull Psychon Soc.* 1991;5(5/6):435–465.

106. Pennebaker JW. *Opening up: The healing power of confiding in others.* New York, NY: Avon Books; 1990.

107. Pennebaker JW. Overcoming inhibition: Rethinking the roles of personality, cognition, and social behavior. In: Traue HC, Pennebaker JW, eds. *Emotion, inhibition, and health.* Seattle, WA: Hogrefe & Huber; 1993:100–115.

108. Horowitz MJ. *Stress Response Syndromes.* New York, NY: Jason Aronson, Inc.; 1976.

109. Wegner DM, Zanakos S. Chronic thought suppression. *J Pers.* 1994;62(4):587–613.

110. Littrell J. Is the reexperience of painful emotion therapeutic? *Clin Psychol Rev.* 1998;18(1):71–102.

111. Greenberg MA, Wortman CB, Stone AA. Emotional expression and physical health: Revising traumatic memories or fostering self-regulation? *J Pers Soc Psychol.* 1996;71(3):588–602.

112. Greenberg MA, Stone AA. Emotional disclosure about traumas and its relation to health: Effects of previous disclosure and trauma severity. *J Pers Soc Psychol.* 1992;63(1):75–84.

113. Hughes CF, Uhlmann C, Pennebaker JW. The body's response to processing emotional trauma: Linking verbal text with autonomic activity. *J Pers.* 1994;62(4):565–585.

114. Pennebaker JW, Kiecolt-Glaser JK, Glaser R. Disclosure of traumas and immune function: Health implications for psychotherapy. *J Consult Clin Psychol.* 1988;56(2):239–245.

115. Mann SJ, Delon M. Improved hypertension control after disclosure of decades-old trauma. *Psychosom Med.* 1995;57(5):501–505.

116. Smyth JM. Written emotional expression: Effect sizes, outcome types, and moderating variables. *J Consult Clin Psychol.* 1998;66(1):174–184.

117. Cohen S, Wills TA. Stress, social support, and the buffering hypothesis. *Psychol Bull.* 1985;98(2):310–357.

118. Kelly AE, McKillop KJ. Consequences of revealing personal secrets. *Psychol Bull.* 1996;120(3):450–465.

119. Shortt JW, Pennebaker JW. Talking versus hearing about Holocaust experiences. *Basic Appl Soc Psych.* 1992;13(2):165–179.

120. Pennebaker JW. Social mechanisms of constraint. In: Wegner DM, Pennebaker JW, eds. *Handbook of mental control.* Englewood Cliffs, NJ: Prentice Hall; 1993.

121. Murray EJ, Segal DL. Emotional processing in vocal and written expression about traumatic experiences. *J Trauma Stress.* 1994;7(3):391–405.

122. Murray EJ, Lamnin AD, Carver CS. Emotional expression in written essays and psychotherapy. *J Soc Clin Psychol.* 1989;8(4):414–429.

123. Ehlers A, Clark DM. Early psychological interventions for adult survivors of trauma: A review. *Biol Psychiatry.* 2003;53:817–826.

124. Rose S, Bisson J, Wessely S. A systematic review of single-session psychological interventions ('debriefing') following trauma. *Psychother Psychosom.* 2003;72(4):176–184.

125. Mayou RA, Ehlers A, Hobbs M. A three-year follow up of psychological debriefing for road traffic accident victims. *Br J Psychiatry.* 2000;176:589–593.

126. Foa EB, Hearst-Ikeda D, Perry KJ. Evaluation of a brief cognitive-behavioral program for the prevention of chronic PTSD in recent assault victims. *J Consult Clin Psychol.* 1995;63:948-955.

127. Bryant RA, Harvey AG, Dang ST, et al. Treatment of acute stress disorder: A comparison of cognitive-behavioral therapy and supportive counseling. *J Consult Clin Psychol.* 1998;66(5):862–866.

128. Bryant RA, Sackville T, Dang ST, et al. Treating acute stress disorder: An evaluation of cognitive behavior therapy and supportive counseling techniques. *Am J Psychiatry.* 1999;156:1780–1786.

129. Bryant RA, Moulds ML, Guthrie RM. Treating acute stress disorder following mild brain injury. *Am J Psychiatry.* 2003;160:585–587.

130. Stein DJ, Zungu-Dirwayi N, Linden GJH, et al. Pharmacotherapy for post-traumatic stress disorder (Review). *Cochrane Database Syst Rev.* 2000;4: CD002795.

131. Sherman JJ. Effects of psychotherapeutic treatments for PTSD: A meta-analysis of controlled clinical trials. *J Trauma Stress.* 1998;11(3):413–435.

132. van Etten M, Taylor S. Comparative efficacy of treatments for posttraumatic stress disorder: A meta-analysis. *Clin Psychol Psychother.* 1998;15:721–738.

133. Deacon BJ, Abramowitz JS. Cognitive and behavioral treatments for anxiety disorders: A review of meta-analytic findings. *J Clin Psychol.* 2004;60(4):429–441.

134. Shapiro F. Eye movement desensitization: A new treatment for posttraumatic stress disorder. *J Behav Ther Exp Psychiatry.* 1989;20(3):211–217.

135. Renfrey G, Spates RC. Eye movement desensitization: A partial dismantling study. *J Behav Ther Exp Psychiatry.* 1994;25(3):231–239.

136. Davidson PR, Parker KC. Eye movement desensitization and reprocessing: A meta-analysis. *J Consult Clin Psychol.* 2001;69(2):305–316.

137. Quirk DA. Motor vehicle accidents and post-traumatic anxiety conditioning. *Ont Psychol.* 1985;17:11–18.

138. Blonstein CH. Treatment of automobile driving phobia through imaginal and in vivo exposure plus response prevention. *Behav Ther.* 1988;11:70–86.

139. Wald J, Taylor S. Preliminary research on the efficacy of virtual reality exposure therapy to treat driving phobia. *Cyberpsychol Behav.* 2003;6(5):459–465.

140. Kidd D, Stewart G, Baldry J, et al. The functional independence measure: A comparative validity and reliability study [see comments]. *Disabil Rehabil.* 1995; 17(1):10–14.

141. Helgeson VS, Cohen S. Social support and adjustment to cancer: Reconciling descriptive, correlational, and intervention research. *Health Psychol.* 1996;15(2): 135–148.

14

Quality Care Indicators for Trauma Rehabilitation

Pamela A. Palmer Smith and Barbara Beach

INTRODUCTION

Historically in the field of trauma rehabilitation, hospital lengths of stay (LOS) and resource utilization were determined by the physician and interprofessional team solely on the basis of patient care needs. Patient goals and expected outcomes were established based on the individual practitioner's clinical experience and knowledge. As care proceeded, resources were used as needed to achieve the goals that would result in the expected outcomes. This model for care delivery included little attention to the cost and charges for providing care because most patient care was reimbursed based on a percentage of charges.

As a result of the changing payment structure in the health care delivery industry, a resource-driven model for care is now the norm. Instead of first establishing goals for the patient in a trauma rehabilitation unit, the first step is to determine the financial resources available to the patient, which are identified prior to admission. Based on the available resources, patient goals are established, which may, and often do, lead to a different set of expected outcomes following inpatient rehabilitation. As a result, physicians and hospital administrators alike have begun to search for ways to determine the effect of these changes on patients and on financial outcomes for health care delivery institutions (Fig. 14–1).

OVERVIEW

Maintaining a system for measuring outcomes has long been a standard in rehabilitation medicine. Since the early 1970s, the Commission on Accreditation of Rehabilitation Facilities (CARF) has required rehabilitation facilities to measure patient care outcomes as a means of determining quality of care and

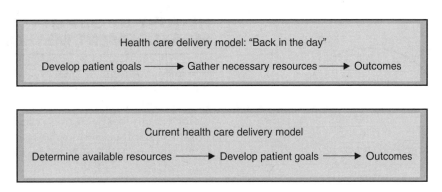

Figure 14–1. Drivers for the health care delivery system.

Rehabilitation examples:

- Underuse of services – patients with spinal cord injuries (SCI) do not get annual physicals, lack of funding for services, many clinics and hospitals no longer taking Medicare, Medicaid, etc.
- Overuse of services – extended lengths of stay (LOS) because of discharge delays, lack of placement options, unnecessary procedures
- Misuse of services – injured by the care received, for example, patients get pressure ulcers while hospitalized
- Variation of services – inpatient rehabilitation unavailable in some communities; variation in outcomes such as the percentage of patients discharged to the community; lack of appropriate equipment, trained staff, residency/physician training, or patient volume to ensure staff skill and competency to treat a more complex or specialized patient population (SCI, brain injury, etc.)

Figure 14–2. Potential barriers to quality in trauma rehabilitation.

services. Only since 2001, however, has reimbursement for inpatient rehabilitation services been linked to outcome measures through the use of a prospective payment system. Previously, most payment for rehabilitation services was based on percentage of charges or per diem rate models. Case rate reimbursement has led to more interest and scrutiny of the costs and results of patient care within rehabilitation facilities.

Who values, needs, or requires information about health care quality measurement and outcomes? Clinicians, hospital administrators, and patients themselves value information on the quality of care. Stakeholders interested in patient care outcomes also include those who pay for health care services, such as Medicare, Medicaid, commercial insurance providers, and workers' compensation programs. Agencies such as the National Committee for Quality Assurance (NCQA), the Joint Commission on Accreditation of Healthcare Organizations (JCAHO), CARF and state Departments of Health are interested in outcomes of care for accreditation of health care organizations.

Business models for quantitative measurement of results and outcomes have been used in the design of quality improvement models in numerous health care delivery organizations. Experts in the field of outcomes measurement such as Deming (1), Drucker (2), and Donabedian (3) have applied concepts and

principles from business models to develop methods for measuring patient care outcomes. For example, the use of data to understand variation in procedures and outcomes has led to significant improvements in care delivery.

In the years before prospective payment was implemented as a model for reimbursement in the health care industry, measurement of patient care outcomes was not a priority for many health care delivery organizations. According to the Agency for Healthcare Research and Quality (AHRQ), misuse, underuse, overuse, and variation are critical problems within the American health care delivery system (4). Significant research and evidence indicate these major problems have led to out of control costs and unsatisfactory results in inpatient care (5) (Fig. 14–2).

The literature is rich with articles, books, and essays related to quality of health care delivery—what it is and what it is not. Consistently, experience shows that after a certain point, more health care does not necessarily produce better outcomes or quality of life, and that doing the right thing the right way is the simple explanation of what quality of health care should aspire to at all levels of care and care delivery settings (Fig. 14–3).

HISTORY OF QUALITY MEASUREMENT METHODS

The measurement of quality in health care delivery has evolved significantly over the past 20 years. Rehabilitation medicine has led other medical specialties in clinical outcomes research and the application of this information to improvements in practice.

As early as 1913, E.A. Codman, MD, a member of the American College of Surgeons, failed in his attempt to begin an outcome assessment method for improving patient care in hospitals (6). Only

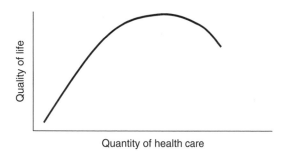

Figure 14–3. Quality of life.

much later has a different health care system been juggling a variety of strategies to monitor and measure the quality of care and patient outcomes. Not until the mid-1980s did our current understanding of outcomes measurement start to enter in earnest.

In 1986, Donebedian proposed that medical care quality be evaluated in three dimensions: structure, process, and outcome (3). We find that in the practice of medicine, it is difficult to separate the outcomes dimension from the process dimension because of the complexity of most patient care processes. Conceptually, outcomes are the end results of care, but in the practice settings, definitions are not always straightforward (7). Consequently, measuring quality in acute trauma rehabilitation medicine remains a challenge.

The concept of outcomes management was proposed by Paul Ellwood, MD, in 1988 as a solution to the unstable and confusing state of modern medicine. Trained as a physiatrist, Ellwood made a landmark lecture to the 99th Annual Meeting of the Massachusetts Medical Society. He cited the emergence of the managed care industry, illustrated consumer and provider dissatisfaction with health care, and challenged physicians to support a national strategy for outcomes management (8).

Described as a technology of patient experience, "outcomes management is designed to help patients, payers, and providers make rational medical care related choices based on better insight into the effect of those choices on the patient's life" (8). He went on to describe the need for an outcomes management system using a common language that is understandable to patients, and a system that compares specific outcome indicators using a national database.

In this chapter, we examine the subject of quality of care in trauma rehabilitation from a variety of perspectives. This chapter discusses strategies and methods for developing a quality model for rehabilitation medicine, as well as offers specific examples of the techniques and technology involved in quality measurement and improvement. In addition, certification and standards pertinent to trauma rehabilitation will be presented.

DEFINITIONS

To facilitate discussion of quality management, we believe it would be helpful to review a number of definitions below.

Quality: In the clinical context, quality can be defined as the degree to which professionals meet the established, explicitly defined, and measurable specifications based on the best available evidence and judgment, while considering the patient's needs, goals, and values (9).

Institute of Medicine (IOM) definition of quality: The degree to which health services for individuals and populations increase the likelihood of desired health outcomes and are consistent with current professional knowledge (10).

Quality measurement: To be useful, quality must be defined by measurement (9).

Continuous Quality Improvement (CQI): A structured organizational process for involving staff in planning and executing a continuous stream of improvements in systems and staff performance in order to provide quality health care that meets or exceeds the customer's expectations (11).

Total Quality Management (TQM): An ongoing process whereby top management takes whatever steps necessary to enable everyone in the organization, in the course of performing all duties, to establish and achieve standards that meet or exceed the needs and expectations of customers, both external and internal (12). The philosophy of an organization should be dedicated to TQM throughout the organization. In TQM, senior management supports project development and inclusion of quality improvement standards in job descriptions; legitimizes time spent on quality improvement, providing resources such as essential training for staff; and formally recognizes quality improvement efforts (13).

Outcomes Management System: A system and methods to collect standardized data about outcomes of care that includes both condition-specific and generic items. Data are collected concurrently and are continuous or periodic. Ongoing, consistent feedback is provided to stakeholders (14).

Value: Appropriateness, quality of outcomes, service, and cost are elements of health care value. The concept of value includes the use of resources expended in health care as part of a definition of quality. The quality of outcomes cannot be separated from the resources used and their costs (14).

The Deming System of Profound Knowledge: W. Edward Deming developed a theory used by many organizations, including hospitals, to transform the people and organization into a optimization model of performance. He described a 14-point method that has been used by many hospitals as a means to improve quality and outcomes. Countless business and hospital administrators have applied such concepts as driving fear out of the workplace, and the use of data to inform decision making (1).

Quality indicator: A quality indicator is a measurable element within a process or an outcome of care whose value suggests one or more dimensions of quality in the care provided, and is amenable to change by the care providers (15,16). Berwick states that patients and families should be actively involved in determining quality of care indicators (17).

Outcomes research: Such research "seeks to understand the end results of particular health care practices and interventions. End results include effects that people experience and care about, such as change in their ability to function; in particular, for individuals with chronic conditions where cure is not always possible and results include quality of life as well as mortality" (4).

Standards: These are "not some rigid laws to be followed blindly forever; they are a starting point—data elements and recommendations that respond continually to what is learned from application and subsequent research" (8). In general, a standard is viewed as a stricter form of a guideline, and an assumption is made that clinical practice guidelines can function as standards. A clinical practice guideline is developed through a formal or informal group process and combines best evidence with expert local and national opinion; clinical practice guidelines are specific and offer a recommended course of action for patients under typical circumstances (16).

Report cards: *Report cards* is a generic term for performance statements pertaining to health care organizations and health care providers. The balanced scorecard offers a proven framework for translating strategic objectives into key performance measurements that evaluate the outcomes of the implemented strategy and provide feedback in the performance of strategic initiatives (18). Baker and Pink were among the first to argue that the theory and concepts of a balanced scorecard were relevant to hospitals (19). In order to connect practices, outcomes, quality, value, and costs, health care organizations must use a balanced scorecard.

A FRAMEWORK FOR MEASURING QUALITY

In health care delivery organizations today, quality of care measurement is a well-established practice among physicians, nurses, and other professional staff. Powerful databases, improved standards, and the speed with which the Internet disseminates information have supported the work of measuring benchmarking and improving the quality of patient care processes and outcomes.

One cannot underestimate the magnitude and variety of resources required to effectively implement a quality measurement model within a health care delivery organization. Significant time must be allowed for education at all levels, development of an overarching philosophy and framework, as well as the time and resources needed to actually implement the model at the trauma rehabilitation department level. Although this task may seem daunting, most likely much of the work is already in place or in process at almost every facility providing trauma rehabilitation services. The purpose of this section of the chapter is to provide sufficient detail to enable the reader to develop, implement, and/or evaluate a quality measurement program that will meet the needs of the leadership, staff, as well as the patients served in a trauma rehabilitation department

Effective systems, such as in most health care delivery institutions, operate as one organism composed of subsystems, each with interdependent components (20). The connections among these subsystems are based on communication and coordination (21). Therefore, patient care quality measurement is not an isolated component of an organized health care delivery system but an interprofessional, collaborative process implemented throughout the organization at many levels.

A systemwide model for quality measurement serves many purposes. A quality model within an organized health care delivery system performs ten central functions, which we summarize below and discuss in greater detail in the following sections.

1. Provides a theoretical framework or conceptual model to management and staff as an overall means of explaining the purpose of patient care quality measurement efforts by defining terms and explaining their relationships.
2. Describes how patient care quality will be measured across the continuum of care and includes guidelines in the selection of useful indicators.
3. Provides education and training for staff at all levels in the organization on quality measurement and improvement.
4. Provides the necessary resources to design, implement, and evaluate a quality measurement program.
5. Directs resources to collect, analyze, and report data.
6. Establishes structures for reporting and disseminating information.
7. Identifies methods for evaluating the department quality measurement program and ensures coordination with the organization's goals, values, and mission.

8. Determines how sensitive data will be disseminated and manages the relationship between the quality function and such issues as patient care risk management and professional credentialing.
9. Defines how the quality measurement function meets the needs of internal customers (e.g., clinical leadership, process improvement teams) and external customers (e.g., CARF, JCAHO) (15,22–24).
10. Designs methods for monitoring the process of implementing programmatic and systematic changes based on results of outcomes measurement and quality indicator data.

PURPOSES AND FUNCTIONS OF AN OUTCOMES MANAGEMENT SYSTEM

1. An outcome management system provides a theoretical framework or conceptual model to management and staff as an overall means of illustrating the purpose of patient care quality measurement efforts by defining terms and describing their relationships.

   When measuring patient care quality, an organizational quality model or conceptual framework is needed before selection of indicators and methods can proceed (25). Donabedian's three-dimensional model for quality measurement provided the foundation for much of the research and development that followed in the field of quality measurement in health care and includes the idea that measuring quality of care cannot be an afterthought, but needs to be part of routine care and service.

   The idea is to build a model for collecting and analyzing data and information that enable staff to identify problems and areas for improvement, thus leading to the creation of sustainable changes and improvements in patient care processes and outcomes. Through continuous monitoring and systematic analysis, quality measurement and improvements in both patient care processes and outcomes become realistic goals.

   At the executive level of most organizations, a model for quality improvement is designed that is meant to lead each department or service line in their particular quality measurement program. This model may come down from the leadership of a multi-organizational structure or the CEO of an independent, community-based specialty facility, such as a rehabilitation medicine facility.

The work of Donabedian (3) is evident in much of the literature on quality measurement that has developed over the past 20 years. For example, the value compass was named to reflect its similarity to a directional compass with four distinct dimensions: (i) costs and finances, (ii) patient/families perception of satisfaction with health care, (iii) patient functional status, risk status, quality of life, and (iv) patient care clinical outcomes. For the purposes of this chapter, the clinical value compass approach (value compass) will be used to illustrate a quality model.

2. An outcome management system also describes how patient care quality will be measured across the continuum of care and includes guidelines in the selection of useful indicators.

   Although an organization may adopt a particular framework, such as the value compass model, each level in the organization, department, or service line is challenged to measure quality in concert with the overall organizational framework. This work requires shared vision, mission, language, and clear expectations for the results expected using the institution's quality model. Building a framework to support a quality model requires staff and leadership to share common knowledge about the concepts and principles of their own quality measurement model and to commit to using the model they choose as an integral component of their work.

   The value compass model is based on the idea that for a particular patient population, certain processes can be identified that lead to expected outcomes. Harborview Medical Center adopted the value compass model in 2000 based on the work of Nelson and others (26). Using the value compass model, the results of the care and services provided to patients at the rehabilitation medicine department level can be measured based on categories, such as clinical quality, operations, satisfaction, and finance. This model provides a 360-degree snapshot of the department's work and quality of care (Fig. 14–4) (27).

   A quality indicator is a measurable element representing a process or an outcome of care whose value suggests one or more dimensions of quality in the care provided and is adaptable by the care providers (15). Selecting useful indicators of quality in patient care should be an interprofessional process and include leadership, management, staff, and patient/family involvement.

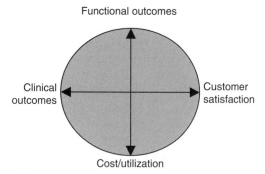

Figure 14–4. The value compass. (From Nelson EC, Mohr JJ, Batalden PB, et al. Improving health care: Part 1. The clinical value compass. *J Qual Improv.* 1996;22[4], with permission.)

The purpose of a quality model is to establish the relationship among its concepts as a guide to selecting specific, measurable indicators. By illustrating the relationships between the various dimensions of quality, a quality model can serve as a guide to selecting specific, measurable indicators, such as the following (Table 14-1):

- high-volume patient care activities or events;
- high-risk or problem-prone;
- high-cost (25);
- high-interest.

The value compass framework can be a model in which indicators of interest are organized and used as a tool for guiding the

work of the leadership team responsible for measuring quality (Fig. 14–5). The effectiveness of the quality improvement program is partially determined by the clarity with which the key indicators and sources are identified. A primary function of the leadership team is to clearly and concisely describe how patient care quality will be measured. This document can serve as a guiding force in the team's work over time.

How one selects the most useful indicators to measure quality of patient care depends on many factors. The quality plan should provide directions for selecting specific indicators that clearly relate to and support the model for quality measurement. Time limits and thresholds should also be determined by the quality plan, with adequate resources allocated for collecting, analyzing, and interpreting data. Equally important is establishing a mind-set in the staff that will enable change in the processes and practice patterns based on the information and analysis of quality indicators.

Is the data available; is it accessible with the resources available? What budget restrictions apply and how does that influence the selection of the most useful indicators? The individuals responsible for the work must answer these questions and others.

3. Additionally, an outcomes measurement system provides education and training for staff at all levels in the organization on the subject of quality measurement and improvement.

Table 14-1 Categories of Indicators Based on the Value Compass Model

	High Volume	High Cost	High Risk	High Interest
Clinical quality	FIM change LOS efficiency	Barriers to discharge	Discharges back to acute care, adverse events, comorbidities associated with each diagnostic group	% of patients discharged to the community; age and LOS for high acuity populations such as patients with burns, SCI ventilator dependent
Satisfaction	Patient satisfaction with pain control	Litigation, insurance denials	Patient complaints surveys	% of patients who would recommend your facility
Operations	Expected vs. actual LOS for the top five diagnoses or volume	Agency costs for staff; % of staff turnover; patient days	% staff vacancy rates	New program utilization such as stroke support group
Finance	% of Medicare (PPS) payer mix	Average daily census	LOS outliers % of uninsured % of cases denied or dollar amount not reimbursed	Cost vs. charges by diagnosis Expected vs. actual LOS by payer

FIM, Functional Independence Measure; LOS, lengths of stay; PPS, prospective payment system; SCI, spinal cord injury.
From Harborview Medical Center Rehabilitation Medicine Department. Quality Model/Dashboards, 2004, with permission.

Value Compass Framework
QUALITY IMPROVEMENT PROGRAM: Dashboards

CLINICAL QUALITY	
INDICATORS	**SOURCE**
FIM score changes total, and TBI, stroke, SCI, multitrauma	UDS M®
% discharged to community	UDS M®
LOS and LOS efficiency	UDS M®
Unexpected discharges to acute care	Care manager's report

SATISFACTION	
INDICATORS	**SOURCE**
Inpatient discharge survey	Patient Relations
Outpatient clinic surveys	Patient Relations/NRC
Patient satisfaction after discharge (telephone)	iT Health Track, Inc.
Patient comments	Letters of recognition/ comment collection

OPERATIONS	
INDICATORS	**SOURCE**
Inpatient LOS, admits	UDS M® Finance reports
Outpatient clinic visits	Appointment software
Staff vacancy rate	Manager's report

FINANCE	
INDICATORS	**SOURCE**
Payer mix	UDS M®
Revenue & expenses	Finance system
Charges vs. reimbursement	Decision support/special reports (UDS M® and finance)
Combined departments (inpatient & therapies) expense report	Decision support/ special reports

Figure 14–5. Value compass dashboards. FIM, Functional Independence Measures; LOS, lengths of stay; SCI, spinal cord injury; TBI, traumatic brain injury. (From Harborview Medical Center. Rehabilitation Medicine Department, 2004, with permission.)

The development of the knowledge worker in the age of information technology (2) has offered health care organizations the capacity to collect clinical, as well as cost accounting, data to help determine the financial and clinical outcomes related to patient care delivery. Organizations must determine the training and educational needs of those involved in quality measurement and improvement. Significant investment in staff education and training is required for the successful implementation of a quality plan. The value of any quality measurement model will be determined by, in part, the knowledge, skill, and investment of those leading the charge and of those staff members responsible for implementing changes in practice based on results of quality measurement.

Starting at the executive level of the organization, education and training in quality measurement are necessary. Common strategies are to present such information at department-level meetings, including meetings of the board of directors or trustees, medical leadership, and senior administrative staff. Use of consultants is often helpful

at this level of training. Caution would be advised not to invite individuals from other organizations who may present their model as the recommendation rather then doing an individualized assessment.

Setting the stage or establishing the context for such presentations is critical to the success of this educational strategy. Often, senior administrators are more likely to want a "unique" model for quality measurement that is consistent with the organization's unique culture, leadership personalities, and available resources, such as information systems, to support the work.

Administrative leadership should also attend local and national conferences on quality measurement to keep abreast of current trends in the field. Clinical leadership is frequently exposed to information on quality measurement as a component of professional organization–sponsored conferences or meetings. Site visits to other facilities may also be used to educate administrators and directors on this subject; however, this is often time consuming and may lead to minimal results. Site visits may be effective if used within an integrated health care delivery system, such as a chain of rehabilitation facilities.

Finally, journal articles, books, and the Internet often serve as legitimate and innovative sources of information that will increase the knowledge of the administration and clinical leadership in a way that is convenient and cost-effective. Englebardt (28) describes technology in distributed education as a means of using Web-based courses and other methods to connect multiple learners with each other, regardless of physical location. This is also an effective strategy for ensuring everyone on the team is exposed to the same information in the same form, which can improve the quality of group discussions, thus improving results of training. One should not a priori assume members of any senior leadership team (administrative and clinical) have the knowledge or experience needed to effectively participate in designing a quality model. The only way to ensure such knowledge and shared understanding is to offer opportunities as part of an organizational commitment to quality.

In an ideal situation, following purposeful education and training, the senior leadership team is able to openly discuss individual views, goals, and ideas for the organization's quality measurement model. Once the model is designed and a plan developed for implementation, the process of educating staff at all levels can begin.

Getting the word out to all employees is the next critical step. Manager's and department director meetings are ideal forums for education and training. Again, this group of staff may have a wide variety of skills and differences in their understanding and experience in quality measurement. Assessment of the group's educational needs is an important step in the educational process. Failure to correctly assess the group's needs could result in gaps in learning and frustration among the management team. For example, it is likely the management team will include members who have years of experience in management, but who completed their education before instruction in quality measurement became a component of the professional training in their field. Instruction in quality measurement has only been included in these schools for the past 10 to 15 years. In contrast, relatively new managers may have been exposed to the subject in school, but lack the experience and skill necessary to implement

the quality measurement model in their department.

Many of the same strategies used for educating senior leadership can be successfully used with managers and department directors. Resources should be available to support the individual's education based on their personal interest, the areas they manage, and their potential to apply the knowledge and skill that will result in successful implementation of a quality model in their area.

New manager training and orientation should include the explicit expectation for participation in implementation of the quality model with clearly described roles and responsibilities related to their department. As an organization embarks on implementing a new or revised quality measurement model, it may be prudent to select specific areas and managers to "pilot" the model. This implementation strategy may help embed the work at the department level by selecting the most capable managers to lead the work. When completed, these managers could serve as mentors or "experts" to other managers who may benefit from their experience. Innovative educational strategies are often the most successful when attempting to improve quality in an organization. Leadership should risk trying new ways to educate and train, while monitoring and evaluating results.

The use of in-house newsletters is another way to educate staff at all levels in the organization, and particularly staff at the clinical practice and support levels (i.e., staff nurses, therapists, and technicians). Well-scripted articles in newsletters or other routine publications can be systematically planned to provide simple to complex information appropriate to the staff. A "series" approach can be an effective way to entice staff into reading the articles and anticipating the next issue. These articles can target different areas of the organization as a way to engage staff in identifying with the content, thus making it of value in their daily work lives. Consider including information about special training that managers have attended and a Frequently Asked Questions (FAQ) section.

In many organizations, Websites may be an effective vehicle for getting information to staff. Again, innovative and diverse strategies are often successful when trying to educate large numbers of staff on the organization's quality measurement model. Attention should be paid to the principles of adult learning, such as the *"what's in it for me?"* approach. This concept should be considered and applied to all educational strategies regardless of the person's position in the organization.

Leadership at the rehabilitation department level should determine the education and training needs of staff at all levels in the department. This process is best decided at the leadership team level following discussion to determine how staff will be involved in data collection and analysis. Once these decisions have been agreed upon, educational strategies can be planned that will result in staff participation and commitment to the department's quality model.

Formal and informal training can be arranged to increase the level of understanding among rehabilitation department level staff. The primary question is, what responsibilities and expectations are identified for each staff member? Once this question is answered, appropriate education and training can be planned. In addition, the department leadership should assess the department quality measurement model and identify the specific work to be accomplished. Is the quality program recently designed by the larger organization, or is the model already embedded in the department but changing direction, leadership, or focus? What new technology is available, such as computerized patient records or UDS M® (29) that will make data more readily available? How do staff currently use information systems, and is there room for improvement such as more robust applications that require training staff? Does the department include new managers, directors, or staff with different interests, experiences, or talents? It is essential for the leadership team to answer these questions before planning for staff education and development in the area of quality measurement.

4. Furthermore, an outcomes management system provides the necessary resources for designing, implementing, and evaluating a quality measurement program.

The organization's senior leadership is responsible and accountable for providing adequate resources that will result in the design, implementation, and evaluation of the quality measurement program, including the department-level program. Annual budgets should include adequate funds to support quality measurement programs at all department levels of operation. In addition, funds in support of education and training, including

travel if needed, must be secured for that purpose. Indirect resources should also be funded adequately, such as production of the numerous publications that are designed to educate staff. At a later date, analyzing the return on investment may be part of the quality measurement program evaluation and an important indicator for its value to the overall organization, as well as the rehabilitation department-level program evaluation.

The organization committed to quality of care measurement and improvement is dedicated to providing resources for training—if necessary, hiring new employees, acquiring new information technology, and purchasing supplies and equipment—that will result in successful quality program operations and lead to measurable improvements in the quality of care provided to patients. Determination of how much money is needed to accomplish this task must be individually determined based on available assets, program expectations, and commitment to other projects, mission, and strategic goals.

Innovative uses of current resources, redirection of current staff, and/or investments in additional resources are successful strategies for organizations and departments alike. In many settings, pockets of unlikely resources in the form of people and materials are available to be redirected into work that supports the quality measurement model. For example, staff at various levels with computer skills or interest in learning new work, such as data management or even training, may prove to be valuable assets in various aspects of operating a quality measurement program.

5. An outcomes management system directs resources to collect, analyze, and report data and information.

Leadership should search for information that may be available from untapped sources. Various types of data may be already collected for reasons other than measuring quality that may then be useful in the quality measurement model. Clearly established department level program goals, in combination with inquisitive investigation, may lead to valuable information from sources beyond the department setting. Effective relationships among managers and staff are needed to enable results such as sharing data across departments. For example, leadership may find it useful to include data collected by case managers related to insurance providers or from risk management or medical records/computerized patient records department.

Department leadership may benefit from sharing staff, technology, and/or information across departments. An open and collaborative culture is necessary for successful sharing among and between departments. In addition, confidence in data quality and integrity is necessary for this approach to be beneficial. Strong and supportive interprofessional relationships are needed when senior leadership or department directors reallocate resources from one area to another for the purpose of operating a quality measurement model. This may take the form of a temporary reassignment of staff, use of office space, computer software, or the shifting of full-time equivalents (FTEs) in support of the program.

6. An outcomes management system also establishes structures for reporting and disseminating information.

Lines of reporting and communication must be clearly defined across the organization, including at the individual department level, in order to effectively implement a quality measurement model. The organizationwide quality of care oversight committee usually includes all dimensions of quality. For example, representatives from risk management, medical staff leadership and credentialing, and the clinical quality measurement program manager and/or executive sponsor should form the group responsible for designing an overall reporting structure for all quality measurement work within the organization. Philosophically, does the leadership view quality measurement as work that is embedded in each department and supported within each department or supported by staff and resources in a centralized department?

Considerations should also be made for the size of the facility/organization, variety of services/departments, areas of focus (i.e., centers of excellence), and reporting relationships among senior leadership and department directors/managers. Is the organization designed using service lines or traditional departments structured by clinical specialty or function? Are senior leaders responsible for services across a continuum or areas offsite or even in a different city or state?

Organizational charts and other diagrams are often helpful in communicating the chain of command and reporting structures related to a quality measurement program. Whatever the reporting structure, it must protect the confidentiality and privacy of information that is part of the quality measurement program. If quality measurement is part of the work of the rehabilitation department leadership/department meetings, minutes and other documents should be identified as "Confidential quality improvement information," in order to be protected from discovery as part of possible legal processes. In addition, the sharing of such information with other groups should be carefully scripted and monitored. For example, when information is presented out of the context for which it was designed, misunderstanding and improper analysis may result. Therefore, when reporting department-level quality information, it is important to present this information from the listener's perspective in order to elicit the expected results.

The reporting structure in many organizations includes a facility/organizationwide senior leadership oversight committee. This group will often include all members of the senior leadership team, other executives, and members of the board of directors/trustees. In addition, each division and/or department will provide committee structures that conduct and monitor the work of quality measurement and report up to the senior level committee. These department-level committees are also responsible for reporting information across all levels of staff within their department. Mechanisms for sharing quality information among staff should again incorporate safeguards to ensure confidentiality and privacy.

Staff should be presented with data gathered as part of the department quality measurement program. In most cases, rehabilitation department staff is interested in learning about patient care outcomes and overall department performance. Members of the department leadership and management team should consistently assess the learning needs of staff and offer educational opportunities as a prerequisite to sharing quality data. In addition, the presentation of such information may differ for each audience. For example, using pie charts and bar graphs may be appropriate for staff, while using spider diagrams may be more appropriate for an audience of senior administrators. Staff will often relate personal stories and examples when describing their work, so including stories and case studies is a way to engage staff in conversations about quality improvement.

The forum, format, timing, audience participation, and skill of the presenter are equally important in relation to gaining expected results when presenting quality program information to staff. Casual, easily accessible settings will make it easier for staff to attend. Publicizing the meeting/forum with a catchy title makes it more appealing to some staff. Spending time up front to state the purpose and goals for the meeting will reinforce the messages and add value for the staff. Leaders often make the mistake to assume staff clinicians, technicians, and others working with rehabilitation patients are not interested in the results of their work. On the contrary, staff provide bedside care 24 hours a day, 7 days a week on the trauma rehabilitation unit. Inherently, their dedication and interest in improving the clinical outcomes for their patients is often a driving force to their work and should not be underestimated. The onus is on the manager to present the information in a clear, meaningful manner, while engaging staff in a conversation that will lead to further investment and loyalty, as well as improved quality of care.

7. An outcomes management system identifies methods for evaluating the department-level quality measurement program and ensures coordination with the organization's goals, values, and mission.

Program evaluation can be used to evaluate the effectiveness of a quality measurement program in many dimensions. For example, besides the actual results of measuring indicators, how did the program fare in terms of training and involving staff? Other elements of evaluation include the costs related to the quality measurement program, including contracts with software vendors or others who perform follow-up phone services for patient satisfaction or functional status changes, for instance. The department-level leadership team most commonly determines the depth to which a program is evaluated. The critical factor in evaluation is a comparison of the program achievements with the initial goals and objectives.

The initial establishment of program goals and objectives is the foundation for evaluation. That is to say, what did the team set out to accomplish, and what were the results? Leaders should strictly adhere to the original goals and objectives throughout the implementation process and trust that the initial work of developing these goals and strategies was legitimate and need not be second-guessed down the road. The leadership team should not waver from using the initial goals and objectives to conduct program evaluation. The team should consider changing the evaluation criteria only after thoughtful analysis of and consensus on how the criteria will change. One reason to adjust criteria for evaluation might be that volumes in a certain patient population did not reach a point that statistical analysis would be valid. In this case, a different target group could be identified. Rationale for changing mid-stream should always be documented in meeting minutes and be included in the final program evaluation document.

An annual program evaluation should be conducted either in sequence with the organization's fiscal year or upon the anniversary of the program's implementation. The evaluation may also be scheduled when the relevant data are available. For example, if patient satisfaction data are always a quarter behind other information, the evaluation may be scheduled to correspond to that date. The intention of annual evaluation is to establish a predictable timeline for analysis of the results that can be repeated year to year.

To develop an outcomes grid, the program objectives and goals should be combined with a specific and realistic target. The grid should also include parameters for weight or the value of each outcome measure with results. An outcomes grid can serve as a road map in conjunction with the dashboard document based on the value compass. All of these documents must be aligned and consistent with the organizationwide goals for quality measurement, as well as realistic and achievable for the rehabilitation department (Table 14-2).

8. An outcomes management system determines how sensitive data will be disseminated and manages the relationship between the quality function and such issues as patient care, risk management, and professional credentialing.

Dissemination of quality measurement data and information is often determined by an organizationwide policy. Organizational charts often illustrate the connection between individual departments and the other levels of committees responsible for quality measurement. Often, the standard is that all information reported at these meetings be considered sensitive and identified as such on all written documents.

Table 14-2 Outcomes Grid Used in Annual Reporting

Weight	Program Objective	Outcome Measure	Apply to:	Document/Data Source	Time Source	Min.	Goal	Facility Data	% of Goal	Performance Index
25%	Maximize independence in self-care, mobility, and social skills	Average FIM gain per person served will be 28 pt gain in FIM admission to discharge	All persons served	UDS M® FIM total motor/cognitive score	a/d FIM d/c FIM	23 pt	28 pt	27.2	97	14.5
		Average FIM gain per person served from discharge f/u will be no <8 pt	All persons served	UDS M® report	f/u FIM	0 pt	8	7.3	91	9.1
20%	Maximize patient/ family satisfaction	90% of persons served/ family are very satisfied with overall program results	All persons served	iTHealthTrack, Inc. report benchmark	f/u	80%	3.78	3.80	100	20
20%	Provide an efficient program of care	Persons served will meet 80% of goal average LOS efficiency.	All persons served	UDS M® report – LOS efficiency	Cal y	80%	2	2.12	100	20
15%	Educate patient and family regarding skills and information to maintain gains	90% of persons served/ family will be very satisfied with the education/ info received	All persons served	iTHealthTrack, Inc. report	d/c	70%	80%	96%	100	15
10%	Minimize re-hospitalization	<10% of persons served will be d/c to acute service during inpatient hospitalization	All persons served	UDS M® report on unplanned discharges	Cal y	<15%	<10%	8%	100	10
10%	Maximize community integration	80% of persons served will be d/c'd back to the "community" defined as home, board and care, or transitional living	All persons served	UDS M® database data fields: admit from, d/c f/u living setting.	a/d d/c f/u	70%	80%	80%	100	10

FIM, Functional Independence Measures; UDS, Uniform Data System; Cal, calendar; pt, point(s); LOS, lengths of stay; a/d, from admission; d/c, to discharge; f/u, to follow up.
From Harborview Medical Center and the University of Washington Medical Center: Department of Rehabilitation Medicine Annual Report. Outcomes Grid, 2004, with permission.

The department leadership team is responsible for determining what information is shared with staff and in what forum. In general, results are shared with staff regularly, such as at an annual staff meeting for that specific purpose. CARF standards require that staff be informed and contribute to discussion regarding patient care outcomes and quality improvement processes. Adequate time should be given to deliver these results and for questions, comments, and suggestions from staff. These meetings should be documented as part of the department's quality measurement program and attendance documented.

Information and results should also be reported up through the organization as indicated by the organizational chart for quality measurement and improvement. The audience should always be considered when reporting department specific information. Additional time might be needed to clarify terms or explain the rationale for measurement of some indicators. In addition, feedback from these outside groups should be brought back to the department-level team for discussion and consideration.

Again, at the organizationwide level, policies often dictate how risk management issues will be documented and communicated. Sentinel events and other unexpected outcomes should always be managed and documented outside the department-level quality measurement program plan. Systems for additional security of information must be maintained in the event of these situations, which include clear directions for reporting, documenting, and investigating.

Professional credentialing is another function that should be managed separately from the organization or department quality measurement program. The details of this work should be under administrative-level support and in line with medical staff bylaws, as well as hospital insurance protocols. Additional discussion on this subject is beyond the scope and purpose of this chapter.

9. An outcomes management system also defines how the quality measurement function meets the needs of internal customers (e.g., clinical leadership, case/care managers, social workers).

The department leadership team should consider internal customers when designing and implementing a quality measurement program. As program goals and specific indicators are identified, consideration should be given to the value of certain information to members of the team, such as social workers or care mangers. For instance, length of stay and denials by payer type may be of interest to the care manager responsible for continued stay insurance authorization. Social workers would probably be interested in the percentage of patients discharged to the community by diagnosis and length of stay for patients discharged to skilled nursing facilities. Based on these data and information, these staff could analyze and adjust processes or systems that could improve results; however, few changes in outcomes are due to the unique work of specific individuals. Thus, there is difficulty in using outcomes to make changes without more comprehensive analysis and assessment of the problems, processes, and program goals.

10. Finally, an outcomes management system designs methods for monitoring the process for implementing programmatic and systematic changes based on results of outcomes measurement and quality indicator data.

The goal for implementing changes in rehabilitation department processes and structures should be to create sustainable results based on reliable data and information. The leadership team responsible for quality measurement and improvement is charged with analysis of these data and application of effective planning within the team and staffs that will result in improvements in patient care quality.

Implementing programmatic and systematic changes in trauma rehabilitation departments may include simple adjustments in the way procedures are performed or more complex changes, such as redesign of care delivery systems. Actually using quality data to implement change is a difficult process in quality measurement programs. These steps require significant resources to design and implement the changes, as well as evaluate results and continue improvement, while preventing people and systems from sliding back into old ways of performing. The leadership team and/or quality measurement group is responsible for working closely and in concert with the unit and department leadership when changes are implemented. The key to success is adequate preparation of the staff involved in the change and the ability of leadership to clearly articulate the reason for the change as well as the expected results.

BUSINESS PRODUCTS FOR MEASURING QUALITY INDICATORS

The following are examples of business products for measuring quality of care and outcomes in rehabilitation medicine:

- **UDS M® (http://www.udsmr.org) (30).** Uniform Data System for Medical Rehabilitation is a widely used system for documenting severity of impairment/disability and outcomes used by inpatient and outpatient facilities. Besides individual patient FIM data, UDS M® services also include data analysis by facility, as well as comparison to regional and national data. Additional products, such as pediatric measures and tools, are also available. Therapists and nurses are recredentialed every 2 years and must pass the test at an 80% level.
- **iTHealthTrack, Inc. (www.ithealthtrack.org) (29).** A business designed to provide telephone follow-up with rehabilitation patients after discharge, providing functional gains post discharge and measures of satisfaction. Provides case-mix adjusted benchmarks to enable comparisons, while ensuring patient privacy and data security.
- **FIM Ware (http://www.udsmr.org) (30).** A uniform method that enables the documentation of severity of patient impairment and the functional results of medical rehabilitation. Provides a common language to promote communication about patient's functional status across disciplines and provides a basis for comparison of rehabilitation outcomes.
- **National Research Corporation (NRC) (www.nationalresearch.com) (31).** A patient satisfaction survey that can be mailed to a patient's residence following discharge. NRC maintains a library of standardized, tested, and reliable questions from which to choose, or customers may write custom questions to be included. NRC provides local benchmark data for >100 metropolitan statistical areas, as well as customer-defined service areas, state, and national benchmarks for a variety of measures.
- **Press-Ganey (www.pressganey.com) (32).** Satisfaction survey that measures satisfaction of internal and external sources with 30% of all hospitals using the measure and opportunity for benchmarking. Provides services to both inpatient and outpatient programs regarding satisfaction with services for more than 6,000 clients with 8 million surveys completed per year. Services include mailing out surveys and extensive benchmarking with real-time online viewing of reports. Press-Ganey began measuring patient satisfaction with the experience of care in 1985 and serve 30% of all hospitals and 40% of all hospitals of more than 100 beds in the United States.

ACCREDITATION AND STANDARDS PERTINENT TO TRAUMA REHABILITATION

COMMISSION ON ACCREDITATION OF REHABILITATION FACILITIES

The Commission on Accreditation of Rehabilitation Facilities (CARF) (33) is an international accrediting body surveying numerous programs including medical rehabilitation. Standards are developed through the National Advisory Committee, which is made up of stakeholders, such as providers, consumers, and purchasers of services. Facilities seeking accreditation are required to meet organizational as well as program specific standards. Surveys are conducted by medical rehabilitation specialists currently working in the field of rehabilitation. Trauma rehabilitation services are surveyed under the Comprehensive Integrated Inpatient Rehabilitation standards for medical programs. Although other states have Emergency Medical Services (EMS) systems and a designation process, Washington State is the only state currently requiring CARF accreditation and adherence to Washington Administrative Codes (WAC) as part of its designation for trauma services.

CARF requirements for accreditation include meeting Business Practice Standards (organization-wide standards) that include leadership, accessibility, patient rights, information management and performance improvement, patient input, legal requirements, safety, financial management and human resources, as well as specific program standards as mentioned in the previous text. CARF standards have included requirements to address the measurement of patient outcomes since the early 1970s.

CARF standards for comprehensive Integrated Inpatient Rehabilitation Programs set a baseline for inpatient services. The following requirements for personnel in inpatient rehabilitation are briefly described here to set the context for comparing CARF standards to the additional requirements mandated by Washington State, which include CARF accreditation and will be addressed later in this chapter.

- Medical direction of the rehabilitation unit may be provided by a physician trained in physical medicine and rehabilitation (physiatrist) or a neurologist, orthopaedist, pediatrician, or other physician, depending on the setting. Physicians must be board certified in their area of specialty and demonstrate appropriate experience and training to provide rehabilitation physician services through one of the following: a formal residency in physical medicine and rehabilitation; a fellowship in rehabilitation for a minimum of 1 year; or a minimum of 2 years experience as a collaborative team member providing rehabilitation services in a comprehensive inpatient rehabilitation program.
- Rehabilitation physician services can be provided by a physical medicine and rehabilitation physician (physiatrist) or neurologist, orthopaedist, pediatrician, or other physician who is qualified by virtue of training and experience in rehabilitation.
- Rehabilitation nursing services must be provided 24 hours per day, 7 days per week, and there must be coverage by registered nurses with rehabilitation experience.
- CARF standards related to allied health professionals, such as occupational therapy, physical therapy, and speech, for example, require that such professionals have the credentials appropriate to their discipline. In addition, the staff needs to be appropriately oriented, maintain specific competencies, and have resources available to foster continuing education.

JOINT COMMISSION ON THE ACCREDITATION OF HOSPITALS ORGANIZATION

JCAHO (National, optional) (34) surveys hospitals and ambulatory care facilities. Surveys encompass standards that focus on hospital and clinical practice, quality improvement, and safety. Surveyors include physicians, nurses, or other clinicians who may work full-time, part-time, or intermittently and must have recent experience in management, but may currently be employed in medicine.

Trauma Designation (Washington State Only)

Trauma designation includes meeting CARF standards and additional requirements mandated by the state that address staffing, services, and participation in a quality assurance program. The trauma designation is regulated by the state Department of Health (DOH).

Department of Health (State)

The Department of Health is required for hospital licensure in all states, but may be specific to certain areas of the hospital in some states, and includes deemed status for serving Medicare patients.

Medicare (Federal)

The Prospective Payment System (PPS) is required for hospitals providing services to Medicare patients as mandated by the Prospective Payment System implemented in 2001 or 2002, depending on the hospital's fiscal year.

WASHINGTON STATE REQUIREMENTS FOR TRAUMA REHABILITATION/LEVEL 1

Washington State is currently the only state that has implemented a special rehabilitation designation for hospitals treating trauma patients that specifically mandates CARF accreditation and Washington Administrative Codes (WAC) that dictate the components of the services to be delivered (35). Such hospitals are required to provide a continuum of care including acute, inpatient rehabilitation services, and outpatient treatment for trauma victims. Harborview Medical Center in Seattle is the only Level 1 acute trauma center serving residents of Washington, Idaho, Alaska, and Montana and is one of three Level 1 trauma rehabilitation units in the state of Washington.

The original intent of the trauma designation was to ensure patients were transferred to the appropriate level of care, such as an acute rehabilitation unit versus a skilled nursing care facility. In the early 1990s, a commission that included local hospital representatives and other stakeholders was established by the governor of Washington to address improving the care provided to patients with spinal cord injuries. A subcommittee included physiatrists and administrators specialized in adult and pediatric rehabilitation whose interest was to ensure the proper treatment for adults and children with spinal cord and other traumatic injuries. CARF standards were identified as the baseline for establishing standards that rehabilitation units within hospitals applying for trauma designation must meet. While the CARF standards are comprehensive in themselves, Washington State adds additional requirements that deepen the standards and further define services and education.

The goals and objectives of the development of the EMS Trauma System in the state of Washington had the following goals and objectives:

- pursue trauma prevention activities to decrease the incidence of trauma;
- provide optimal care for the trauma victim;
- prevent unnecessary death and disability from trauma and emergency illness;
- contain costs of trauma care and trauma system implementation.

Trauma designation is contingent upon the execution of a contract between the hospital and the state Department of Health. The process for application and survey is executed through the DOH Office of Emergency Medical and Trauma Prevention. Hospitals are surveyed every 2 years.

Level 1 designated trauma rehabilitation programs must treat trauma inpatients and outpatients, regardless of disability or level of service or complexity, who are 15 years or older. The adolescent patient's educational goals, premorbid learning or developmental status, social or family needs, and other factors indicate whether they are treated in an adult or pediatric rehabilitation setting.

Washington State requires that inpatient rehabilitation services must be available as part of the trauma designation and includes specific details related to nursing hours per patient day (HPPD) and certification of staff in the nursing specialty of rehabilitation.

The following are requirements for trauma rehabilitation Level 1 designation:

- Patients must receive services on a designated rehabilitation-nursing unit. A peer group for persons with similar disabilities must be provided. An initial care plan and weekly update must be reviewed and approved by a Certified Rehabilitation Registered Nurse (CRRN).
- Medical services require direction by a physiatrist who is in-house or on-call and responsible for rehabilitation issues 24 hours per day.
- A registered nurse must manage the unit; rehabilitation nursing personnel must provide services 24 hours per day, and at least one CRRN must be on duty each day and evening shift when a trauma patient is present. There must be orientation and training for all levels of rehabilitation nursing personnel. Six hours of clinical nursing care per patient per day must be provided.

- Health personnel and services must be available 24 hours per day. Pharmaceuticals with an on-call pharmacist must be available for consultation and with the capability of immediate access to patient and pharmacy databases within 5 minutes notification. Personnel trained in intermittent urinary catheterization and respiratory must be available.
- Staff registered or certified and in-house or available for treatment every day, as is indicated in the rehabilitation plan, must include the following: occupational therapy; physical therapy; psychology including neuropsychological services; and clinical psychological services, including testing and counseling, substance abuse counseling, social services, and speech language pathology.
- The following services must be provided in-house or through affiliation or consultation arrangements with staff who are licensed, registered, certified, or degreed: communication augmentation; driver evaluation and training; orthotics; prosthetics; rehabilitation engineering; therapeutic recreation; and vocational rehabilitation.
- Diagnostic services must be provided in-house or through affiliation or consultative arrangements with staff that are licensed, registered, certified, or degreed. The following services are included: diagnostic imaging and electrophysiologic testing.
- The trauma center must serve as a regional referral center for patients in their geographical area needing Levels 2 and 3 rehabilitation care.
- The facility must have outreach programs regarding trauma care, consisting of telephone and on-site consultation with physicians and other health care professionals in the community and outlying areas.
- The facility must provide a formal program of continuing education both in-house and through outreach, which is provided by nurses and allied health care professionals.
- An ongoing structured program for conducting clinical studies, applied research, or analysis in rehabilitation of trauma patients, and for reporting results within a peer review process must be in place.
- A Level 1 trauma rehabilitation service shall have a quality assurance improvement program.
- The trauma center must participate in a trauma registry.
- Levels 1 through 5 and pediatric Levels 1 through 3 must participate in a quality assurance program.

Table 14-3	Private and Government Agency Comparison	
	CARF/JCAHO	**Department of Health**
	Survey to Standards	**Survey to Regulations**
Purpose	Performance improvement	Licensure and/or Medicare/Medicaid provider certificate
Emphasis	Evaluation	Inspection
Value	Improvement	Enforcement
Expectations	Achievable standards	Minimum standards
Approach	Education/consultation	Sanctions/penalties/fines
Findings	Recommendations for improvement	Citations
Award	Accreditation	Licensure/certification
Compliance	Voluntary	Mandatory
Oversight	Private/not for profit	Government entity

Trauma rehabilitation facilities may be reviewed by numerous accrediting organizations such as JCAHO or state agencies such as the DOH. While many of the standards or regulations are similar, the purpose for each survey is different. Rehabilitation facilities are also required to meet conditions of participation and the newly implemented PPS to allow reimbursement for treatment and services to patients insured by Medicare (Table 14-3).

SUMMARY

This chapter has provided a historical perspective on the development of quality measures, a definition of terms, strategies, and methods for developing a quality measurement model, and the components of an outcomes management system. An example of one possible method of gathering and reporting data was illustrated with the value compass model. Products for measurement were reviewed along with accreditation options and the model currently used by the state of Washington for Level 1 trauma rehabilitation designation.

Quality measurement and outcomes research will play a significant role in planning for the future. Since the implementation of PPS, rehabilitation facilities have seen a decrease in their lengths of stay nationwide. By applying a quality measurement and outcomes model, leaders in rehabilitation facilities will have the difficult task of determining how decreased length of stay really affects patient outcomes. The following questions remain:

- Can patients learn everything that they used to learn and practice in the hospital over the course of several months?
- Are outpatient clinics capable of continuing the learning process begun in the inpatient program?
- Can the patient actually ever attain the high level of independence they were once able to achieve due to the length of treatment and opportunity for 24/7 access to the interdisciplinary team and the ability to practice newly learned skills, in the hospital, on home passes, and on recreational outings?
- What is the floor for the reimbursement hospitals can afford to accept and how low can they go before it becomes impossible to continue to operate an inpatient rehabilitation unit?

Other research questions:

- What will be the effect on patient's long-term quality of health and life functioning as related to changes in insurance coverage for rehabilitation hospitals, both for outpatient and inpatient?
- Without a national health care plan to address the needs of the uninsured, how will rehabilitation facilities continue to afford to care for patients with limited or no health care insurance?
- With shrinking resources, rehabilitation services are under scrutiny and are often labeled "elective rather than essential" to improving function and getting patients back to work after an injury or illness. How will reductions in financial support for trauma funding and changes in private insurance authorization criteria affect rehabilitation facility admissions?
- What are the effects of continued efforts to reduce lengths of stay on long-term recovery and continued improvement in patient function?

REFERENCES

1. Deming WE. *Out of the crisis*. Cambridge, MA: Massachusetts Institute of Technology, Center for Advanced Educational Study; 1986.
2. Drucker PF. *Post-capitalist society*. New York, NY: Truman Talley Books/Dutton; 1992.
3. Donabedian AA. Criteria and standard for quality assessment and monitoring. *QRB Qual Rev Bull*. 1986;12:99–108.
4. Agency for Healthcare Research and Quality (AHRQ). Available at: www.ahrq.gov. Accessed 2003.
5. Institute of Medicine of the National Academies (IOM). The quality chasm, 2003.
6. Stevens R. *Sickness and in wealth: American Hospitals in the Twentieth Century*. New York, NY: Basic Books Inc; 1989.
7. Hegyvary ST. Patient care outcomes related to management of symptoms. In: Fitzpatrick JJ, Stevenson JS, eds. *Annual review of nursing research*. New York, NY: Springer-Verlag; 1993:145–168.
8. Ellwood PM. Shattuck lecture-outcomes management: A technology of patient experience. *N Engl J Med*. 1988;23:1549–1556.
9. Ross, A, Fenster, LF. The dilemma of managing value. *Front Health Serv Manage*. 1996;12(1):3–32.
10. Institute of Medicine of the National Academies (IOM). Available at: http://www.iom.edu. Accessed November 11, 2003.
11. McLaughlin C, Kaluzny A. *Continuous quality improvement in health care*. Gaithersberg, MD: Aspen Inc; 1994.
12. Miller WJ. A working definition for total quality management. *J Qual Mange*. 1996;1(2):149–159.
13. Slee VN, Slee DA, Schmidt HJ. Slee's health care terms. *Comprehensive Edition*. 3rd ed. St. Paul, MN: Tringa Press; 1996.
14. Fenster LF. *Bringing order to a chaotic system by defining and measuring quality and outcomes*. Seattle, WA: Northwest Organization of Nurse Executives, Regional Meeting; October 1991.
15. Donabedian A. Specialization in clinical performance monitoring: what it is, and how to achiever it. In: Couch J, ed. *Health care quality management in the 21st century*. Tampa, FL: The American College of Physician Executives, Hillsboro Printing Co; 1991:417–430.
16. Berstein SJ, Hilborne L. Clinical indicators: The road to quality care? *Jt Comm J Qual Improv*. 1993;19(11):501–509.
17. Berwick DM. Eleven worthy aims for clinical leadership of health system reform. *J Am Med Assoc*. 1994;272:797–802.
18. Oliveira J. The balanced scorecard: An integrative approach to performance evaluation. *Healthc Financ Manage*. 2001;55(5):42–46.
19. Baker GR, Pink GH. A balanced scorecard for Canadian hospitals. *Healthc Manage Forum*. 1995;8(4):7–21.
20. McKay R. Theories, models, and systems for nursing. In: Nicoll LH, ed. *Perspectives on nursing theory*. 2nd ed. Philadelphia, PA: JB Lippincott Co; 1992.
21. Morgan, G. *Images of organizations*. Thousand Oaks, CA: Sage Publications Inc; 1997.
22. Genovich-Richards J. Designing quality management programs for today and tomorrow. In: Kazandjian VA, ed. *The epidemiology of quality*. Gaithesburg, MD: Aspen Publishers; 1995:55–83.
23. Kazandjian VA. Indicators of performance or the search for the best pointer dog. *The epidemiology of quality*. Gaithersburg, MD: Aspen Publishers; 1995:25–37.
24. Warwick AM, Landford AM, Reitz JA. Hospital use of clinical and organizational performance indicators. In: Kazandijan WA, ed. *The epidemiology of quality*. Gaithersburg, MD: Aspen Publishers; 1995:123–143.
25. Enthoven AC, Vorhaus CB. A vision of quality in health care delivery. *Health Aff*. 1997;16(3):44–57.
26. Nelson EC, Mohr JJ, Batalden PB, et al. Improving health care: Part 1. The clinical value compass. *J Qual Improv*. 1996;22(4).
27. Gooding T. Harborview Medical Center. *The compass*. October Edition. Seattle, WA; 2000.
28. Englebardt SP, Nelson R, eds. Health care informatics: An interdisciplinary approach. *Technology and Distributed Education*. St. Louis, MO: Mosby; 2002.
29. iTHealthTrack, Inc. Available at: www.ithealthtrack.org. Accessed 2005.
30. Uniform Data System for Medical Rehabilitation (UDS M®). Available at: www.udsmr.org. Accessed 2005.
31. National Research Corporation (NRC). Available at:www.nationalresearch.com. Accessed 2005.
32. Press-Ganey. Available at: www.pressganey.com. Accessed 2005.
33. Commission on Accreditation of Rehabilitation Facilities (CARF) *Standards manual*. Tucson, AZ: CARF; 2003.
34. Joint Commission on Accreditation of Healthcare Organizations (JCAHO). Available at: www.jcaho.org. Accessed 2005.
35. Washington State Department of Health. Available at: www.doh.wa.gov. Accessed 2005.

15

Special Consideration for Pediatric Patients with Disability Due to Trauma

Teresa Massagli and Joyce M. Engel

Injuries are the most significant cause of morbidity in children after infancy. National Health Interview Survey data show that each year 25% of children in the United States experience a nonfatal injury that requires medical attention or limits the child's activity (1). The nonfatal injury rate for children 0 to 4 years old is 20 per 100,000 and increases with age to 31 per 100,000 in children 15 to 19 years old. Nonfatal injuries are more common in families with lower income and in nonmetropolitan areas. Injuries more commonly occur in the home in younger children, and on roads, in schools, and in industrial centers in teenagers (1).

The National Pediatric Trauma Registry has collected data from 55 pediatric trauma centers in the United States and Canada and provides some information on the types of injuries that lead to disability in children, though it does not include burns (2). For children with residual disability, the mechanism of injury is more often blunt trauma (84%) and unintentional (93%) than a penetrating injury (13%) or intentional (6%). Fall from a height, pedestrian versus vehicle, motor vehicle crash, bicycle crash, gunshot wound, motorcycle crash, and stab wound are the most common injury mechanisms in children that lead to disability (3). Rates of disability at 6 months postinjury vary from 7% to 54% of injured children treated in trauma centers, with head, spine, and extremity injuries being the most common causes of disability (4–6).

INTERVENTIONS IN THE ACUTE CARE SETTING

Children with significant injuries are ideally admitted to regional pediatric trauma centers, or to Level 1 or Level 2 adult trauma centers. In the trauma setting, it is critical to include rehabilitation early on to identify appropriate preventive measures, and to plan for following treatment in an intensive care unit (ICU) or postacute care. In the ICU, the rehabilitation team can instruct family members on appropriate interaction with the child and preventative care measures, such as passive range of motion (PROM) therapy and can begin discussions about the postacute care the child may need. When interviewing or counseling parents, one needs to be sensitive to the parents' readiness to receive information about the child's injury, prognosis, or anticipated treatments or disposition.

When assessing a child in the acute care setting, there are a number of positioning and skin issues to consider. Children in traction or wearing cervical collars are prone to development of pressure ulcers over the occiput, which can be difficult to visualize beneath the hair. For children with a prolonged ICU course, or in whom paresis, paralysis, or spasticity is present, early intervention with passive range of motion should be implemented to prevent later muscle shortening or joint contractures. If spasticity is severe or if decorticate or decerebrate rigidity is present, serial casting may be necessary to prevent plantar flexion or elbow flexion contractures (7). Before embarking on a casting protocol, the ICU team needs to verify that the extremity is not needed for arterial or venous access, and emergency plans should be in place to remove the cast at any time should questions of skin integrity or need to access the limb occur.

Once the acutely injured child is stabilized, planning needs to be started for disposition after acute care. Physiatrists are important members of the discharge planning team in the trauma setting. Physiatrists will determine if the child will need further rehabilitative care and if so, in what setting. If the child has simple lower-extremity fractures, the child may learn to ambulate with an assistive device in the trauma hospital and be discharged directly to home, with planning for return to school, such as transportation, pain medication use at school, and early dismissal from classes to avoid moving through crowded hallways. At the other end of the spectrum is the child with a devastating brain injury who remains unresponsive but no longer requires acute care. The disposition of such a child is always challenging, whether discharged to a skilled nursing facility or to home after extensive family training. Plans should be made for ongoing rehabilitation follow-up to monitor equipment needs, range of motion (ROM), nutrition, skin, and neurologic change. Family training can sometimes be a justification for admission to rehabilitation even if the child would not otherwise meet criteria for inpatient rehabilitation, as might happen in infants, children who are unresponsive, or children with multiple extremity fractures. In such cases, the rehabilitation team is ideally suited to train the family in managing transfers, wheelchair use, hygiene, toileting, dressing, use of gastrostomy tubes, splinting, and passive range of motion, and to identify resources for ongoing therapies, in-home care, and education.

Children and young teens who require inpatient rehabilitation should go to a specialized pediatric rehabilitation program whenever possible. Special expertise of pediatric team members and the pediatric milieu can be recognized by accrediting agencies such as the Commission on Accreditation of Rehabilitation Facilities (CARF). Children >15 years of age often go to adult rehabilitation programs, but if a pediatric rehabilitation program is available, it may be beneficial for the older teen who is still in high school to go to the pediatric program. Such programs often have hospital-based teachers who can help to assess for educational needs, provide ongoing tutorial support during the hospitalization, and recommend or help negotiate support from the school when the child returns. The parents of an older teen may benefit from touring both pediatric and adult facilities to help decide the placement of their child.

THE PEDIATRIC REHABILITATION ASSESSMENT

The general components of a rehabilitation assessment of a child are the same as for an adult but require some modifications depending on age. When considering a patient's medical history, the birth history and early developmental milestones are important, especially for infants and young children. The social history for school age children should assess educational performance. It is not always helpful to ask about a child's grades because of wide variations in standards. Instead, one should inquire about performance on standardized tests, learning difficulties, special education, or behavioral concerns. In teenagers, the history should include inquiries about risk-taking behavior and drug and alcohol use.

The neurologic exam and assessment of mental status may need to be adjusted for young children. Examination of passive range of motion, spasticity, deep tendon reflexes, and some cranial nerves require little modification. Infants will normally track a bright light or object (red is a good color) to midline by 1 month of age and by 3 months will track a full arc. From birth to about 3 months of age, infants may have limitations in elbow extension and hip extension and tight popliteal angles, due to fetal positioning. Manual muscle testing and the sensory exam are rarely reliable in children <4 to 5 years old. In young children, much of the exam is by observation of the child in supine, prone, sitting, and standing positions to look for symmetry of movement, weight support, synergistic patterns, balance, and gait. Assessment of coordination is also difficult in young children and is best done by observation. However, by 4 to 5 years of age, the child should normally be able to perform rapid alternating movements, and by the age of 5 should be able to walk in a tandem gait. The sensory exam in infants and toddlers may be limited to observing response to pinprick, such as grimacing or withdrawal of the limb. Cortical sensory function (stereognosis, 2-point discrimination) can be done as for adults in children >5 to 6 years of age. If the child does not know numbers, graphesthesia can be assessed by drawing a simple shape such as a square (8). Knowledge of development is useful when assessing function (9–11), and some key milestones that are practical to observe during a physiatric assessment are shown in Table 15-1.

Table 15-1	Selected Motor and Language Milestones in Early Childhood (9–11)	

Age in Mo	Milestones
3	Rolls prone to supine
	Follows visually past midline through 180 degree arc
6	Sits unsupported
	Transfers objects between hands
9	Cruising
	Finger feeding
	Looks for toys dropped over edge
	Uses *mama* and *dada*
	Understands *no*
12	Walks without support
	Uses 1–2 words
15	Walks with foot flat contact
	Speaks 4–6 words; understands simple commands
	Scribbles in imitation
18	Walks with heel strike; walks backwards
	Recognizes 8 body parts
	Scribbles spontaneously
21	Uses 50 words
24	Runs
	Walks up and down stairs alone
	Able to walk on toes
	Hand dominance established
	Uses spoon well
	Starting toilet training
	Uses 2-word phrases
30	Makes horizontal and vertical strokes with pencil
36	Pedals tricycle
	Walks up stairs with alternating feet
	Able to stand on one leg
	Copies circle
	Names 1 color; knows 250 words; uses 3-word sentences; gives age, sex, name
	Toilet trained day and night
48	Walks down stairs with alternating feet
	Able to walk on heels
	Dresses and undresses with supervision; buttoning
	Asks questions; can describe recent experiences
	Draws square
60	Skips
	Can walk on tiptoes
	Balances 10 s on each foot
	Able to hop on one leg
	Draws person with head, body, and limbs
	Knows address; follows 3-step commands

PAIN ASSESSMENT

Because of concerns that pain is often underrecognized, hospital-accrediting organizations have begun placing increased emphasis on pain assessment in hospitalized patients in recent years. The Joint Commission on Accreditation of Hospitals Organization (JCAHO), for example, considers pain measures the "fifth vital sign."

Children with traumatic injuries often undergo multiple painful surgical, medical, and rehabilitative procedures. Untreated pain can leave the child at risk for reduced activity level and participation, resultant physical decline, and emotional and social difficulties, over and above the other effects of trauma. Trauma-related pain can contribute to reduced quality of life for the child and family (12). Untreated pain may also exacerbate injury, prevent wound healing, lead to infection, prolong hospitalization, and even contribute to mortality (13). The assistive devices for mobility (e.g., wheelchairs, crutches, prosthetics) required by many survivors of trauma are also associated with increased risk of chronic pain (e.g., shoulder pain from repetitive stress, back pain caused by changes in gait patterns). Moreover, data suggest childhood pain is a determinant of later pain responses and chronic pain in general (14).

The International Association for the Study of Pain defines pain as an unpleasant sensory and emotional experience associated with actual or potential tissue damage or described in terms of such damage (15). Differentiating acute from chronic pain is essential for using the appropriate evaluation and intervention strategies. Acute pain and its associated physiologic, psychological, and behavioral responses are almost invariably caused by tissue damage or irritating stimulation in relation to bodily insult (e.g., burn, fracture). In acute pain, the intensity of pain typically decreases over a period of days to weeks (13). When pain from an injury persists beyond the anticipated healing time, it is classified as chronic (16). Chronic pain does not appear to serve a biologic purpose and is often experienced in the presence of minimal or no apparent tissue damage. Chronic pain exists without a known time limit.

Pain appears to be a serious problem after trauma for many pediatric rehabilitation patients. Children with traumatic brain injury (TBI) may experience pain from headaches and from associated musculoskeletal injuries (17). Children can develop headaches after TBI from trauma to the head itself or from tension headaches. They may also experience head and neck pain from whiplash injuries or migraines triggered by the head trauma.

Pain is reported to be a significant problem for most youths that sustain a spinal cord injury (SCI) (18,19). SCI-related pain may result from spinal deformities, postural instability, long bone fractures, hip dislocation, pressure sores, urinary tract infections, and spasticity (20–22). Neuropathic or deafferentation pain can also result from the neurologic injury. Aggressive treatment for pain in children with SCI is warranted because, in adults, SCI-related pain is particularly refractory to treatment (23).

Children aged 5 to 19 years with acquired amputation experience phantom limb and residual limb pain as frequently as adults with amputation (24–26). Other areas of pain (e.g., headache) are also common in this population (26).

Burn injury is believed to be one of the most painful of all conditions, regardless of age. Acute pain at the site of the burn injury occurs immediately. Additionally, there is a rapid neuronal up-regulation at multiple levels of the sensory pathway that may exacerbate the acute pain and increase risk of the development of chronic pain. The amount of acute local pain in burns is a function of the wound's depth. Pain may also occur with healing due to nerve regeneration and tissue reinnervation. Pain may arise not only in the burned area but also at donor sites harvested for skin closure (27). The pain from nursing or rehabilitative procedures (e.g., dressing changes, splinting) may exacerbate existing pain caused by the initial burn injury or subsequent surgeries (28), and special care needs to be taken to both prevent and control these exacerbations.

Successful pain interventions are predicated on accurate evaluation of pain (29). If pain is assessed in a manner similar to that for assessing vital signs, more effective treatment may result (30). Adequate pain evaluation allows the clinician to assess pain characteristics, to decide whether or not intervention is needed, and to determine its effectiveness (31). Interview of the child or parent, observation of possible pain behaviors, and measurement of physiologic responses may all help to identify and quantify pain in children (Table 15-2).

Table 15-2 Assessment of Pain and Pain Behaviors in Children

Covert	Overt	Physiological
(Child/Parent Report or Interview)		
• Occurrence of episode • Location (e.g., body outline) • Frequency • Duration • Exacerbating/relieving factors • Quality (e.g., burning) • Severity: visual analogue scale or graphic rating scale • Numerical rating scale • Picture scales (e.g., Oucher) • Faces rating scales (e.g., Faces Pain Scale) • Verbal rating scale (e.g., "none" to "very severe")	• Facial expressions (e.g., grimacing) • Crying • Postural guarding • Antalgic gait or rest position • Body movements • Torso rigidity or arching • Legs rigidly extended or legs drawn to chest • Squirming/kicking • Touching or holding painful body part(s) • Social withdrawal/lack of interest in surroundings	• Increased heart rate • Mixed evidence of increased/decreased respiratory rate • Increased blood pressure • Decreased vagal tone • Increased cortisol/cortisone levels • Mixed evidence of increased/decreased oxygen saturation • Increased skin blood flow • Increased palmar sweating

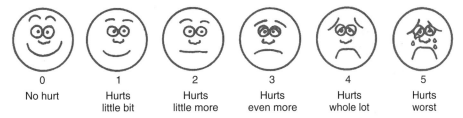

Figure 15–1. Wong-Baker Faces Scale. The Faces Scale is recommended for use in children 3 years or older. The assessor points to each face, using the words to describe the pain intensity. The child selects the face that best describes his or her pain intensity and the number of the face is recorded by the assessor. (From Wong DL, Hockenberry-Eaton M, Wilson D, et al. *Wong's essentials of pediatric nursing.* 6th ed. St. Louis, MO: Mosby, Inc.; 2001:1301, with permission.)

However pediatric pain is measured, the youth's level of cognitive development must be considered. Children as young as 4 years old can provide reliable self-reports of pain occurrence, location, and intensity. Self-report (covert behavior), the gold standard for pain assessment, could include verbal, gestural, numeric, pictorial, tactile, mechanical, or electronic modes of communication (31). Numerous standardized self-report measures like the poker-chip tool (32), the Wong-Baker Faces Pain Scale (33) (Fig. 15–1), the Oucher Scale (34) (Fig. 15–2), and a visual analog scale have been used successfully for the child that is 4 to 8 years old to describe his or her pain intensity. Use of the child's own language will facilitate ongoing communication. A child's distractibility and lack of familiarity with health care providers can affect self-reports. Older children (10 years or older) can often record numerical pain intensity ratings along with other relevant information (e.g., activity level) in a pain diary. Worry about the significance of pain in terms of disability and disfigurement may influence pain reports in the adolescent (31).

Parents can also provide valuable information about their child's pain. Parents of young children are often able to observe and describe components of their child's pain experience that the child may not be aware of or that he or she may be unable to articulate. In older children and adolescents, the congruence between the child's self-reports and the parents' can be compared and any discrepancies explored. Dahlquist (35) recommends the clinician ask the parents to provide information about the current pain episode and to obtain as much information as possible about this episode, then discuss previous pain experiences. Basic questions to ask the parent include, When does the child have pain? Where is the pain? Under what conditions does the pain occur? What is the quality (e.g., cramping), intensity, frequency, and duration of the pain? How does the pain affect the child? What exacerbates the pain? Does anything help relieve the pain (35)?

Overt motor behavior or observable pain responses (e.g., postural guarding, antalgic gait) are commonly used as indicators of pain. Distress behaviors (e.g., crying, grimacing, arching) can also serve as proxy measures of pain magnitude and are often used in evaluating pain in youth, especially those with limited communication skills (36). The assessment of overt pain behaviors in youth, however, may be problematic. Distress behaviors could be expressed in response to anxiety, fatigue, frustration, or hunger instead of pain. In addition, the child's medication intake may be minimized by the fear of needles that may be more aversive than the pain itself (37). Finally, the youth's activity level may not be an accurate indicator of pain, since many children experiencing mild-to-moderate-intensity or chronic pain will still engage in play or leisure activities (38).

Physiological pain responses are the third major category used in the assessment of pain. Potential indicators of pain include changes in heart rate, respiratory rate, blood pressure, cortisol and cortisone levels, oxygen saturation, vagal tone, endorphin levels, and palmar sweating. Changes in these physiologic measures are sometimes used to make indirect inferences about pain (36). Similar to overt pain behaviors, hyperactivity of the sympathetic nervous system can occur in response to other forms of stress to the body besides pain. Biologic measures of presumed pain such as heart rate, respiratory rate, and blood pressure may be most helpful in infants experiencing short, sharp pain (31).

Cultural, spiritual, and familial influences are other important factors to be considered in pediatric pain assessment and treatment, especially when the pain etiology is unclear (39). These influences may include the child's and parents' beliefs about the causes and implications of pain, use of pain remedies, acceptability of various types of pain interventions (e.g., acupuncture, hypnosis), and the quality of the child–parent–health care provider interactions (40).

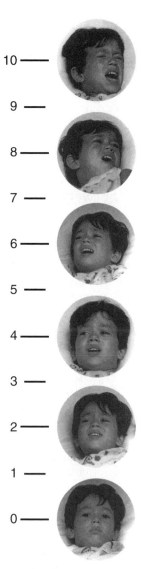

Figure 15–2. Oucher Scale. The Oucher Scale is appropriate for children aged 3 to 12 years old. The scale has six pictures of a 4-year-old boy expressing a range of pain severity from no pain to the worst unbearable pain. Pictures of white, African-American, and Hispanic children are available. The pictures are arranged alongside a scale numbered from 0 ("no hurt") to 10 ("biggest hurt you could ever have"). The child points to the picture that best describes his or her current pain. The assessor records the associated number. Children who can count to ten can use the numeric scale directly. (From Beyer J. The Oucher: A user's manual and technical report. Denver, CO: University of Colorado Health Sciences Center; 1988, with permission.)

PAIN MANAGEMENT

Pain management is considered a basic human right, regardless of age (13). Since health care providers often fail to assess and measure pain routinely, especially in youth (41), pain may be undertreated. The reasons for undertreatment of pain include the low priority of providing pain relief in the health care system, lack of knowledge of pain interventions among health professionals and consumers, and fear of opioid addiction (42). In addition, children and their parents may deny or underreport pain because they are unable to assess it, are fearful of the pain interventions, or want to avoid further hospitalization (13).

The choice of pain intervention depends upon objective findings, type of pain, pain characteristics, pain behaviors, the child's stage in development, his or her energy level and interests, practicality, time constraints, and costs, in addition to the parents' and child's wishes (43). Pain interventions must also accommodate medical challenges the rehabilitation patient may have and the child's natural environments (home, school). Parents and youth should be involved in treatment planning to the maximum extent that is feasible. The child and family members need information about treatment options and what to expect from treatment. They should be presented with a rationale for treatment and be informed of any possible discomfort associated with treatment. Information on what the child might experience may reduce anxiety, and, consequently, discomfort. In the young child, dolls or drawings can be used to explain treatment procedures, answer questions, and express feelings. Engaging the child in decision making can promote cooperation as well as lessen discomfort by increasing the child's sense of control (41,44). Among adolescents, the long-term health benefits of rehabilitation procedures can be emphasized. Participation of the child and parents in goal setting often promotes understanding of interventions and compliance.

Pain control is typically achieved through a combination of pharmacologic and nonpharmacologic approaches. The World Health Organization (WHO) analgesic ladder is well established in adult pain management as a stepwise approach for choosing an analgesic and is believed appropriate for youth (45). Scheduled use of medications or other nonpharmacologic interventions such as hypnosis or virtual reality before therapies or procedures is often helpful (46,47). A detailed review of pharmacologic interventions is beyond the scope of this chapter.

Pain management from birth through 2 years of age emphasizes pharmacologic interventions and environmental adaptations. The child may be comforted with swaddling, neutral warmth, environmental consistency, low lighting, and contact with familiar objects (e.g., toys, blanket) or persons. Often the presence of parents during rehabilitative procedures is recommended as a means to establishing a therapeutic atmosphere of trust among the child, parent, and health care provider (44,48). Parents may also serve as coaches and distracters and not necessarily as restrainers during medical and rehabilitative procedures (49).

Resting and splinting are often sufficient for reducing pain from minor injuries (50). If needed, physical agent modalities may also be used for pain reduction. Transcutaneous nerve stimulation (TENS) is a method of afferent stimulation designed to control pain by passing electricity through electrodes placed on the skin. Clinical indications for TENS include low back pain, inflammatory disorders of soft tissues, and postoperative pain (51). TENS has been used successfully in children with intact cognition as young as age 8. TENS can be used in a variety of settings and during routine activities. Written instructions, including illustrations of proper electrode placement, should be given to the child and family (52).

Massage is an almost instinctual approach to pain relief through rubbing or kneading of a body part. The regulation of muscle tone through reflex and mechanical action can induce muscle relaxation and sedation. Massage can enhance muscle flexibility, promote the loosening of scar tissue, provide analgesia, and increase feelings of well-being. Clinical indications for massage include musculoskeletal complaints of discomfort or pain. Such complaints include discomfort or pain secondary to an injury or from other trauma, such as postsurgery pain. Massage may also be used to prepare patients for exercise and to improve their functional performance by reducing edema and increasing range of motion.

Pain relief and improved functional performance may also be achieved through the use of heat (e.g., hydrocollator packs, heating pad, ultrasound, fluidotherapy, chemical pack). Mild heat can induce muscle relaxation and sedate sensory nerve endings. Heat is indicated for subacute and chronic traumatic and inflammatory conditions (e.g., muscle spasms). Acute inflammatory conditions may be aggravated by heat and active bleeding prolonged. Heat treatments are not recommended for youth younger than 4 years of age, owing to their unreliable thermoregulatory systems, which could produce fever or burns. Ultrasound is a deep-heating modality to treat deeper structures. Ultrasound is indicated for swelling, scar tissue, and adhesions (53). Ultrasound is contraindicated over areas of thrombophlebitis and epiphyses of growing bone and over the spinal cord in cases of laminectomy that reduce protection of the spinal cord (54).

The application of cold (e.g., ice packs, cold immersion baths or whirlpools, vapocoolant sprays) can reduce muscle spasm and exercise-induced muscle soreness and has been associated with quicker return to activity.

Therapeutic exercise programs can improve movement, increase range of motion, strengthen muscles, increase endurance, correct posture and gait abnormalities, improve circulation, and enhance bone density that may subsequently reduce discomfort and increase participation. A progressive quota-based exercise program can facilitate goal attainment. Treatment times should be coordinated with pain medication administration so as to reduce any discomfort associated with exercise or functional activities (52). Exercise may also provide pain relief through the production of endorphins (55).

Thermal biofeedback consists of measuring surface skin temperature so the child can learn to increase peripheral body temperature, a presumed indicator of reduced sympathetic nervous system activity and hence of generalized relaxation. Electromyographic (EMG) biofeedback of facial and neck muscle activity allows the child to learn how to relax muscles that might induce headache (56). Biofeedback is typically used in conjunction with relaxation training (52). Relaxation techniques include abdominal breathing (57), progressive muscle relaxation (58), autogenics (59), guided imagery (60), and Benson's relaxation response (61). There is evidence to support the use of relaxation in relieving headaches (62) and procedure-related pain (63). Distraction techniques (e.g., listening to favorite stories or music, television watching, art, play) have also demonstrated efficacy in relieving pain associated with medical procedures (13).

Hypnotherapy can be used to alter the child's perception of pain by providing suggestions for analgesia or amnesia (64). Virtual reality and hypnosis have been helpful in the reduction of narcotics and pain intensity in youths with burn pain (46,47,65).

TRAUMATIC BRAIN INJURY

In 1995, the incidence of TBI resulting in hospitalization of children 0 to 4 and 5 to 14 years old was estimated to be 75 to 105 per 100,000 per year, with most of these hospitalizations for moderate and severe injuries (66). The etiology of TBI in children varies with age. Infants and toddlers are more likely to be injured from falls or child abuse. Child abuse may involve repeated injuries, delays in accessing health care, and anoxia, which compounds the initial brain injury. Young children are frequently injured as pedestrians or in bike crashes. Adolescents are more likely to be injured as motor vehicle occupants and in sports activities (67).

Children experience diffuse axonal injury more often than focal injuries, in part because of the relatively large size of the head and relatively weaker neck musculature than in adults, with less restraint of motion. Children also tend to have a higher frequency of epidural hematomas and fewer subdural hematomas, possibly due to greater flexibility of the immature skull and lack of dural adhesions (68). Children <3 years old who experience a linear skull fracture should be monitored for the development of a growing skull fracture and leptomeningeal cyst. This is a very rare complication and occurs most commonly when the fracture is diastatic, with separation of the edges of >3 mm. The fracture "grows" as a result of a tear in the dura, which allows pulsation of the cerebrospinal fluid, or herniation of the meninges into the fracture. The resulting pressure causes remodeling of the bone over months to years and results in a skull defect that usually requires surgical repair (69). Clinicians should palpate the area of known skull fractures in young children to monitor for this rare complication.

The risk of late posttraumatic seizures (after the first week) is related to brain injury severity. In children, only those with severe injuries appear to have a risk above baseline, with about 7.5% of children developing late seizures. While children have a lower incidence of late seizures than do adults, they have a higher incidence of immediate or impact seizures and early seizures. Early seizures (in the first week) occur in 30% of children with severe injuries but in only 10% of adults with severe injuries. However, neither immediate nor early seizures are predictive of late seizures in children (70).

In the ICU setting, children are likely to have an indwelling bladder catheter for careful monitoring of fluid status. Once the child no longer requires ICU care, the indwelling catheter should be discontinued and the child placed in diapers until he or she is alert enough to begin voiding trials. After severe TBI, it is common for children to have a disinhibited spastic bladder, with frequent small-volume voiding. Postvoid residual urine volumes are not often encountered, except when children are on high doses of narcotic pain medications. When the child becomes more alert, frequent void trials during the day should be employed but diapers (or condom catheters for teenage males) may be needed at night for some time. Discontinuing fluid intake after dinner and awakening the child during the night to void are frequently employed but may have limited success, as voiding can be triggered with only a small amount of urine present in the bladder. In this phase of recovery, it may be more therapeutic for children to have uninterrupted sleep than to attempt to achieve nighttime continence by waking them.

Children with mild TBI do not appear to have significant neurobehavioral sequelae at 1 year after injury. Using a subsample of the 1970 birth cohort, Bijur found that children with mild TBI 1 to 5 years prior to assessment were indistinguishable from uninjured children on measures of cognition, achievement, and behavior with the exception of teacher ratings of hyperactivity (71). Because of the timing of follow-up, this study may have missed early sequelae that later resolved. A more recent prospective cohort study of children with mild TBI found an increased risk of psychiatric illness, particularly hyperactivity, during the first year after TBI in children who had no prior psychiatric history. Prior psychiatric illness conferred a significant independent risk for psychiatric illness after mild TBI (72). While mild TBI and concussion do not appear to cause long-term problems, they may cause temporary symptoms of fatigue, irritability, emotional lability, sleep disturbance, headache, and reduced attention and short-term memory. If a child with mild or moderate TBI has any neurologic or behavioral signs or symptoms such as balance impairment, short-term memory impairment, slow response speed, or excessive sleepiness at the time of discharge from the trauma hospital to home, we recommend follow-up in 3 to 4 weeks with brief language and cognitive assessments and a neurologic and mental status exam. In most children, symptoms resolve by then, but we have found that up to one third of children with moderate TBI still have ongoing concerns that may influence school performance (73). Babies and toddlers with mild TBI present a special challenge because the examination and screening measures are limited. Tools such as the Bayley Scales of Infant Development or the Peabody Developmental Motor Scales, administered by specially trained occupational or physical therapists, can be used to assess gross motor (Peabody and Bayley) and cognitive (Bayley) skills (74,75). They can be administered initially to establish a baseline and repeated after a period of time, such as 6 months, to see if the child has continued to develop new skills at an appropriate rate.

A variety of early measures can offer prognostic information for children who suffer moderate to severe TBI. The admission Glasgow Coma Score (GCS), the GCS over time, the duration of time until the child reliably follows commands, and the duration of posttraumatic amnesia (PTA) are useful indicators of prognosis after severe TBI in children. In a case control study of children with TBI, children with an initial GCS of 3 to 8 scored 1.1 standard deviations below controls on neurobehavioral measures 1 year after injury. Those in the most severe group, with an initial GCS of 3 to 5, performed from

2 to 4 standard deviations below controls on testing 1 year after TBI (76). Another study of consecutive admissions of children with an initial GCS of 3 to 8 found that only 27% had good recovery on the Glasgow Outcome Scale at 5 to 7 years after injury. Nearly 70% were receiving some special education services at school. If the GCS remained 8 or less at 24 or 72 hours, the numbers achieving good recovery dropped to 14% and 8%, respectively (77).

In a study of 344 children with a median duration of coma of 5 to 6 weeks, Brink found that at 1 year after injury, 73% of the children were independent in activities of daily living (ADL) and mobility, but only 28% scored within 1 standard deviation of 100 on intellectual quotient testing, and 46% had significant behavior problems. Children had persistent cognitive deficits if coma lasted longer than 1.7 weeks. For those children with coma of up to 6 weeks' duration, 94% were independent in ADL and mobility at 1 year after injury. If coma lasted more than 12 weeks, only 38% were independent (78,79).

The Children's Orientation and Amnesia Test was developed as a way to assess posttraumatic amnesia in children with TBI. Duration of PTA has been found to correlate with outcome. In children with PTA lasting <1 week, 67% had good recovery at 1 year. With PTA lasting 8 to 14 days, 43% had good recovery, and with PTA of >14 days, only 11% had good recovery as measured by the Glasgow Outcome Scale (80).

Children with moderate and severe TBI who are admitted to inpatient rehabilitation programs should have comprehensive neuropsychological, educational, and language testing done prior to discharge to assist with school planning. It is better for the rehabilitation program than for the school district to do this for several reasons. The testing typically done by school districts to evaluate children for special education may not be sensitive to the deficits seen after TBI. It can take the school several weeks to pull together a team to do the assessment, thus delaying the child's return to school. Finally, the rehabilitation team has the expertise in deficits after TBI to interpret the results for the school. School personnel may not have had much exposure to children with TBI, whose deficits change and tend to improve over time in contrast to children with static disabilities. While the rehabilitation team can identify the deficits and suggest strategies to manage them, it is up to the school to determine what resources they have and how they will use them for the child. For instance, in a medical rehabilitation setting, a speech therapist may work on reading skills, but in the school, a special education teacher may take on this task. While special services such as physical therapy (PT), occupational therapy (OT),

and speech can be provided at school, the amount of therapy time is limited, and some children may need both outpatient clinic-based therapies as well as school-based therapies. It is very important for the two groups to work together to maximize the child's function at school.

Family members need support and education during rehabilitation. It is helpful to provide written information about brain injury, typical deficits, the time course of improvement, and the special education system (81). Few school districts have significant exposure to children with TBI, so preparation of the parent for expectations about school reintegration and education of the school team about disabilities and accommodations are key components of discharge planning.

SPINAL CORD INJURY

Traumatic spinal cord injury is uncommon in children <16 years old. This age group accounts for only 4.5% of new cases of SCI in the United States each year. Motor vehicle crashes are the leading cause of SCI throughout childhood. Young children may be injured when unrestrained or by inappropriate placement of vehicle restraints. Lap belts worn above the pelvis can result in lumbar SCI through flexion-distraction injuries (Chance fractures). Shoulder harnesses crossing too high across the neck can cause odontoid fractures. Violence-related and sports-related injuries tend to occur more often in older children and adolescents (82). Birth trauma can produce cervicothoracic SCI with breech presentations, or upper cervical SCI in forceps or manual rotation deliveries. Developmental abnormalities of the cervical spine can place the spinal cord at increased risk of injury. Such abnormalities include instability of the atlantoaxial joint, as seen in Down syndrome, juvenile rheumatoid arthritis or os odontoideum; and dysplasia of the base of the skull, as seen in achondroplasia.

From birth to 3 years old, males and females are affected by SCI with equal frequency, but beyond the age of 3, such injuries occur predominantly in males. The male-to-female ratio becomes 60:40 in children 4 to 8, 70:30 in children 9 to 15, and 85:15 in teenagers 16 to 20 years old (83). Children with SCIs who are younger than 8 years old are more likely to have paraplegia (70%) than tetraplegia (30%), but in the 9- to 15-year-old age group, 53% have tetraplegia and 47% have paraplegia (83). The cervical spine and ligaments of children under 8 to 10 years of age are not as stable as in older children and adults. This difference in younger children is due to greater elasticity of their ligaments, a more horizontal orientation of their facet joints, incomplete ossification of vertebrae with relative anterior wedging, and the relatively large size of the head compared to the strength of their cervical muscles (84). As a result, few cervical injuries are incomplete in this age group, and injury is more likely at C1 to C3 than at lower levels as for adults (83). The greater mobility of the spinal column may also produce SCI without any findings on radiographs or computed tomography (CT) scans, a phenomenon referred to as "SCIWORA" (spinal cord injury without radiographic abnormality) (85). Only about 65% of these cases will have abnormalities on magnetic resonance imaging (MRI) (86). SCIWORA occurs in 60% of children <10 but in only 20% of older children with more mature spinal columns. Most cases of SCIWORA result in complete SCI.

Children with SCI are at risk for a host of medical and musculoskeletal complications. Autonomic dysreflexia can be difficult to diagnose in children for two reasons. First, infants and young children may not complain of any symptoms, and second, there is no clear blood pressure that signifies dysreflexia. Practice guidelines recommend using a blood pressure elevation of 20 to 40 mm Hg over baseline as a possible sign of dysreflexia (87). Initial management is as for adults, but if refractory to physical measures, nifedipine may be administered at a dosage of 0.25 mg/kg/dose, or 10 mg for children >40 kg. Spasticity is reported to occur less commonly in children with SCI compared to adults (88). If spasticity is bothersome and unresponsive to typical conservative measures, baclofen may be initiated at 0.125 mg/kg/dose (up to 5 mg) two to three times a day and increased periodically to a maximum of 1 to 2 mg/kg/day or 80 mg in children aged 12 years and older (89). Latex allergy was first described as a complication in children with myelomeningocele but has been reported in children with SCI (90). In the absence of known prior latex allergy, it is reasonable to use regular sterile catheters during the acute hospitalization but then switch to latex-free catheters when beginning clean intermittent catheterization (CIC). Immobilization hypercalcemia is a complication seen more often in children than adults. Especially at risk are males, adolescents, and those with higher levels of SCI. It can present with vague symptoms that mimic infection or depression, so a high index of suspicion is necessary when children present with fatigue, constipation, anorexia, nausea, vomiting, or apathy during the first several months after SCI. Diagnosis is made by obtaining an ionized calcium level, or total serum calcium corrected for albumin. Treatment with intravenous saline and intravenous pamidronate can result in prompt resolution of symptoms (91). The incidence of deep venous thrombosis (DVT) has been reported to be 13% in children younger than 15 years old in Model SCI Systems data, but the numbers of children included were small (92). Children should have similar prophylactic measures as adults, unless they are too small to wear compression hose. Low–molecular weight heparin can be administered at a dose of 0.5 mg per kg subcutaneously twice a day for children >2 months of age, and 0.75 mg per kg twice daily in those younger than 2 months (89).

Musculoskeletal complications typically develop over time and should be monitored at outpatient follow-up visits. Heterotopic ossification is reported to affect only about 3% of children with SCI (93). Both indomethacin and etidronate have been used to treat heterotopic ossification in children, but etidronate has caused rickets when used in children (94). Virtually all children with SCI prior to puberty develop scoliosis, and about two thirds require surgery. When SCI occurs after skeletal maturity, only 20% develop scoliosis and only 5% require surgery (95). The use of orthoses is controversial because the potential benefit of slowing progression of the curve must be weighed against the interference with wheelchair mobility and self-care. However, it is desirable to delay posterior spine fusion as long as possible, because the fusion arrests spine growth and can limit the ultimate growth of chest height if done in early childhood. Spine fusion can also change the child's trunk mobility and ability to do self-care such as a bowel program or catheterization. Hip instability is common after SCI, especially in those injured prior to the age of 5 years. A dislocated hip may affect sitting posture or require accommodation in the wheelchair seat. Young children with tetraplegia should have close follow-up of finger range of motion. They can develop severe extension contractures of the metacarpal phalangeal joints of digits 2 through 5, which are nearly impossible to treat with splints once they develop. The consequence is that the child with functional wrist extension will not be able to use a tenodesis grasp.

In children with SCI, expectations for functional outcome are influenced by more than just the child's level and completeness of SCI. A child's ability to be independent is also influenced by age and level of cognitive development, the power of "normal" strength muscles, the relative length of arms to trunk height, the presence of a spinal orthosis, and the family's expectations for the child. It can be difficult to even determine the motor and sensory level of SCI in infants. Repeated observations may be needed to distinguish reflex movements from voluntary control. Manual muscle testing is not generally reliable in children <5 years of age (8,96).

It is difficult to train children <3 to 4 years of age with tetraplegia or high paraplegia to develop sitting balance, yet many age-appropriate activities for these children happen on the floor. A soft thoracolumbosacral orthosis can facilitate sitting, leaving hands free for play activities. Children <4 years old generally lack upper-body power to transfer independently and are usually lifted by the caregiver. Children can master a sliding board at 5 to 7 years of age. Young children have difficulty lifting themselves to do pressure releases and may require a tiltback by a caregiver. Infants and toddlers do not often get pressure sores, in part because of their lesser weight, frequent handling by caregivers, and the unlikelihood of remaining in wheelchairs for prolonged periods of time. Pressure relief training should be incorporated into therapies for children at the age of about 5 years, depending on upper-body strength. Children can learn more advanced wheelchair skills like wheelies to manage curbs at about 8 years of age.

Age, cognitive level, upper body strength, and the environments in which the child will spend time also influence wheelchair prescription. A stroller for passive mobility is usually all that is needed in children up to 18 to 24 months of age, but after this time it is appropriate to consider wheelchair prescription. Some children as young as 18 to 24 months can learn to use a power wheelchair but will require adult supervision. Children <6 to 8 years old with low cervical or even high thoracic injuries may not have sufficient upper-body strength to propel a manual wheelchair in the community and may need a power chair in childhood to access school campuses and playgrounds or other environments. Manual and power wheelchairs should use seating components that can be adjusted for growth to allow for at least 3 to 5 years of use. A solid seat and back are prescribed until the child is skeletally mature. At that time, teenagers with low thoracic or lumbar level SCI can change to a taut sling seat and low sling back.

Neurogenic bladder is managed with diapers until the age of about 3 years, the time when a child would usually be working on toilet training. Parents need to do catheterization at this age. Children can learn the techniques of clean intermittent catheterization (CIC) at about 5 years of age but need supervision, reminders, and assistance with cleanup for many more years. The young child's bladder capacity is very small, and it is not uncommon for them to need CIC as often as every 3 to 4 hours to stay dry. In the absence of urodynamics, bladder capacity can be estimated from a formula: bladder capacity

(ounces) = age (in years) + 2 (97). Therefore, a 2-year-old child would have an expected bladder capacity of 4 ounces or 120 cc. In children who experience SCI at a young age, the bladder may never grow to typical adult capacity. In late childhood or early adolescence, bladder augmentation may need to be considered if the child cannot stay continent with a reasonable CIC frequency. For children with C6 or C7 levels of injury who have difficulty transferring to a toilet, rearranging clothing to expose the urethra, or holding a catheter, a continent diversion procedure should be considered. The appendix or another piece of bowel is used to create a catheterizable stoma through the umbilicus to the bladder (98). The umbilical location is easier to access for self-catheterization than the perineum. This procedure can also benefit some with higher levels of SCI who are catheterized by others, sparing the need for transfer from the wheelchair to another surface.

Neurogenic bowel is also typically managed with diapers until the child is about 3 years old. Some young children may need stool softeners or glycerin suppositories if they have constipation that cannot be managed with increased fluids or dietary changes. Liquid docusate has a somewhat soapy taste that many children find unpalatable, so other medications may be tried including senna (liquid or granules) and mineral oil. Although concerns have been expressed about the use of these medications in chronic bowel programs (99,100), they appear to be unfounded. Senna was implicated in loss of myenteric plexus neurons in mice models in studies in the 1970s, but there have been no confirming human data documenting adverse effects on the myenteric plexus from use of senna in the last 30 years (101), possibly because the original formulations are no longer in use. Mineral oil was reputed to cause malabsorption of fat-soluble vitamins, but studies of long-term use of mineral oil have shown no such problems, and mineral oil is very well tolerated with few side effects (102). Training to have regular bowel movements on the toilet should begin at the age of about 3 years, and in order to produce results at a regular time, will usually require digital stimulation and/or use of a bisacodyl suppository. Children can learn their own bowel management at age 5 years if they can reach the rectum and maintain sitting balance, but few children reliably do their own bowel program until later in childhood.

Ongoing re-examination and assessment of function as the child matures are key to ensuring the best outcome. Physical abilities for transfers and wheelchair use change with age. The child may need encouragement to take responsibility for self-care. Driving, sexuality, sports participation, cardiovascular fitness, avoidance of repetitive stress injuries, and planning for postsecondary education are important issues to address with adolescents.

It is helpful for the medical rehabilitation team to involve the school in ongoing management. Teaching of some skills, such as pressure releases or transfers, can be incorporated in therapies provided at school as part of an individualized education plan. School-based physical and occupational therapists can help assess barriers in the school environment, consult with physical education teachers on adaptive activities, monitor fit of the wheelchair or orthoses, and train the child in assistive technology such as computers. Education is a strong predictor of employment after SCI, but only 51% of secondary students who sustain SCI complete high school, compared with 75% to 80% of uninjured secondary students (103). Unfortunately, employment rates for adults with pediatric-onset SCI are lower than for the general population, even for those with postsecondary education (104,105). Identified barriers to employment include medical complications, transportation issues, and loss of financial benefits. The importance of facilitating successful education and employment is highlighted by research demonstrating that education, income, recreation opportunities, and avoidance of medical complications are all related to life satisfaction in adults with pediatric-onset SCI but that level of SCI, age at SCI, and time since SCI are not related to life satisfaction (105).

TRAUMATIC AMPUTATIONS

The incidence of acquired amputation in children is unknown. Most studies reporting on epidemiology have relied on case series from prosthetic clinics, with strong selection bias. One retrospective study from a trauma center examined all children younger than 18 years of age who had traumatic amputations over a 10-year period. In this study of 74 children, power lawn mower injuries had the highest incidence (21.6%), and the average age of children with lawn mower injuries was 4.6 years. All of these patients had extensive injuries, resulting in limbs that could not be salvaged. Motor vehicle crashes (16.2%) and farm or power tools (13.5%) were the next most common, with injuries occurring in children with mean age of 11 to 12 years old. One third of patients had isolated digit amputation, and 76% of these digits were salvaged. Twenty-eight percent had upper-extremity amputation, but the limb was salvaged in only one injury proximal to the wrist. Thirty-eight percent had lower-extremity amputations with 14% of the amputated limbs salvaged (106).

Power mower injuries usually result from children riding on a mower with a parent. The injuries usually result in very contaminated and crushed wounds, precluding replantation. Partial foot amputations are the most common type of power mower injury. Amputation due to motor vehicle crashes usually result in transtibial or knee disarticulation levels of amputation in children. Farm machinery accidents often involve entanglement in equipment that is powerful and not easily stalled. Thus, amputation levels tend to be high with severe trauma to the limb. Power tools more commonly result in injury to the hands or digits. Severe burns rarely result in major amputation but often lead to loss of digits of the hands or feet (107).

Some of the special considerations for children with acquired amputations include future growth, developmental stage of the child, complications such as terminal overgrowth, and psychological adaptations. When planning the level of amputation, surgeons should attempt to preserve as much length of the residual limb as possible. Although initial prosthetic fitting may be more complicated, disarticulation is preferable to long bone resection in growing children to preserve the growth plate and avoid future problems with terminal overgrowth, but not if it results in a higher level of amputation than a transdiaphyseal amputation (108). In the upper limb, most growth occurs at the shoulder and wrist, whereas in the lower extremity, it is the epiphyses at the knee that account for most of the growth. The distal femoral epiphysis accounts for 70% of the longitudinal growth of the femur. If this epiphysis is lost in an infant or young child, the residual limb may be quite short by the time of adolescence (108,109).

Because young children may not be compliant with weight-bearing restrictions, some surgeons advocate for delayed prosthetic fitting after lower-extremity amputation. A soft dressing or cast is used for the first week, then replaced by a rigid dressing with pylon and foot. Gait training is started and gradually increased over 6 to 8 weeks (108). Following lower-extremity amputation, the child may need an assistive device for ambulation. Children as young as 12 to 15 months who were previously ambulatory can be trained to use a walker. Children can be taught to use crutches at about 8 to 9 years, or as early as 6 to 7 years if they are very coordinated. However, they may not be able to master stair use with only one crutch at this age, and they should be taught to scoot up and down stairs on their buttocks. Young children also need parental supervision at the start of crutch use for ambulation, until they are safe users.

A complication unique to amputations in skeletally immature children is terminal overgrowth. It can occur in both acquired limb loss and in congenital limb deficiency, but it does not occur after skeletal maturity or in patients with disarticulations. Terminal overgrowth most commonly occurs in the tibia, fibula, and humerus and rarely in the femur. It has not been reported in the radius or ulna (110). The cause is not clear and has been hypothesized to be due to disproportional growth of the bone versus soft tissue, contracture of the soft tissue envelope, or excessive bone remodeling during wound healing (111). Terminal overgrowth should be suspected in diaphyseal or metaphyseal amputations when the child complains of pain, warmth, and swelling at the end of the residual limb. Socket modification may help temporarily, but the condition usually requires surgical revision. It may reoccur up until the child is skeletally mature. Other complications seen in older patients, such as neuromas and painful phantom sensation, are reportedly uncommon in young children, but it must be acknowledged that children <5 years old may have difficulty reporting such symptoms (109). Painful phantom sensation has been reported in older children and adolescents (109). Physical measures such as massaging the uninvolved limb at a similar point, use of medications such as gabapentin, and use of a prosthesis in functional activities may reduce the persistence and severity of phantom pain (112,113).

The developmental stage of the child helps determine which prosthetic components to prescribe. Children are hard on prosthetic components, hence simple but durable components are best. In infants, an upper-extremity prosthesis is prescribed when the child is able to sit, and a lower-extremity prosthesis should be prescribed when the child is pulling up to standing position. If the child has a transfemoral amputation, an articulated knee is not usually prescribed until the child is 3 to 4 years old with a unilateral amputation and even later if the child has bilateral transfemoral amputations. The sockets and components need frequent modifications in growing children and may need to be adjusted several times a year. Starting with a larger socket and thicker socks at first and gradually decreasing sock thickness with growth can increase the lifespan of the socket. Other methods to prolong the use of a socket in a growing child include a slip socket, with one or more inner layers that can be peeled out of the outer socket with growth, and use of adjustable flexible inner sockets with an outer frame. The inner socket can be heat modified to accommodate changes in shape (Fig. 15–3). Suspension systems like neoprene sleeves are preferred to those that require a rigid grip over growing bony prominences. In transtibial amputees, supracondylar suprapatellar

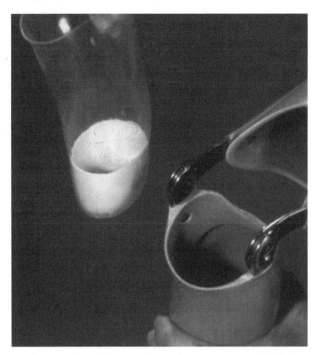

Figure 15–3. Removable, adjustable flexible socket in a laminated frame with a custom-molded distal end pad.

sockets are sometimes avoided by prosthetists because of the need for frequent modifications to accommodate the growth of the femoral condyles. Prostheses may need adjustment three to four times a year and generally require replacement every 1 to 1.5 years in young children, and every 1 to 3 years in teens (114).

There have been no long-term follow-up studies on functional outcome or prosthesis use in children with traumatic amputations. Research on psychosocial outcome of children with limb deficiency has primarily studied those with congenital limb deficiency. A comparison of teens with congenital versus acquired limb deficiency showed no difference in depressive symptoms, anxiety, or general self-esteem. The degree of limb loss was related to self-esteem but not to depressive symptoms in these teenagers (115). Family functioning, parental adjustment, and classmate social support are all important predictors of emotional and behavioral adjustment in children with congenital and acquired limb deficiencies (116).

BURNS

Burn injuries are the leading cause of accidental death in children <2 years old and the second highest cause of accidental death in children <14 years old (117). More than half of all burns occur in children <4 years old. In toddlers, burns typically occur indoors and are usually due to scalds. In older children, most burns occur outdoors, and scalds are less frequent (117).

It is estimated that 10% to 20% of pediatric burns occur as a result of nonaccidental trauma (118), but abuse or neglect can be difficult to prove. A pattern of burns on the feet, buttocks, and perineum with sparing of the back of the knees and anterior hips is suspicious for a child being placed in hot water. Abused burn victims are typically young (about 2 years of age), have an inconsistent described mechanism of injury, and may have a prior history of abuse or stigmata of abuse on exam. They remain at risk for abuse and neglect after discharge. Neglected patients who return to home after discharge have a high rate of noncompliance with ongoing rehabilitation management and clinic visits and must be monitored very closely (119).

Skin varies in thickness with age. In young children, the dermis is not fully developed and a more severe burn may occur than in an adult exposed to the same heat intensity. The American Burn Association classifies injury severity as minor in children with <10% total body surface area (TBSA) partial-thickness burns, moderate with 10% to 20% partial-thickness or 2% to 10% full-thickness, and major with >20% partial-thickness or 10% full-thickness burns (120). Burns to the face, eyes, ears, feet, and perineum are all considered major burns. The rule of nines for determining the extent of surface area burned is unreliable in children <15 years of age, because it underestimates burns to the head and neck and overestimates burns to the legs. Methods to correct for differences in the percentage of body surface area by age have been developed (121).

The majority of children who sustain burns do not require inpatient rehabilitation. However, those with >20% TBSA burns, those with burns of the face and neck, or those with circumferential-extremity burns may require intensive occupational and physical therapy of sufficient duration to warrant treatment in an inpatient rehabilitation unit. As with adult burn rehabilitation, therapy is directed at prevention of contractures, reconditioning, scar management, and psychological treatment. Children have a higher frequency than adults of contractures requiring surgical releases, especially around the hands, head, and axilla (122). Heterotopic ossification is rare in children but occurs in adolescents. The elbow is the most common site, as in adults with burns. Cases with heterotopic ossification in multiple extremities and even the ribs have been reported (123). Face masks and pressure garments can affect facial growth in children, particularly in the maxilla and mandible,

so these pressure management devices should be remeasured more frequently than for adults (124,125). Burns can have long-lasting effects on growth and development. In the first year after a burn, children may develop a profound growth arrest despite adequate nutrition that can last up to 3 years (126). Burns near an epiphysis can cause local growth delay. Scoliosis and kyphosis can occur with burns to the chest and back. Delayed development of language has been noted in young children aged 6 months to 6 years followed for 1 year after injury (127).

In preparation for discharge from the hospital, families and caregivers should receive extensive training. A care manual with written instructions and pictures of splints and exercises can be very helpful, not only for parents, but for outpatient therapists and school personnel as well. Like adult burn patients, pediatric patients should wear pressure garments at all times except during bathing until the scar matures, at 1 to 1.5 years after the burn. Children have difficulty understanding the long-term benefits of their garments, splints, or range of motion programs, so an adult who can supervise these treatments is crucial. The success of outpatient rehabilitation depends on the dedication of the parents. Depending on the extent of the burns, a parent may need to devote 2 to 4 or more hours per day to the child for bathing, wound care, stretching, application of splints and garments, and attending therapies. Prospective research has shown that early reintegration (by 4 months after discharge) to preburn activities was correlated with better health and physical functioning at follow-up as much as 14 years after injury. Those children followed in multidisciplinary clinics for at least 2 years after discharge had better physical function than those who did not follow up in clinic (128). When children are the victims of abuse or neglect, it is important to educate child protective services personnel on the intense special needs of these children, so that resources can be provided to help families comply with garment and splint use, stretching exercises, and attendance at therapies and clinic visits.

The long-term physical and psychological outcome of children with burns appears to be fairly good. In a study of children with a mean age of 7 years at the time of the burn and a mean of 88% TBSA burns, most children were independent in basic ADL at 5-year follow-up. Those who were not independent had finger amputations, joint fusions, or brain anoxia. The children had no more behavior problems than comparison groups of children without burns (129). In another study, children with 80% TBSA burns showed no differences from nonburned children on psychological assessment and were able to develop positive feelings about themselves (130). In contrast to the good outcomes reported in older children, parents of children who sustained burns at ages 2 and 3 years old reported the children to be more depressed, with somatic complaints, sleep problems, and social withdrawal (131). Such outcomes could reflect a developmental response to trauma, or because of the high incidence of abuse and neglect as causes of burns in this age group, could represent pre-existing behavior patterns. This group of younger children may need careful follow-up and treatment to avoid effects on socialization and school performance in later years.

RETURN TO SCHOOL AFTER TRAUMATIC INJURY

A major difference between adult and pediatric rehabilitation after trauma is the prominence that return to school issues must take. Preparation for school re-entry after traumatic injury should begin as soon as possible. Parents should be encouraged to sign consents for mutual exchange of information between the school and the rehabilitation team. These consents allow the team to obtain school records, which can give important information about pre-injury attendance, performance, standardized testing, and prior accommodations or special education services. Provision of education services in the hospital can include assessment of the child's current abilities, the child's ongoing tutoring, and training to use adaptive devices. The school should receive information about the child's expected health status and health maintenance needs at school (e.g., medications, need for CIC, physical restrictions, status of vision and hearing), the child's cognitive and social abilities, the child's ability to tolerate a full day of school, whether the child's condition is expected to change or improve, special transportation needs, and the need for occupational, physical, or speech therapies at school (132). Prekindergarten children who were never enrolled in school can be served through public programs as well, typically programs for infants and toddlers from birth to 3 years of age and through the public school system for children 3 years old and older.

Two laws provide for children with disabilities to receive a free appropriate public education in the least restrictive environment. The Individuals with Disabilities Education Act (IDEA) protects children with 1 or more of 13 disabilities (including speech or language impairments, traumatic brain injury, orthopaedic impairment, and other health impairment) who need special education services and

related services, such as speech pathology, occupational and physical therapy, and transportation (133). The related services can only be provided to assist the child to benefit from special education. IDEA requires that the school, parent, and student develop a written Individualized Education Plan (IEP) with annual goals and objectives, evaluation criteria, and the services to be provided. When a child is served under an IEP, the district receives additional funds. Section 504 of the Rehabilitation Act of 1973 protects a broader group of students than IDEA (134). It includes students with impairments that limit a major life activity such as walking, seeing, hearing, speaking, breathing, learning, working, caring for oneself, and performing manual tasks. Under a 504 plan, students can receive accommodations or related services even if they are not provided any special education. It does not require a written IEP or parental participation and no additional funds are provided to schools. How the child is served depends on the local resources of the school, the child's disabilities, and child/parent preference. If little assistance and monitoring by the school are needed, section 504 may be more appropriate. For instance, a child may need door-to-door transportation, early dismissal from classes to avoid crowded hallways, a study hall time to complete assignments, or a key to an elevator or an accessible bathroom. However, when accountability for provision of services and meeting goals is important, an IEP is more appropriate.

RESTRICTION AND RESUMPTION OF ACTIVITIES

Discharge from the acute care setting or from rehabilitation is an excellent time to review safety precautions and activity restrictions with patients and their parents. The specific activities requiring supervision can often be identified through therapy sessions, community outings, and overnight passes. In the case of TBI, children can be expected to show ongoing improvements, and parents should be empowered to decrease supervision based on their real-life observations at home.

Deciding when to allow a teenager to start driver training or resume driving after an injury requires consideration of the physical and cognitive impairments, the local resources, and family preferences. A teen with physical impairments may need a specialized driving evaluation for adaptive equipment. If the teen has not yet been licensed, he or she could participate in a regular driver education program and be referred for an adaptive equipment evaluation. Some school districts offer driver education programs that will assist with funding for the adaptive equipment evaluation. When a teenager has cognitive impairments, it is prudent to avoid resumption of driving or initiation of driver training until the recovery has stabilized and some assessment of how the child performs in the "real world" can be made. In questionable cases, the teen could be referred to specialized driver evaluation programs, but even if he or she is given clearance to resume driving, there is no guarantee of safety in nontesting situations. For teens yet to be licensed, participation in a driver education program gives the opportunity to see how the child learns the rules of the road and how they perform in on-the-road training.

Children with physical disabilities after trauma can participate in a wide variety of athletic activities (135). A significant challenge to physiatrists is deciding when or if a child who has sustained a moderate or severe brain injury can return to sports, particularly contact and collision sports (136). Specific recommendations for return to collision, contact, and noncollision sports after epidural hematoma, subdural hematoma, intracerebral hematoma, subarachnoid hemorrhage, or diffuse axonal injury have been made by Cantu based on reasoned consideration, not clinical evidence. Cantu has recommended that an athlete who experienced any of these brain injuries cannot return to contact sports if he or she has persistent postconcussion symptoms, permanent neurologic sequelae, hydrocephalus, or spontaneous subarachnoid hemorrhage from any cause. If the athlete has none of these and makes a complete neurologic recovery, he or she could return to contact sports after 1 year and after intensive deliberation. Since few patients with diffuse axonal injury recover without some neurologic residua, return to contact sports is nearly virtually precluded. If the brain injury required surgery for anything other than an epidural hematoma evacuation, the subdural space is theoretically traumatized, thus setting up scarring of the pia arachnoid of the brain to

---

Table 15-3 Classification of Sports by Contact

Contact or Collision	Limited Contact	Noncontact
Basketball	Baseball	Archery
Boxing[a]	Bicycling	Badminton
Diving	Cheerleading	Bodybuilding
Field hockey	Canoeing or kayaking (white water)	Bowling
Football (tackle)	Fencing	Canoeing or kayaking (flat water)
Ice hockey[b]	Field events	Crew or rowing
Lacrosse	High jump	Curling
Martial arts	Pole vault	Dancing
Rodeo	Floor hockey	Ballet
Rugby	Football	Modern
Ski jumping	Flag	Jazz
Soccer	Gymnastics	Field events
Team handball	Handball	Discus
Water polo	Horseback riding	Javelin
Wrestling	Racquetball	Shot put
	Skating	Golf
	Ice	Orienteering
	In-line	Power lifting
	Roller	Race walking
	Skiing	Riflery
	Cross-country	Rope jumping
	Downhill	Running
	Water	Sailing
	Skateboarding	Scuba diving
	Snowboarding	Swimming
	Softball	Table tennis
	Squash	Tennis
	Ultimate frisbee	Track
	Volleyball	Weight lifting
	Windsurfing or surfing	

[a]Participation not recommended by the American Academy of Pediatrics.
[b]The American Academy of Pediatrics recommends limiting the amount of body checking allowed for hockey players 15 years and younger to reduce injuries.
From American Academy of Pediatrics. Committee on Sports Medicine & Fitness. Medical conditions affecting sports participation. *Pediatrics*. 2001;107:1205–1209, with permission.

Table 15-4	Recommendations for Return to Play after a Brain Injury

Brain injury diagnoses: SAH from ruptured congenital vascular lesion or TBI with EDH, SDH, ICH, and/or DAI

Return to Collision or Contact Sports

1. Collision/contact sports are discouraged on a permanent basis even if neurologic recovery is complete if the child had SDH, ICH, SAH requiring surgery (because of scarring of the pia arachnoid to the brain with loss of the normal cushioning effect of the CSF).
2. For all others, no collision or contact sports for 1-y minimum.
3. After 1 year, collision/contact sports are prohibited if:
    a. Original injury was spontaneous subarachnoid hemorrhage from any cause.
    b. Persistent postconcussion symptoms are present.
    c. Permanent neurologic sequelae are present (e.g., cognitive impairment, hemiplegia, hemianopsia).
    d. Hydrocephalus or VP shunt is present.
    e. Symptomatic neurologic or pain-producing abnormalities are present about the foramen magnum.

If the patient had EDH without brain injury or any other condition in which surgery was not required *and* has complete neurologic recovery, return to contact/collision sports may be permitted in select cases after intensive deliberation and informed discussion with the athlete and family.

Return to Limited Contact Sports

1. If neurologic recovery is complete, return to limited contact sports can be considered after deliberation and informed discussion with the athlete and family. The specific sport, the cause of injury (i.e., spontaneous SAH), and the history of surgery with possible resultant scarring should be considered.
2. The timing for return to limited contact sports in children with recent TBI or with residual long-term deficits should be determined on an individual basis. The specific impairments/deficits of the patient and the demands and risks of the sport should be considered. A qualified recommendation to participate may be given after deliberation and informed discussion with the family.

Return to Noncontact Sports

1. There are no contraindications to noncontact sports for any of the brain injuries if neurologic recovery is complete.
2. The timing for return to noncontact sports in children with recent TBI or with residual long-term deficits should be determined on an individual basis. The specific impairments/deficits of the patient and the demands and risks of the sport should be considered. A qualified recommendation to participate may be given after deliberation and informed discussion with the family.

SAH, spontaneous subarachnoid hemorrhage; TBI, traumatic brain injury; EDH, epidural hematoma; SDH, subdural hematoma; ICH, intracerebral hemorrhage; DAI, diffuse axonal injury; CSF, cerebrospinal fluid; VP, ventriculoperitoneal.
From Cantu RC. Return to play guidelines after a head injury. *Clin Sports Med.* 1998;17:45–60, with permission.

the dura and causing loss of the normal cushioning effect of the cerebrospinal fluid (CSF). In this situation, return to a collision sport is discouraged even if the athlete experiences complete recovery (137).

The American Academy of Pediatrics (AAP) has defined collision sports (e.g., boxing, ice hockey, football, rodeo) as those in which athletes hit or collide with one another, the ground, or another object with great force (138). Contact sports (e.g., basketball, soccer) are those in which athletes make contact with each other or inanimate objects, but with less force than in collision sports. However, there is no clear dividing line between the two, so the AAP does not distinguish between collision and contact sports for recommendations regarding participation. In limited contact sports, contact with other athletes or inanimate objects is infrequent or inadvertent. However, some limited contact sports such as downhill skiing can be as dangerous as collision or contact sports. The AAP's classification of sports by contact is shown in Table 15-3. The guidelines for return to play after TBI in Table 15-4 are based upon those of Cantu but do not distinguish between collision and contact

sports. Discussions with patients and families about returning to sports after TBI should include consideration of the child's physical impairments, endurance, reaction time, judgment, cognitive abilities, and the specific sport and circumstances in which the child will participate.

In the case of children who have experienced mild to moderate brain injuries with good outcomes or children with severe injuries who have recovered, once the child is asymptomatic, physical activities can progress to cardiovascular fitness exercises, followed by sport-specific exercises before actual return to team practice and competitive activities. The timing of the progression depends on the nature of the injury, the sport and the symptoms, and the fitness of the athlete (139).

CONCLUSION

Rehabilitation of the child with trauma requires consideration of growth and development, family support, and educational impact. Traumatic injuries can result in pain requiring modifications of traditional approaches in the pediatric patient. Unique medical and musculoskeletal complications also occur in the pediatric trauma patient. Rehabilitation begins in the trauma hospital and continues after discharge to enhance functional independence, academic achievement, and psychosocial functioning.

REFERENCES

1. Danesco ER, Miller TR, Spicer RS. Incidence and costs of 1987-1994 childhood injuries: Demographic breakdowns. *Pediatrics*. 2000;105:e27.
2. Tepas JJ, Ramenofsky ML, Barlow B, et al. National pediatric trauma registry. *J Pediatr Surg*. 1989;24:156–158.
3. Gans BM, DiScala C. Rehabilitation of severely injured children. *West J Med*. 1991;154:566–568.
4. Wesson DE, Williams JI, Spence LJ, et al. Functional outcome in pediatric trauma. *J Trauma*. 1989;29:589–592.
5. Colombani PM, Buck JR, Dudgeon DL, et al. One-year experience in a regional pediatric trauma center. *J Pediatr Surg*. 1985;20:8–13.
6. Potoka DA, Schall LC, Ford HR. Improved functional outcome for severely injured children treated at pediatric trauma centers. *J Trauma*. 2001;51:824–834.
7. Lehmkuhl LD, Thoi LL, Baize C, et al. Multimodality treatment of joint contractures in patients with severe brain injury: Cost, effectiveness, and integration of therapies in the application of serial/inhibitive casts. *J Head Trauma Rehabil*. 1990;5(4):23–42.
8. Alexander MA, Molnar GE. History and examination. In: Molnar GE, Alexander MA, eds. *Pediatric Rehabilitation*. 3rd ed. Philadelphia, PA: Hanley and Belfus; 1999:1–12.
9. Capute AJ, Accardo PJ. A neurodevelopmental perspective on the continuum of developmental disabilities. In: Capute AJ, Accardo PJ, eds. *Developmental disabilities in infancy and childhood*. 2nd ed. Baltimore, MD: Paul H. Brookes; 1996:1–24.
10. Harder JA. Gait analysis of the child with a lower limb deficiency. In: Herring JA, Birch JG, eds. *The child with a limb deficiency*. Rosemont, IL: American Academy of Orthopaedic Surgeons; 1998:331–344.
11. Molnar GE, Sobus KM. Growth and development. In: Molnar GE, Alexander MA, eds. *Pediatric rehabilitation*. 3rd ed. Philadelphia, PA: Hanley and Belfus; 1999:13–28.
12. Zager R, Marquette C. Developmental considerations in children and early adolescents with spinal cord injury. *Arch Phys Med Rehabil*. 1981;62:423–427.
13. Schechter NL, Berde CB, Yaster M. Pain in infants, children, and adolescents. In: Schechter NL, Berde CB, Yaster M, eds. *Pain in Infants and Adolescents*. 2nd ed. Philadelphia, PA: Lippincott Williams & Wilkins; 2003:3–18.
14. Anand KJS. Long-term effects of pain in neonates and infants. In: Jensen TS, Turner JA, Wiesenfeld-Hallen Z, eds. *Progress in Pain, Research, and Management*. Vol 3. Seattle, WA: IASP Press; 1997:881–892.
15. Mersky H, Bogduk N, eds. *Classification of chronic pain: Descriptions of chronic pain syndromes and definitions of pain terms*. 2nd ed. Seattle, WA: IASP Press; 1994.
16. Turk DC, Melzack R. The measurement of pain and the assessment of people experiencing pain. In: Turk DC, Melzack R, eds. *Handbook of pain assessment*. New York, NY: Guilford Press; 1992:3–12.
17. Greenspan AI, MacKenzie EJ. Functional outcome after pediatric head injury. *Pediatrics*. 1994;94:425–432.
18. Jarosz DA. Pediatric spinal cord injuries: A case presentation. *Crit Care Nurs Q*. 1999;22(2):8–13.
19. Reynolds R. Pediatric spinal injury. *Curr Opin Pediatr*. 2000;12:67–71.
20. Campbell J, Bonnett C. Spinal cord injury in children. *Clin Orthop Relat Res*. 1975;112:114–123.
21. Vogel L, Mulcahy MJ, Betz RR. The child with spinal cord injury. *Dev Med Child Neurol*. 1997;39:202–207.
22. Yoshimura O, Takyanagi K, Kawaguchi K, et al. Spinal cord injuries in children observed over many years. *J Med Sci*. 1996;45:37–41.
23. Kennedy P, Frankel H, Gardner B, et al. Factors associated with acute and chronic pain following traumatic spinal cord injuries. *Spinal Cord*. 1997;35:814–817.
24. Brazeal TC, Behrends L, Rosenberg L, et al. Phantom limb sensations and pain in youth burn survivors. Poster Session Presented at the 5th International Symposium on Paediatric Pain. London; June 2000.
25. Krane EJ, Heller LB. The prevalence of phantom sensation and pain in pediatric amputees. *J Pain Symptom Manage*. 1995;10:21–29.
26. Wilkins KL, McGrath PJ, Finley GA, et al. Phantom limb sensations and phantom limb pain in child and adolescent amputees. *Pain*. 1998;78:7–12.
27. Kahana MD. Burn pain management: Avoiding the "private nightmare." In: Schechter NL, Berde CB, Yaster M, eds. *Pain in infants and adolescents*. 2nd ed. Philadelphia, PA: Lippincott Williams & Wilkins; 2003:642–650.
28. Melchert-McKearnan K, Deitz J, Engel JM, et al. Children with burn injuries: Purposeful activity versus rote exercise. *Am J Occup Ther*. 2000;54:381–390.
29. Patterson DR, Jensen M, Engel-Knowles J. Pain and its influence on assistive technology use. In: Scherer MJ, ed. *Assistive technology: Matching device and consumer for successful rehabilitation*. Washington, DC: American Psychological Association; 2002:59–76.
30. American Pain Society. Pain: The fifth vital sign. Available at: http://www.ampainsoc.org/advocacy/fifth.htm. Accessed 2003.
31. Gaffney A, McGrath PJ, Dick B. Measuring pain in children: Developmental and instrument issues. In: Schechter NL, Berde CB, Yaster M, eds. *Pain in infants and adolescents*. 2nd ed. Philadelphia, PA: Lippincott Williams & Wilkins; 2003:128–141.
32. Hester NO, Foster R, Kristensen K. Measurement of pain in children: Generalizability and validity of the pain ladder and the poker-chip tool. In: Tyler DC, Krane EJ, eds. *Advances in pain research and therapy. Vol. 15: Pediatric pain*. New York, NY: Raven Press; 1990:79–84.
33. Bieri D, Reeve RA, Champion GD, et al. The faces pain scale for the self-assessment of the severity of pain experienced by children: Development, initial validation, and preliminary investigation for ratio scale properties. *Pain*. 1990;41:139–150.

34. Beyer J. *The Oucher: A user's manual and technical report*. Denver, CO: University of Colorado Health Sciences Center; 1988.

35. Dahlquist LM. *Pediatric pain management*. New York, NY: Kluwer Academic/Plenum Publishers; 1999.

36. McGrath PA, Gillespie J. Pain assessment in children and adolescents. In: Turk DC, Melzack R, eds. *Handbook of pain assessment*. 2nd ed. New York, NY: Guilford Press; 2001:97–118.

37. Eland JM, Anderson JE. The experience of pain in children. In: Jacox AK, ed. *Pain: A source book for nurses and other health professionals*. Boston, MA: Little, Brown and Company; 1977:453–473.

38. Jay SM, Elliott C. Behavioral observation scales for measuring children's distress: The effects of increased methodological rigor. *J Consult Clin Psychol*. 1984;52(6):1106–1107.

39. Parker LH, Cinciripini PM. Behavioral medicine with children: Applications in chronic disease. *Prog Behav Modif*. 1984;17:136–165.

40. Bernstein BA, Pachter LM. Cultural considerations in children's pain. In: Schechter NL, Berde CB, Yaster M, eds. *Pain in infants and adolescents*. 2nd ed. Philadelphia, PA: Lippincott Williams & Wilkins; 2003:142–156.

41. McGrath PJ, Unruh AM. Psychological treatment of pain in children and adolescents. In: Schechter NL, Berde CB, Yaster M, eds. *Pain in infants, children, and adolescents*. Baltimore, MD: Williams & Wilkins; 1993:219.

42. American Academy of Pain Medicine. FAQs about pain. Available at: http://www.painmed.org/faqs/pain_faqs.html. Accessed 2001.

43. Goldman A, Frager G, Pomietto M. Pain and palliative care. In: Schechter NL, Berde CB, Yaster M, eds. *Pain in infants and adolescents*. 2nd ed. Philadelphia, PA: Lippincott Williams & Wilkins; 2003:539–562.

44. Engel JM. Physical therapy and occupational therapy for pain management in children. *Child Adolesc Psychiatr Clin N Am*. 1997;6:817–828.

45. World Health Organization. *Cancer pain relief and palliative care in children*. Geneva, Switzerland: World Health Organization; 1998.

46. Patterson DR, Everett J, Burns G, et al. Hypnosis for the treatment of burn pain. *J Consult Clin Psychol*. 1992;60:713–717.

47. Hoffman HG, Doctor JN, Patterson DR, et al. Virtual reality as an adjunctive pain control during burn wound care in adolescent patients. *Pain*. 2000;85:305–309.

48. McCaffery M, Wong DL. Nursing interventions for pain control in children. In: Schechter NL, Berde CB, Yaster M, eds. *Pain in infants, children, and adolescents*. Baltimore, MD: Williams & Wilkins; 1993:295–316.

49. Schechter NL. Management of common pain problems in the primary care pediatric setting. In: Schechter NL, Berde CB, Yaster M, eds. *Pain in infants and adolescents*. 2nd ed. Philadelphia, PA: Lippincott Williams & Wilkins; 2003:693–706.

50. Selbst SM, Zempsky WT. Sedation and analgesia in the emergency department. In: Schechter NL, Berde CB, Yaster M, eds. *Pain in infants and adolescents*. 2nd ed. Philadelphia, PA: Lippincott Williams & Wilkins; 2003:651–668.

51. Epstein M, Harris J. Children with chronic pain—can they be helped? *Pediatr Nurs*. 1978;4:42–44.

52. McCarthy CF, Shea AM, Sullivan P. Physical therapy management of pain in children. In: Schechter NL, Berde CB, Yaster M, eds. *Pain in infants and adolescents*. 2nd ed. Philadelphia, PA: Lippincott Williams & Wilkins; 2003:434–448.

53. Long TM, Harp KA. Pain in children. *Orthop Phys Ther Clin N Am*. 1995;4:503–517.

54. Sweitzer RW. Ultrasound. In: Hecox B, Mehreteab TA, Weisberg J, eds. *Physical agents: A comprehensive text for physical therapists*. Norwalk, CT: Appleton & Lange; 1994:163–192.

55. McGrath PJ, Dick B, Unruh AM. Psychologic and behavioral treatment of pain in children and adolescents. In: Schechter NL, Berde CB, Yaster M, eds. *Pain in infants and adolescents*. 2nd ed. Philadelphia, PA: Lippincott Williams & Wilkins; 2003:303–316.

56. Hamalainen M, Masek BJ. Diagnosis, classification, and medical management of headache in children and adolescents. In: Schechter NL, Berde CB, Yaster M, eds. *Pain in infants and adolescents*. 2nd ed. Philadelphia, PA: Lippincott Williams & Wilkins; 2003:707–718.

57. Payne RA. *Relaxation techniques*. 2nd ed. New York, NY: Churchill Livingstone; 2000.

58. Jacobson E. *You must relax*. New York, NY: McGraw-Hill; 1957.

59. Schultz JH, Luthe W. *Autogenic training: A psychophysiologic approach to psychotherapy*. New York, NY: Grune & Stratton; 1959.

60. Townsend MC. Therapeutic approaches in psychiatric nursing care. *Psychiatric mental health nursing: Concepts of care*. 3rd ed. Philadelphia, PA: F. A. Davis; 2000:177–186.

61. Benson H. *The relaxation response*. New York, NY: Times Books; 1975.

62. McGrath P, Larsson B. Headache in children and adolescents. *Child Adolesc Psychiatr Clin N Am*. 1997; 6:843–861.

63. Powers SW. Empirically supported treatment in pediatric psychology: Procedure-related pain. *J Pediatr Psychol*. 1999;24:131–145.

64. Kuttner L, Solomon R. Hypnotherapy and imagery for managing children's pain. In: Schechter NL, Berde CB, Yaster M, eds. *Pain in infants and adolescents*. 2nd ed. Philadelphia, PA: Lippincott Williams & Wilkins; 2003:317–328.

65. Patterson DR. Non-opiod based approaches to burn pain. *J Burn Care Rehabil*. 1995;16:372–376.

66. Thurman DJ, Finkelstein B, Leadbetter SL. A proposed classification of traumatic brain injury severity for surveillance systems. Proceedings of the Annual Meeting of the American Public Health Association. New York; November 21, 1996.

67. Krauss JF, Rock A, Hemyari P. Brain injuries among infants, children, adolescents and young adults. *Am J Dis Child*. 1990;144:684–691.

68. Kaufman BA, Dacey RG. Acute care management of closed head injury in childhood. *Pediatr Ann*. 1994; 23:18–28.

69. Muhonen MG, Piper JG, Menezes AH. Pathogenesis and treatment of growing skull fractures. *Surg Neurol*. 1995;43:367–372.

70. Annegers JF, Grabow JD, Groover RV, et al. Seizures after head trauma: A population study. *Neurology*. 1980;30:683–689.

71. Bijur PE, Haslum M, Golding J. Cognitive and behavioral sequelae of mild head injury in children. *Pediatrics*. 1990;86:337–344.

72. Massagli TL, Fann JR, Burington BE, et al. Psychiatric illness after mild traumatic brain injury in children. *Arch Phys Med Rehabil.* 2004;85(9):1428–1434.

73. Shurtleff HA, Massagli TL, Hays RM, et al. Screening children and adolescents with mild or moderate traumatic brain injury to assist school reentry. *J Head Trauma Rehabil.* 1995;10(5):64–79.

74. Bayley N. *Bayley II.* San Antonio, TX: Psychological Corporation; 1993.

75. Folio M, Fewell R. *Peabody developmental motor scales and activity cards.* Allen, TX: DLM Teaching Resources; 1983.

76. Massagli TL, Jaffe KM, Fay GC, et al. Neurobehavioral sequelae of severe pediatric traumatic brain injury: A cohort study. *Arch Phys Med Rehabil.* 1996; 77:223–231.

77. Massagli TL, Michaud LJ, Rivara FP. Association between injury indices and outcome after severe traumatic brain injury in children. *Arch Phys Med Rehabil.* 1996;77:125–132.

78. Brink JD, Garrett AL, Hale WR, et al. Recovery of motor and intellectual function in children sustaining severe head injuries. *Dev Med Child Neurol.* 1970; 12:565–571.

79. Brink JD, Imbus C, Woo-Sam J. Physical recovery after severe closed head trauma in children and adolescents. *J Pediatr.* 1980;97:721–727.

80. Ewing-Cobbs L, Levin HS, Fletcher JM, et al. The children's orientation and amnesia test: Relationship to severity of acute head injury and to recovery of memory. *Neurosurgery.* 1990;27:683–691.

81. Schoenbrodt L, ed. *Children with traumatic brain injury: A parent's guide.* Bethesda, MD: Woodbine House; 2001.

82. Go BK, DeVivo M, Richards JS. The epidemiology of spinal cord injury. In: Stover SL, Delisa JA, Whiteneck GG, eds. *Spinal cord injury: Clinical outcomes from the model systems.* Gaithersburg, MD: Aspen Publications; 1995:21–25.

83. Vogel LC, DeVivo MJ. Etiology and demographics. In: Betz RR, Mulcahey MJ, eds. *The child with a spinal cord injury.* Rosemont, IL: American Academy of Orthopaedic Surgeons; 1996:3–12.

84. Wilberger JE. Anatomy and biomechanics of the immature spine. In: Wilberger JE, ed. *Spinal cord injuries in children.* New York, NY: Futura Publishing; 1986:1–20.

85. Pang D, Wilberger JE. Spinal cord injury without radiographic abnormalities in children. *J Neurosurg.* 1982;57:114–129.

86. Grabb PA, Pang D. Magnetic resonance imaging in the evaluation of spinal cord injury without radiographic abnormality in children. *Neurosurgery.* 1994;35:406–414.

87. Consortium for Spinal Cord Medicine. Acute management of autonomic dysreflexia: Individuals with spinal cord injury presenting to health care facilities. *J Spinal Cord Med.* 2002;25:S67–S88.

88. Vogel LC. Spasticity: Diagnostic workup and medical management. In: Betz RR, Mulcahey MJ, eds. *The child with a spinal cord injury.* Rosemont, IL: American Academy of Orthopaedic Surgeons; 1996: 261–268.

89. Vogel LC, Anderson CJ. Spinal cord injuries in children and adolescents: A review. *J Spinal Cord Med.* 2003;26:193–203.

90. Vogel LC, Schrader T, Lubicky JP. Latex allergy in children and adolescents with spinal cord injuries. *J Pediatr Orthop.* 1995;15:517–520.

91. Massagli TL, Cardenas DC. Treatment of immobilization hypercalcemia after spinal cord injury with pamidronate disodium. *Arch Phys Med Rehabil.* 1999;80:998–1000.

92. Waring WP, Karunas RS. Acute spinal cord injuries and the incidence of clinically occurring thromboembolic disease. *Paraplegia.* 1991;29:8–16.

93. Betz RR. Heterotopic ossification. In: Betz RR, Mulcahey MJ, eds. *The child with a spinal cord injury.* Rosemont, IL: American Academy of Orthopedic Surgeons; 1996:345–351.

94. Silverman SL, Hurvitz EA, Nelson VS, et al. Rachitic syndrome after disodium etidronate therapy in an adolescent. *Arch Phys Med Rehabil.* 1994;75:118–120.

95. Dearolf WW, Betz RR, Vogel LC, et al. Scoliosis in pediatric spinal cord injured patients. *J Pediatr Orthop.* 1990;10:214–218.

96. McDonald CM, Jaffe KM, Shurtleff DB. Assessment of muscle strength in children with meningomyelocele: Accuracy and stability of measurements over time. *Arch Phys Med Rehabil.* 1986;67:855–861.

97. Koff SA. Estimating bladder capacity in children. *Urology.* 1983;21:248.

98. Peters CA. Bladder reconstruction in children. *Curr Opin Pediatr.* 1994;6:183–193.

99. Stiens SA, Goetz LL. Neurogenic bowel dysfunction: Evaluation and adaptive management. In Young BJ, Young MA, Stiens SA, eds. *Physical medicine and rehabilitation secrets.* 2nd ed. Philadelphia, PA: Hanley and Balfus; 2002:469.

100. Curtis AC, Ballmer RS. The prevention of carotene absorption by liquid petrolatum. *JAMA.* 1939;113: 1785–1788.

101. Muller-Lissner SA. Adverse effects of laxatives: Fact and fiction. *Pharmacology.* 1993;47:138–145.

102. Sharif F, Crushel E, O'Driscoll K, et al. Liquid paraffin: A reappraisal of its role in the treatment of constipation. *Arch Dis Child.* 2001;85:121–124.

103. DeVivo MJ, Richards JS, Stover SL, et al. Spinal cord injury: Rehabilitation adds life to years. *West J Med.* 1991;154:602–606.

104. Massagli TL, Dudgeon BJ, Ross BW. Educational performance and vocational participation after spinal cord injury in childhood. *Arch Phys Med Rehabil.* 1996;77:995–999.

105. Vogel LC, Klass SJ, Lubicky JP, et al. Long-term outcomes and life satisfaction of adults who had pediatric spinal cord injuries. *Arch Phys Med Rehabil.* 1998;79:1496–1503.

106. Trautwein LC, Smith DG, Rivara FP. Pediatric amputation injuries: Etiology, cost, and outcome. *J Trauma.* 1996;41:831–838.

107. Letts M, Davidson D. Epidemiology and prevention of traumatic amputations in children. In: Herring JA, Birch JG, eds. *The child with a limb deficiency.* Rosemont, IL: American Academy of Orthopaedic Surgeons; 1998:235–251.

108. Dormans JP. Management of pediatric mutilating extremity injuries and traumatic amputations. In: Herring JA, Birch JG, eds. *The child with a limb deficiency.* Rosemont, IL: American Academy of Orthopaedic Surgeons; 1998:253–265.

109. Bryant PR, Pandian G. Acquired limb deficiencies. 1. Acquired limb deficiencies in children and young adults. *Arch Phys Med Rehabil.* 2001;82(Suppl. 1): S3–S8.

110. Davids JR. Terminal bony overgrowth of the residual limb: Current management strategies. In: Herring JA, Birch JG, eds. *The child with a limb deficiency.* Rosemont, IL: American Academy of Orthopaedic Surgeons; 1998:269–280.

111. Speer DP. The pathogenesis of amputation stump overgrowth. *Clin Orthop.* 1981;159:294–307.

112. Stanger M. Limb deficiencies and amputations. In: Campbell SK, Vander Linden DW, Palisano RJ, eds. *Physical therapy for children.* 2nd ed. Philadelphia, PA: WB Saunders; 2000:370–397.

113. Lotze M, Grodd W, Birbaumer N, et al. Does use of a myoelectric prosthesis prevent cortical reorganization and phantom limb pain? *Nat Neurosci.* 1999;2: 501–502.

114. Cummings DR. Pediatric prosthetics: Current trends and future possibilities. *Phys Med Rehabil Clin N Am.* 2000;11:653–679.

115. Varni JW, Setoguchi Y. Perceived physical appearance and adjustment of adolescents with congenital/acquired limb deficiencies: A path-analytic model. *J Clin Child Psychol.* 1996;25:201–208.

116. Varni JW, Pruitt SD, Seid M. Health related quality of life in pediatric limb deficiency. In: Herring JA, Birch JG, eds. *The child with a limb deficiency.* Rosemont, IL: American Academy of Orthopaedic Surgeons; 1998:457–473.

117. Purdue GF, Hunt JL, Burris AM. Pediatric burn care. *Clin Ped Emerg Med.* 2002;3:76–82.

118. Bennett B, Gamelli R. Profile of an abused burned child. *J Burn Care Rehabil.* 1998;19:88–94.

119. Hultman CS, Priolo D, Cairns BA, et al. Return to jeopardy: The fate of pediatric burn patients who are victims of abuse and neglect. *J Burn Care Rehabil.* 1998;19:367–376.

120. American Burn Association. Hospital and prehospital resources for optimal care of patients with burn injury: Guidelines for development and operation of burn centers. *J Burn Care Rehabil.* 1990;11:98–104.

121. Lund C, Browder NC. The estimation of areas of burns. *Surg Gynecol Obstet.* 1944;79:352–358.

122. Kramer MD, Jones T, Deitch EA. Burn contractures: Incidence, predisposing factors, and results of surgical therapy. *J Burn Care Rehabil.* 1988;9:261–265.

123. Koch BM, Wu CM, Randolph J, et al. Heterotopic ossification in children with burns: Two case reports. *Arch Phys Med Rehabil.* 1992;73:1104–1106.

124. Fricke NB, Omnell ML, Dutcher KA, et al. Skeletal and dental disturbances in children after facial burns and pressure garment use: A 4-year follow-up. *J Burn Care Rehabil.* 1999;20:239–249.

125. Staley M, Richard R, Billlmire D, et al. Head/face/neck burns: Therapist considerations for the pediatric patient. *J Burn Care Rehabil.* 1997;18:164–171.

126. Rutan RL, Herndon DN. Growth delay in postburn pediatric patients. *Arch Surg.* 1990;125:392–395.

127. Gorga D, Johnson J, Bentley A, et al. The physical, functional, and developmental outcome of pediatric burn survivors from 1 to 12 months post injury. *J Burn Care Rehabil.* 1999;20:171–178.

128. Sheridan RL, Hinson MI, Liang MH, et al. Long-term outcome of children suffering massive burns. *JAMA.* 2000;283:69–73.

129. Meyers-Paal R, Blakeney P, Robert R, et al. Physical and psychological rehabilitation outcomes for pediatric patients who suffer 80% or more TBSA, 70% or more third degree burns. *J Burn Care Rehabil.* 2000; 21:43–49.

130. Blakeney P, Meyer W, Moore P, et al. Psychosocial sequelae of pediatric burns involving 80% or greater total body surface area. *J Burn Care Rehabil.* 1993;14: 684–689.

131. Meyer WJ, Robert R, Murphy L, et al. Evaluating the psychosocial adjustment of 2- and 3-year-old pediatric burn survivors. *J Burn Care Rehabil.* 2000;21: 179–184.

132. Ross B. Meeting the educational needs of children with disabilities: A collaborative management approach. *Phys Med Rehabil Clin N Am.* 1991;2(4): 781–800.

133. The Individuals with Disabilities Education Act (IDEA). 20 USC b1400 et seq, June 4, 1997.

134. Rehabilitation Act of 1973, Pub L No. 93–112, section 504.

135. Chang FM. Physically challenged athletes. In: Sullivan JA, Anderson SJ, eds. *Care of the young athlete.* Rosemont, IL: American Academy of Orthopaedic Surgeons and the American Academy of Pediatrics; 2000:149–161.

136. Barrett JR, Kuhlman GS, Stanitski CL, et al. The preparticipation physical evaluation. In: Sullivan JA, Anderson SJ, eds. *Care of the young athlete.* Rosemont, IL: American Academy of Orthopaedic Surgeons and the American Academy of Pediatrics; 2000, 43–56.

137. Cantu RC. Return to play guidelines after a head injury. *Clin Sports Med.* 1998;17:45–60.

138. American Academy of Pediatrics, Committee on Sports Medicine & Fitness. Medical conditions affecting sports participation. *Pediatrics.* 2001;107: 1205–1209.

139. Putakian M, Harmon KG. Head injuries. In: Birrer RB, Griesemer BA, Cataletto MB, eds. *Pediatric sports medicine for primary care.* Philadelphia, PA: Lippincott Williams & Wilkins; 2002:266–290.

16

Prevention of Disability Secondary to Trauma

David C. Grossman

INJURY CONTROL AS A PUBLIC HEALTH DISCIPLINE

HISTORY OF INJURY CONTROL

Injury control is now widely accepted as a scientific discipline that integrates the fields of public health, trauma care, rehabilitation medicine, and biomechanics.

The exact origins of injury control as a scientific discipline are unclear, but two clinical aspects of injury control, acute care and rehabilitation, are as old as the field of medicine itself. The public health dimensions of injury control are far younger and probably have their deepest roots in occupational safety. Starting in the late 17th century, Bernadina Ramazzini of Italy, the father of occupational medicine, also took a strong interest in the science and practice of preventing occupational injury (1). The public health paradigm for injury prevention for nonoccupational injury took root much later and initially focused on poisoning prevention among children. In the United States, an epidemic of aspirin poisonings among children led to important changes in the packaging of medications and the innovation of the child-proof cap, which subsequently was associated with a dramatic decline in the rate of unintentional poisoning deaths. Perhaps the most significant advance for injury prevention in the United States in this field took place as a result of advocacy for improved automobile safety. The publication of Ralph Nader's book, *Unsafe at Any Speed: The Designed-in Dangers of the American Automobile*, about automobile design flaws associated with increased risk of injury, led to passage of the National Traffic and Motor Vehicle Safety Act and the Highway Safety Act in 1966 by the United States Congress. These legislative acts led to historic and extensive collaborations among physicians, mechanical and biomechanical engineers, and statisticians in order to improve the design of autos and highways and reduce the risk of injury from crashes.

PARADIGMS OF INJURY PREVENTION

Before this watershed period of motor vehicle safety, most injuries, especially motor vehicle crashes, were viewed largely as having a behavioral origin—whether it was driver inattention, drinking, fatigue, or "carelessness." The solution for most of these incidents was also thought to be behavioral interventions. Little attention was paid to potential environmental or vehicle solutions. For public health professionals, the triad of *host*, *agent*, and *environment* was a long-standing paradigm in domains such as infectious disease and environmental health. William Haddon, a physician and the first head of the US Highway Safety Bureau, incorporated these concepts into the work and vision for his agency. During Haddon's tenure, injury control truly became a public health discipline. Haddon took the triad model of public health and modified it to reflect the short time frame of injury causation. Injuries are caused by the deposition of kinetic and thermal energy into the human body. Haddon's approach to injury control extended

		Epidemiological Dimension			
		Human Factors	**Agent or Vehicle**	**Physical Environment**	**Sociocultural Environment**
Event Dimension	**Pre-event**	Intoxicated pedestrian	Speeding vehicle	Intersection with poor lighting	Low rate of enforcement of yield laws
	Event	Osteoporosis in elderly pedestrians	Car front-end profile	Road surface characteristics	Speed limits
	Post-event	Elderly pedestrian	Crash investigation with vehicle inspection	Distance to trauma care facility	Regionalized trauma care

Figure 16–1. Haddon's matrix, pedestrian injury example.

beyond primary crash prevention to finding ways to reduce this energy transmission from the car to the occupant's body during impact and to prevent secondary injuries after the crash.

Haddon's matrix (Fig. 16–1), now the most widely accepted paradigm for injury control, illustrates these concepts by placing time periods under each of the triad categories. These three temporal dimensions, precrash, during crash, and postcrash, each provide different windows of opportunity to intervene and prevent primary and secondary injury. As illustrated in the figure, seat belts and airbags are both interventions that reduce the risk of crash *injury* during the crash phase but that clearly are not associated with crash prevention. This matrix provided a breakthrough in the science of motor vehicle injury but has been generalized for use in other types of injuries, including drowning, firearm injuries, fires, and other injury mechanisms. It also defined a clear role for trauma care teams, emergency medical service providers, and physiatrists in the prevention of injury, largely in the prevention of secondary effects of injury during medical care.

A second paradigm in the field of injury control is the concept that the most powerful interventions integrate the three Es on injury prevention: Education, Enforcement, and Engineering. Rarely, one can succeed with only interventions of a single dimension, but most require a combination of *education* (at the individual or community level), *enforcement* of laws to reinforce behavior change, and *engineering* technical interventions. One of the clearest examples of the use of this strategy combination has occurred with the promotion of seat belts. For example, in the early 1980s, <20% of passengers and drivers regularly used seat belts, compared to current

usage rates of approximately 80% in 2004. These changes in belt use occurred as a result of changing normative behaviors regarding driving. Steady, ongoing community education efforts accompanied by laws and enforcement, and continuing technical improvements in belt design, have all played a role in the improvements in belt usage.

APPROACHES TO PREVENTION OF SPECIFIC INJURIES

MOTOR VEHICLE INJURY

Motor vehicle crashes are the leading cause of mortality from the ages of 1 to 34 years, leading to more than 41,000 deaths and 500,000 hospitalizations annually. Occupant injuries account for approximately 85% of crash deaths, and pedestrians account for slightly >10%. In Haddon's matrix, risk factors for mortality and injury can be classified as being related to the driver, the vehicle, or the physical and social environment. Similarly, countermeasures for crash-related injuries can be classified by the cells in the matrix. In fact, crash injuries often result from a combination of risk factors (e.g., lack of seat belt use and speeding), and intervention strategies may need to be multifocal. In subsequent sections, we will enumerate potential countermeasures for crash injuries and the evidence for their potential effectiveness.

Drunk Driving

Rates of drunk driving remain unacceptably high in the United States and are one of the most important preventable factors associated with the risk of crashes. Recent systematic reviews of the literature, especially those from the Task Force on Community Preventive Service (sponsored by the Centers for Disease Control and Prevention [CDC]), have concluded that there are a number of proven strategies to reduce injuries from alcohol-associated crashes. These include the following:

- Promptly suspending the driver's licenses of people who drive while intoxicated (2). Administrative revocation of licenses has been implemented in many communities with varying levels of penalty depending on the number of offenses.
- Conducting sobriety tests at highway checkpoints, especially if they are unannounced and conducted in a random fashion with regard to time and geography (3).
- Lowering the permissible levels of blood alcohol concentration (BAC) for adults to 0.08 mg% in all states (3). Thirty-one states in the United States now have these "per se" laws set at 0.08% and receive special incentive grants from the federal government for passing them. Most of the remaining states have set their laws at the 0.1% level. Establishing an even lower acceptable blood alcohol concentration (e.g., 0.05%), as some nations have done, would likely lead to lower rates of death.
- Zero tolerance laws for drivers <21 years old in all states (3). Zero tolerance laws are passed by states and establish special rules with regard to permissible alcohol levels for drivers <21 years old. Any detectable alcohol level is illegal and can result in severe penalties. The enactment of these laws has resulted in a substantial reduction in alcohol-related crash deaths among teenagers.
- Mandatory substance abuse assessment and treatment for driving-under-the-influence offenders (4). This measure can be particularly effective for offenders who do not have a chronic history of drunk driving arrests and abuse. Recent evidence regarding brief interventions, also known as motivational interviewing, suggests that it can lead to an approximate 50% reduction in repeat offenses among alcohol-impaired drivers in the first year after injury.

Teen Drivers

Teenaged drivers are at very high risk of crashes, and this risk is further modified by the time of day (day versus night), alcohol use, teen driver experience, and the presence of other teens in the car when a teen is driving. The major intervention for this constellation of risk factors has been the introduction of graduated driver licensing laws in a number of states. The laws define a specific pathway for young drivers, starting out with a learner's permit, moving to an intermediate driver's license with restrictions, and progressing to a full license. Though the specific rules vary by state, most states have enacted similar laws. For example, the states of Washington and Michigan both require that before a license is granted, a teenage driver must spend at least 50 hours driving under the supervision of an adult, 10 of which must be at night. Newly licensed drivers with intermediate licenses are restricted from late-night driving and can only be accompanied by older adults or family members when driving. After 6 to 12 months, these restrictions are lifted and the license converts to a full license when the driver reaches the age of 18 years. A recent systematic review evaluating 13 studies found that the median decrease in teen crash rates during the first year was 31% (range 26% to 41%). Graduated driver licensing remains a very promising intervention for this age group.

Restraint Use

Restraint systems are now thought to be an integrated set of devices designed to decelerate occupants with minimal interior collisions. These devices include seat belts, airbags, and, in some cars, seat belt pretensioners. One of the most effective interventions to mitigate injury during a motor vehicle crash is the use of seat belts. Studies have shown injury and death was reduced in approximately 45% to 60% of accidents in which the occupants were wearing seat belts (5).

Late-model cars are now designed such that the restraint system includes the seat belt as well as an airbag and, perhaps, belt pretensioners. These components of the system interact to decelerate occupants more slowly than they would if no restraint system was available. Seat belts have been mandatory in cars since the late 1960s, but use rates remained at about 10% to 15% in the United States until the late 1980s. Because of a combination of factors, such as intensive community-based education campaigns (education), the passage of mandatory seat belt usage laws (enforcement), and improved belt designs (engineering), seat belt use in the United States in 2004 is at about 80%. The passage of primary seat belt laws (which permit police to stop cars and issue fines solely for lack of belt use) has been associated with higher belt use rates (6). Some states and provinces, such as California and Washington, have achieved belt use rates close to 95%, among the highest in the world.

A special case of restraints relates to child passenger safety. Infants, toddlers, and children should use specially designed restraint devices that accommodate their smaller size. Infants <1 year old should use a rear-facing infant or convertible car seat; toddlers weighing between 20 and 40 pounds should use a forward-facing harness car seat as long as the child is at least 1 year of age; and children weighing between 40 and 80 pounds should use a booster seat. Young children who are unrestrained or who use regular seat belts are at much higher risk of ejection or injuries to the neck, abdomen, and spine caused by seat belt compression. The effectiveness of these devices overall is estimated at about 54% (7), but little is known about the differential effectiveness of different types of seats.

The CDC Community Preventive Services Task Force has also conducted systematic reviews of the literature regarding child passenger safety and has found "strong evidence" to support child safety seat laws that mandate child restraints for children up to the age of 8 and safety seat distribution and education campaigns. Incentive campaigns and enforcement campaigns are also recommended. Rates of child safety seat use in the United States vary considerably by developmental age with the highest usage rates seen among infants and the lowest among older toddlers and school-aged children. Increasing the use of booster seats has become a major focus for advocates of child passenger safety, as has passing laws that raise the age threshold for which seats are mandated.

Vehicle Crashworthiness

Though vehicle design and crashworthiness are beyond the direct control of the medical community, they are very important factors related to the risk of crash (e.g., rollover risks) and the risk of injury during crash. The role of the National Highway Traffic Safety Administration (NHTSA) is to conduct rule-making activities and to develop safety standards for new motor vehicles. The full scope of these activities is beyond the scope of this chapter, but NHTSA (www.nhtsa.gov) and the Insurance Institute for Highway Safety (www.iihs.org) provide extensive consumer-friendly information regarding safety of specific vehicles. Physicians and other health care providers can help consumers access objective information regarding the crash and injury risks associated with new and used cars being evaluated for purchase.

Pedestrian Injuries

Pedestrian injuries comprise a relatively small proportion of motor vehicle injury overall, but young children and elderly adults are at particularly high absolute and proportionate risk. The prevention strategy for this type of injury varies by age group, but most experts now agree that primary environmental interventions are likely to bring the greatest net reduction in crashes with pedestrians. Examples of effective environmental interventions include traffic calming devices (e.g., speed bumps) (8) and the physical separation of vehicle and pedestrian traffic. Crosswalks have been shown to elevate the risk of injury among the elderly, probably because they induce a false sense of security and insufficient signal timing for this population (9).

Educational group programs for children have demonstrated increased gains in knowledge and observed crossing skills, but it is unknown whether these gains translate into reduced injury (10). Ensuring close supervision of young children around traffic areas is probably a very important intervention, but there have been very few studies regarding this. There is great interest in designing front-end profiles of cars that minimize injury to pedestrians in the event of collision, and some evidence exists that this can reduce the severity of injury and mortality (11,12). Using visibility aids (such as reflective strips on coats or shoes) to increase the visibility of pedestrians has been frequently mentioned as a potential approach to preventing these injuries, though there have not been any trials to see if they can reduce collisions with cars.

Motorcycle Collisions

Compared to passenger vehicles, motorcycles carry a much higher risk of injury and death. The mortality rate for motorcycle travel is >35 times that for traveling in cars. One modifiable factor that can reduce head injuries from these types of collisions is the wearing of motorcycle helmets that meet safety standards set by federal traffic safety agencies. The passage of helmet laws by states and provinces has been shown in multiple studies to lead to much higher rates of helmet use and to reduce the risk of death by 26% in California (13). A recent case-control study also showed that increasing the visibility of motorcycles and their drivers may be associated with a reduced risk of crash (14).

DROWNING

During 2001, a total of 3,372 persons suffered fatal, unintentional drowning in recreational settings. Nonfatal and fatal injury rates were highest for children aged <4 years and for males of all ages. Drowning is the most common type of injury death among children <5 years of age and the second most common for adolescents in the United States.

For every ten children who drown, 36 are hospitalized and many of the nonfatal injuries result in extreme disability from asphyxia. Drowning mortality rates have fallen steadily over the past several decades, though it is unclear whether this trend is related to interventions or changes in exposure to water over the past decades. Since drowning results from a heterogeneous set of circumstances, prevention strategies vary by both the age group as well as by the setting and circumstances. Young children usually drown in pools, lakes, rivers, and drainage ditches, often while unsupervised. Adolescents often drown in open water (such as the ocean, lakes, bays) while swimming or boating. There are very few case-control studies or controlled trials to provide guidance on the relative risks and protective effects of risk and protective factors. For pool drowning, four-sided fencing has clearly been shown to be effective. One study estimated that this intervention can lead to a 75% reduction in this type of drowning, compared to no fencing or a three-sided fence (15).

In the category of open-water drownings, flotation devices offer the most promising intervention. Personal flotation devices (PFD), or lifejackets, are thought to be highly protective against drowning, but the exact magnitude of their effect is unknown. There have been no case-control studies, but case-series studies of the association of PFD use suggest a strong protective effect. An important barrier related to PFD use appears to be their bulky fit and appearance, as well as lack of comfort in hot weather. Anecdotal reports of a community-based campaign in Alaska to promote the use of "float-coats," which combine a cold weather coat with built-in flotation material, have demonstrated a marked increase in the use of devices, since these devices served a dual purpose. Newer devices being marketed include PFDs in small waist-packs that open with a pull of a rip cord or inflate spontaneously by gas cartridge when they contact water. These newer approaches to PFD design may lead to improved compliance with their use.

Alcohol is also strongly associated with open-water drowning, and strategies to reduce alcohol intoxication while boating could have a significant impact on boating-related injuries, especially drowning. Alcohol intoxication also may interfere with a person's response to submersion, as well as exacerbate hypothermia. There is a paucity of evidenced-based approaches to this particular problem, though some of the same strategies used to prevent drunk driving could potentially be employed with boaters. These include the establishment of "per se" laws that specify a legal limit for blood alcohol concentration, the use of random Breathalyzer checks of boaters, and the impoundment of boats of violators of these laws.

FIRES AND BURNS

House fires are the major source of burn-related morbidity and mortality in the United States. In 2002, fire departments responded to 401,000 home fires in the United States, which claimed the lives of an estimated 2,670 people (not including firefighters) and injured another 14,050. The morbidity associated with extensive flame burns is well documented and is associated with lengthy hospital stays, multiple surgeries, and extensive psychological morbidity. The rates of fire injury are highest among the elderly and young children and are probably related with the ability of these age groups to respond and escape from a dwelling on fire. Rates of fire deaths have dropped significantly over the past several decades, but much additional work can be done to reduce this rate further.

About 75% of house fire deaths result from asphyxiation and are not associated with extensive burns. Therefore, advanced burn care, though important in the treatment of nonfatal burns, will have a limited role in further reducing fire deaths. The primary prevention strategy for house fires is partly embedded in building and electrical codes (since faulty heating and electrical systems are a major cause of house fires) and also in preventing cooking fires and cigarette-related fires in the home, the major cause of house fires. Though no clear public health strategies are available to prevent cooking fires, significant progress has been made in reducing cigarette ignition fires. Cigarette ignition fires usually start when a smoldering cigarette drops from the hand or mouth of a smoker who is either asleep or inebriated, causing ignition of a carpet, upholstery, or other flammable fabric. One approach to the prevention of ignition is the fire-safe cigarette (16). Though the technology is relatively old, this type of cigarette has recently been mandated in the state of New York. A fire-safe cigarette self-extinguishes after a short period of time if it has not been used. Extensive laboratory testing of its ability to self-extinguish has made this technology very promising, though its limited market penetration has made rigorous field evaluations difficult to conduct.

Smoke alarms are another very important source of protection from house fire. Since a large proportion of injured persons are sleeping during the ignition of fires, smoke alarms provide an opportunity to awaken and escape from fire. Several case-control studies have estimated that, when used, smoke alarms reduce the incidence of death and injury from house fire by 50% to 70% (17). More than 90% of homes in the United States already have detectors present, but only about one half to three quarters of these are in working condition (18).

One of the most common reasons for nonfunctional detectors is the removal of their batteries or their disconnection from the electrical supply. Batteries may be removed from some types of smoke detectors because of their propensity to have false alarms associated with cooking or other activities (19).

The public health challenge for fire protection in this century will be to ensure that all homes have *functional* detectors with minimal frequency of false alarms. Photoelectric detectors, which appear to have far fewer alarms, with 10-year lithium batteries may provide this level of improvement.

Flame burns can also occur when clothing ignites from a source such as a campfire or candle. Clothing burns are most commonly seen among children and became relatively unusual after the passage of the US Flammable Fabrics Act of 1953. This act mandated that sleepwear for children contain flame-retardants or be composed of nonflammable fabric. Cotton and nylon clothing is especially prone to rapid inflammation. Fires of this type caused deep full-thickness burns in young children. Despite attempts to regulate this type of burn out of existence, they still occur since loopholes have allowed some manufacturers to sell cotton nightwear for another ostensible purpose.

Another major type of burns results from scalding liquids, such as coffee or boiling water. These burns can also result in deep wounds and are the leading cause of burn hospitalizations for children <5 years old. These burns were, at one time, commonly a result of tap water. However, after regulations were passed that mandated water heater thermostats be set to 120°, the incidence of these types of burns fell dramatically (20).

FALLS

Falls are the leading cause of injury leading to hospitalization and pose a vexing problem for public health strategists. This type of injury is a heterogeneous category of incidents that require different interventions, depending on the developmental age of the victim, the circumstances, and the environment in which they occur. Falls are common. More than one third of adults >65 years fall each year, and >1.5 million seniors were treated in a hospital emergency room in 2001 for fall-related injuries. Most intervention trials on falls have been conducted in the elderly population, but much more work is needed to understand risk and protective factors for falls in other age groups.

Potentially modifiable risk factors associated with falls in the elderly include lower-body strength, unsteady gait and balance, adverse effects of medications, and the friction coefficient of shoe wear and floors. Osteoporosis is perhaps the most important risk factor associated with fractures resulting

from falls. A recent systematic review of the prevention of falls among the elderly emphasized that much more is known about the primary prevention of falls in this population compared to the prevention of injuries (especially hip fractures) when falls occur. A large number of potentially promising interventions with efficacy shown to date include exercise and balance training with a trained professional, nutritional supplementation with calcium and vitamin D, withdrawal of psychotropic medications, and home hazard assessment and modification. Hip protectors have been studied as a strategy for preventing hip fractures once a fall has occurred. These protectors provide substantial cushion over a large energy-absorbing surface to reduce the incidence of femoral neck fractures. A recent Cochrane systematic review of trials that employed hip protectors found that there appeared to be no important protective effect when trials randomized individual patients by institution or studied patients within their own homes. Clustered trials of institutionalized elderly with a high background incidence of falls appeared to have some beneficial effect (21).

Children are also at high risk of falls, and the circumstances of these falls vary with their developmental age. Some of the most serious types of falls usually occur during recreation or from heights, such as the upper floors of buildings. Factors that influence the severity of the fall include the height of the fall and the energy absorbing capacity of the fall surface. Playground falls from heights >1.5 meters are associated with a fourfold increase in the risk of injury, compared with falls from elevations lower than this (22). Modifying the surfacing of playgrounds is another important strategy for reducing injuries; asphalt surface is associated with a sixfold increase in the risk of injury compared to sand surfacing (23). More research is needed regarding risk and protective factors for window falls, but there is some evidence that the placement of horizontal window guards on the windows of high-rise apartment buildings can lead to a substantially decreased risk of falls for toddlers and children.

FIREARM INJURIES

Firearm injuries are a leading cause of injury and death among adolescents and young adults. More than 90% of firearm injuries are intentional and thus are usually classified by the intent, as homicides, suicides, or legal intervention. When grouped together as a single mechanism, firearms emerge as the second leading cause of death overall after motor vehicle crashes for persons between the ages of 15 and 34 years. The prevention of firearm injuries also depends on the age of the victim and shooter and the circumstances surrounding the injury. For example, the approach to the prevention of homicide is quite different from that to suicide prevention. The science of prevention for this mechanism is still in its infancy and we still know relatively little about how best to stem these injuries. As with all injuries, key strategies include policy and legislation, education, and technological innovation. The direct prevention of *firearm homicide* is beyond the scope of this chapter and primarily relies on key law enforcement and criminal justice approaches to minimizing access to guns by criminals and the interdiction of illegal guns from illegal sources. Firearm suicide is much more closely intertwined with public health, and mental health and health providers have a stronger role in prevention. There is ample evidence from multiple case-control studies that the presence of a firearm in a household is strongly associated with occupant death by suicide and that recent acquisition of a gun is temporally associated with an increased risk of firearm injury (24–27). Restricting access to lethal means of suicide, for example, outlawing sales of firearms to persons with mental illness, has often been proposed as one strategy to reduce this type of injury. However, convincing evidence is lacking for adults that this will not result in substitution of another method. However, restricting the access of children and adolescents to firearms may be a more promising approach, since this age group has much lower degree of intent, and restricting access may be easier with children than with adults. The most practical ways that families can restrict access to guns are by either eliminating them from the home or by securing them in a locked, enclosed container such as a safe or lockbox. Preliminary evidence from a recent study suggests that locking guns is strongly associated with a reduced risk of suicide and unintentional injuries from firearms. There is also evidence that if law mandates such storage, they can lead to a reduced rate of suicide and unintentional gun injuries (28).

Changing the design of firearms so that they cannot be fired without explicit owner permission could also prevent some types of unintentional gun injuries (29). Such "smart" firearms use advanced technology to lock the trigger unless the gun "recognizes" its owner's unique identity. The technology for these modifications is already available and on the market, but they have yet to be widely adopted, partly because of the increased costs associated with this design.

Contrary to widespread popular opinion, firearm injuries among children cannot be prevented solely by behavior modification. The effectiveness of using school-based curricula to instruct young children on firearm safety rules is unproven. Several studies have demonstrated that explicit one-on-one and small-group training of children that warns against touching or playing with guns does not reduce their propensity to touch and handle guns (30).

Given the high frequency of firearm injuries, there is an urgent need to identify other prevention strategies for reducing the rate of these types of injuries.

RECREATIONAL AND SPORTS INJURIES

Important preventable causes of recreational injuries include those resulting from bicycle crashes, equestrian injuries, animal bites, skiing, boating, and the use of motorized craft, such as snowmobiles, all terrain vehicles (ATV), and personal watercraft. These diverse mechanisms of trauma, though not important causes of mortality, do contribute substantially to the burden of nonfatal injury and disability.

A review of prevention strategies for each of these mechanisms is beyond the scope of this chapter, and in fact, there are few proven strategies for many of them. One common prevention strategy for many of them is the promotion of helmet use for bicycles, equestrians, skiing, and the use of snowmobiles and ATV. Traumatic brain injury is the most severe consequence from all of these mechanisms and preventing this outcome is paramount. Extensive evidence has accumulated regarding the effectiveness of helmets as a measure to prevent brain injury and regarding the impact of promotion campaigns on rates of head injuries in the community. Bicycle helmets are thought to be about 63% to 88% protective against severe or fatal brain injuries, and motorcycle helmets reduce the risk of head injury by 72% (OR 0.28, 95% CI 0.23, 0.35) (31).

There is far less firm evidence regarding the efficacy of helmets in other recreational pursuits such as skiing or equestrianism, but since the mechanisms and forces are likely to be similar, their promotion is fully sensible, pending additional evidence.

Like other injury prevention efforts, successful campaigns to increase helmet wearing must include health promotion components, policy, and enforcement, as well as the reasonable economic incentives to change behavior. There are now multiple examples of population-based efforts throughout the world to promote helmet wearing that have been associated with large increases in helmet use and subsequent declines in rates of head injury in various communities.

In addition to causing head injuries, snow sports result in high rates of lower- and upper-extremity injuries, particularly fractures and severe ligamentous injuries. One unpublished systematic review concluded that ski injuries could potentially be reduced by improving the binding technology of ski boots and releases, and by improvements in skier education. Promoting the use of wrist guards could reduce snowboarding injuries of the upper extremities.

Injuries from organized recreational sports are another important source of nonfatal but disabling injuries. However, well-executed, controlled trials of prevention strategies are relatively uncommon, perhaps because a clear understanding of the underlying risk factors for these injuries is lacking. The primary prevention of musculoskeletal injuries in contact sports, especially in soccer and football, is especially challenging, given that the magnitude and direction of forces applied to players is not always predictable or controllable. A better understanding of the biomechanical mechanisms of soft tissue and boney injuries would help define forms of prohibited contact between players and perhaps have an effect on contact-related injuries. Other primary approaches, such as prophylactic stretching or taping and splinting, have not been shown to be effective in noninjured players.

ALCOHOL-RELATED INJURIES

Alcohol plays an enormous role in the mechanism of many types of injuries involving adults and adolescents. More than 40% of fatal motor vehicle crashes and pedestrian injuries are alcohol-related. Similarly strong associations with alcohol exist with fire deaths, homicides, suicides, drowning, and virtually every mechanism. Since alcohol is not associated with the risk of survival in trauma patients, similar associations are seen with patients in trauma centers who suffer nonfatal injuries. It is estimated that up to 40% to 50% of trauma patients have a history of alcohol problems, making them a target for possible secondary prevention. Approaches to primary prevention of some types of alcohol-related injuries, such as motor vehicle injury and boating, are discussed in the previous text. However, it is also important to consider secondary prevention measures, since there is considerable recidivism among trauma patients with alcohol-related injuries. Trauma centers and rehabilitation units should be viewed as important nodes of clinical recognition where alcoholism can be recognized (with screening) and treated in its earliest stages. In fact, a number of trauma centers are already engaged in this practice, since there is evidence that blood alcohol screening and treatment of affected patients can lead to a 50% reduction in trauma recidivism in the first year after the index injury (32). The primary approach to the treatment of these patients rests on motivational interviewing, also known as a brief intervention, and has been endorsed by the US Preventive Services Task Force as an effective approach to the reduction of risky and harmful alcohol use by adults (33).

INTENTIONAL INJURIES

Intentional injuries include fatal (homicides and suicides) and nonfatal (assault, suicide attempts) injuries. Assaults are also commonly classified by the victim-perpetrator relationship, such as child abuse, domestic violence, or youth violence. Though once viewed as mainly criminal justice or mental health problems, violence and suicide are increasingly incorporated into the model of public health (34).

The primary prevention of these outcomes is particularly well suited for the public health paradigm and theoretical models of prevention. Assault and self-inflicted injuries represent domains of *intent*, rather than specific mechanisms. For example, poisonings, motor vehicle crashes, and falls could all either be unintentional or intentional. Thus, developing prevention strategies for intentional injuries could be focused on the underlying behavior, the mechanism employed, or both. Because of the intent associated with these injuries, fully passive approaches to primary prevention are often difficult to develop.

An exhaustive discussion of the prevention of violence and suicide is beyond the scope of this chapter. Earlier sections of this chapter specifically refer to prevention strategies for firearm injuries, an important mechanism of intentional injury. Brief mention will be made regarding the prevention of two particularly commonly encountered presentations of violence to clinicians: family violence experienced by children and that experienced by women.

Approaches to the recognition and treatment of child abuse have advanced considerably, but prevention approaches to this problem are much further behind. C. Henry Kempe, the pediatrician who was responsible for bringing child abuse into the medical domain, was also one of the first to write about using home visitors to prevent child abuse. Several decades after his proposals first emerged, there is now convincing evidence regarding the protective value of having home visitation by nurses (35). A systematic review of 26 trials by the Task Force on Community Preventive Services found that the median decrease in measures of child abuse and neglect among those receiving home visitation was 39% (24% to 74%). Most of these programs involve frequent visitation over a several-year period, making them costly to implement. Secondary prevention of child abuse represents another potential opportunity to intervene. Commonly, clinicians depend on encounters to recognize physical signs of abuse and neglect. Screening of all patients in a clinical or other setting could be a more sensitive mechanism, but there have not been trials of screening for this condition (36).

Violence against children and intimate partners was only a relatively recent addition to the recognized list of syndromes viewed by clinicians (37,38). The primary prevention of violence against women, also known as domestic violence, is a formidable challenge and extends well beyond the boundaries of public health and medicine. However, there is increasing interest in the role of clinicians in the recognition and treatment of women assaulted by intimate partners, since secondary prevention of this type of injury is increasingly viewed as feasible and effective. A recent review by the US Preventive Services Task Force concluded that there was insufficient evidence to recommend systematic screening for family and intimate partner violence in clinical settings. Another review performed for the Cochrane database similarly concluded that no randomized controlled trials of screening instruments have been performed to evaluate the effectiveness of screening in preventing further injury (39,40). At least one trial found that when at-risk women can be identified, civil protection orders are effective in preventing future police reports of violence (41).

ROLE OF CLINICIANS IN INJURY PREVENTION

Prevention is only one phase of injury control. The control of injury is a multidisciplinary effort that requires the skills and expertise of a wide variety of professionals from biomechanical engineers to behavioral scientists. Each phase of injury control— biomechanics, acute care, rehabilitation, and prevention—is an integral component of approaches to primary and secondary prevention. Acute care brings together the skills of trauma care providers with prehospital personnel and is usually focused on secondary prevention; rehabilitation efforts also focus on preventing secondary injury from causing further disability. But clinicians play an important role in primary prevention, too.

Clinicians can play important roles in injury prevention through patient care and education by developing and establishing policies at an institutional or regional level, by conducting research on primary prevention, and by advocating legislative and administrative rulings to prevent injury. Clinicians can also become active in professional societies and other organizations that work to promote injury prevention at local, state, and national levels.

Clinical encounters also provide valuable opportunities for clinicians to proactively screen, counsel, and intervene as appropriate to reduce and prevent injury, and when there is sufficient evidence to justify these activities. These activities can occur in a variety of settings, including primary care, inpatient wards, and rehabilitation units.

The science of injury prevention has advanced considerably over the past 40 years, and the falling rates of many types of injury are a direct result of the employment of effective interventions. Continued efforts to advance the science will depend on the continued generation of high-quality research on the efficacy and dissemination of injury control strategies.

REFERENCES

1. Franco G. Ramazzini and workers' health. *Lancet.* 1999;354(9181):858–861.
2. DeJong W, Hingson R. Strategies to reduce driving under the influence of alcohol. *Annu Rev Public Health.* 1998;19:359–378.
3. Shults RA, Elder RW, Sleet DA, et al. Reviews of evidence regarding interventions to reduce alcohol-impaired driving. *Am J Prev Med.* 2001;21(4 Suppl. 1): 66–88.
4. Wells-Parker E, Bangert-Drowns R, McMillen R, et al. Final results from a meta-analysis of remedial interventions with drink/drive offenders. *Addiction.* 1995; 90(7):907–926.
5. Cummings P, Rivara FP. Car occupant death according to the restraint use of other occupants: A matched cohort study. *JAMA.* 2004;291(3):343–349.
6. Rivara FP, Thompson DC, Cummings P. Effectiveness of primary and secondary enforced seat belt laws. *Am J Prev Med.* 1999;16(Suppl. 1):30–39.
7. National Highway Traffic Safety Administration. *Traffic safety facts 2000.* DOT HS 809. Washington, DC: National Highway Traffic Safety Administration; 2000:324.
8. Bunn F, Collier T, Frost C, et al. Area-wide traffic calming for preventing traffic related injuries. *Cochrane Database Syst Rev.* 2003;(1):CD003110.
9. Koepsell T, McCloskey L, Wolf M, et al. Crosswalk markings and the risk of pedestrian-motor vehicle collisions in older pedestrians. *JAMA.* 2002;288(17): 2136–2143.
10. Duperrex O, Roberts I, Bunn F. Safety education of pedestrians for injury prevention. *Cochrane Database Syst Rev.* 2002;(2):CD001531.
11. Robertson LS. Car design and risk of pedestrian deaths. *Am J Public Health.* 1990;80(5):609–610.
12. Roudsari BS, Mock CN, Kaufman R, et al. Pedestrian crashes: Higher injury severity and mortality rate for

light truck vehicles compared with passenger vehicles. *Inj Prev.* 2004;10(3):154–158.

13. Kraus JF, Peek C, McArthur DL, et al. The effect of the 1992 California motorcycle helmet use law on motorcycle crash fatalities and injuries. *JAMA.* 1994; 272(19):1506–1511.

14. Wells S, Mullin B, Norton R, et al. Motorcycle rider conspicuity and crash related injury: Case-control study. *BMJ.* 2004;328(7444):857.

15. Pitt WR, Balanda KP. Childhood drowning and near-drowning in Brisbane: The contribution of domestic pools. *Med J Aust.* 1991;154(10):661–665.

16. Brigham PA, McGuire A. Progress towards a fire-safe cigarette. *J Public Health Policy.* 1995;16(4):433–439.

17. Runyan CW, Bangdiwala SI, Linzer MA, et al. Risk factors for fatal residential fires. *N Engl J Med.* 1992; 327(12):859–863.

18. Rowland D, DiGuiseppi C, Roberts I, et al. Prevalence of working smoke alarms in local authority inner city housing: Randomised controlled trial. *BMJ.* 2002;325 (7371):998–1001.

19. Fazzini TM, Perkins R, Grossman D. Ionization and photoelectric smoke alarms in rural Alaskan homes. *West J Med.* 2000;173(2):89–92.

20. Feldman KW, Schaller RT, Feldman JA, et al. Tap water scald burns in children. *Pediatrics.* 1978;62(1): 1–7.

21. Parker M, Gillespie L, Gillespie W. Hip protectors for preventing hip fractures in the elderly. *Cochrane Database Syst Rev.* 2004;3:CD001255.

22. Chalmers DJ, Marshall SW, Langley JD, et al. Height and surfacing as risk factors for injury in falls from playground equipment: A case-control study. *Inj Prev.* 1996;2(2):98–104.

23. Sosin DM, Keller P, Sacks JJ, et al. Surface-specific fall injury rates on Utah school playgrounds. *Am J Public Health.* 1993;83(5):733–735.

24. Brent DA, Baugher M, Birmaher B, et al. Compliance with recommendations to remove firearms in families participating in a clinical trial for adolescent depression. *J Am Acad Child Adolesc Psychiatry.* 2000; 39(10):1220–1226.

25. Cummings P, Koepsell TD, Grossman DC, et al. The association between the purchase of a handgun and homicide or suicide. *Am J Public Health.* 1997;87(6): 974–978.

26. Kellermann AL, Rivara FP, Rushforth NB, et al. Gun ownership as a risk factor for homicide in the home. *N Engl J Med.* 1993;329(15):1084–1091.

27. Kellermann AL, Rivara FP, Somes G, et al. Suicide in the home in relation to gun ownership. *N Engl J Med.* 1913;327(7):467–472.

28. Cummings P, Grossman DC, Rivara FP, et al. State gun safe storage laws and child mortality due to firearms. *JAMA.* 1997;278(13):1084–1086.

29. Teret SP, Culross Pl. Product-oriented approaches to reducing youth gun violence. *Future Child.* 2002;12(2): 118–131.

30. Jackman GA, Farah MM, Kellermann AL, et al. Seeing is believing: What do boys do when they find a real gun? *Pediatrics.* 2001;107(6):1247–1250.

31. Thompson DC, Rivara FP, Thompson R. Helmets for preventing head and facial injuries in bicyclists. *Cochrane Database Syst Rev.* 2000;(2):CD001855.

32. Gentilello LM, Rivara FP, Donovan DM, et al. Alcohol interventions in a trauma center as a means of reducing the risk of injury recurrence. *Ann Surg.* 1999; 230(4):473–480; discussion 480–483.

33. Whitlock EP, Polen MR, Green CA, et al. Behavioral counseling interventions in primary care to reduce risky/harmful alcohol use by adults: A summary of the evidence for the US Preventive Services Task Force. *Ann Intern Med.* 2004;140(7):557–568.

34. Foege WH, Rosenberg ML, Mercy JA. Public health and violence prevention. *Curr Issues Public Health.* 1995;1:2–9.

35. Hahn RA, Bilukha OO, Crosby A, et al. First reports evaluating the effectiveness of strategies for preventing violence: Early childhood home visitation. Findings from the Task Force on Community Preventive Services. *MMWR Recomm Rep.* 2003;52(RR-14):1–9.

36. Nygren P, Nelson HD, Klein J. Screening children for family violence: A review of the evidence for the US Preventive Services Task Force. *Ann Fam Med.* 2004; 2(2):161–169.

37. Kempe CH. Paediatric implications of the battered baby syndrome. *Arch Dis Child.* 1971;46(245):28–37.

38. Appleton W. The battered woman syndrome. *Ann Emerg Med.* 1980;9(2):84–91.

39. Nelson HD, Nygren P, McInerney Y, et al. Screening women and elderly adults for family and intimate partner violence: A review of the evidence for the US Preventive Services Task Force. *Ann Intern Med.* 2004; 140(5):387–396.

40. Coulthard P, Yong S, Adamson L, et al. Domestic violence screening and intervention programmes for adults with dental or facial injury. *Cochrane Database Syst Rev.* 2004;(2):CD004486.

41. Holt VL, Kernic MA, Lumley T, et al. Civil protection orders and risk of subsequent police-reported violence. *JAMA.* 2002;288(5):589–594.

INDEX

Page numbers followed by *f* indicate figures; page numbers followed by *t* indicate tables

A

Abbreviated Injury Scale (AIS)
  and ISS calculations, 28, 31
  as rehabilitation predictor, 11, 14
  score assignment, 28
Acticoat, 185
Acute respiratory distress syndrome (ARDS), 45
Acute stress disorder (ASD), 248, 254, 255*t*
Addiction Severity Index (ASI), 234
ADL (activities of daily living) evaluation, 42
Adrenocortical insufficiency, acute, 94
Aeromedical helicopters, 20
Agency for Healthcare Research and Quality (AHRQ), 274
Agitated Behavior Scale, 102
Agitation, posttraumatic, 101–102
Airlift Northwest, 22
Alcohol Dependence Scale (ADS), 233
Alcohol Use Disorders Identification Test (AUDIT), 232
Alcohol Use Inventory (AUI), 234
Alcoholics Anonymous (AA), 229–230, 236–238
Alcoholism. *See* Substance abuse, TBI and SCI patients
Allograft, 184
American Board of Medical Specialties (ABMS), 3
American Board of Physical Medicine, 3
American Burn Association, 184
American College of Surgeons (ACS), 21, 274
  Early Care of the Injured Patient, 21
  Resources for Optimal Care of the Injured Patient, 21, 27–30
American Congress of Physical Therapy (1921), 3
American Medical Association (AMA), 3, 200
American National Standards Institute (ANSI) Standards A117.1-1986, 133
American Spinal Injury Association (ASIA), 115–116, 121
  International Standards for Neurological and Functional Classification of Spinal Cord Injury, 116
  International Standards for Neurological and Functional Classification of Spinal Cord Injury Patients, 121
Americans with Disabilities Act, 131, 133

Amputations
  Symes, 151–152
  traumatic, 143
    epidemiology, 143
    versus nontraumatic, 2
    requiring rehabilitation, 15, 16*f*
  traumatic lower extremity
    age and gender, 143
    amputation level distribution, 143
    burns and, 188–189
    decision making, amputation versus salvage, 144, 145–146
    degenerative arthritis, 148
    Ertl procedure, 152
    immediate postoperative prosthesis (IPOP) technique, 147
    informed consent, 144–145
    knee joints, prosthetic, 155–156
    knee pain, 148–149
    limb salvage, outcomes after, 149–150
    low back pain, 148
    mechanical skin injury, 148
    myodesis, 154
    myoplasty, 154
    narrow mediolateral (M/L) prosthetic socket, 155
    outcomes, 148–149
    patient education, 146
    phantom limb pain, 148
    pneumatic compressive devices, 147
    preoperative period, 144
    prosthetic fitting, 150–156. *See also* Prosthetic fitting, lower extremity amputations
    psychological issues, 146
    removable rigid dressing, 147
    residual limb management, 146–148
    residual limb pain, 148
    return to work, 148
    rigid dressings, 147
    Silesian bandage suspension, 155
    soft dressings, 146–147
    suction suspension system, 155
    Unna dressings, 147
Anterior spinal artery syndrome, 117
Antibiotics, use of in Korean War, 3
Apraxia, 94
Arizona Battery for Communication Disorders (ABCD), 44
Arterial lines, 56
Ashworth scale, 118
Assistive technology devices, 132–133
Atelectasis, 50–51, 133

ATLS (advanced trauma life support) course, 21
Autonomic dysreflexia (AD), 134
Axillary abduction pillow, 193
Axonotmesis
  compound motor action potential (CMAP), 162–163
  defined, 160
  needle electomyography (EMG), 164–165
  nerve and muscle, effects on, 161–162
  prognosis for recovery, 167–168
  SNAP, 163–164
Azulay, J., 106

B

BADLs (basic activities of daily living), 35, 37, 53
Balance screening, 43
Barrie, P. S., 45
Baryza, M. J., 190
Batalden, P. B., 277
Baumgarten, A., 238
Bayley Scales of Infant Development, 298
Beck Depression Inventory, 246
Bed positioning, 45
Behavioral theories, 249
Bell-Krotoski, J. A., 170
Benign positional paroxysmal vertigo (BPPV), 95
Berg Balance Scale, 43
Bernat, James, 144–145
Best, A. K., 144
Bilevel positive airway pressure (BiPAP), 122, 134
Blackerby, W. F., 238
Blackwell, S. J., 193
Body weight support system (BWSS), 131
Bohannon, R. W., 52
Bolt, 56
Bombardier, C. H., 226, 232, 238, 253, 254
Bonanni, F., 144
Bonanno, G. A., 245
Bones. *See also* Musculoskeletal injuries
  blood supply to, 80
  cancellous, 79–80
  cortical, 79, 80
  fracture types, 80
  healing, primary and secondary, 80
  ligaments, 80
  osteons, 80
  tendons, 80